NurseNotes

Medical–Surgical

Core Content At-A-Glance

NurseNotes

Medical–Surgical
Core Content At-A-Glance

Robyn M. Nelson, RN, DNSc
Professor of Nursing
California State University
Sacramento, California

Janice Horman Stecchi, RN, EdD
Dean, College of Health Professions
University of Massachusetts Lowell
Lowell, Massachusetts

Edited by
Sally Lambert Lagerquist, RN, MS
Former Instructor of Undergraduate and Graduate Programs
  and Continuing Education in Nursing
University of California, San Francisco, School of Nursing
President, Review for Nurses, Inc., and RN Tapes Company
San Francisco, California

Lippincott
Philadelphia • New York

Acquisitions Editor: Susan Glover
Assistant Editor: Bridget Blatteau
Project Editor: Tom Gibbons
Production Manager: Helen Ewan
Production Coordinator: Nannette Winski
Design Coordinator: Doug Smock
Indexer: Nancy Newman

Library of Congress Cataloging in Publications Data

Nelson, Robyn M.
    Nurse notes : medical-surgical / Robyn M. Nelson, Janice Horman
Stecchi ; edited by Sally Lambert Lagerquist.
        p.   cm.
    Includes bibliographical references and index.
    ISBN 0-7817-1130-4
    1. Nursing—Outlines, syllabi, etc. 2. Nursing—Examinations,
questions, etc. I. Stecchi, Janice Horman. II. Lagerquist, Sally L. III. Title.
    [DNLM: 1. Perioperative Nursing—examination questions.
2. Perioperative Nursing—outlines. WY 18.2 N429n 1997]
RT52.N45   1997
610.73′076—dc20
DNLM/DLC
for Library of Congress   96-23717
                                                                         CIP

Care has been taken to confirm the accuracy of the information presented and to describe generally accepted practices. However, the authors, editors, and publisher are not responsible for errors or omissions or for any consequences from application of the information in this book and make no warranty, express or implied, with respect to the contents of the publication.

The authors, editors and publisher have exerted every effort to ensure that drug selection and dosage set forth in this text are in accordance with current recommendations and practice at the time of publication. However, in view of ongoing research, changes in government regulations, and the constant flow of information relating to drug therapy and drug reactions, the reader is urged to check the package insert for each drug for any change in indications and dosage and for added warnings and precautions. This is particularly important when the recommended agent is a new or infrequently employed drug.

Some drugs and medical devices presented in this publication have Food and Drug Administration (FDA) clearance for limited use in restricted research settings. It is the responsibility of the health care provider to ascertain the FDA status of each drug or device planned for use in their clinical practice.

9 8 7 6 5 4 3 2 1

Any publication project is a joint effort—made possible by the mutual support and respect of a coauthor, the inspiration of past and present nursing students, seemingly tireless and deadline-driven editorial staff, the understanding of family and friends, and a personal commitment to the profession of nursing and the quality of patient care. Thank you for the opportunity.

Robyn Nelson

To all my colleagues, past, present and those in the future, who have made or will make a difference in a patient's life. The facts contained in this book will help you to know what to do, but it takes a great deal more than that to be a nurse. You have to care enough to function in an ever-changing environment. You must listen to the concerns of patients and their families and help them through difficult times. Your greatest reward will come when you know *you* have made the difference.

A special thanks to my family—husband Dave; sons Dave, Bill, and Joe; and my dad—for being so understanding of my time away from you as I also try to make a difference in people's lives.

Janice Stecchi

To Tom, my husband

Thank you for 31 years of hearing you speak gently and laughing often; of giving freely of yourself; of thinking deeply, working hard side by side, and loving much.

To Elana, our daughter
To Kalen, our son

Thank you for your patience, your caring, your actions in giving me the "space" to work on this book, and the needed support in family matters and in keeping our nursing review office running during the final 3 months of this project. This book wouldn't have been "airborne" without you! You were there when we needed you the most!

Sally Lagerquist

Preface

There are numerous outstanding, comprehensive medical-surgical textbooks on the market today—some over 2000 pages long! Nursing students preparing for professional nursing practice must understand the "art and science" of nursing—the theory and techniques—that can be covered thoroughly only in a textbook. However, students frequently ask for help to *focus* their studying and preparation before caring for patients in the clinical setting. Review books used to prepare for the nursing licensure examination, particularly *NCLEX-RN Examination Review*, have successfully condensed the world of nursing practice in all clinical areas, but several trends in nursing have led to the need to provide students with condensed review material specific to just one clinical area.

Intended Audience

NurseNotes: Medical-Surgical will be particularly useful to students in nursing programs who spend the greatest amount of clinical time in medical-surgical settings, including acute care and long-term care. The book concisely presents selected clinical disorders for each body system within the nursing process framework. A brief overview of the *pathophysiologic* basis for each disorder is followed by *risk factors*, *objective* and *subjective* physical assessment findings, NANDA-approved *nursing diagnoses*, current approaches to *nursing care*, and criteria to determine achievement of desired patient *outcomes*. Common *pharmacologic* therapies, recommended *diets*, and *diagnostic procedures* are integrated with the discussion of the clinical disorder. Students no longer have to refer to separate chapters for this information.

Although the NCLEX tests knowledge of all clinical areas, a major focus of the exam is physiologic integrity and safe and effective nursing care. A student may feel the need to review only medical-surgical nursing care in preparation for the test. *NurseNotes: Medical-Surgical* may also be helpful to nurses facing work transformation or job redesign who must move to a new clinical unit or in preparation for certification exams.

Features

Special added features include end-of-chapter *Study and Memory Aids, Summary of Key Points,* and *questions and answers* covering the five steps of the nursing process with fact-packed *rationale.* Also included is a disk containing additional questions with answers.

Unique to this book are visual features that include numerous text figures (30), easy-to-read charts (81), shaded boxes for emphasis, and special symbols to highlight phases of the nursing process (▶◀), hands-on nursing care (☞), diagnostic tests and procedures ([▟▙▜]), laboratory data (▰▰▰), and medications (●). *Diets* (●), *positions,* and *tubes* appear in italics. **Health teaching** (▩) sections stand out in bold face.

How to Benefit from This Book

The extensive *appendices* should be very useful in providing even more study and review material under one cover. They include over 300 need-to-know common *acronyms* and *abbreviations*; review of *nutrition* and *pharmacology* (over 300 drugs are reviewed); *indices* to quickly locate 60 *diets*, 105 common diagnostic studies and procedures, lab data, 25 common tubes, a checklist of over 100 need-to-know hands-on nursing treatments/care, 40 examples of *positioning* of the patient, and questions and answers related to the steps of the nursing process as well as 4 client needs and 8 categories of human function; an index to 28 *mnemonics/memory aids* for various conditions; quick guide to 25 *common clinical signs*; *home health care* situations; NCLEX-RN test plan; and health and welfare agencies and *resources* for patient education.

Preparation of care plans and test review will be easier with this clinically focused book. The authors and editor of this book have brought together their 100 years of combined clinical expertise and nursing education experience to assist the nursing student, new graduate, re-entry nurse, or foreign graduate in achieving theoretical and clinical competence in the care of medical-surgical patients as easily as possible.

Robyn M. Nelson, RN, DNSc
Coauthor of *NurseNotes: Medical–Surgical*

Janice Horman Stecchi, RN, EdD
Coauthor of *NurseNotes: Medical–Surgical*

Sally Lambert Lagerquist, RN, MS
Editor, *NurseNotes* series

Acknowledgments

A number of individuals have contributed their experience, ideas, and energies to all phases in the development of *NurseNotes: Medical–Surgical*.

Foremost, I wish to thank Bonnie Bergstrom for her invaluable help with the entire *NurseNotes* series, and particularly for the preliminary compilation of this longest of all four manuscripts. She did an amazing job in coordinating the diverse styles of the coauthors and the editor and incorporating the critiques of several reviewers. Her editing and organizational skills helped greatly in the process of translating our intent into a meaningful format, especially in the practice questions and answers sections.

Eileen Hackett, RN, MA, Associate Professor, College of the Desert, Palm Springs, California, and Lynda Schweid, RN, Assistant Dean, Health Sciences, Contra Costa College, California, contributed most of the helpful modifications that were incorporated into the final form of the 500 exam questions and answers. Their expertise in the manuscript review process helped us to meet our requirements for clarity, up-to-date context and relevance in the selection of the 250 questions and rationale for the book, as well as for the 250 additional questions on disk.

Tom Gibbons, Associate Managing Editor at Lippincott-Raven, helped greatly with the process of translating complex information from several most undecodable handwritings into a printed form that everyone can understand and benefit from. What perseverance in an eye-straining task!

Sue Glover, Senior Nursing Editor, has our appreciation for helping this book "mature" from an incomplete manuscript to the finished form.

Sally Lagerquist
Editor, *NurseNotes* series

Contents

List of Illustrations

List of Tables

Nursing Assessment of the Adult

Chapter Outline

Assessment, Analysis, and Nursing Diagnosis of the Adult

Assessment is the process of gathering a comprehensive database about the patient's present, past, and potential health problems, as well as a description of the patient as a whole in the context of his or her environment. It includes a comprehensive nursing history, a physical examination, and laboratory/x-ray data, and it concludes with the formulation of nursing diagnoses. In the following units, possible nursing diagnoses are listed under each disorder.

Subjective Data

Nursing History

The nursing history obtains data for the planning and implementation of nursing actions.

 I. **General information:** reason for admission; duration of present illness; previous hospitalization; history of illnesses; diagnostic procedures prior to admission; allergies—type and severity of reactions; medications taken at home—over-the-counter and prescription.

 II. **Information relative to growth and development:** age; menarche—age at onset; heavy menses; dysmenorrhea; vaginal discharge; date of last Papanicolaou smear; pregnancies; abortions; miscarriages.

 III. **Information relative to psychosocial functions:** feelings (anger, denial, fear, anxiety, guilt, life-style changes); language barriers; family support; spiritual needs; history of trauma/rape.

 IV. **Information relative to nutrition:** appetite—normal, changes; dietary habits; food preferences or intolerances; difficulty swallowing or chewing; dentures; use of caffeine/alcohol; weight changes; excessive thirst, hunger, sweating.

 V. **Information relative to fluid and gas transport:** difficulty breathing; shortness of breath; history of cough/smoking; colds; sputum; swelling of extremities; chest pain; palpitations; varicosities; excessive bruising; blood transfusions; excessive bleeding.

 VI. **Information relative to protective functions:** skin problems—rash, itch; current treatment; unusual hair loss.

 VII. **Information relative to comfort, rest, activity, mobility:** usual activity (ADL); present ability and restrictions; rest and sleep pattern; weakness; joint or muscle stiffness, pain, or swelling; occupation; interests.

 VIII. **Information relative to elimination:** bowel habits; changes—constipation, diarrhea; ostomy; emesis; nausea; voiding—retention, frequency, dysuria, incontinence.

 IX. **Information relative to sensory/perceptual functions:** pain—verbal report; quality, location; precipitating factors; duration; limitations in vision (glasses), hearing, touch, smell; orientation to person, place, time; confusion; headaches; fainting; dizziness; convulsions.

Objective Data
Physical Assessment

▶ **I. Physical assessment**—requires knowledge of normal findings, organization, and keen senses, i.e., visual, auditory, touch, smell. For abnormal findings, refer to the *Assessment* section of each health problem discussed under the categories of human functioning.

  A. Components

    1. Inspection—uses observations to detect deviations from normal.

    2. Auscultation—to perceive and interpret sounds arising from various organs, particularly heart, lungs, and bowel.

    3. Palpation—to assess for discomfort, temperature, pulsations, size, consistency, and texture.

    4. Percussion—to elicit vibrations produced by underlying organ structures; used less frequently in nursing practice.

      a. *Flat*—normal percussion sound over muscle or bone.

      b. *Dull*—normal percussion sound over organs such as liver.

      c. *Resonance*—normal percussion sound over lungs.

      d. *Tympany*—normal percussion sound over stomach or bowel.

  B. Sequence°

    1. *General appearance*—well or poorly developed or nourished. Color (black, white, jaundiced, pale). In distress (acutely or chronically)?

    2. *Vital signs*—blood pressure (which arm or both, orthostatic change). *Pulse* (regular or irregular, orthostatic change). *Respirations* (labored or unlabored, wheeze). *Temperature* (axillary, rectal, or oral). Weight. Height.

    3. *Skin, hair, and nails*—pigmentation, scars, lesions, bruises, turgor. Describe or draw rashes.

      a. *Skin color:*
        Red—fever, allergic reaction, CO poisoning.

°From Judge R, Zuidema G, Fitzgerald F. *Clinical Diagnosis* (5th ed). Boston; Little, Brown, 1989. Pp. 30–31.

        White (pallor)—excessive blood loss, fright.
        Blue (cyanosis)—hypoxemia, peripheral vasoconstriction.
        Mottled—cardiovascular embarrassment.

      b. *Skin temperature:*
        Hot, dry—excessive body heat (heat stroke).
        Hot, wet—reaction to increased internal or external temperature.
        Cool, dry—exposure to cold.
        Cool, clammy—shock.

    4. *Nodes*—any cervical, supraclavicular, axillary, epitrochlear, inguinal lymphadenopathy? If so, size of nodes (in cm), consistency (firm, rubbery, tender), mobile or fixed.

    5. *Head*—scalp, skull (configuration), scars, tenderness, bruits.

    6. *Eyes:*

      a. External eye: conjunctivae, sclerae, lids, cornea, pupils (including reflexes), visual fields, extraocular motions.

      b. Fundus: disk, blood vessels, pigmentation.

    7. *Ears*—shape of pinnae, external canal, tympanic membrane, acuity, air conduction versus bone conduction (Rinne test), lateralization (Weber's test).

    8. *Nose*—septum, mucosa, polyps.

    9. *Mouth and throat*—lips, teeth, tongue (size, papillation), buccal mucosa, palate, tonsils, oropharynx.

    10. *Neck*—suppleness; trachea, larynx, thyroid, blood vessels (jugular veins, carotid arteries).

    11. *Chest and lungs:*

      a. Inspection: contour, symmetry, expansion.

      b. Palpation: expansion, rib tenderness, tactile fremitus.

      c. Percussion: diaphragmatic excursion, dullness.

      d. Auscultation: crackles, rubs, wheezes, egophony, pectoriloquy.

        (1) Use diaphragm or bell. Normal sounds over alveoli—*vesicular*. Large airway or abnormal sounds—*bronchial or bronchovesicular*. Adventitious sounds—*crackles or wheezes*.

        (2) *Crackles*—discontinuous noises heard on auscultation; caused by popping open of air spaces; usually associated with increased fluid in the lungs; *formerly* called *rales*.

        (3) *Wheezes*—high-pitched, whistling sounds made by air flowing through narrowed airways; formerly called rhonchi.

    12. *Heart:*

      a. Inspection: point maximal impulse, chest contour.

      b. Palpation: point maximal impulse, thrills, lifts, thrusts.

      c. Auscultation: heart sounds, gallops, murmurs, rubs. Use diaphragm for high-pitched sounds of normal heart sounds (S_1 and S_2) and bell for abnormal sounds (S_3 and S_4).

13. *Breasts*—symmetry, retraction, lesions, nipples (inverted, everted), masses, tenderness, discharge.

14. *Abdomen:*
   a. **Inspection:** scars (draw these), contour, masses, vein pattern.
   b. **Auscultation:** bowel sounds, rubs, bruits. Use diaphragm. Auscultate after inspection and before palpation and percussion. Listen to each quadrant for at least 1 min. If bowel sounds are present, they will be heard in lower right quadrant (area of ileocecal valve).
   c. **Percussion:** organomegaly, hepatic dullness.
   d. **Palpation:** tenderness, masses, rigidity, liver, spleen, kidneys.
   e. **Hernia:** femoral, inguinal, ventral.

15. *Genitalia:*
   a. **Male:** penile lesions, scrotum, testes. Circumcised?
   b. **Female:** labia, Bartholin's and Skene's glands, vagina, cervix. Bimanual examination of internal genitalia.

16. *Rectum*—perianal lesions, sphincter tone, tenderness, masses, prostate, stool color, occult blood.

17. *Extremities*—pulses (symmetry, bruits, perfusion). Joints (mobility, deformity). Cyanosis, edema. Varicosities. Muscle mass.

18. *Back*—contour spine, tenderness. Sacral edema.

19. *Neurologic:*
   a. **Mental status:** alertness, memory, judgment, mood.
   b. **Cranial nerves:** (I–XII).
   c. **Cerebellum:** gait, finger-nose, heel-shin, tremors.
   d. **Motor:** muscle mass, strength, deep-tendon reflexes. Pathologic or primitive reflexes.
   e. **Sensory:** touch, pain, vibration. Heat and cold as indicated.

II. **General assessment**—provides information on the patient as a whole.
   A. *Race, sex, apparent age* in relation to stated age.
   B. *Nutritional status*—well hydrated and developed or obesity, cachexia—include weight.
   C. *Apparent health status*—general good health or mild, moderate, severe debilitation.
   D. *Posture and motor activity*—erect, symmetric, and balanced gait and muscle development or ataxic, circumducted, scissor, or spastic gait; slumped or bent-over posture; mild, moderate, or hyperactive motor responses.
   E. *Behavior*—alert; oriented to person, time, place; hears and comprehends instructions, or tense, anxious, angry; uses abusive language; slightly or largely unresponsive; delusions, hallucinations.

   F. *Odors*—noncontributory, or acetone, alcohol, fetid breath, incontinent of urine or feces.

▶ III. **Health assessment of the older adult**
   A. *Skin:*
   1. Decrease in elasticity → wrinkles and lines, dryness.
   2. Loss of fullness → sagging.
   3. Wasting appearance due to generalized loss of adipose and muscle tissue.
   4. Decrease of adipose tissue on extremities, redistributed to hips and abdomen in middle age.
   5. Bony prominences become visible.
   6. Excessive pigmentation → age spots.
   7. Dry skin and deterioration of nerve fibers and sensory endings → pruritus.
   8. Pallor and blotchiness because of decreased blood flow.
   9. Overgrowth of epidermal tissue leads to lesions (some benign, some premalignant, some malignant).

   B. *Nails:*
   1. Dry, brittle.
   2. Increased susceptibility to fungal infections.
   3. Decreased growth rate.
   4. Toenails thick, difficult to cut.

   C. *Hair:*
   1. Loss of pigment → graying, white.
   2. Decreased density of hair follicles → thinning of hair.
   3. Baldness due to decreased blood flow to skin and decreased estrogen production.
      a. Hair distribution thin on scalp, axilla, pubic area, upper and lower extremities.
      b. Decreased facial hair in *men.*
   4. Increased facial (chin, upper lip) hair in *women* due to decreased estrogen production.

   D. *Eyes:*
   1. Loss of soluble protein with loss of lens transparency → development of *cataracts.*
   2. Decrease in pupil size limits amount of light entering the eye → elderly need more light to see.
   3. Decreased pupil reactivity → decrease in rate of light changes to which a person can readily adapt.
   4. Diminished night vision due to decreased accommodation to darkness and dim light.
   5. Shrunken appearance due to loss of orbital fat.
   6. Blink reflex—slowed.
   7. Eyelids—loose.
   8. Visual acuity—decreased.
   9. Peripheral vision—diminished.
   10. Visual fields—diminished.
   11. Lens accommodation—decreased; requires corrective lenses.
   12. *Presbyopia*—lens may lose ability to become convex enough to accommodate to nearby objects; starts at age 40 (*farsightedness*).
   13. Color of iris—fades.
   14. Conjunctiva—thins, looks yellow.

15. Increased intraocular pressure leads to glaucoma.
  E. *Ears:*
    1. Changes in cochlea: decrease in average pitch of sound.
    2. Hearing loss: greater in left ear than right; greater in higher frequencies than in lower.
    3. Tympanic membrane: atrophied, thickened, causing hearing loss.
    4. *Presbycusis*—progressive loss of hearing in old age.
  F. *Mouth:*
    1. Dental caries.
    2. Poorly fitting dentures.
    3. Cancer of the mouth—increased risk.
    4. Decrease in taste buds → inability to taste sweet/salty foods.
    5. Olfactory bulb atrophies → decreased ability to smell.
  G. *Cardiovascular:*
    1. Blood pressure increased due to lack of elasticity of vessels → increased resistance to blood flow; decreased diameter of arteries.
    2. Atherosclerotic plaques → thrombosis.
    3. Valves become sclerotic, less pliable → reduced filling and emptying.
    4. Diastolic murmurs heard at base of heart.
    5. Loss of elasticity, decreased contractility → decreased cardiac output.
    6. Pumping action of the heart is reduced due to changes in the coronary arteries → pooling of blood in systemic veins and shortness of breath.
    7. Dysrhythmias due to disturbance of the autonomic nervous system.
    8. Extremities—pedal pulses weaker due to arteriosclerotic changes; colder extremities, mottled color.
  H. *Respiratory:*
    1. Efficiency reduced with age.
    2. Greater residual air in lungs after expiration.
    3. Decreased vital capacity.
    4. Decreased capacity to cough because of weaker expiratory muscles.
    5. Decreased ciliary activity → stasis of secretions → susceptibility to infections.
    6. Dyspnea on exertion (DOE) due to oxygen debt in the muscles.
    7. Reduced chest wall compliance.
  I. *Breasts:*
    1. Atrophy.
    2. Cancer risk—increased with age.
  J. *Gastrointestinal:*
    1. Pernicious anemia due to lack of intrinsic factor.
    2. Gastric motility—decreased.
    3. Esophageal peristalsis—decreased.
    4. Hiatal hernia—increased incidence.
    5. Digestive enzymes—gradual decrease of ptyalin (which converts starch), pepsin and trypsin

(which digest protein), lipase (fat-splitting enzyme).
    6. Absorption—decreased.
    7. Constipation due to improper diet.
  K. *Endocrine:*
    1. Basal metabolism rate lowered → decreased temperature.
    2. Cold intolerance.
    3. *Women:* decreased ovarian function → increased gonadotropins.
    4. Decreased renal sensitivity to ADH → unable to concentrate urine as effectively as younger persons.
    5. Decreased clearance of blood glucose after meals → elevated postprandial blood glucose
    6. Risk of diabetes mellitus increased with age.
  L. *Urinary:*
    1. Renal function—impaired due to poor perfusion.
    2. Filtration—impaired due to reduction in number of functioning nephrons.
    3. Urgency and frequency: *men*—often due to prostatic hypertrophy; *women*—due to perineal muscle weakness.
    4. Nocturia—both men and women.
    5. Urinary tract infection—increased incidence.
    6. Incontinence—especially with dementia.
  M. *Musculoskeletal:*
    1. Muscle mass—decreased.
    2. Bony prominences—increased.
    3. Demineralization of bone.
    4. Shortening of trunk due to narrowing of intervertebral space.
    5. Posture—normal; some kyphosis.
    6. Range of motion—limited.
    7. Osteoarthritis—related to extensive physical activities and joint use.
    8. Gait—altered.
    9. Osteoporosis related to menopause, immobilization, elevated levels of cortisone.
    10. Calcium, phosphorus, and vitamin D levels decreased.
  N. *Neurologic:*
    1. Voluntary, automatic reflexes—slowed.
    2. Sleep pattern—changes.
    3. Mental acuity—changes.
    4. Sensory interpretation and movement—changes.
    5. Pain perception—diminished.
    6. Dexterity and agility—lessened.
    7. Reaction time—slowed.
    8. Memory—past more vivid than recent memory.
    9. Depression.
    10. Alzheimer's disease.
  O. *Sexuality:*
    1. *Women*
      a. Estrogen production—decreased with menopause.
      b. Breasts atrophy.
      c. Vaginal secretions—reduced lubricants.

d. Sexuality—drive continues; sexual activity declines.

2. *Men*

    a. Testosterone production—decreased.

    b. Testes—decrease in size; decreased sperm count.

    c. Libido and sexual satisfaction—no changes.

IV. Routine laboratory studies—see Appendix G for normal ranges.

  A. *Hematology:*

    1. *Complete blood count*—detects presence of anemia, infection, allergy, and leukemia.

    2. *Prothrombin time*—increase may indicate need for vitamin K therapy.

    3. *Serology* (VDRL)—determines presence of syphilis; false positives may indicate collagen dysfunctions.

  B. *Urinalysis:*

    1. *Physical*—color, appearance, odor, specific gravity.

    2. *Chemical*—pH, protein, glucose, ketones, bilirubin.

    3. *Microscopic*—RBC, WBC, casts, crystals, bacteria.

  C. *Chest x-ray*—detects tuberculosis or other pulmonary dysfunctions, as well as changes in size and/or configuration of heart.

  D. *Electrocardiogram*—detects rhythm and conduction disturbances, presence of myocardial ischemia or necrosis, and ventricular hypertrophy.

  E. *Blood chemistries*—detect deviation in electrolyte balance, presence of tissue damage, and adequacy of glomerular filtration.

V. Common diagnostic procedures

  A. Noninvasive diagnostic procedures—procedures that provide an indirect assessment of organ size, shape, and/or function; these procedures are considered safe, are easily reproducible, need less complex equipment for recording, and generally do not require the written consent of patient and/or guardian.

    1. General nursing responsibilities:

      a. Reduce patient's anxieties and provide emotional support by:

        (1) Explaining purpose and procedure of test.

        (2) Answering questions regarding safety of the procedure, as indicated.

        (3) Remaining with patient during procedure when possible.

      b. Utilize procedures in the collection of specimens that prevent contamination and facilitate diagnosis—clean-catch urine and sputum specimens after deep breathing and coughing, for example.

  B. Invasive diagnostic procedures—procedures that directly record the size, shape, or function of an organ and that are often complex or expensive or that need to be performed by highly trained personnel; these procedures may result in morbidity and occasionally mortality of the patient and therefore require the written consent of the patient or guardian.

    1. General nursing responsibilities:

      a. *Prior to procedure:* institute measures to provide for patient's safety and emotional comfort.

        (1) Have patient sign permit for procedure.

        (2) Ascertain and report any patient history of allergy or allergic reactions.

        (3) Explain procedure briefly, and accurately advise patient of any possible sensations, such as flushing or a warm feeling, when a contrast medium is injected.

        (4) Keep patient *NPO* 6–12 h before procedure if anesthesia is to be used.

        (5) Allow patient to verbalize concerns, and note attitude toward procedure.

        (6) Administer preprocedure sedative, as ordered.

        (7) If procedure done at bedside:

          (a) Remain with patient, offering frequent reassurance.

          (b) Assist with optional positioning of patient.

          (c) Observe for indications of complications—shock, pain, or dyspnea.

      b. *Following procedure:* institute measures to prevent complications and promote physical and emotional comfort.

        (1) Observe and record vital signs.

        (2) Check injection cut-down or biopsy sites for bleeding, infection, tenderness, or thrombosis.

          (a) Report untoward reactions to physician.

          (b) Apply warm compresses to ease discomfort, as ordered.

        (3) If topical anesthetic is used during procedure (e.g., gastroscopy, bronchoscopy), do *not* give food or fluid until gag reflex returns.

        (4) Encourage relaxation by allowing patient to discuss experience and verbalize feelings.

Growth and Development*

Young Adulthood (20–30 Years of Age)

I. Stage of development—psychosocial stage: *intimacy versus isolation.*

II. Physical development

  A. At the *height* of bodily vigor.

---

*Adapted from Saxton D, et al. *Addison-Wesley Manual of Nursing Practice.* Menlo Park, CA: Addison-Wesley, 1983.

B. *Maximum* level of strength, muscular development, height, and cardiac and respiratory capacity; also, period of peak sexual capacity for men.

III. Cognitive development
   A. Close to *peak* of intelligence, memory, and abstract thought.
   B. Maximum ability to solve problems and learn new skills.

IV. Socialization
   A. Has a vision of the future and imagines various possibilities for self.
   B. Defines and tests out what can be accomplished.
   C. Seeks out a mentor to emulate as a guiding, though transitional, figure; the mentor is usually a mixture of parent, teacher, and friend who serves as a role model to support and facilitate the developing vision of self.
   D. Grows from a beginning to a fuller understanding of own authority and autonomy.
   E. Transfers an interest into an occupation or profession; crucial work choice may be made after one has knowledge, judgment, and self-understanding, usually at the end of young adulthood; when the choice is deferred beyond these years, valuable time is lost.
   F. Experiments with and chooses a life-style.
   G. Forms mature peer relationships with the opposite sex.
   H. Overcomes guilt and anxiety about the opposite sex and learns to understand the masculine and feminine aspects of self as well as the adult concept of roles.
   I. Learns to take the opposite sex seriously and may choose someone for a long-term relationship.
   J. Accepts the responsibilities and pleasures of parenthood.

Adulthood (31–45 Years of Age)

   I. Stage of development—psychosocial stage: *generativity versus self-absorption.*
   II. Physical development
   A. Gradual decline in biologic functioning, although in the late 30s the individual is still near peak.
   B. Period of peak sexual capacity for women occurs during the mid-30s.
   C. Distinct sense of bodily decline occurs around 40 years of age.
   D. *Circulatory* system begins to slow somewhat after 40 years of age.

III. Cognitive development
   A. Takes longer to memorize.
   B. Still at peak in abstract thinking and problem solving.
   C. Generates new levels of awareness.
   D. Gives more meaning to complex tasks.

IV. Socialization
   A. Achieves a realistic self-identity.
   B. Perceptions are based on reality.
   C. Acts on decisions and assumes responsibility for actions.

D. Accepts limitations while developing assets.
E. Delays immediate gratification in favor of future satisfaction.
F. Evaluates mistakes, determines reasons and causes, and learns new behavior.
G. Struggles to establish a place in society.
   1. Begins to settle down.
   2. Pursues long-range plans and goals.
   3. Has a stronger need to be responsible.
   4. Invests self as fully as possible in social structure, including work, family, and community.
H. Seeks advancement by improving and using skills, becoming more creative, and pursuing ambitions.

Middle Life (46–64 Years of Age)

   I. Stage of development—psychosocial stage: *continuation of generativity versus self-absorption.*
   II. Physical development
   A. Failing *eyesight,* especially for close vision, may be one of the first symptoms of aging.
   B. Hearing loss is very gradual, especially for low sounds; hearing for *high-pitched* sounds is impaired more readily.
   C. There is a gradual loss of *taste* buds in the 50s and gradual loss of sense of *smell* in the 60s, causing the individual to have a diminished sense of taste.
   D. *Muscle strength* declines because of decreased levels of estrogen and testosterone; it takes more time to accomplish the same physical task.
   E. *Lung* capacity is impaired, which adds to decreased endurance.
   F. The *skin* begins to wrinkle, and hair begins to gray.
   G. *Postural changes* take place because of loss of calcium and reduced activity.

III. Cognitive development
   A. *Memory* begins to decline slowly around 50 years of age.
   B. It takes longer to *learn* new tasks, and old tasks take longer to perform.
   C. *Practical judgment* is increased due to experiential background.
   D. May tend to withdraw from mental activity or overcompensate by trying the impossible.

IV. Socialization
   A. The middle years can be very rewarding if previous stages have been fulfilled.
   B. The years of responsibility for raising children are over.
   C. Husbands and wives usually find a closer bond.
   D. There is less financial strain for those with steady employment.
   E. Individuals are usually at the height of their careers; most leaders in their field are in this age group.
   F. Self-realization is achieved.
   1. There is more inner direction.
   2. There is no longer a need to please everyone.
   3. Individual is less likely to compare self with others.

    4. Individual approves of self without being dependent on standards of others.
    5. There is less fear of failure in life because past failures have been met and dealt with.

Early Late Years
(65–79 Years of Age)

  I. **Stage of development**—psychosocial stage: *ego integrity and acceptance versus despair and disgust.*
 II. **Physical development**
    A. Continues to decrease in vigor and capacity.
    B. Has more frequent aches and pains.
    C. Likely to have at least one major illness.
III. **Cognitive development**
    A. Mental acuity continues to slow down.
    B. Judgment and problem solving remain intact, but the processes may take longer.
    C. May have problems in remembering *names* and *dates.*
IV. **Socialization**
    A. Individual is faced with the reality of the experience of physical decline.
    B. Physical and mental changes intensify the feelings of aging and mortality.
    C. Increasing frequency of death and serious illness among friends, relatives, and associates reinforces further the concept of mortality.
    D. Constant reception of medical warnings to follow certain precautions or to run serious risks otherwise adds to general feeling of decline.
    E. Individual is less interested in obtaining the rewards of society and is more interested in utilizing own inner resources.
    F. Individuals feel that they have earned the right to do what is important for self-satisfaction.
    G. Retirement allows time for expression of own creative energies.
    H. Overcomes the splitting of youth and age; gets along well with adolescents.
    I. Learns to deal with the reality that only old age remains.
    J. Provides moral support to grandchildren; more tolerant of grandchildren than was of own children.
    K. Tends to release major authority of family to children while holding self in the role of consultant.

Late Years
(80 Years of Age and Older)

  I. **Stage of development**—psychosocial stage: *continuation of ego integrity and acceptance versus despair and disgust.*
 II. **Physical development**
    A. Additional sensory problems occur, including diminished sensation to *touch and pain.*
    B. Increase in loss of muscle tone occurs, including *sphincter* (urinary and anal) control.

    C. Individual is insecure and unsure about orientation to *space* and sense of *balance,* which may result in falls and injury.
III. **Cognitive development**
    A. Has better memory for the *past* than the present.
    B. *Repetition* of memories occurs.
    C. Individual may use *confabulation* to fill in memory gaps.
    D. Forgetfulness may lead to serious *safety* problems, and individual may require constant supervision.
    E. Increased arteriosclerosis may lead to mental illness (dementia and other cognitive disorders).
IV. **Socialization**
    A. Few significant relationships are maintained; deaths of friends, family, and associates cause isolation.
    B. Individual may be preoccupied with immediate bodily needs and personal comforts; the *gastrointestinal tract* frequently becomes the major focus.
    C. Individuals see they can provide others with an example of wisdom and courage.
    D. Individuals come to terms with themselves.
    E. Individuals are concerned with own mortality.
    F. Individuals come to terms with the process of dying and prepare for own death.

⌖ Summary of Key Points

1. Avoid bias, prejudice, or stereotyping during an assessment. For example, a 34-year-old man complaining of chest pain on exertion is not too young to have severe coronary artery disease.
2. Use an organized approach for completing an assessment (e.g., head-to-toe, systems).
3. Subjective data are the information given by the patient or family member.
4. Objective data consist of what the nurse observes, hears on auscultation or percussion, feels during palpation, or smells. These data validate the subjective findings.
5. Assessment always begins with inspection.

Questions

  1. Which information about a patient is an example of subjective data?
    1. Vital signs
    2. Reason for admission
    3. Chest x-ray
    4. Color of urine
  2. The first step in performing a physical assessment is:
    1. Inspection
    2. Palpation
    3. Percussion
    4. Auscultation
  3. On auscultation of the lungs the nurse hears a popping sound. The correct assessment would most likely be:
    1. Fremitus

2. Crepitus
3. Crackles
4. Wheezes

4. A normal physical assessment finding in the older adult would be:
   1. Increased taste
   2. Thinning of toenails
   3. Increased lung compliance
   4. Decreased elasticity of skin

Answers/Rationale

1. **(2)** Subjective data includes what the patient or family members tell the nurse. The information gathered during the nursing history is subjective data. Objective data are observations made during physical assessment or the results from laboratory/diagnostic tests **(1,3,4)**. **AS, 5, SECE**

2. **(1)** Regardless of the system being assessed, the sequence *always* begins with inspection or observation. The *next* step is usually palpation **(2)**, followed by percussion **(3)**, and finally auscultation **(4)**. The *exception* is the GI system, where auscultation *follows* inspection. **AS, 5, SECE**

3. **(3)** Crackles (*formerly* called rales) are the discontinuous sounds heard on auscultation, produced by the popping open of airways; usually associated with fluid accumulation in the lungs. Fremitus **(1)** is sound vibration felt with the hand placed on the chest. Crepitus **(2)** is the crackling sound of air in the subcutaneous tissue when palpation is done. Wheezes **(4)** are high-pitched sounds produced by air through narrowed airways. **AS, 6, PhI**

4. **(4)** With aging, the skin loses moisture and elasticity, developing wrinkles and lines. Taste buds **(1)** decrease, *not* increase; in particular there is a decrease in the ability to taste salt and sweet. Toenails **(2)** thicken, *not* thin, as peripheral circulation decreases. Lung compliance **(3)** decreases with age; consequently, the older adult tends to hypoventilate and is at greater risk for pulmonary problems. **AS, 5, PhI**

Key to Codes

Nursing process: AS, assessment; **AN,** analysis; **PL,** planning; **IMP,** implementation; **EV,** evaluation. (See Appendix M for explanation of nursing process steps.)

Category of human function: 1, protective; **2,** sensory-perceptual; **3,** comfort, rest, activity, and mobility; **4,** nutrition; **5,** growth and development; **6,** fluid-gas transport; **7,** psychosocial-cultural; **8,** elimination. (See Appendix O for explanation.)

Client need: SECE, safe, effective care environment; **PhI,** physiological integrity; **PsI,** psychosocial integrity; **HPM,** health promotion/maintenance. (See Appendix P for explanation.)

Peripheral Vascular Disorders

Chapter Outline

- Hypertension
- Arteriosclerosis
- Arteriosclerosis Obliterans
- Aneurysms
- Varicose Veins
- Vein Ligation and Stripping
- Thrombophlebitis
- Peripheral Embolism

- Summary of Key Points
- Study and Memory Aids
  - Positioning
  - Diagnostic Study
- Diets
- Drug Review
- Questions
- Answers/Rationale

Hypertension

Defined as a sustained, elevated systemic arterial blood pressure. A diastolic elevation is more serious, reflecting pressure on arterial wall during the resting phase of the cardiac cycle (Table 2.1).

I. Pathophysiology: increased peripheral resistance leading to thickened arteriole walls and left ventricular hypertrophy.

II. Risk factors:
- **A.** African-Americans (2:1).
- **B.** Use of birth control pills.
- **C.** Overweight.
- **D.** Smoking.
- **E.** Stress.
- **F.** Excessive sodium intake.
- **G.** Lack of activity.

III. Classifications:
- **A.** *Primary* (essential): occurs in 90% of patients; etiology unknown; diastolic pressure is ≥90 mm Hg, and other causes of hypertension are absent. *Benign* hypertension (diastolic pressure ≤120 mm Hg) is considered controllable; *malignant* hypertension (diastolic >140 − 150 mm Hg) is uncontrollable.
- **B.** *Secondary:* occurs in remaining 10%; usually renal, endocrine, neurogenic, and/or cardiac in origin.
- **C.** *Labile* (prehypertensive): a fluctuating blood pressure; increases during stress, otherwise normal or near normal.
- **D.** See Table 2.1 for comparison of hypertension and hypotension.

IV. Assessment
- **A.** *Subjective data:*
  1. Early-morning headache, usually occipital.
  2. Light-headedness, tinnitus.
  3. Palpitations.
  4. Fatigue, insomnia.
  5. Forgetfulness, irritability.
  6. Altered vision: white spots, blurring, or loss.
- **B.** *Objective data:*
  1. Epistaxis (nosebleeds).
  2. Elevated blood pressure: systolic >140 mm Hg, diastolic >90 mm Hg; narrowed pulse pressure.
  3. Retinal changes; papilledema.
  4. Shortness of breath on slight exertion.
  5. Cardiac, cerebral, and renal changes.

V. Analysis/nursing diagnosis
- **A.** *Altered peripheral tissue perfusion* related to increased peripheral resistance.
- **B.** *Decreased cardiac output* related to ventricular hypertrophy.
- **C.** *Risk for injury* related to altered vision.
- **D.** *Risk for activity intolerance* related to inadequate oxygenation.
- **E.** *Fatigue* related to poor perfusion.

VI. Nursing care plan/implementation
- **A.** Goal: *provide for physical and emotional rest.*
  1. Rest periods before/after eating, visiting hours; *avoid* upsetting situations.
  2. Give tranquilizers, sedatives, as ordered.
- **B.** Goal: *provide for special safety needs.*
  1. Monitor blood pressure: both arms; *standing, sitting, lying positions.*

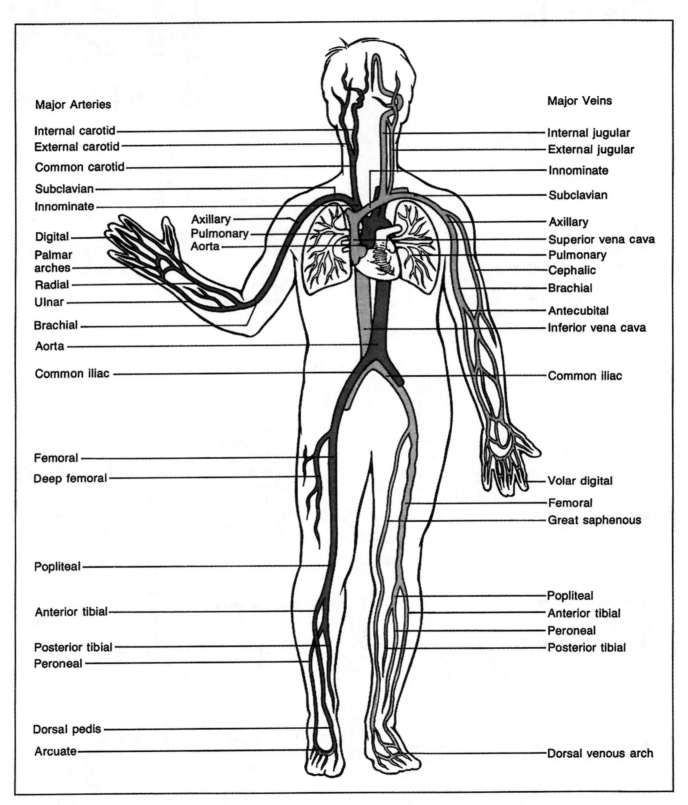

Major Arteries

Internal carotid
External carotid
Common carotid
Subclavian
Innominate
Digital
Palmar arches
Radial
Ulnar
Brachial
Aorta
Common iliac
Femoral
Deep femoral
Popliteal
Anterior tibial
Posterior tibial
Peroneal
Dorsal pedis
Arcuate

Axillary
Pulmonary
Aorta

Major Veins

Internal jugular
External jugular
Innominate
Subclavian
Axillary
Superior vena cava
Pulmonary
Cephalic
Brachial
Antecubital
Inferior vena cava
Common iliac
Volar digital
Femoral
Great saphenous
Popliteal
Anterior tibial
Peroneal
Posterior tibial
Dorsal venous arch

Peripheral vascular system: major arteries and major veins.

TABLE 2.1   **IMBALANCES IN BLOOD PRESSURE: COMPARATIVE ASSESSMENT OF HYPOTENSION AND HYPERTENSION**

	Hypotension	*Hypertension*
Common causes	Angina pectoris Myocardial infarction Acute and chronic pericarditis Valvular defects Heart failure	Essential hypertension Iron deficiency anemia Pernicious anemia Arteriosclerosis obliterans Polycythemia vera
⋈ Assessment		
Behavior	Anxiety, apprehension, decreasing mentation, confusion	Nervousness, mood swings, irritability, difficulty with memory, depression, confusion
Neurologic	Essentially noncontributory	Decreased vibratory sensations, increased/decreased reflexes, *Babinski* reflex, changes in coordination
Head/neck	Distended neck veins, worried expression	Bruits over carotids, distended neck veins, epistaxis, diplopia, ringing in ears, dull occipital headaches on arising
Skin	Pale, cool, moist	Dry, pale, glossy, flaky, cold; decreased or absent hair
GI	Anorexia, nausea, vomiting, constipation	Anorexia, flatulence, diarrhea, constipation
Respiratory	Dyspnea, orthopnea, paroxysmal nocturnal dyspnea, tachypnea, moist crackles, cough	Dyspnea, orthopnea, moist crackles
Cardiovascular	Tires easily	Decreased exercise tolerance, weakness, palpitations
	Blood pressure—decreased systolic, decreased systolic/diastolic	Blood pressure—increased systolic, increased systolic and diastolic
	Pulse—increased/decreased, weak, thready, irregular, arrhythmias	Decreased or absent pedal pulses
Renal	Oliguria	Oliguria, nocturia, proteinuria
Extremities	Dependent edema	Tingling, numbness, or cold hands and feet, dependent edema, ulcers of legs or feet

Source: Lagerquist, SL: *Little, Brown's NCLEX-RN Examination Review.* Boston: Little, Brown, 1996. P. 50.

2. Limit/prevent activities that increase pressure (anxiety, anger, frustration, upsetting visitors, fatigue).

3. Assist with ambulation; change position gradually to prevent dizziness and light-headedness (postural hypotension).

4. Monitor for electrolyte imbalance when on *low-sodium diet, diuretic therapy;* monitor intake and output to prevent fluid depletion and arrhythmias resulting from potassium loss.

5. Observe for signs of hemorrhage, shock, and stroke, which may occur after surgery.

C. Goal: **health teaching** (patient and family).

1. Procedures to decrease anxiety; relaxation techniques, stress management.

2. Importance of taking meds as prescribed for most rapid improvement of condition.

3. Side effects of: hypotensive drugs, diuretics, adrenergic blockers, vasodilators, calcium channel blockers (faintness, nausea, vomiting, postural hypotension, sexual dysfunction). See Appendix D for specific pharmacologic actions.

4. Weight control to reduce arterial pressure.

5. *Restrictions:* stimulants (tea, coffee, tobacco), sodium, calories, fat.

6. Life-style adjustments: daily exercise needed; reduce occupational and environmental stress; importance of rest.

7. Blood pressure measurement: daily, same conditions, position preference of physician.

8. Signs, symptoms, complications of disease (headache, confusion, visual changes, nausea/vomiting, convulsions).

9. Causes of intermittent hypotension: alcohol, hot weather, exercise, febrile illness, hot bath.

⋈ **VII. Evaluation/outcome criteria**

A. Blood pressure within normal range for age (diastolic <90 mm Hg)—stable.

B. Minimal or no pathophysiologic or therapeutic

complications (e.g., visual changes, CVA, drug side effects).

C. Reduces weight to reasonable level for height, bone structure.

D. *Takes prescribed medications* regularly, even when symptoms have resolved.

E. Complies with restrictions: no smoking; restricted sodium, fat.

F. Exercises regularly—program compatible with personal and health care goals.

Arteriosclerosis

Arteriosclerosis is a loss of elasticity, thickening, and hardening of arterial walls. The common type is atherosclerosis. Arteriosclerosis precedes angina pectoris and myocardial infarction.

    I. Pathophysiology

      A. Atherosclerotic plaque, discrete lumpy thickening of arterial wall.

      B. Narrows lumen, can occlude vessel.

   II. Risk factors

      A. Increased serum cholesterol (low-density lipids) level.

      B. Hypertension.

      C. Cigarette smoking.

      D. Diabetes mellitus.

(See Angina pectoris, p. 32–35, and Myocardial infarction, pp. 35–38, for nursing implications.)

Arteriosclerosis Obliterans

Arteriosclerosis obliterans is the most common obstructive disorder of the arterial system (aorta, large and medium-size arteries). It frequently involves the femoral artery.

    I. Pathophysiology: fatty deposits in intimal, medial layer of arterial walls; plaque formation → narrowed arterial lumens; decreased distensibility → decreased blood flow; ischemic changes in tissues.

   II. Risk factors

      A. Age (>50).

      B. Sex (men).

      C. Diabetes mellitus.

      D. Hyperlipidemia—obesity.

      E. Cigarette smoking.

      F. Hypertension.

      G. Polycythemia vera.

  III. Assessment

      A. *Subjective data:*

        1. Pain:

          a. *Type*—cramplike.

          b. *Location*—foot, calf, thigh, buttocks.

          c. *Duration*—variable, may be relieved by rest.

          d. *Precipitating causes*—exercise (intermittent claudication), but occasionally may occur when at rest.

        2. Tingling, numbness in toes, feet.

        3. Persistent coldness of one or both lower extremities.

      B. *Objective data:*

        1. Lower extremities:

          a. Pedal pulses—absent or diminished.

          b. Skin—shiny, glossy, dry, cold, chalky white, decreased/absent hair, ulcers, gangrene.

        2. Lab data: increased serum cholesterol, triglycerides, CBC, platelets.

        3. *Angiography*—indicates location, nature of occlusion.

  IV. Analysis/nursing diagnosis

      A. *Altered tissue perfusion* related to peripheral vascular disease.

      B. *Risk for activity intolerance* related to pain and sensory changes.

      C. *Pain* related to ischemia.

      D. *Risk for impaired skin integrity* related to poor circulation.

      E. *Risk for injury* related to numbness of extremities.

   V. Nursing care plan/implementation

      A. Goal: *promote circulation; decrease discomfort.*

        1. *Position:* elevate *head* of bed on blocks (3–6 in.), as gravity aids perfusion to thighs, legs; elevating legs increases pain.

        2. Comfort: keep warm; *avoid* chilling or use of heating pads, which may burn skin; apply bed socks.

        3. Circulation: check pedal pulses, skin color, temperature qid.

        4. Medications:

          a. *Vasodilators.*

          b. *Anticoagulants*—heparin sodium, dicumarol, ASA.

          c. *Antihyperlipidemics*—clofibrate, cholestyramine resin, nicotinic acid.

      B. Goal: *prevent infection, injury.*

        1. Skin care: use bed cradle; sheepskin; heel pads; mild soap, dry thoroughly; lotion; do *not* massage, so as to prevent release of thrombus.

        2. Foot care: wear properly fitting shoes, slippers when out of bed; inspect for injury or pressure areas; nail care by podiatrist.

        3. *Diet:* high in vitamins B and C to improve cardiovascular functioning and skin integrity; low fat

      c. Goal: *health teaching.*

        1. Skin care; inspect daily.

        2. Activity: balance exercise, rest to increase collateral circulation; walk only until painful.

        3. Exercises: walking, Buerger-Allen exercises (gravity alternately fills and empties blood vessels).

        4. *Avoid* smoking.

        5. Recognizes and reports signs of occlusion (e.g., pain, cramping, numbness in extremities, color changes—white or blue, temperature changes—cool to cold).

VI. Evaluation/outcome criteria
   A. Decreased pain.
   B. Skin integrity preserved; no loss of limb.
   C. Quits smoking.
   D. Does exercises to increase collateral circulation.

Aneurysms

Aneurysms can form in either the thoracic or abdominal aorta and are defined as localized or diffuse dilatations or outpouchings of a vessel wall, usually an artery, that exert pressure on adjacent structures. They primarily occur in men over 60 years of age and are resected surgically. This involves reconstruction with a synthetic or vascular graft.

I. Risk factors
   A. Atherosclerosis.
   B. Trauma.
   C. Syphilis.
   D. Congenital weakness.
   E. Local infection.

II. Assessment
   A. *Subjective data:*
     1. Pain:
       a. Constant, boring, neuralgic, intermittent—low back, abdominal.
       b. Angina—sudden onset may mean rupture or dissection, which are **emergency** conditions.
     2. Dyspnea; orthopnea.
     3. Dysphagia.
   B. *Objective data:*
     1. Vital signs:
       a. Radial pulses differ.
       b. Tachycardia.
       c. Hypotension after rupture, leading to shock.
     2. Pulsating mass: abdominal, chest wall pulsation; edema of chest wall (thoracic aneurysm); periumbilical pulsation (abdominal aneurysm); audible bruit over aorta.
     3. Cyanosis, mottled below level of aneurysm.
     4. Veins: dilated, superficial—neck, chest, arms.
     5. Cough: paroxysmal, brassy.
     6. Diaphoresis, pallor, fainting after rupture.
     7. Peripheral pulses:
       a. Femoral present.
       b. Pedal weak or absent.
     8. Stool bloody from irritation.

III. Analysis/nursing diagnosis
   A. *Altered peripheral tissue perfusion* related to distal arterial emboli.
   B. *Pain* related to pressure on lumbar nerves.
   C. *Anxiety* related to risk of rupture.

IV. Nursing care plan/implementation
   A. Goal: *provide emergency care prior to surgery for dissection or rupture.*
     1. *Vital signs:* at least every 5 min (systolic blood pressure <100 mm Hg and pulse >100 beats/min with rupture).

     2. *IVs:* may have 2–4 sites; lactated Ringer's may be ordered.
     3. *Urine output:* monitored every 15–30 min.
     4. *O$_2$:* usually via nasal prongs.
     5. Medications as ordered: antihypertensives to prevent extension of dissection.
     6. Transport to operating room quickly.
     7. See The Perioperative Experience, p. 111, for general preoperative care.
   B. Goal: *prevent complications postoperatively.*
     1. *Position:* initially flat in bed; *avoid* sharp flexion of hip and knee, which places pressure on femoral and popliteal arteries; turn gently side to side; note erythema on back from pooled blood.
     2. *Vital signs:* CVP; hourly peripheral pulses distal to graft site, including neurovascular check of lower extremities; absent pulses for 6–12 h indicates occlusion; *Doppler blood flow* instrument.
     3. Urine output: hourly from indwelling catheter.
       a. Immediately report anuria or oliguria (<30 mL/h).
       b. Check color for hematuria.
       c. Monitor daily blood urea nitrogen and creatinine levels.
     4. Observe for *signs of atheroembolization* (patchy areas of ischemia); report change in color, motor ability, or sensation of lower extremities.
     5. Observe for *signs of bowel ischemia* (decreased/absent bowel sounds, pain, *guaiac*-positive diarrhea, abdominal distention); may have *nasogastric tube.*
     6. Measure abdominal girth; increase seen with graft leakage.
   C. Goal: *promote comfort.*
     1. *Position:* alignment, comfort; prevent heel ulcers.
     2. *Medication:* narcotics.
   D. Goal: **health teaching.**
     1. Minimize recurrence; *avoid* trauma, infection, smoking, *high-cholesterol diet,* obesity.
     2. Regular medical supervision.

V. Evaluation/outcome criteria
   1. Surgical intervention before rupture.
   2. No loss of renal function.

Varicose Veins

Varicose veins are abnormally lengthened, tortuous, dilated superficial veins (saphenous) and result from incompetent valves, especially in lower extremities. The process is irreversible.

I. Pathophysiology: dilated vein → venous stasis → edema; fibrotic changes; pigmentation of skin; lowered resistance to trauma.

II. Risk factors
   A. Congenital defect of venous valves.
   B. Trauma.

C. Deep-vein thrombosis.
D. Pregnancy.
E. Abdominal tumors.
F. Chronic disease (heart, liver).
G. Occupations requiring long periods of standing.

▶ **III. Assessment**
  A. *Subjective data:*
    1. Dull aches; heaviness in legs.
    2. Pain; muscle cramping.
    3. Fatigue in lower extremities, increased with hot weather, high altitude; history of risk factors.
  B. *Objective data:*
    1. Nodular protrusions along veins.
    2. Edema.
    3. Diagnostic tests: *Trendelenburg* test; *phlebography*; *Doppler* blood flow measurement.

▶ **IV. Analysis/nursing diagnosis**
  A. *Altered tissue perfusion* related to venous valve incompetence.
  B. *Pain* related to edema and muscle cramping.
  C. *Risk for activity intolerance* related to leg discomfort.
  D. *Body image disturbance* related to disfigurement of leg.

▶ **V. Nursing care plan/implementation**
  A. Goal: *promote venous return from lower extremities.*
    1. Activity: walk every hour.
    2. Discourage prolonged sitting, standing, sitting with crossed legs.
    3. *Position:* elevate legs q2–3h; elastic stockings or Ace wraps.
  B. Goal: *provide for safety.*
    1. Assist with early ambulation.
    2. Surgical asepsis with wounds, leg ulcers.
    3. Observe for hemorrhage—if occurs: *elevate leg,* apply pressure, notify physician.
    4. Observe for allergic reactions if sclerosing drugs used; have *antihistamine* available.
  C. Goal: **health teaching.**
    1. Weight-reducing techniques, dietary approaches if indicated.
    2. Preventive measures: *leg elevation; avoid* prolonged standing, sitting, high chairs, tight girdles, constrictive clothing; wear support hose.
    3. Expectations for *Trendelenburg test.*
      a. While patient is lying down, elevate leg 65 degrees to empty veins.
      b. Apply tourniquet high on upper thigh (do not constrict deep veins).
      c. Patient stands with tourniquet in place.
      d. Filling of veins is observed.
      e. Normal response is slow filling from below in 20–30 sec, with no change in rate when tourniquet is removed.
      f. Incompetent veins distend very quickly with back flow.
    4. Prepare for vein ligation and stripping.

▶ **VI. Evaluation/outcome criteria**
  A. Relief or control of symptoms.
  B. Activity without pain.

Vein Ligation and Stripping

Vein ligation and stripping is the surgical intervention used for the treatment of advancing varicosities, stasis ulcerations, and cosmetic needs of patient. The procedure involves ligation of the saphenous vein at the groin, where it joins the femoral vein, and saphenous stripping from the groin to the ankle. The legs are then wrapped with a pressure bandage.

▶ **I.** See Varicose veins, pp. 13–14, for assessment data and nursing diagnosis of the patient requiring surgery.

▶ **II. Nursing care plan/implementation**
  A. Goal: *prevent complications.*
    1. *Position: elevate* legs 18 out of 24 h above level of heart, for 1 wk. (See *Positioning Box* at end of unit.)
    2. Activity:
      a. Assist with early, frequent ambulation; medicate for pain before ambulation.
      b. *No* chair sitting to prevent venous pooling, thrombus formation.
    3. Bleeding: check elastic bandages, dressings several times a day.
  B. Goal: **health teaching** to prevent recurrence.
    1. Weight reduction.
    2. *Avoid* constricting garments.
    3. Change positions frequently.
    4. Wear support hose/stockings to enhance venous return.
    5. *No* crossing legs at knees.

▶ **III. Evaluation/outcome criteria**
  A. No complications—hemorrhage, infection, nerve damage, deep-vein thrombosis.
  B. No recurrence of varicosities.
  C. Adequate circulation to legs: strong pedal pulses.
  D. Resumes daily activities; free of pain.

Thrombophlebitis

Thrombophlebitis is the formation of a blood clot in an inflamed vein, secondary to phlebitis or partial obstruction. It may lead to venous insufficiency and pulmonary embolism.

  I. Pathophysiology: endothelial inflammation → formation of platelet plug (blood clot) → slowing of blood flow → increase in procoagulants in local area → initiation of clotting mechanisms.

  II. Risk factors
    A. Immobility.
    B. Venous disease.
    C. Prolonged sitting—knees bent.
    D. Childbirth.
    E. Hypercoagulability of blood.
    F. Venous trauma (IVs).
    G. Fractures.

▶ **III. Assessment**
  A. *Subjective data:*
    1. Calf stiffness, soreness.
    2. Severe pain: walking, dorsiflexion of foot (*Homans' sign*).

TABLE 2.2 ⋈ NURSING RESPONSIBILITIES WITH ANTICOAGULANT THERAPY

	Heparin	*Warfarin (Coumadin)*
Monitor	aPTT (25–38 sec); therapeutic level usually 1.5–2.0 times control (50–80 sec)	PT (11–15 sec); therapeutic level—International Normalized Ratio (INR): 2–3 (sample/control)
Inspect	Ecchymosis, bleeding gums, petechiae, hematuria	Bleeding, ecchymosis
Administer	With an infusion pump; never mix with other drugs; *never* aspirate; *avoid* massaging site	Same time every day; PO
Avoid	Salicylates and other anticoagulants, e.g., non-steroidal anti-inflammatory agents, corticosteroids, some penicillins	Same as heparin
Antidote	Protamine sulfate	Vitamin K

Source: Lagerquist, SL: *Little, Brown's NCLEX-RN Examination Review.* Boston: Little, Brown, 1996. P. 70.

B. *Objective data:*
    1. Vein: red, hot, hard, thready.
    2. Limb: swollen, pale, cold.
    3. Vital signs: low-grade fever.

⋈ **IV. Analysis/nursing diagnosis**
    A. *Altered peripheral tissue perfusion* related to venous stasis.
    B. *Pain* related to inflammation.
    C. *Activity intolerance* related to leg pain.

⋈ **V. Nursing care plan/implementation**
    A. Goal: *provide rest, comfort, and relief from pain.*
        1. Bedrest.
        2. *Position:* as ordered; usually extremity *elevated;* watch for pressure points.
        3. Apply warm, moist heat to affected area as prescribed (cold may also be ordered).
        4. Assess progress of affected area: swelling, pain, soreness, temperature, color.
        5. Administer *analgesics* as ordered.
    B. Goal: *prevent complications.*
        1. Observe for signs of embolism (pain at site of embolism); allergic reaction (anaphylactic shock) with streptokinase.
        2. *Precautions: no* rubbing or massage of limb.
        3. *Medications:* anticoagulants (sodium heparin, coumadin); streptokinase (*Streptase*). (Table 2.2)
        4. *Bleeding:* hematuria, epistaxis, ecchymosis.
        5. Skin care, to relieve increased redness/maceration from hot or cold applications.
        6. Range of motion: unaffected limb.
    C. Goal: **health teaching.**
        1. *Precautions:* tight garters, girdles; sitting with legs crossed; oral contraceptives.
        2. *Preventive measures:* walking daily, swimming several times weekly if possible, wading, rest periods—with legs *elevated,* elastic stockings (may remove at bedtime).
        3. *Medication side effects:* anticoagulants—pink toothbrush, hematuria, easily bruised.
            a. Carry MedicAlert card/bracelet.
            b. *Contraindicated drugs,* which increase or decrease anticoagulant effects—aspirin, glutethimide (Doriden), cefamandole, cefotetan, plicamycin, chloramphenicol (Chloromycetin), neomycin, phenylbutazone (Butazolidin), barbiturates.
        4. Prepare for surgery (thrombectomy, vein ligation).

⋈ **VI. Evaluation/outcome criteria**
    A. No complications (e.g., embolism).
    B. No recurrence of symptoms.
    C. Free of pain—ambulates without discomfort.

Peripheral Embolism

A peripheral embolism is made up of fragments of thrombi, globules of fat, clumps of tissue, calcified plaques, or air that moves in the circulation and lodges in a vessel, obstructing blood flow. Thrombic emboli are the most common. They may be venous or arterial.

☞ Summary of Key Points

1. The pain associated with **arterial disease** is provoked by exercise/activity, relieved by rest, and worsens with elevation.
2. Concepts important to understand about **maintaining adequate circulation** include: autoregulation, coagulation, hydration, vessel size (inflammation, vasoconstriction, or vasodilation), viscosity of blood, vascular resistance, and venous valve competence.
3. Prevention of **hypertension** should focus on recognizing risk factors and managing modifiable risks. For example, weight loss may be one of the most effective ways to lower blood pressure.
4. **Disorders of the peripheral vascular system** involve narrowing, obstruction, or damage to arteries or veins, resulting in ischemia, or a lack of blood flow to the tissues or organs involved.
5. A patient with **thrombophlebitis** may be asymptomatic.

⚲ Study and Memory Aids

POSTOPERATIVE POSITIONING OF PATIENT WITH VASCULAR CONDITION

Condition	Position	Purpose
Iliofemoral bypass; Arterial insufficiency	1. Do *not* elevate legs. 2. *Avoid* hip flexion—walk or stand, but do *not* sit.	1. Arterial flow is helped by gravity. 2. Flexion of the hip compresses the vessels of the extremity.
Vein strippings; vein ligations	1. Keep legs elevated. 2. Do *not* stand or sit for long periods.	1. Prevents venous stasis. 2. Prevents venous pooling.

Source: Jane Vincent Corbett, RN, MS, Ed.D., Professor, School of Nursing, University of San Francisco. Used with permission.

Diagnostic Study

Phlebography (lower limb venography)—determines patency of the tibial-popliteal, superficial femoral—common femoral, and saphenous veins. A contrast medium is injected into the superficial and/or deep veins of the involved extremity, followed by acquisition of x-ray studies, while the leg is placed in a variety of positions; *used to* detect deep-vein thrombosis and to select a vein for use in arterial bypass grafting; localized clotting may result.

Assessment of Hypertension: "Elevated"

E xertional SOB
L ack of activity
E arly-morning headache
V ascular changes
A nxiety increased
T ired
E pistaxis
D iastolic pressure elevated

Hypertension: Complications—4 Cs

CHF (congestive heart failure)
CVA (cerebrovascular accident)
CD (coronary artery disease)
CRF (chronic renal failure)

**No Smoking
with hypertension**

Central Venous Pressure

Determined by vascular tone, blood volume, and the ability of the heart to receive and pump blood. Measured using a central venous catheter placed in the superior vena cava; normal value: 2–12 mm Hg.

Varicose Veins Assessment: "Twisted"

T wisted
W ork posture
I rreversible process
S welling
T rendelenburg test result positive
E xtremities—lower
D ull aches

Vein Ligation and Stripping

No sitting

Diets

Hypertension

↓Na
↓Calories
↓Cholesterol
 No caffeine

Arteriosclerosis Obliterans

↑ Vitamin B & C
↓ Fat

Aneurysms

↓ Cholesterol
↓ Caloric intake

◦ Drug Review

Hypertension

Adrenergic blockers—Atenolol (*Tenormin*), 50–150 mg qd
  Propranolol hydrochloride (*Inderal*), 80–240 mg bid
Angiotensin converting enzyme (ACE) inhibitor—Enalapril (*Vasotec*), 10–40 mg daily
Calcium channel blockers—Verapamil (*Calan*), 80–120 mg tid
Diuretics—Furosemide (*Lasix*), 20–80 mg daily
Sedatives/tranquilizers
  Chlordiazepoxide HCl (*Librium*), 5–10 mg PO
  Diazepam (*Valium*), 2–10 mg PO
Vasodilators—Diazoxide (*Hyperstat*), 1–3 mg/kg IV q 5–15 min
  Hydralazine (*Apresoline*), 10–50 mg q.i.d.

Note: See also aneurysm medications.

Arteriosclerosis Obliterans

Anticoagulants
  Heparin sodium, IV 5,000 U. IV to start followed by 20,000–40,000 U infusion over 24 hours SC 8000–10,000 units q8h adjusted according to partial thromboplastin time (PTT)
  Warfarin (*Coumadin*), 10 mg daily adjusted according to prothrombin time (PT)
Antihyperlipidemics
  Clofibrate (*Atromid* S) 2 g/d in 2–4 divided doses
  Cholestyramine (*Questran*), 4 g 1–6 times daily
  Colestipol (*Colestid*), 5–30 g daily
  Nicotinic acid (*Nicobid*), 500 mg daily up to 2 g tid
Antiplatelet—Aspirin, 1–3 g daily in 2–4 divided doses
Hemorheologic agents—Pentoxifylline (Trental), 400 mg tid with meals

Aneurysms

Antihypertensive: Angiotensin-converting enzyme (ACE) inhibitor—Catopril (*Capoten*), 12.5–25 mg tid

Thrombophlebitis/Peripheral Embolism

Anticoagulants
  Heparin sodium, IV 1000 units/hr; SC 8000–10,000 units q8h adjusted according to PTT
  Warfarin (*Coumadin*), 10 mg daily adjusted according to PT
Thrombolytic agents—Streptokinase (*Streptase*), IV 250,000 IU loading dose followed by 100,000 IU/h for 24 h

Note: Give with no other anticoagulants, aspirin, large doses of penicillin or penicillin-like drugs, some cephalosporins, plicamycin or valproic acid, which may increase risk of bleeding.

Questions

1. Which vital sign change is the most likely indicator of hypertension?
  1. A narrowing pulse pressure.
  2. Irregular pulse.
  3. Fluctuating systolic pressure.
  4. Diastolic pressure exceeding 90 mm Hg.
2. After a month of treatment for hypertension, a patient returns for a clinical follow-up and is found to have a blood pressure of 190/130 mm Hg. The nurse should first seek information on the patient's:
  1. Stress level at work.
  2. Progress with relaxation techniques.
  3. Compliance with prescribed drug therapy.
  4. Success with a weight-loss program.
3. A patient is to receive atenolol (Tenormin) PO. Which existing condition should the nurse assess for that may be adversely affected by this drug?
  1. Diabetes mellitus.
  2. Cholecystitis.
  3. Duodenal ulcer.
  4. Diverticulosis.
4. To evaluate the effectiveness of a low-sodium diet in a patient with hypertension, the nurse should check:
  1. Serum sodium levels.
  2. Changes in body weight.
  3. Appearance of ankles.
  4. Breath sounds.
5. Patient teaching for a hypertensive patient receiving captopril (Capoten) should include which point?
  1. The need for more potassium in the diet.
  2. The need to limit fluid intake to increase drug effectiveness.
  3. The fact that taste perception may be decreased.
  4. The need to test the urine for glucose.
6. Which abnormal laboratory result would the nurse likely in a patient taking captopril (Capoten)?
  1. Hypokalemia.
  2. Hyperkalemia.
  3. Leukocytosis.
  4. Hypernatremia.

7. To promote optimal rest at night in a patient taking a diuretic, the patient should be instructed to:
   1. Restrict daytime fluid intake to prevent nocturia.
   2. Take the diuretic in the morning with food.
   3. Drink a hot beverage before bedtime to relax.
   4. Sleep with the head elevated to promote breathing.

8. A patient admitted to the emergency room with a BP of 240/180 mmHg receives diazoxide (Hyperstat) IV. The nurse would monitor this patient for which adverse effect?
   1. Rebound hypertension.
   2. Chest pain.
   3. Reflex bradycardia.
   4. Pallor and sweating.

9. The nurse should advise a patient who is on a salt-restricted diet to avoid eating:
   1. Eggs and milk.
   2. Potatoes and rice.
   3. Apples and plums.
   4. Carrots and spinach.

10. The activated partial thromboplastin time (aPTT) in a patient on heparin is 75 seconds. The most appropriate nursing action would be to:
    1. Prepare an injection of vitamin K and notify the physician.
    2. Discuss with the MD the need to discontinue the drug.
    3. Observe for signs of bleeding during the shift.
    4. Continue treatment: this lab result is desirable.

11. The best explanation for the nurse to give a patient who asks why he is receiving both heparin and warfarin sodium (Coumadin) to achieve anticoagulation is that:
    1. Anticoagulation occurs faster when both are taken.
    2. There is less chance of bleeding when both are taken.
    3. Heparin treatment will be stopped once the Coumadin is working.
    4. Coumadin speeds up the effects of heparin.

12. Discharge teaching for a patient receiving Coumadin should include the need to avoid eating:
    1. Citrus fruits.
    2. Green leafy vegetables.
    3. Potatoes and rice.
    3. Dairy products.

13. A patient with thrombophlebitis must be observed closely for the occurrence of which complication?
    1. Dyspnea.
    2. Petechiae.
    3. Hematuria.
    4. Tetany.

14. Physical assessment in a patient with arterial insufficiency of the lower extremities would reveal:
    1. Thickened skin on the soles of the feet.
    2. Prominent superficial blood vessels in the legs.
    3. Diminished dorsalis pedis pulses.
    4. Excessive hair on legs above ankles.

15. Which lab test finding would be abnormal in a patient with deep-vein thrombosis?
    1. Red blood cell count (RBC).
    2. Prothrombin time (PT).
    3. Hematocrit value (HCT).
    4. Activated partial thromboplastin time (aPTT).

Answers/Rationale

1. **(4)** The classic blood pressure reading denoting hypertension is a systolic pressure of 140 mm Hg or greater and a diastolic pressure of 90 mm Hg or greater. The diastolic pressure increases as vascular resistance increases. A narrowing of the pulse pressure **(1)** occurs with hypovolemic shock, because the systolic pressure decreases initially with decreased volume. An irregular pulse **(2)** may occur with heart failure and electrical conduction abnormalities. Fluctuations in the systolic pressure **(3)** often occur with for example, stress, anxiety, and fluid volume changes. **AN, 6, PhI**

2. **(3)** The patient's blood pressure indicates a poor response to pharmacotherapy. It would be important to *first* determine whether the patient is taking the medication as prescribed, because drug therapy would have the most immediate effect. Job stress **(1)** may *then* be considered as a possible cause of increased pressure, if it is determined that the patient is complying with drug therapy. Relaxation techniques **(2)** and weight loss **(4)** would be useful in reducing the BP but they would not likely be as effective as drug therapy after only 1 month. **EV, 6, PhI**

3. **(1)** Atenolol, a beta-blocker used in the treatment of hypertension or angina, may mask the symptoms of hypoglycemia and can produce hyperglycemia. There are no known contraindications to its use in patients with gallbladder disease **(2)**, ulcers **(3)**, or intestinal disorders **(4)**. **AS, 6, PhI**

4. **(2)** The purpose of a low-sodium diet in a patient with hypertension is to minimize fluid retention. The best indication of fluid status and fluid loss is a reduction in body weight. The serum sodium level **(1)** may be normal and would not reflect changes in the fluid status. Ankle swelling **(3)** would indicate heart failure or venous pooling. Although the swelling should be less if the patient is observing a low-sodium diet, it may not reflect a true reduction in the fluid level. If breath sounds **(4)** become congested, this *may* indicate that the heart is not handling the circulating volume (which should decrease with a low-sodium diet); however, the breath sounds may also be congested as a result of other causes, such as pneumonia. **EV, 6, PhI**

5. **(3)** The patient should be advised that captopril may cause taste to be impaired, but the problem generally disappears within 8 to 12 weeks after the start of ther-

---

Key to Codes

Nursing process: AS, assessment; **AN,** analysis; **PL,** planning; **IMP,** implementation; **EV,** evaluation. (See Appendix M for explanation of nursing process steps.)

Category of human function: 1, protective; **2,** sensory-perceptual; **3,** comfort, rest, activity, and mobility; **4,** nutrition; **5,** growth and development; **6,** fluid-gas transport; **7,** psychosocial-cultural; **8,** elimination. (See Appendix O for explanation.)

Client need: SECE, safe, effective care environment; **PhI,** physiological integrity; **PsI,** psychosocial integrity; **HPM,** health promotion/maintenance. (See Appendix P for explanation.)

apy. Potassium (1), as well as sodium, must be *avoided*, unless the MD directs otherwise, because of the risk for electrolyte imbalance. Captopril prevents the production of angiotensin II, resulting in vasodilation. Restricting fluid intake (2) may contribute to more severe hypotensive episodes. *Protein, not* glucose (4), may be found in the urine of a patient taking captopril. **IMP, 6, PhI**

6. **(2)** The serum potassium level may be increased. The serum potassium level would *not* be decreased (1), and the sodium level would be decreased, *not* increased (4), because the drug blocks the effects of the aldosterone mechanism, which normally conserves sodium and excretes potassium. The white blood cell count would be decreased, *not* increased (3). **AN, 6, PhI**

7. **(2)** Diuretics should be taken in the morning so the patient is not awakened at night by the need to urinate. Generally, fluid intake is not restricted (1) as long as the kidneys are working to eliminate any excess fluid. Drinking a beverage (3) before bedtime would only increase the likelihood of nocturia. Sleeping with the head elevated (4) would help a patient breathe more easily if there were problems with heart failure; it would have no bearing on the effects of a diuretic. **IMP, 6, HPM**

8. **(2)** Diazoxide is a vasodilator that produces reflex tachycardia, increased cardiac output, and possibly angina (chest pain). The patient should be monitored for hypotension, *not* hypertension (1), and tachycardia, *not* bradycardia (3). The patient may appear flushed, *not* pale (4). **EV, 6, PhI**

9. **(1)** Milk contains the most sodium of the food choices listed. By themselves eggs are not higher in sodium than spinach (4), but the combination of eggs and milk should be avoided. Potatoes and rice (2), apples and plums (3), and carrots (4) are very low in sodium. **PL, 6, HPM**

10. **(4)** The normal aPTT is 25 to 38 seconds; the desired time is 1½ to 2 times the control (usually 50 to 80 seconds). A time of 75 seconds would therefore be desired. Vitamin K (1) is not the antidote to heparin; protamine sulfate would be given to control excessive anticoagulation resulting from heparin therapy. Heparin treatment should *not* be discontinued (2). Observing for bleeding (3) is important, because bleeding is al-

ways a risk of anticoagulation therapy, but the best action to take in this patient is to continue therapy. **EV, 6, SECE**

11. **(3)** Heparin is given IV or subcutaneously and is more rapid acting than Coumadin. Coumadin is taken PO, and it takes days for a therapeutic blood level of the agent to be reached. Once the prothrombin level is high enough, the patient will be discharged home on a regimen of Coumadin. The two drugs do not potentiate each other's effects (1 and 4). Each drug affects a different clotting component, and the risk of bleeding associated with treatment with either agent alone is as great as, not less than (2), that associated with treatment with the two together. **IMP, 6, PhI**

12. **(2)** Green leafy vegetables are high in vitamin K, which would interfere with the anticoagulant effects of Coumadin. The other foods (1, 3, and 4) *may* be eaten by patients taking Coumadin. **IMP, 6, HPM**

13. **(1)** The greatest concern in a patient with thrombophlebitis is that a clot may be dislodged from the vein and migrate to the lungs (pulmonary emboli), causing respiratory distress, or to the brain, causing a stroke. Dyspnea is a symptom of a pulmonary embolus. Petechiae (2) are pinpoint hemorrhages on the skin and mucous membranes and result from fat emboli or bleeding disorders. Hematuria (3), or blood in the urine, would be a side effect of anticoagulant therapy or indicate the presence of bladder or kidney disease. Tetany (4), or carpopedal spasms, is associated with, for example, a low calcium level resulting from hypoparathyroidism. **AS, 6, PhI**

14. **(3)** A hallmark of arterial insufficiency is decreased or absent arterial pulses; the pedal pulse is one. The toenails, *not* the soles (1) thicken in arterial insufficiency. The condition in option 2 is seen in venous insufficiency. The limb would be hairless, *not* hairy (4), in arterial insufficiency. **AS, 6, PhI**

15. **(4)** The aPTT is an important and very sensitive way of screening for coagulation disorders. It is also used to monitor the effects of heparin therapy. The red blood cell count (1) and hematocrit (3) are *not* coagulation studies. The prothrombin time (2) is also used in diagnostic coagulation studies, but the aPTT is *more* sensitive. The prothrombin time is used to monitor the effects of Coumadin therapy. **AS, 6, PhI**

Cardiac Structure Disorders

Chapter Outline

Cardiac Valvular Defects

Alteration in the structure of a valve; impedes flow of blood or permits regurgitation; often associated with an inflammatory response resulting from an infection.

I. Pathophysiology
- **A.** *Stenosis*—narrowing of valvular opening due to adherence, thickening, and rigidity of valve cusp.
- **B.** *Insufficiency* (incompetence)—incomplete closure of valve due to contraction of chordae tendineae, papillary muscles, or to calcification, scarring of leaflets.
- **C. Mitral stenosis:**
  1. Most common residual cardiac lesion of rheumatic fever.
  2. Affects *women* <45 yr more often than men.
  3. Narrowing of mitral valve.
  4. Interferes with filling of left ventricle.
  5. Produces pulmonary hypertension, right-ventricular failure.
- **D. Mitral insufficiency** (incompetence):
  1. Leaking/regurgitation of blood back into left atrium.
  2. Results from rheumatic fever, bacterial endocarditis; less common.
  3. Affects *men* more often.
  4. Produces pulmonary congestion, ventricular heart failure.
- **E. Aortic stenosis:**
  1. Fusion of valve flaps between left ventricle and aorta.
  2. Congenital or acquired from atherosclerosis or from rheumatic fever and bacterial endocardi-

tis; seen in *men* more often; pulmonary circulation congested, cardiac output decreased.
- **F. Aortic insufficiency:**
  1. Incomplete closure of valve between left ventricle and aorta (regurgitation).
  2. Left ventricular failure leading to right ventricular failure.

II. Risk factors
- **A.** Congenital abnormality.
- **B.** History of rheumatic fever.
- **C.** Atherosclerosis.

⋈ III. Assessment: Table 3.1.

⋈ IV. Analysis/nursing diagnosis
- **A.** *Decreased cardiac output* related to inadequate ventricular filling.
- **B.** *Fluid volume excess* related to compensatory response to decreased cardiac output.
- **C.** *Impaired gas exchange* related to pulmonary congestion.
- **D.** *Activity intolerance* related to impaired cardiac function.
- **E.** *Fatigue* related to poor oxygenation.

⋈ V. Nursing care plan/implementation
- **A.** Goal: *reduce cardiac workload.*
- **B.** Goal: *promote physical comfort and psychological support.*
- **C.** Goal: *prevent complications.*
- **D.** Goal: *prepare patient for surgery* (commissurotomy, valvuloplasty, or valvular replacement, depending on defect and severity of condition).
- **E.** See Cardiac Surgery, pp. 24–25, for specific nursing actions.

⋈ VI. Evaluation/outcome criteria
- **A.** Relief of symptoms.

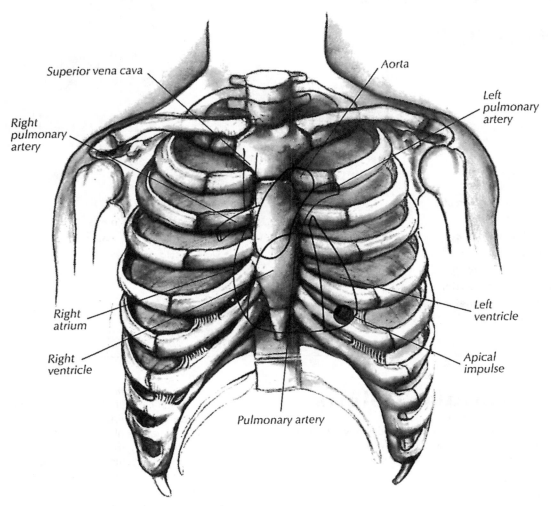

Surface projection of the heart and great vessels on the anterior body wall.

B. Increase in activity level.

C. No complications following surgery.

Cardiac Catheterization

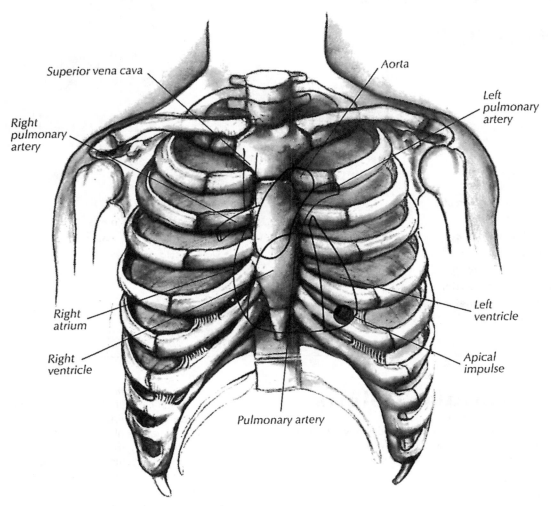 A diagnostic procedure to evaluate cardiac status. Introduces a catheter into the heart, blood vessels; analyzes blood samples for oxygen content, cardiac output, pulmonary artery blood flow; done prior to heart surgery; frequently combined with angiography to visualize coronary arteries; also provides access for specialized cardiac techniques (e.g., internal pacing and coronary angioplasty).

I. Approaches:

  A. *Right-heart* catheterization—venous approach (antecubital or femoral) → right atrium → right ventricle → pulmonary artery.

  B. *Left-heart* catheterization—retrograde approach: right brachial artery or percutaneous puncture of femoral artery → ascending aorta → left ventricle.

    1. Transseptal: femoral vein → right atrium → septum → left atrium → left ventricle.

    2. *Angiography/arteriography:* done during left-heart catheterization.

II. Precatheterization

  A. Assessment

    1. *Subjective data:*

      a. Allergies: iodine, seafood.

      b. Anxiety.

    2. *Objective data:*

      a. Vital signs: baseline data.

      b. Distal pulses: mark for reference after catheterization.

  B. Analysis/nursing diagnosis

    1. *Anxiety* related to fear of unknown.

    2. *Knowledge deficit* related to difficulty learning or limited exposure to information.

  C. Nursing care plan/implementation

    1. Goal: *provide for safety, comfort.*

      a. Signed informed consent.

      b. *NPO* (except for medications 6–8 h before).

      c. Have patient urinate before going to lab.

      d. Give sedatives, as ordered, 30 min before procedure (e.g., midazolam HCl [Versed]).

TABLE 3.1   COMPARISON OF SYMPTOMATOLOGY OF VALVULAR DEFECTS

✉ Assessment	Mitral Stenosis	Mitral Insufficiency	Aortic Stenosis	Aortic Insufficiency
Subjective Data				
Fatigue	✓	✓	✓	✓
Shortness of breath	✓			
Orthopnea	✓		✓	✓
Paroxysmal nocturnal dyspnea (PND)	✓		✓	✓
Cough	✓	✓		
Dyspnea on exertion (DOE)		✓	✓	✓
Palpitations		✓	✓	
Syncope on exertion			✓	
Angina			✓	✓
Weight loss		✓		
Objective Data				
Vital signs				
Blood pressure:				
Low or normal	✓	✓		
Normal or elevated			✓	✓
Pulse:				
Weak, irregular	✓	✓		
Rapid, "waterhammer"				✓
Respirations: Increased, shallow	✓			
Cyanosis	✓			
Jugular vein distention	✓			
Enlarged liver	✓			
Dependent edema	✓		✓	
Murmur	✓	✓	✓	✓

Source: Lagerquist, SL: *Little, Brown's NCLEX-RN Examination Review.* Boston: Little, Brown, 1996. P. 58.

2. Goal: **health teaching.**
    a. Procedure: duration (1–3 h).
    b. Expectations (strapped to table for safety, must lie still, awake but mildly sedated).
    c. Sensations (hot, flushed feeling in head with injection of contrast medium; thudding in chest from premature beats during catheter manipulation; desire to cough, particularly with right-heart angiography and contrast medium injection).
    d. Alert physician to unusual sensations (coolness, numbness, paresthesia).

III. **Postcatheterization**
✉ A. **Assessment** (potential complications):
    1. *Subjective data:*
        a. Puncture site: increasing pain, tenderness.
        b. Palpitations.
        c. Affected extremity: tingling numbness, pain from hematoma or nerve damage.
    2. *Objective data:*
        a. Vital signs: shock, respiratory distress (related to pulmonary emboli, allergic reaction).
        b. Puncture site: bleeding (hematoma).
        〰️ c. ECG: arrhythmias, signs of MI.
    d. Affected extremity: color, temperature, peripheral pulses.
✉ B. **Analysis/nursing diagnosis**
    1. *Decreased cardiac output* related to arrhythmias or MI.
    2. *Altered tissue perfusion* related to bleeding following procedure.
    3. *Pain* related to puncture site tenderness.
✉ C. **Nursing care plan/implementation**
    1. Goal: *prevent complications.*
        a. Bed rest: 3–6 h; with femoral approach, *supine position,* 12–24 h on bed rest; encourage ankle flexion, extension, and rotation.
        b. Vital signs: record q15 min for 1 h, q30 min for 3 h or until stable; check BP on opposite extremity.
        c. Puncture site: observe for bleeding, swelling, inflammation, or tenderness; check pulse distal to insertion site to determine patency of artery; report complaints of coolness, numbness, or paresthesia in extremity.
        〰️ d. ECG: monitor, document rhythm.
        💊 e. Give medications as ordered: sedatives, mild narcotics, antiarrhythmics.

2. Goal: _provide emotional support._
   a. Explanations: brief, accurate; patient anxious to learn results of test.
   b. Counseling: refer as indicated.
3. Goal: **health teaching.**
   a. Late complications: infection.
   b. Prepare for surgery if indicated.
   c. Follow-up medical care.
D. **Evaluation/outcome criteria:** no complications (e.g., cardiac arrest, hematoma at insertion site).

Percutaneous Transluminal Coronary Angioplasty (PTCA)

A balloon-tipped catheter is threaded to site of coronary occlusion and inflated repeatedly until blood flow increases distal to the obstruction; a nonsurgical alternative to bypass surgery for coronary artery occlusion; recommended in patients with poorly controlled angina, mild or no symptoms, multiple- or single-vessel disease with a noncalcified, discrete, and proximal lesion that can be reached by the catheter; costs less and requires shorter hospitalization and rehabilitation period (see Cardiac Catherization, for nursing process). **Atherectomy** may also be done. In this procedure a cutter is positioned against the blockage and mechanically debrides the plaque. An **intravascular stent,** a coilspring tube, may be placed in the coronary artery, and the stent acts as a mechanical scaffold to reopen the blocked artery. The patient will receive anticoagulant and antiplatelet therapy following the procedure.

Cardiac Surgery

Done to alter the structure of the heart or vessels when the following congenital or acquired disorders interfere with cardiac functioning: septal defects; transposition of great vessels; tetralogy of Fallot; pulmonary/aortic stenosis; coronary artery bypass; valve replacement.

Cardiopulmonary bypass (used in open-heart surgery): blood from cardiac chambers and great vessels is diverted into a pump oxygenator; allows full visualization of heart during surgery; maintains perfusion and body functioning.

I. Preoperative care
A. Assessment:
1. See specific conditions for preoperative signs and symptoms (i.e., valvular defects, angina, MI); see also Preoperative Preparation, p. 111.
2. Establish complete baseline: daily weight; vital signs—integrity of all pulses, BP both arms; central venous pressure (CVP) or pulmonary artery pressures (_Swan-Ganz catheter_); neurologic status; emotional status; nutritional and elimination patterns.
3. Lab values—urine, electrolytes, enzymes, coagulation studies.

4. Pulmonary function studies.
B. Analysis/nursing diagnosis (see also Myocardial Infarction, p. 35):
1. _Decreased cardiac output_ related to myocardial damage.
2. _Activity intolerance_ related to poor cardiac function.
3. _Knowledge deficit_ related to insufficient time for teaching.
4. _Anxiety_ related to fear of unknown.
5. _Fear_ related to possible death.
6. _Spiritual distress_ related to possible death.
C. Nursing care plan/implementation
1. Goal: _provide emotional and spiritual support._
   a. Arrange for religious consultation if desired.
   b. Provide opportunity for family visit morning of surgery.
   c. Encourage verbalization/questions: fear, depression, despair frequently occur.
2. Goal: **health teaching.**
   a. Diagnostic procedures, treatments, specifics for surgery (i.e., leg incision with use of saphenous vein in coronary artery bypass surgery).
   b. Postoperative regimen: turn, cough, deep breathe, ROM, equipment used, medication for pain.
   c. Tour ICU; meet personnel.
   d. Alternative method of communication while intubated.
D. Evaluation/outcome criteria
1. Displays moderate anxiety level.
2. Verbalizes/demonstrates postoperative expectations.
3. Quits smoking before surgery.

II. Postoperative care
A. Assessment:
1. _Subjective data:_
   a. Pain.
   b. Fatigue—sleep deprivation.
2. _Objective data:_
   a. **Neurologic:** level of consciousness; pupillary reactions; movement of limbs (purposeful, spontaneous).
   b. **Respiratory:** rate changes (_increases_ occur with obstruction, pain; _decreases_ occur with CO_2 retention); depth (shallow with pain, atelectasis); symmetry; skin _color;_ patency/_drainage_ from chest tubes; _sputum_ (amount, color); endotracheal tube placement (bilateral breath sounds).
   c. **Cardiovascular:**
      (1) BP—_hypotension_ may indicate heart failure, tamponade, hemorrhage, arrhythmias, or thrombosis; _hypertension_ may indicate anxiety, hypervolemia.
      (2) Pulse: radial, apical, pedal; rate (>100 beats/min may indicate shock, fever, hypoxia, arrhythmias); rhythm, quality.

(3) CVP or *Swan-Ganz* (elevated in cardiac failure); temperature (normal post-op: 98.6°–101.6°F oral).

d. **Gastrointestinal (GI):** nausea, vomiting, distention.

e. **Renal:** urine—minimum output (30 mL/h); color; specific gravity (<1.010 occurs with *overhydration*, renal tubular damage; >1.020 present with *dehydration*, oliguria, blood in urine).

B. Analysis/nursing diagnosis

1. *Decreased cardiac output* related to decreased myocardial contractility or postoperative hypothermia.
2. *Pain* related to incision.
3. *Ineffective airway clearance* related to effects of general anesthesia.
4. *Altered tissue perfusion* related to postoperative bleeding or thromboemboli.
5. *Fluid volume deficit* related to blood loss.
6. *Risk for infection* related to wound contamination.
7. *Altered thought processes* related to anesthesia or stress.
8. *Body image disturbance* related to incision or limitations.
9. *Sleep pattern disturbance* related to ICU environment or pain.

C. Nursing care plan/implementation

1. Goal: *provide constant monitoring to prevent complications.*
   a. Respiratory:
      (1) Observe for respiratory distress: restlessness, nasal flaring, *Cheyne-Stokes respiration,* dusky/cyanotic skin; assisted or controlled ventilation via *endotracheal* tube common first 24 h; supplemental O_2 after extubation.
      (2) *Suctioning;* cough, deep breathe.
      (3) *Elevate* head of bed.
      (4) Position chest tube to facilitate drainage; mediastinal sump tube maintains patency—"milking" not necessary. See also chest tube care in Chap. 6, p. 68.
   b. *Cardiovascular:*
      (1) *Vital signs:* BP > 80–90 mm Hg systolic; *CVP:* range 5–15 cm H_2O unless otherwise ordered; pulmonary artery line (*Swan-Ganz*): mean pressure 4–12 mm Hg; I&O: report <30 mL of urine/h from indwelling urinary catheter.
      (2) ECG; PVCs occur most frequently following aortic valve replacement and bypass surgery.
      (3) Peripheral pulses if leg veins used for grafting.
      (4) Activity: turn q2h; ROM; progressive, early ambulation.
   c. Inspect dressing for bleeding.
   d. Medications according to therapeutic directives—cardiotonics (digoxin); coronary vasodilators (nitrates); antibiotics (penicillin); analgesics; anticoagulants (with valve replacements); antiarrhythmics (quinidine, procainamide HCl [Pronestyl]).

2. Goal: *promote comfort, pain relief.*
   a. Medicate: *Demerol or morphine* sulfate, as severe pain lasts 2–3 d.
   b. Splint incision when moving or coughing.
   c. Mouth care: keep lips moist.
   d. *Position:* use pillows to prevent tension on chest tubes, incision.

3. Goal: *maintain fluid, electrolyte, nutritional balance.*
   a. I&O; urine specific gravity.
   b. Measure chest tube drainage—should not exceed 200 mL/h for first 4–6 h.
   c. Give fluids as ordered; maintain *IV patency.*
   d. *Diet:* clear fluids → solid food if no nausea, GI distention; sodium intake restricted, low fat intake.

4. Goal: *promote emotional adjustment.*
   a. Anticipate behavior disturbances (depression, disorientation often occur 3 d postop) related to medications, fear, sleep deprivation.
   b. Calm, oriented, supportive environment, as personalized as possible.
   c. Encourage verbalization of feelings (family and patient).
   d. Encourage independence to avoid cardiac-cripple role.

5. Goal: **health teaching.**
   a. Alterations in life-style, activity, diet, work.
   b. Available community resources for cardiac rehabilitation (e.g., American Heart Association, Mended Hearts).
   c. Drug regimen: purpose, side effects.
   d. Potential complications: dyspnea, pain, palpitations common postoperatively.

D. Evaluation/outcome criteria

1. No complications; incision heals.
2. Activity level increases—no signs of overexertion (e.g., fatigue, dyspnea, pain).
3. Relief of symptoms.
4. Returns for follow-up medical care.
5. Takes prescribed medications; knows purposes and side effects.

Pericarditis

Inflammation of parietal and/or visceral pericardium; acute or chronic condition; may occur with or without effusion.

I. Pathophysiology: fibrosis or accumulation of fluid in pericardium → compression of cardiac pumping → decreased cardiac output → increased systemic, pulmonic venous pressure.

II. Risk factors

A. Bacterial, viral, and/or fungal infections.
B. Tuberculosis.

C. Collagen diseases.
D. Uremia.
E. Transmural MI.
F. Trauma.

III. Assessment
   A. *Subjective data:*
      1. Pain:
         a. *Type*—sharp, moderate to severe.
         b. *Location*—wide area of pericardium, may radiate; right arm, jaw/teeth.
         c. *Precipitating factors*—movement, deep inspiration, swallowing.
      2. Chills; sweating.
      3. Apprehension; anxiety.
      4. Fatigue.
      5. Abdominal pain.
      6. Shortness of breath.
   B. *Objective data:*
      1. Vital signs:
         a. BP: decreased pulse pressure; pulsus paradoxus—abnormal drop in systemic BP of >8–10 mm Hg during inspiration.
         b. Pulse: tachycardia.
         c. Temperature: elevated; erratic course; low grade.
      2. Pericardial friction rub.
      3. Increased CVP, distended neck veins, dependent pitting edema, liver engorgement.
      4. Restlessness.
      5. Lab data: elevated AST(SGOT); WBC; chest x-ray—cardiac enlargement.

IV. Analysis/nursing diagnosis
   A. *Decreased cardiac output* related to impaired cardiac muscle contraction.
   B. *Pain* related to pericardial inflammation.
   C. *Anxiety* related to unknown outcome.
   D. *Fatigue* related to inadequate oxygenation.
   E. *Ineffective breathing pattern* related to discomfort during inspiration.

V. Nursing care plan/implementation
   A. Goal: *promote physical and emotional comfort.*
      1. *Position:* semi-Fowler's (upright or sitting); bed rest.
      2. Vital signs: q2–4h and prn: *apical* and *radial* pulse; notify physician if heart sounds decrease in amplitude or if pulse pressure *narrows,* indicating cardiac tamponade; cooling measures as indicated.
      3. O₂ as ordered.
      4. Medications as ordered:
         a. *Analgesics*—aspirin, morphine sulfate.
         b. *Nonsteroidal anti-inflammatory agents (NSAIs).*
         c. *Antibiotics.*
         d. *Digitalis* and *diuretics,* if heart failure present.
      5. Assist with aspiration of pericardial sac (pericardiocentesis) if needed: medicate as ordered; *elevate head* 60 degrees; monitor ECG; have defibrillator and pacemaker available.

      6. Prepare for pericardiectomy (excision of constricting pericardium) as ordered.
      7. Continual emotional support.
      8. Enhance effects of analgesics: positioning; turning; warm drinks.
      9. Monitor for *signs of cardiac tamponade:* tachycardia; tachypnea; hypotension; pallor; narrowed pulse pressure; pulsus paradoxus; distended neck veins.
   B. Goal: *maintain fluid, electrolyte balance.*
      1. Parenteral fluids as ordered; strict I&O.
      2. Assist with feedings; *low-sodium diet* may be ordered.

VI. Evaluation/outcome criteria
   A. Relief of pain, dyspnea.
   B. No complications (e.g., cardiac tamponade).
   C. Return of normal cardiac functioning.

☞ Summary of Key Points

1. Structural damage is often associated with an inflammatory response resulting from an infection.
2. A **mitral valve** defect is the most prevalent valvular disorder.
3. A **murmur** will be found on auscultation if valvular stenosis or regurgitation is present.
4. Pericardial friction rub and fever are classic signs of **acute pericarditis.**
5. Coronary arteries are assessed during **left-heart catheterization.**
6. **Normal heart sounds** (high pitched) are best heard with the diaphragm of the stethoscope, and abnormal sounds such as gallops (low pitched) are best heard with the bell.

☼ Study and Memory Aids

Prior to cardiac catheterization: ✔ for shellfish or iodine allergy.

Cardiac Surgery: Behavior Modification

Diagnostic Studies

[MWM] Noninvasive Diagnostic Procedures

Multiple-gated acquisition scan (MUGA)—also known as *blood pool imaging.* Red blood cells are tagged with a radioactive isotope. A computer-operated camera takes sequential pictures of actual heart-wall motion; *complement* to cardiac catheterization; *used to:* determine valvular effectiveness, follow progress of heart disease, diagnose cardiac aneurysms, detect coronary artery disease, determine effects of cardiovascular drug therapy. No special preparation. Painless, except for injections. Wear *gloves* if contact with patient urine occurs within 24 h after scan.

Doppler ultrasonography—*used to* measure blood flow in the major veins and arteries. The transducer of the test instrument is placed on the skin, sending out bursts of ultra-high-frequency sound. The ratio of ankle to brachial systolic pressure (API ≥ 1) provides information about vascular insufficiency. Sound varies with respiration and the Valsalva maneuver. No discomfort to the patient.

[MWM] Invasive Diagnostic Procedures

Cardiac catheterization—insertion of a radiopaque catheter into a vein to study the heart and great vessels.

Right-heart catheterization—catheter is inserted through a cutdown in the antecubital vein into the superior vena cava and through the right atrium, ventricle, and into the pulmonary artery.

Left-heart catheterization—catheter may be passed retrogradely to the left ventricle through the brachial or femoral artery; it can be passed into the left atrium after right-heart catheterization by means of a special needle that punctures the septa; or it may be passed directly into the left ventricle by means of a posterior or anterior chest puncture.

Cardiac catheterization is *used to:*
Confirm diagnosis of heart disease and determine the extent of disease.
Determine existence and extent of congenital abnormalities.
Measure pressures in the heart chambers and great vessels.
Obtain estimate of cardiac output.
Obtain blood samples to measure oxygen content and determine presence of cardiac shunts.

▷ *Specific Nursing Interventions*

Preprocedure patient teaching:
Fatigue due to lying still for 3 h or more is a common complaint.
Some fluttery sensations may be felt—occurs as catheter is passed backward into the left ventricle.
Flushed, warm feeling may occur when contrast medium is injected.

☞ *Postprocedure observations:*
[MWM] Monitor ECG pattern for arrhythmias.
Check extremities for color and temperature, peripheral pulses (femoral and dorsalis pedis) for quality.

● Drug Review

Cardiac Valvular Defects

Mitral stenosis
Anticoagulants
Beta-blockers
Digitalis
Diuretics

Mitral regurgitation
Angiotensin-converting enzyme
Nitrates

Mitral valve prolapse
Antibiotics
Beta-blockers

Aortic stenosis
Antibiotic before invasive procedures
Digitalis
Diuretics

Cardiac Catheterization

Antiarrhythmics—Procainamide (Pronestyl).
Local anesthesia
Sedative for relaxation before procedure.

Percutaneous Transluminal Coronary Angioplasty

Anticoagulation therapy during procedure.
Aspirin or dipyridamole (Persantine) for long-term use after procedure.

Pericarditis

Antibiotic therapy
Aspirin
Nonsteroidal anti-inflammatory agent

Questions

1. The nurse knows that a patient understands what to expect after open-heart surgery if he says:
   1. "I won't be able to have sexual intercourse for 6 months after the surgery."
   2. "I will be on a ventilator for a while after the surgery."
   3. "I can't return to work as a carpenter after the surgery."
   4. "After the surgery I won't have to take any of my cardiac medications."

2. The nurse would expect urine output to be significantly increased in a patient who undergoes urine output cardiac catheterization because:
   1. Cardiac output would be improved.
   2. The contrast medium used has a diuretic effect.
   3. Myocardial perfusion would be restored.
   4. Fluids are given IV during the procedure.

3. A patient who undergoes angioplasty and stent placement to eliminate a blockage in the left coronary artery is given one enteric-coated aspirin daily for its:
   1. Antipyretic action.
   2. Analgesic effect.
   3. Anticoagulatant action.
   4. Anti-inflammatory effect.

4. A patient who has undergone a femoropopliteal bypass graft complains of pain and appears restless; nail beds and lips are slightly cyanotic, and skin is cool. What should the nurse do first?
   1. Check the vital signs.
   2. Elevate the affected leg.
   3. Assess the level of consciousness.
   4. Call the MD immediately.

Answers/Rationale

1. **(2)** All patients who undergo open-heart surgery are mechanically ventilated for a while after the surgery to reduce the effort of breathing and the work of the heart. The resumption of sexual activity **(1)**, the ability to return to work **(3)**, and the medication regimen **(4)** would be all "unknowns" at the time of preoperative teaching. **EV, 6, SECE**

2. **(2)** The contrast medium, which usually has an iodine base, produces diuresis. The test is done to determine the status of cardiac function. The test does not cause cardiac output **(1)** or myocardial perfusion **(3)** to be improved. The amount of fluids infused IV during the procedure **(4)** is not significant enough to cause an increase in urine output. **AN, 6, PhI**

3. **(3)** A low dose of aspirin is prescribed for its anticoagulatant action; aspirin has this effect because it interferes with the adherence of platelets. The other actions **(1, 2, and 4)** are also properties of aspirin but not ones that constitute the reason for *this* patient needing to take an aspirin daily. **IMP, 6, HPM**

4. **(1)** These are symptoms of poor perfusion and hypoxemia. Vital signs should therefore be assessed to determine whether shock has occurred. If shock is diagnosed, the head of the patient's bed should be lowered and the leg, or legs, elevated **(2)**, as appropriate. The level of consciousness **(3)** has already changed. The MD should be called **(4)** *after* the data are gathered. **PL, 6, PhI**

Key to Codes

Nursing process: AS, assessment; **AN,** analysis; **PL,** planning; **IMP,** implementation; **EV,** evaluation. (See Appendix M for explanation of nursing process steps.)

Category of human function: 1, protective; **2,** sensory-perceptual; **3,** comfort, rest, activity, and mobility; **4,** nutrition; **5,** growth and development; **6,** fluid-gas transport; **7,** psychosocial-cultural; **8,** elimination. (See Appendix O for explanation.)

Client need: SECE, safe, effective care environment; **PhI,** physiological integrity; **PsI,** psychosocial integrity; **HPM,** health promotion/maintenance. (See Appendix P for explanation.)

Cardiac Function Disorders

Chapter Outline

Cardiac Dysrhythmias

Any variation in normal rate, rhythm, or configuration of waves on ECG (Figure 4.1).

I. Pathophysiology
  A. Dysfunction of SA node, atria, AV node, or ventricular conduction.
  B. Primary heart problem or secondary systemic problem.

II. Risk factors
  A. Myocardial infarction (MI).
  B. Drug toxicity.
  C. Stress.
  D. Cardiac surgery.
  E. Hypoxia.
  F. See also Table 4.1.

III. Assessment: see Table 4.1 for specific dysrhythmias.

IV. Analysis/nursing diagnosis
  A. *Decreased cardiac output* related to abnormal ventricular function.
  B. *Altered tissue perfusion* related to inadequate cardiac functioning.
  C. *Risk for injury* (death) related to improper cardiac function.
  D. *Risk for activity intolerance* related to inadequate oxygenation.
  E. Anxiety related to dependence, fear of death.

V. Nursing care plan/implementation
  A. Goal: *provide for emotional and safety needs.*
    1. Obtain ECG to document dysrhythmia
    2. Encourage discussion of fears, feelings.
    3. *Bed rest,* restricted activities, quiet environment, limit visitors.
    4. Oxygen, if ordered.
    5. Check vital signs frequently for shock, heart failure (HF), drug toxicity.
    6. Prepare for cardiac emergency: CPR.
    7. Give *cardiac* medications; check lab results for digitalis and potassium levels, to prevent drug toxicity.
  B. Goal: *prevent thromboemboli.*
    1. Apply antiembolic stockings (TED hose).
    2. Give *anticoagulants* as ordered
      a. Check for bleeding—gums, urine.
      b. Monitor lab results—Lee White clotting time and activated partial thromboplastin time [aPTT] with heparin; prothrombin time [PT] with coumadin.
    3. Encourage flexion-extension of feet.
  C. Goal: *provide for physical and emotional needs with pacemaker insertion.*
    1. *General concerns:*
      a. Report excessive bleeding/infection at insertion site—hematoma may contribute to wound infection.
      b. Encourage verbalization of feelings.
      c. Report prolonged hiccoughs, which may indicate pacemaker failure.
      d. Know pacing mode: fixed-rate or demand (most common).
    2. **Temporary pacemaker:**
      a. *Limit excessive activity of extremity* if antecubital insertion, to prevent displacement; subclavian insertion increases catheter stability.
      b. Secure wires to chest to prevent tension on catheter.

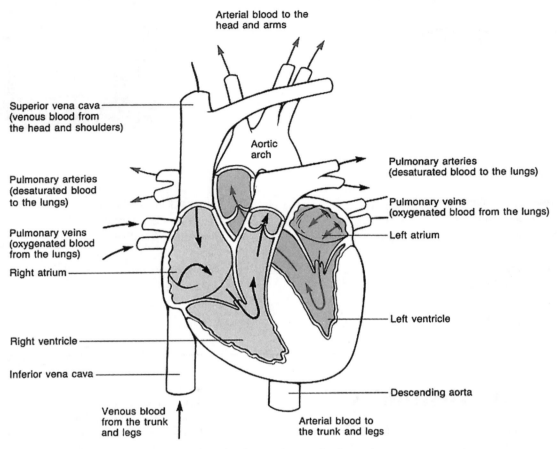

Arterial blood to the
head and arms

Superior vena cava
(venous blood from
the head and shoulders)

Aortic
arch

Pulmonary arteries
(desaturated blood
to the lungs)

Pulmonary arteries
(desaturated blood to the lungs)

Pulmonary veins
(oxygenated blood
from the lungs)

Pulmonary veins
(oxygenated blood from the lungs)

Right atrium

Left atrium

Right ventricle

Left ventricle

Inferior vena cava

Descending aorta

Venous blood
from the trunk
and legs

Arterial blood to
the trunk and legs

Blood Flow Through the Heart.

c. Do *not* defibrillate over insertion site, to avoid electrical hazards.

☞ d. Electrical safety (grounding; disconnect electric beds/call lights; use battery-operated equipment).

3. Permanent pacemaker:

a. *Limit activity of shoulder* for 48–72 h with transvenous catheter to prevent dislodgement.

☞ b. Postinsertion ROM (passive) at least once per shift after 48 h to prevent frozen shoulder.

4. Health teaching following permanent pacemaker:

a. Explain procedure: duration, equipment, purpose, type of pacemaker.

b. MedicAlert bracelet; pacemaker information card.

c. Daily pulse-taking upon arising (report variation of ±5 beats).

d. Signs, symptoms of: *malfunction* (vertigo, syncope, dyspnea, slowed speech, confusion, fluid retention); *infection* (fever, heat, pain, skin breakdown at insertion site).

e. *Restrictions:* contact sports; electromagnetic interferences (few)—TV/radio transmitters, improperly functioning microwave ovens, certain cautery machines; may trigger airport metal-detector alarm.

◀ **VI. Evaluation/outcome criteria**

A. Regular cardiac rhythm; monitors own radial pulse.

B. No complications (e.g., pacemaker malfunction).

C. Returns for regular follow-up of pacemaker function.

D. Tolerates physical or sexual activity.

E. Wears identification bracelet; carries pacemaker identification card.

Cardiac Arrest

Sudden, unexpected cessation of heartbeats and effective circulation, leading to inadequate perfusion and sudden death.

I. Risk factors

A. MI.

B. Multiple traumas.

C. Respiratory arrest.

D. Drowning.

E. Electric shock.

F. Drug reactions.

NORMAL SINUS RHYTHM

Rhythm: Regular.
Rate: 60 to 100 per minute.
P waves: Normal, preceding every QRS.
Pacemaker site: SA node.
P–R interval: Normal (0.12–0.20 sec).
QRS complexes: Normal, each preceded by a P wave.
Clinical significance: Normal rhythm.
Treatment: None.

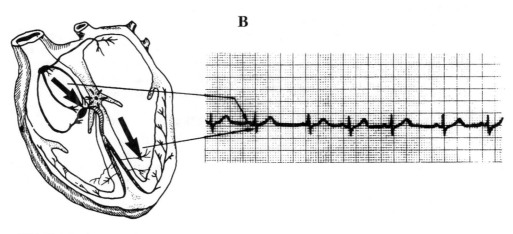

SINUS ARRHYTHMIA

Rhythm: Regularly irregular.
Rate: Normal.
P waves: Normal, preceding every QRS.
Pacemaker site: SA node.
P–R interval: Normal (0.12–0.20 sec).
QRS complexes: Normal, each QRS preceded by a P wave.
Clinical significance: Sinus arrhythmia is a normal phenomenon, caused by the effects of the parasympathetic nervous system of breathing.
Treatment: None.

FIGURE 4.1   NORMAL SINUS RHYTHM AND ABNORMALITIES. (A) NORMAL SINUS RHYTHM, (B) SINUS ARRHYTHMIA.

SINUS ARREST

Rhythm: Irregular.

Rate: May be normal to slow.

P waves: Normal, where present, preceding each QRS. However, if the SA node does not discharge or is blocked, the entire P–QRS–T complex is absent.

Pacemaker site: SA node.

P–R interval: Normal (0.12–0.20 sec).

QRS complexes: Normal, each preceded by a P wave.

Clinical significance: Occasional episodes are not significant; however, if the heart rate is reduced below 30 to 50 per minute, cardiac output may fall and an ectopic focus in the ventricles may take over.

Treatment:

• None necessary if the patient is asymptomatic, blood pressure is well maintained, and there is no evidence of ventricular irritability.

• Treatment to increase the heart rate must be undertaken if there are signs of hypoperfusion or atrial or ventricular ectopic arrhythmias. In those instances, ATROPINE SULFATE, 0.5 mg, is given by IV bolus. The dose may be repeated at 5- to 10-minute intervals until the heart rate has increased to 70 or more per minute or until a maximum dose of 2.0 mg of atropine has been given.

FIGURE 4.1   (CONTINUED) (C) SINUS ARREST.

II. Assessment—*objective data:*
   A. Unresponsive to stimuli (i.e., verbal, painful).
   B. Absence of breathing, carotid pulse.
   C. Pale or bluish: lips, fingernails, skin.
   D. Pupils: dilated.

III. Analysis/nursing diagnosis
   A. *Decreased cardiac output* related to heart failure.
   B. *Impaired gas exchange* related to breathlessness.
   C. *Altered tissue perfusion* related to pulselessness.

IV. Nursing care plan/implementation
   A. Goal: *prevent irreversible cerebral anoxic damage:* initiate **CPR** within 4–6 min; continue until relieved; document assessment factors, effectiveness of actions; presence or absence of pulse at 1 min and every 4–5 min.
   B. Goal: *establish effective circulation, respiration:* see Emergency Nursing Procedures, Chapter 25 pp. 301–318, for complete protocols.

V. Evaluation/outcome criteria:
   A. Carotid pulse present; check after 1 min and every few minutes thereafter.
   B. Responds to verbal stimuli.
   C. Pupils constrict in response to light.
   D. Return of spontaneous respiration; adequate ventilation.

Angina Pectoris

Transient paroxysmal episodes of substernal or precordial pain.

   I. Pathophysiology
   A. Insufficient blood flow through coronary arteries.
   B. Temporary myocardial ischemia.

   II. Risk factors
   A. *Cardiovascular:*
      1. Atherosclerosis.
      2. Thromboangiitis obliterans.
      3. Aortic regurgitation.
      4. Hypertension.
   B. *Hormonal:*
      1. Hyperthyroidism.
      2. Diabetes mellitus.

TABLE 4.1 COMPARISON OF SELECTED CARDIAC DYSRHYTHMIAS

Dysrhythmia	Description	Etiology	Symptoms/Consequences	Treatment
Dysrhythmias of Sinus Node				
Sinus dysrhythmia	Phasic shortening then lengthening of P-P and R-R interval	Respiratory variation in impulse initiation by SA node	Usually none	Usually none
Sinus tachycardia	P waves present followed by QRS Rhythm regular Heart rate 100–150 beats/min	Increased metabolic demands Decreased oxygen delivery, heart failure, shock, hemorrhage, anemia	May produce palpitations Prolonged episodes may lead to decreased cardiac output	Treat underlying cause Occasionally sedatives
Sinus bradycardia	P waves present followed by QRS Rhythm regular Heart rate <60 beats/min	Physical fitness Parasympathetic stimulation (sleep) Brain lesions Sinus dysfunction Digitalis excess	Very low rates may cause decreased cardiac output: light-headedness, faintness, chest pain	⬤ Atropine if cardiac output is decreased Pacemaker Treat underlying cause if necessary
Atrial Dysrhythmias				
Premature atrial beats	Early P wave QRS may or may not be normal Rhythm irregular	Stress Ischemia Atrial enlargement Caffeine Nicotine	May produce palpitations Frequent episodes may decrease cardiac output Is sign of chamber irritability	Sedation ⬤ Quinidine May require no other treatment
Atrial tachycardia	P wave present (may merge into previous T wave QRS usually normal Rapid heart rate usually >150 beats/min)	Sympathetic stimulation Chemical stimuli (caffeine, nicotine) Drug toxicity	Palpitations Possible anxiety	Usually none Prolonged episodes may require carotid artery pressure, vagal stimulation, *verapamil*, digitalis, or beta-bockers ⬤
Atrial fibrillation	Rapid, irregular P waves (>350/min) Ventricular rhythm irregularly irregular Ventricular rate varies, may increase to 120–150 beats/min if untreated	Rheumatic heart disease Mitral stenosis Atrial infarction Coronary atherosclerotic heart disease Hypertensive heart disease Thyrotoxicosis	Pulse deficit Decreased cardiac output if rate is rapid Promotes thrombus formation in atria	⬤ Digitalis ⬤ Quinidine Cardioversion

(continued)

C. *Blood disorders:*
1. Anemia.
2. Polycythemia vera.

◀ **III. Assessment**
   A. *Subjective data:*
      1. Pain (Table 4.2, p. 36).
         a. *Type:* squeezing, pressing, burning.

         b. *Location:* retrosternal, substernal, left of sternum, radiates to left arm.
         c. *Duration:* short, usually 3–5 min, <30 min.
         d. *Cause:* emotional stress, overeating, physical exertion, exposure to cold.
         e. *Relief:* rest, nitroglycerin.
      2. Dyspnea.

TABLE 4.1   COMPARISON OF SELECTED CARDIAC DYSRHYTHMIAS (CONTINUED)

Dysrhythmia	Description	Etiology	Symptoms/Consequences	Treatment
Ventricular Dysrhythmias				
Premature ventricular beats (PVBs)	Early wide bizarre QRS, not associated with a P wave Rhythm irregular	Stress Acidosis Ventricular enlargement Electrolyte imbalance Myocardial infarction Digitalis toxicity Hypoxemia, hypercapnia	Same as for premature atrial beats	Medications: 　Disopyramide (Norpace) 　Lidocaine 　Mexiletine 　Potassium 　Procainamide 　Quinidine 　Sodium bicarbonate ☞ Oxygen Treat heart failure
Ventricular tachycardia	No P wave before QRS QRS wide and bizarre Ventricular rate >100, usually 140–240 beats/min	PVB striking during vulnerable period Hypoxemia Drug toxicity Electrolyte imbalance Bradycardia	Decreased cardiac output Hypotension Loss of consciousness Respiratory arrest	Medications: 　Bretylium 　Lidocaine 　Mexiletine 　Procainamide Cardioversion
Ventricular fibrillation	Chaotic electrical activity No recognizable QRS complex	Myocardial infarction Electrocution Freshwater drowning Drug toxicity	No cardiac output Absent pulse or respiration Cardiac arrest	Defibrillation Bretylium Epinephrine Sodium bicarbonate ☞ CPR
Ventricular standstill	Can be distinguished from ventricular fibrillation only by ECG P waves *may* be present No QRS "Straight line"	Myocardial infarction Chronic diseaes of conducting system	Same as for ventricular fibrillation	☞ CPR Pacemaker ⬭ Intracardiac epinephrine ⬭ Isoproterenol

(continued)

3. Palpitations.
4. Dizziness, faintness.
5. Epigastric distress, indigestion, belching.
B. *Objective data:*
　1. Tachycardia.
　2. Pallor.
　3. Diaphoresis.
▨ **IV. Analysis/nursing diagnosis**
　A. *Altered cardiopulmonary tissue perfusion* related to insufficient blood flow.
　B. *Pain* related to myocardial ischemia.
　C. *Activity intolerance* related to onset of pain.
▨ **V. Nursing care plan/implementation**
　A. Goal: *provide relief from pain.*
　　1. Rest until pain subsides.
　⬭ **2.** Nitroglycerin or amyl nitrite, as ordered.
　　3. Identify precipitating factors: large meals, heavy exercise, stimulants (coffee, smoking), sex when fatigued, cold air.

　4. Vital signs: hypotension.
　5. Assist with ambulation; dizziness, flushing occur with nitroglycerin.
B. Goal: *provide emotional support.*
　1. Encourage verbalization of feelings, fears.
　2. Reassurance; positive self-concept.
　3. Acceptance of limitations.
🏠 **C.** Goal: **health teaching.**
　1. *Pain:* alleviation, differentiation of angina from myocardial infarction, precipitating factors (see Table 4.2).
　⬭ **2.** *Medication:* frequency, expected effects (headache, flushing); carry fresh *nitroglycerin;* loses potency after 6 mo ("stings" under tongue when potent); may use nitroglycerin paste—instruct how to apply.
　🍎 **3.** *Diet:* restrict calories if weight loss indicated; restrict fat, cholesterol, gas-producing foods; small, frequent meals.

TABLE 4.1   COMPARISON OF SELECTED CARDIAC DYSRHYTHMIAS (CONTINUED)

Dysrhythmia	*Description*	*Etiology*	*Symptoms/ Consequences*	*Treatment*
Impulse Conduction Deficits				
First-degree AV block	PR interval prolonged, >0.20 sec	Rheumatic fever Digitalis toxicity Degenerative changes of coronary atherosclerotic heart disease Infections Decreased oxygen in AV node	Warns of impaired conduction	Usually none as long as it occurs as an isolated deficit
Bundle-branch block	Same as normal sinus rhythm except QRS see duration >0.10 sec	Hypoxia Acute myocardial infarction Heart failure Coronary atherosclerotic heart disease Pulmonary embolus Hypertension	Same as first-degree AV block	Usually none unless severe blockage of left posterior division (see text)
Second-degree AV blocks	P waves usually occur regularly at rates consistent with SA node initiation (not all P waves followed by QRS; PR interval may lengthen before nonconducted P wave or may be consistent; QRS may be widened)	Acute myocardial infarction	Serious dysrhythmia that may lead to decreased heart rate and cardiac output	May require temporary pacemaker
Complete third-degree AV block	Atria and ventricles beat independently P waves have no relation to QRS Ventricular rate may be as low as 20–40 beats/min	Digitalis toxicity Infectious disease Coronary artery disease Myocardial infarction	Very low rates may cause decreased cardiac output: light-headedness, fainting, chest pain	Pacemaker ⊃ Epinephrine if isoproterenol ineffective ⊃ Isoproterenol to increase heart rate

Source: Phipps W, Long B, Woods N, Cassmeyer V. (eds.) *Medical-Surgical Nursing* (5th ed), St. Louis: Mosby, 1995.

AV = atrioventricular; CPR = cardiopulmonary resuscitation; ECG = electrocardiogram; PVB = premature ventricular beat; SA = sinoatrial node.

4. Diagnostic tests if ordered (e.g., cardiac catheterization; see Chap. 3, Diagnostic Studies Box).
5. *Exercise:* regular, graded, to promote coronary circulation.
6. Prepare for coronary artery bypass surgery, if necessary.
7. Behavior modification to assist with life-style changes, (i.e., stress reduction, stop smoking).

VI. Evaluation/outcome criteria
   A. Relief from pain.

B. Fewer attacks.
C. No MI.
D. Alters life-style; complies with limitations.
E. No smoking.

Myocardial Infarction

Localized area of necrotic tissue in the myocardium from cessation of blood flow; leading cause of death in North America.

TABLE 4.2 ◼ **COMPARISON OF PHYSICAL CAUSES OF CHEST PAIN: ASSESSMENT**

Characteristic	Myocardial Infarction	Pericarditis	Gastric Disorders	Angina Pectoris	Dissecting Aneurysm	Pulmonary Embolism
Onset	Gradual or sudden	Sudden	Gradual or sudden	Gradual or sudden	Abrupt, without prodromal symptoms	Gradual or sudden
Precipitating factors	Can occur at rest or after exercise or emotional stress	Breathing deeply, rotating trunk, recumbency, swallowing or yawning	Inflammation of stomach or esophagus; hypersecretion of gastric juices; some medications	Usually after physical exertion, emotional stress, eating, exposure to cold or defecation; unstable angina occurs at rest	Hypertension	Immobility or prolonged bed rest following surgery, trauma, hip fracture, heart failure, malignancy, oral contraceptives
Location	Substernal, anterior chest, or midline; rarely back; radiates to jaw or neck	Precordial; radiates to neck or left shoulder and arm	Xiphoid to umbilicus	Substernal, anterior chest; poorly localized	Correlates with site of intimal rupture; anterior chest or back; between shoulder blades	Pleural area, retrosternal area
Quality	Crushing, burning, stabbing, squeezing or vicelike	Pleuritic, sharp	Aching, burning, cramp-like gnawing	Squeezing, feeling of heavy pressure; burning	Sharp, tearing or ripping sensation	Sharp, stabbing
Intensity	Asymptomatic to severe; increases with time	Mild to severe	Mild to severe	Mild to moderate	Severe and unbearable; maximal from onset	Aggravated by breathing
Duration	30 min to 1–2 h; may wax and wane	Continuous	Periodic	Usually 2–10 min; average 3–5 min	Continuous; does not abate once started	Variable
Relief	Narcotics	*Sitting up,* leaning forward	Physical and emotional *rest,* food, antacids, H₂-receptor antagonists	Nitroglycerin, *rest*	Large, repeated doses of narcotics	O₂; *sitting up;* morphine
Associated symptoms	Nausea, fatigue, heart-burn; peripheral pulses equal	Fever, dyspnea, nausea, anorexia, anxiety	Nausea, vomiting, dysphagia, anorexia, weight loss	Belching, indigestion, dizziness	Syncope, loss of sensations or pulses, oliguria; discrepancy between BP in arms; decrease in femoral or carotid pulse	Dyspnea, tachypnea, diaphoresis, hemoptysis, cough, apprehension

I. Pathophysiology

A. Coronary occlusion due to thrombosis, embolism, or hemorrhage adjacent to atherosclerotic plaque.

B. Insufficient blood flow from cardiac hypertrophy, hemorrhage, shock, or severe dehydration.

II. Risk factors

A. Age (35–70 yr).

B. Men more than women until menopause.

C. Life-style.

D. Stress.

E. High-cholesterol diet (specifically low-density lipoproteins).

F. Chronic illness (diabetes, hypertension).

III. Assessment

A. *Subjective data:*

1. Pain (see Table 4.2).

a. *Type:* sudden, severe, crushing, heavy tightness.

b. *Location:* substernal; radiates to one or both arms, jaw, neck.

c. *Duration:* >30 min.

d. *Cause:* unrelated to exercise; frequently occurs when sleeping (REM stage).

e. *Relief:* oxygen, narcotics; *not* relieved by rest or nitroglycerin.

2. Nausea.

3. Shortness of breath.

4. Apprehension, fear of impending death.

5. History of cardiac disease (family); occupational stress.

B. *Objective data:*

1. Vital signs: shock; rapid (>100 beats/min), thready pulse; fall in blood pressure (BP); tachypnea, shallow respirations; elevated temperature within 24 h (100°–103°F).

2. Skin: cyanotic, ashen or clammy; diaphoretic.

3. Emotional: restless.

4. Lab data: *increased*—WBC (12,000–15,000/ μL), serum enzymes (CK-MB, LDH_1, $>LDH_2$ "flipped LDH"); *changes*—ECG (elevated ST segment, inverted T wave, arrhythmia).

IV. Analysis/nursing diagnosis

A. *Decreased cardiac output* related to myocardial damage.

B. *Impaired gas exchange* related to poor perfusion, shock.

C. *Pain* related to myocardial ischemia.

D. *Activity intolerance* related to pain or inadequate oxygenation.

E. *Fear* related to possibility of death.

V. Nursing care plan/implementation

A. Goal: *reduce pain, discomfort.*

1. *Narcotics*—morphine, meperidine HCl (Demerol); note response.

2. Humidified oxygen; mouth care—oxygen is drying.

3. *Position:* semi-Fowler's to improve ventilation.

B. Goal: *maintain adequate circulation.*

1. Monitor vital signs and urine output; observe for cardiogenic shock.

2. Monitor ECG for arrhythmias.

3. Give medications as ordered: *antiarrhythmics* —lidocaine HCl, quinidine HCl, procainamide (Pronestyl), bretylium (Bretylol); propranolol (Inderal); verapamil; *anticoagulants* —heparin sodium, bishydroxycoumarin (Dicoumarin); *thrombolytic agents*—streptokinase, tissue plasminogen activator(t-PA), AP-SAC/anistreplase (Eminase).

4. Recognize HF: edema, cyanosis, dyspnea, cough, crackles.

5. Check lab data—normal: serum enzymes (CK 0–7 IU/LDH <115 IU/L; LDH_1 <LDH_2); *blood gases* (pH 7.35–7.45; Pco_2 35–45 mEq/L; Po_2 80–100 mm Hg; HCO_3, 22–26); *electrolytes* (K^+ 3.5–5.0 mEq/L); *clotting time* (aPTT 25–33 sec; PT 11–15 sec).

6. Central venous pressure (CVP)—zero level at right atrium; fluctuates with respiration; normal range 5–15 cm H_2O; note trend; *increases* with heart failure.

7. ROM of lower extremities; TED hose/antiembolic stockings.

C. Goal: *decrease oxygen demand/promote oxygenation.*

1. Oxygen as ordered.

2. Activity: *bed rest* (24–48 h); planned rest periods; control visitors.

3. *Position:* semi-Fowler's to facilitate lung expansion and decrease venous return.

4. Anticipate needs of patient: call light, water.

5. Assist with feeding, turning.

6. Environment: quiet, comfortable.

7. Reassurance; stay with anxious patient.

8. Give medications as ordered: *cardiotonics, calcium channel blockers, vasodilators, vasopressors.*

D. Goal: *maintain fluid, electrolyte, nutritional status.*

1. IV (keep vein open); CVP; vital signs; urine output—30 mL/h.

2. Lab data within normal limits (Na^+ 135–145 mEq/L; K^+ 3.5–5.0 mEq/L).

3. Monitor ECG—*hyperkalemia:* peaked T wave; *hypokalemia:* depressed T wave.

4. *Diet:* progressive low calorie, low sodium, low cholesterol, low fat.

E. Goal: *facilitate fecal elimination.*

1. Medications: *stool softeners* to prevent Valsalva (straining); mouth breathing during bowel movement; recognize **complications of Valsalva**—chest pain, cyanosis, diaphoresis, arrhythmias.

2. Bedside commode if possible.

F. Goal: *provide emotional support.*

1. Recognize fear of dying: denial, anger, withdrawal.

2. Encourage expression of feelings, fears, concerns.

3. Discuss rehabilitation, life-style changes; prevent cardiac-invalid syndrome by promoting self-care activities, independence.

G. Goal: *promote sexual functioning.*
  1. Encourage discussion of concerns re: activity, inadequacy, limitations, expectations—include partner (usually resume activity 5–8 wk following uncomplicated MI).
  2. Identify need for referral for sexual counseling.

H. Goal: **health teaching.**
  1. Diagnosis and treatment regimen.
  2. *Caution* about when to *avoid* sexual activity: following heavy meal, alcohol ingestion; when fatigued, tense, under stress; with unfamiliar partners; in extreme temperatures.
  3. Information about sexual activity: less fatiguing positions (side to side; noncardiac on top); vasodilators, if ordered, prior to intercourse; select comfortable, familiar environment.
  4. Available community resources for information, support groups (e.g., American Heart Association, Stop Smoking Clinics).
  5. Medications: administration, importance, untoward effects, pulse taking.
  6. Control risk factors: rest, diet, exercise, no smoking, weight control, stress-reduction techniques.
  7. Need for follow-up care for regulation of medications, evaluating risk factors.
  8. Prepare for coronary bypass if planned.

VI. Evaluation/outcome criteria
  A. No complications: stable vital signs; relief of pain.
  B. Adheres to prescribed medication regimen, demonstrates knowledge about medications.
  C. Activity tolerance is increased, participates in program of progressive activity.
  D. Reduction or modification of risk factors. Plans to alter life-style (e.g., loses weight, quits smoking).

Heart Failure

Inability of the heart to meet the peripheral circulatory demands of body; cardiac decompensation; combined right and left ventricular HF.

I. Pathophysiology: increased cardiac workload or decreased effective myocardial contractility → decreased cardiac output (forward effects). Left ventricular failure → pulmonary congestion; right atrial and right ventricular failure → systemic congestion → peripheral edema (backward effects). Compensatory mechanisms in HF include tachycardia, ventricular dilatation, and hypertrophy of the myocardium; compensatory mechanisms develop in 50%–60% of heart disease patients.

II. Risk factors
  A. Decreased myocardial contractility:
    1. Myocarditis.
    2. MI.
    3. Tachyarrhythmias.
    4. Bacterial endocarditis.
    5. Acute rheumatic fever.
  B. Increased cardiac workload:
    1. Elevated temperature.
    2. Physical/emotional stress.

    3. Anemia.
    4. Hyperthyroidism (thyrotoxicosis).
    5. Valvular defects.

III. Assessment
  A. *Subjective data:*
    1. Shortness of breath:
      a. Orthopnea (sleeps on two or more pillows).
      b. Paroxysmal nocturnal dyspnea (sudden breathlessness during sleep).
      c. Dyspnea on exertion (climbing stairs).
    2. Apprehension, anxiety, irritability.
    3. Fatigue, weakness.
    4. Reported weight gain, feeling of puffiness.
  B. *Objective data:*
    1. Vital signs:
      a. BP: decreasing systolic; narrowing pulse pressure.
      b. Pulse: *pulsus alternans* (alternating strong-weak-strong cardiac contraction), increased.
      c. Respirations: crackles.
    2. Edema: dependent, pitting (1+ to 4+ mm).
    3. Liver: enlarged, tender.
    4. Neck veins: distended.
    5. Chest x-ray:
      a. Cardiac enlargement.
      b. Dilated pulmonary vessels.
      c. Diffuse interstitial lung edema.

IV. Analysis/nursing diagnosis
  A. *Decreased cardiac output* related to decreased myocardial contractility.
  B. *Activity intolerance* related to generalized weakness and inadequate oxygenation.
  C. *Fatigue* related to edema and poor oxygenation.
  D. *Altered tissue perfusion* related to peripheral edema and inadequate blood flow.
  E. *Fluid volume excess* related to compensatory mechanisms.
  F. *Impaired gas exchange* related to pulmonary congestion.
  G. *Anxiety* related to shortness of breath.
  H. *Sleep pattern disturbance* related to paroxysmal nocturnal dyspnea.

V. Nursing care plan/implementation
  A. Goal: *provide physical rest/reduce emotional stimuli.*
    1. *Position:* sitting or semi-Fowler's until tachycardia, dyspnea, edema resolved; change position frequently; pillows for support.
    2. Rest: planned periods; limit visitors, activity, noise.
    3. Support: stay with anxious patient; have supportive family member present; administer *sedatives/tranquilizers* as ordered.
    4. Warm fluids if appropriate.
  B. Goal: *provide for relief of respiratory distress; reduce cardiac workload.*
    1. Oxygen: low flow rate; encourage deep breathing (5–10 min q2h); auscultate breath sounds for congestion, pulmonary edema.

2. *Position:* head of bed 20–25 cm (8–10 in.) alleviates pulmonary congestion.

3. Medications as ordered:

    a. *Digitalis* preparations.

    b. *Inotropic Agents*—dobutamine, dopamine.

    c. *Vasodilators*—ACE inhibitors, nitrates, calcium channel blockers.

    d. *Diuretics*—thiazides, furosemide, ethacrynic acid.

    e. *Tranquilizers*—phenobarbital, diazepam (Valium), chlordiazepoxide HCl (Librium).

    f. *Stool softeners* to prevent Valsalva maneuver.

C. Goal: *provide for special safety needs.*

    1. Skin care:

        a. Inspect, massage, lubricate bony prominences.

        b. Use foot cradle, heel protectors; sheepskin.

    2. Siderails up if hypoxic (disoriented).

    3. Vital signs: monitor for signs of fatigue, pulmonary emboli.

    4. ROM: active, passive; elastic stockings.

D. Goal: *maintain fluid and electrolyte balance, nutritional status.*

    1. Urine output: 30 mL/h minimum; estimate insensible loss in diaphoretic client.

    2. Daily weight; same time, clothes, scale.

    3. IV: use microdrip to prevent circulatory overloading.

    4. *Diet:*

        a. Low sodium as ordered.

        b. Small, frequent feedings.

        c. Discuss food preferences with patient.

E. Goal: **health teaching.**

    1. Diet restrictions; meal preparation.

    2. Activity restrictions, if any; planned rest periods.

    3. Medications: schedule, purpose, dosage, side effects (importance of daily pulse taking, daily weights, intake of *potassium*-containing foods).

    4. Available community resources for dietary assistance, weight reduction, exercise program.

VI. **Evaluation/outcome criteria**

A. Increase in activity level tolerance—fatigue decreased.

B. No complications—pulmonary edema, respiratory distress.

C. Reduction in dependent edema.

Pulmonary Edema

Sudden transudation of fluid from pulmonary capillaries into alveoli.

I. **Pathophysiology:** increased pulmonary capillary permeability; increased hydrostatic pressure (pulmonary hypertension); and/or decreased blood colloidal osmotic pressure; fluid accumulation in alveoli → decreased compliance → decreased diffusion of gas → hypoxia, hypercapnea.

II. **Risk factors**

A. Left ventricular HF.

B. Pulmonary embolism.

C. Drug overdose.

D. Smoke inhalation.

E. Central nervous system (CNS) damage.

F. Fluid overload.

III. **Assessment**

A. *Subjective data:*

    1. Anxiety.

    2. Restlessness at onset progressing to agitation.

    3. Stark fear.

    4. Intense dyspnea, orthopnea, fatigue.

B. *Objective data:*

    1. Vital signs:

        a. Pulse: tachycardia, gallop rhythm.

        b. Respiration: tachypnea; moist, bubbling wheezing.

        c. Temperature: normal to subnormal.

    2. Skin: pale, cool, diaphoretic, cyanotic.

    3. Auscultation: crackles, wheezes.

    4. Cough: productive of large quantities of pink, frothy sputum.

    5. Right ventricular HF: distended neck veins, peripheral edema, hepatomegaly, ascites. (Note: Left-sided failure can cause right-sided failure.)

    6. Mental status: restless, confused, stuporous.

IV. **Analysis/nursing diagnosis**

A. *Decreased cardiac output* related to decreased myocardial contractility.

B. *Impaired gas exchange* related to pulmonary congestion.

C. *Altered tissue perfusion* related to inadequate blood flow.

D. *Anxiety,* severe, related to difficulty breathing.

E. *Fear* related to pulmonary congestion.

V. **Nursing care plan/implementation**

A. Goal: *promote physical, psychological relaxation measures to relieve anxiety.*

    1. Slow respirations: morphine sulfate, as ordered, to reduce respiratory rate, to sedate, and to produce vasodilation.

    2. Remain with patient.

    3. Encourage slow, deep breathing; assist with coughing.

    4. Work calmly, confidently, unhurriedly.

    5. Frequent rest periods.

B. Goal: *improve cardiac function, reduce venous return, relieve hypoxia.*

    1. Oxygen: 100%, preferably by demand valve to slow respiratory rate, provide uniform ventilation, reduce venous return, and inhibit "leaky capillary" syndrome.

    2. IV: 5% dextrose in water.

    3. Give aminophylline, as ordered, to lower venous pressure and increase cardiac output.

    4. *Position:* high Fowler's; extremities in dependent position to reduce venous return and facilitate breathing.

5. Medications as ordered: digitalis; diuretics—furosemide (Lasix); inotropic agents—dobutamine (Dobutrex), dopamine; nitroglycerin.
        6. Vital signs; auscultate breath sounds.
        7. *Diet:* low sodium; fluid restriction as ordered.
    C. Goal: **health teaching** (include family or significant other).
        1. Medications.
            a. Side effects.
            b. Potassium supplements if indicated.
            c. Pulse taking.
        2. Exercise, rest.
        3. *Diet:* low sodium.
        4. Signs of complications: edema; weight gain of 2–3 lb (0.9–1.4 kg) in a few days; dyspnea.
VI. **Evaluation/outcome criteria**
    A. No complications; vital signs stable; clear breath sounds.
    B. No weight gain; weight loss if indicated.
    C. Alert, oriented, calm.

☞ Summary of Key Points

1. Functional disorders of the heart are associated with coronary artery disease.
2. Cardiac pain is diffuse; a patient is usually unable to point to one location, unlike respiratory pain, which is more defined or localized.
3. Establish unresponsiveness before beginning CPR. Call for help, then remember your ABCs—**a**irway, **b**reathing, and **c**irculation.
4. Not all chest pain is brought on by exertion, eating, or emotion. Unstable angina occurs at rest.
5. Left ventricular failure (pulmonary edema) is a more severe condition than right ventricular failure.

💡 Study and Memory Aids

CPR—Remember the "ABCs"

AIRWAY
BREATHING
CIRCULATION

Angina: Pain Pattern

Exertion → Pain
Rest + nitroglycerin → relief

Angina: Precipitating Factors—"3 E's"

E ating
E motion
E xertion (Exercise)

Myocardial Infarction: "INTENSE PAIN"

I schemia
N ecrotic cardiac tissue
T ightness in chest
E xtended duration
N ausea
S evere pain
E CG changes

P revent Valsalva manuever
A nxiety
I ntense
N ot relieved by rest

Heart Failure: "OVERLOAD"

O rthopnea
V entricular failure
E nlarged heart
R eported weight gain
L ungs congested
O utput decreased
A pprehension
D ependent edema

Pulmonary Edema: "Fowlers"

F ailure—left ventricular
O rthopnea
W heezing
L ung congestion
E mergency
R estlessness
S kin—cyanotic

〰 Diagnostic Studies

Graphic Studies of Heart
Electrocardiography—graphic record of electrical activity generated by the heart during depolarization and repolarization; *used to* diagnose abnormal cardiac rhythms and heart disease.
Echocardiography (ultrasound cardiography)—graphic record of motions produced by cardiac structures as high-frequency sound vibrations are echoed through chest wall into the heart; transesophageal echocardiography produces a clearer image, particularly in obese, barrel-chested, or COPD patients; *used to* dem-

onstrate valvular or other structural deformities, detect pericardial effusion, diagnose tumors and cardiomegaly, or evaluate prosthetic valve function.

Phonocardiography—graphic record of heart sounds; *used to* keep a permanent record of patient's heart sounds before and after cardiac surgery.

Procedures to Evaluate the Cardiovascular System

Angiocardiography—intravenous injection of a radiopaque solution or medium for the purpose of studying its circulation through the patient's heart, lungs, and great vessels; *used to* check the competency of heart valves, diagnose congenital septal defects, detect occlusions of coronary arteries, confirm suspected diagnoses, and study heart function and structure prior to cardiac surgery.

Angiography (arteriography)—injection of a contrast medium into the arteries to study the vascular tree; *used to* determine obstructions or narrowing of peripheral arteries.

Pericardiocentesis (pericardial aspiration)—puncture of the pericardial sac is performed to remove fluid accumulating with pericardial effusion. The goal is to prevent cardiac tamponade (compression of the heart). **Nursing responsibilities:** monitor ECG and CVP *during the procedure*, have resuscitative equipment ready. *Head of bed elevated to 45–60 degrees.* Maintain peripheral IV with saline or glucose. *Following the procedure: monitor BP, CVP, and heart* sounds for recurrence of tamponade (pulsus paradoxus).

Diets

Angina Pectoris

↓ Calories
↓ Cholesterol
↓ Fat
↓ Gas-forming foods

Heart Failure

Low sodium
Small frequent feedings

Pulmonary Edema

↓ Sodium
↓ Fluids

Review of Physiology: Blood Flow

Vena cava
↓
Right atrium
↓
Tricuspid valve
↓
Right ventricle
↓
Pulmonary valve
↓
Right and left pulmonary arteries
↓
Lung/oxygenation
↓
Pulmonary veins
↓
Left atrium
↓
Bicuspid (mitral) valve
↓
Left ventricle
↓
Aortic valve
↓
Aorta

Drug Review

Cardiac Dysrhythmias

Anticholinergics: atropine
Antidysrhythmics
    Class IA Quinidine
          IB Lidocaine (xylocaine)
          IC (Tambocor) (Hecainide acetate)
          II Propranolol (Inderal)
          III Bretylium tosylate (Bretylol)
          IV Verapamil (Calan)

Beta-adrenergics
    Dobutamine (Dobutrex)
    Dopamine hydrochloride (Intropin)
    Epinephrine
    Isoproterenol (Isuprel)
    Norepinephrine (Levophed)

Cardiac Arrest/CPR: Medications Used, Depending on Symptoms and Response

Antiarrhythmic
    Adenosine
    Bretylium
    Isoproterenol
    Lidocaine
    Procainamide hydrochloride

Anticholinergic
  Atropine
Beta-adrenergic blocker
  Propranolol
Calcium channel blocker
  Verapamil
Cardiac glycoside
  Digoxin
Cardiac stimulant
  Epinephrine
Diuretic
  Furosemide
Electrolyte modifier
  Calcium
  Sodium bicarbonate
Inotropic Agent
  Dobutamine
  Dopamine
Vasodilator
  Nitroglycerin
Vasopressor
  Dopamine
  Norepinephrine

Angina Pectoris

Beta-blockers
  Atenolol (Tenorim): 25–50 mg/d
  Metoprolol (Lopressor): 100–450 mg/d
  Propranolol (Inderal): 40 mg bid
Calcium channel blockers
  Diltiazem (Cardizem): 30–120 mg 3–4 times daily.
  Nifedipine (Procardia): 10–30 mg tid
  Verapamil (Calan): 80–120 mg tid
Vasodilators
  Isosorbide dinitrate (Isordil): 2.5–10 mg po q2–3 h
    for acute attack
  Nitroglycerine: 0.15–0.6 mg repeated q5min for 15
    min for acute attacks
  Nitroglycerin long-acting preparations ointment
    1–2 inches q8h
  Nitroglycerin *patch:* 0.1–0.6 mg/h up to 0.8 mg/h
    worn 12–14 h/d

Acute Myocardial Infarction

Analgesics
  Meperidine (Demerol): 50–150 mg q3–4 h as
    needed; IV, 15–35 mg/h as a continuous
    infusion.
  Morphine: IV, 2.5–15 q4 h or loading dose of 15
    mg with 0.8–10 mg/h, rate increased as needed;
    SC, 5–20 mg q4 h as needed.
Anticoagulants
  Heparin sodium: IV, 5,000 U IV to start, followed
    by 20,000–40,000 U IV infusion over 24 hours;
    SC, 8000–10,000 U q8h, adjusted according to
    aPTT

  Warfarin (Coumadin): 10 mg daily, adjusted
    according to PT
  Bishydroxycoumarin (Dicumarol): 200–300 mg to
    start, then 25–200 mg based on PT
Antiarrhythmics (some of the drugs used)
  Bretylium (Bretylol): 5 mg/kg bolus over 15–30
    sec, not to exceed 30 mg/kg/d
  Lidocaine HCl: IV 50–100 mg (1 mg/kg) bolus;
    may be repeated in 5 min, then 1–4 mg/min
    infusion.
  Procainamide (Pronestyl): 50 mg/kg/d
  Propranolol (Inderal): 0.5–3 mg; repeat once in 2
    min if needed; 180–240 mg/d in divided doses
    starting 5–21 days post MI.
  Quinidine: 400–600 mg q2–3h, not to exceed 4 g/d.
Calcium channel blockers: Verapamil (Calan): 80–
  120 mg tid
Cardiac glycoside: Digoxin (Lanoxin): digitalizing
  dose: IV, 10–15 µg/kg over 24 h; or PO, 10–15 µg/
  kg over 24 h; maintenance dose, 0.1–0.375 mg/d.
  (Take apical pulse before administering drug)
Lipid-Lowering:
  Cholestyramine (Questran): 4 g 1–6 times daily
  Gemfibrozil (Lopid): 600 mg bid 30 min before
    breakfast and dinner
  Lovastatin (Mevacor): 20 mg qd with evening meal
  Niacin: 10–20 mg qd
Thrombolytic agents
  Alteplase (Activase t-PA) 100 mg over 90 min. 15
    mg bolus given over 1–2 min, then, 50 mg over
    30 min; then 35 mg over 60 min.
  Anistreplase (Eminase): IV, 30 U over 2–5 min
  Streptokinase (Streptase): 1.5 million U diluted to
    45 ml infused over 60 minutes
Vasodilators: Hydralazine (Apresoline): 10–100 mg
  qid
Vasopressors: Dopamine (Intropin): 1–5 µg/kg/min;
  gradually increase in 1–4 µg/kg/min increments at
  10–30 min intervals until optimum response. Most
  patients are maintained on dose of 20 µg/kg/min or
  less

Heart Failure

Cardiac glycosides
  Digoxin (Lanoxin): 0.1–0.375 mg/d
  Dobutamine (Dobutrex): IV, 2.5–15 µg/kg/min
  Dopamine (Intropin): IV, 0.5–5 µg/kg/min initially;
    increase to 50 µg/kg/min
Diuretics
  Furosemide (Lasix): 20–80 mg/d
  Hydrochlorothiazide (HydroDIURIL, Esidrix): 25–
    100 mg/d
Inotropic
  Dobutamine (Dobutrex): IV, 2.5–15 µg/kg/min
  Dopamine (Intropin): IV, 0.5–5 µg/kg/min initially;
    increase to 50 µg/kg/min
Stool softeners
  Docusate (Colace): 50–500 mg/d

Tranquilizers

Chlordiazepoxide HCl (Librium): 5–25 mg 3–4
   times daily
Diazepam (Valium): 2–10 mg 2–4 times daily
Phenobarbital Sodium (Luminal): 30–120 mg/d in
   divided doses.

Vasodilators

Captopril (Capoten): 6.25–12.5 mg 3 times daily
Isosorbide dinitrate (Isordil): 10–40 mg q 6h.
Nifedipine (Procardia): 10–30 mg 3 times daily
Verapamil (Calan): 80–120 mg 3 times daily

Pulmonary Edema

Aminophylline: loading dose of 500 mg followed by
   250–500 mg q6–8 h. Note: monitor theophylline
   levels
Digoxin (Lanoxin): 0.1–0.375 mg/d
Dobutamine (Dobutrex): IV, 2.5–15 µg/kg/min
Dopamine (Intropin): IV, 0.5–5 µg/kg/min initially;
   increase in 5–10 µg/kg/min increments up to rate
   of 20–50 µg/kg/min
Furosemide (Lasix): 20–80 mg/d
Morphine: IV, 2.5–15 q4h or loading dose of 15 mg
   with 0.8–10 mg/h, rate increased as needed; SC,
   5–20 mg q4h as needed
Nitroglycerin: 0.15–0.6 mg sublingual repeated q5min
   for 15 min for acute attacks

Questions

1. When resuming activities that require physical exertion,
   a patient who has had a myocardial infarction (MI)
   should be advised to take nitroglycerin (NTG):
   1. When any chest pain develops.
   2. As soon as any pressure or discomfort is felt.
   3. Before engaging in activities known to involve exer-
      tion.
   4. If the pain does not go away with rest.

2. What most common side effects would a nurse look for
   in a patient receiving atenolol (Tenormin), a beta-
   blocker used to manage angina pectoris?
   1. Bradycardia and hypotension.
   2. Fatigue and weakness.
   3. Bronchospasm and wheezing.
   4. Dry eyes and blurred vision.

3. Which statement by a patient scheduled for a treadmill
   test would be of greatest concern to the nurse?
   1. "I drank coffee this morning."
   2. "I took my propranolol (Inderal) this morning."
   3. "I slept 10 hours last night."
   4. "I've been having indigestion this morning."

4. A patient has been admitted to the telemetry unit to
   undergo testing to rule out an MI. The lab reports that
   the CK-MB is elevated. The most appropriate nursing
   action would be to:
   1. Give the patient 10 mEq/L of potassium to prevent
      arrhythmias.
   2. Prepare the patient for transfer to the CCU.
   3. Continue to monitor the lab results.
   4. Increase the amount of O_2 being administered to de-
      crease the ischemia.

5. Furosemide (Lasix) has been given IV to treat a patient
   with fluid retention. The best indicator of drug effectiveness is:
   1. Hourly urine output.
   2. Daily weight.
   3. Urine specific gravity.
   4. Serum sodium level.

6. The nurse instructs a patient to take lovastatin (Mevacor) with meals because taking it on an empty stomach
   will:
   1. Increase gastric irritation.
   2. Decrease drug absorption.
   3. Cause constipation or diarrhea.
   4. Lead to drug toxicity.

7. Which nursing action would be most helpful in reducing anxiety in a patient being admitted for evaluation
   and treatment of a possible MI?
   1. Explain the equipment being used.
   2. Pull the curtain around the bed for privacy.
   3. Offer the patient literature on unit policies.
   4. Explain use of the call light, and put it within reach.

8. Which laboratory test provides the most specific information about cardiac damage?
   1. ALT; (SGPT).
   2. CK-MB.
   3. LDH.
   4. AST; (SGOT).

9. The nurse should assess a patient with right ventricular
   failure for the presence of:
   1. Orthopnea and difficulty breathing at night.
   2. Weight gain and jugular venous distention.
   3. Confusion and apathy.
   4. Chest pain and elevated temperature.

10. Which foods should the nurse suggest to a patient who
    is on digoxin to minimize the risk of digitalis toxicity?
    1. Turkey, green beans, and French bread.
    2. Cottage cheese, cooked broccoli, and fish.
    3. Beef, green peas, and sweet corn.
    4. Whole grain cereal, orange juice, and apricots.

11. Which statement by the patient would indicate an accu-
    rate understanding of the teaching regarding adverse
    effects of digoxin?
    1. "I will call the MD if I become nauseated."
    2. "I will report my weight to the MD daily."
    3. "My gums may get puffy."
    4. "Hives or a rash may occur."

12. Which is the correct method for checking the pulse in a
    patient receiving digoxin?
    1. Taking the apical-radial pulses at the same time.
    2. Comparing the apical pulse with the pulse from the
       previous week.
    3. Counting the apical pulse for a full minute.
    4. Counting the apical pulse for 15 seconds and multi-
       plying it by 4.

13. A patient receiving digoxin has an apical pulse of 100
    beats/min. The appropriate nursing response would
    be to:

1. Record the rate and call the MD.
2. Record the rate and give the next dose of digoxin.
3. Give the medication and recheck the pulse in 15 minutes.
4. Hold the medication and check the pulse in 30 minutes.

Answers/Rationale

1. **(3)** Exertion, which includes sexual activity, increases cardiac workload. Taking NTG before engaging in activities that involve exertion should prevent any ischemia. Ischemia has already occurred once pain develops **(1)** and pressure is felt **(2)**. Rest **(4)** is important, but NTG should be taken before or during rest if chest pain arises unexpectedly with exertion. **IMP, 6, HPM**

2. **(2)** All of the choices are adverse or side effects of atenolol, but the *most common* are fatigue and weakness. If the more serious (and less common) side effects **(1 and 3)** occurred regularly in a patient, it is unlikely that treatment with the drug would be continued in that person. The visual problems **(4)** are also less common; a person suffering from them would be prone to have accidents, and for this reason, the drug would probably be changed. **AS, 6, PhI**

3. **(4)** Indigestion or epigastric pain may indicate the presence of myocardial ischemia. The patient should be given an antacid, and if this produces no relief, the patient should be given NTG to see if this relieves the pain. The test would not be done if the patient were having chest pain as the result of ischemia, even if it were relieved by NTG. Coffee **(1)** may cause the heart rate to increase, and the test may have to be interrupted if this should happen, but it can still be started. Patients usually take their cardiac drugs **(2)** the day of a treadmill test, and a restful night's sleep **(3)** would be desirable. **EV, 6, PhI**

4. **(2)** CK-MB is the specific isoenzyme for cardiac muscle; the normal value is 0.0 to 4.7 μg/mL, and an elevation is an indicator of an MI. The CCU is the best place for this patient to receive care. A low potassium level may cause arrhythmias, but there are no data to indicate the need for potassium supplements **(1)** to prevent arrhythmias in patients in the acute stage of an MI. Any arrhythmias in this patient would most likely be due to myocardial ischemia. Although it would not be wrong to continue to monitor **(3)** the patient, the diagnosis is established if the CK-MB level is raised 4 to 6 hours after the infarction. The only question is the extent of damage; the level peaks in 18 to 24 hours. O_2 **(4)** would be given, and most likely the patient would already be receiving it. However, the deciding factor here is the priority of the action. In this instance, the most important priority is to transfer the patient to a unit where closer supervision is possible until his/her condition is stable. **IMP, 6, SECE**

5. **(2)** All of the choices will provide data on the hydration or fluid status of the patient, but daily weight is the *best* indicator. Lasix, a loop diuretic, is used for the management of the acute stage of a condition such as pulmonary edema and for chronic heart failure if less potent diuretics, for example, a thiazide, have not worked. The patient's weight should decrease if the drug is effective. The urine volume **(1)** should increase, specific gravity **(3)** decrease, and the serum sodium level **(4)** increase in a patient with pulmonary edema who is receiving Lasix. **EV, 6, PhI**

6. **(2)** Lovastatin is a lipid-lowering agent, and absorption is decreased by 30% if it is not taken with food. Drug side effects include numerous symptoms of GI tract irritation **(1)**, and these occur if the drug is taken *with* food. These side effects include constipation or diarrhea **(3)**, dyspepsia, nausea, and heartburn. These effects are less severe if lovastatin is taken on an empty stomach, and taking the agent on an empty stomach would also lower the risk of toxicity **(4)**. However, optimal absorption is the highest priority. These other side effects, although unpleasant, can be managed by other means. **IMP, 6, PhI**

7. **(4)** The call light is a way for the patient to get help if needed, and its availability can help allay a patient's anxiety. Anxiety would impair any learning **(1 and 3)**; isolating the patient **(2)** would only increase the patient's anxiety. **IMP, 7, PsI**

8. **(2)** CK-MB is the cardiac-specific isoenzyme. The level is elevated 4 to 6 hours after an MI. The ALT level **(1)** is more specific to liver damage. The LDH level **(3)** also increases with cardiac damage, but not until much later. The AST level **(4)** would be elevated around the same time as the CK-MB level, but it is also elevated in other types of muscle damage. **AS, 6, SECE**

9. **(2)** The backward flow of blood caused by right-sided (right ventricular) heart failure leads to venous distention, organomegaly, and weight gain as the result of sodium and water retention. Orthopnea and difficulty breathing at right **(1)** are symptoms of *left* ventricular failure. Confusion and apathy **(3)** are rather inconclusive findings, but electrolyte imbalance or hypoxia stemming from many different causes may produce these symptoms. Chest pain and elevated temperature **(4)** are characteristic of an MI. **AS, 6, PhI**

10. **(4)** Digitalis toxicity is likely to develop when the potassium level is low. This risk is heightened in many patients receiving digoxin because they are also taking a diuretic, which depletes the serum potassium store. Foods high in potassium include: the whole grains, citrus fruits, apricots, bananas, and potatoes. The other foods **(1, 2, and 3)** are not sources of potassium. **IMP, 4, SECE**

Key to Codes

Nursing process: AS, assessment; **AN,** analysis; **PL,** planning; **IMP,** implementation; **EV,** evaluation. (See Appendix M for explanation of nursing process steps.)

Category of human function: 1, protective; **2,** sensory-perceptual; **3,** comfort, rest, activity, and mobility; **4,** nutrition; **5,** growth and development; **6,** fluid-gas transport; **7,** psychosocial-cultural; **8,** elimination. (See Appendix O for explanation.)

Client need: SECE, safe, effective care environment; **PhI,** physiologic integrity; **PsI,** psychosocial integrity; **HPM,** health promotion/maintenance. (See Appendix P for explanation.)

11. **(1)** The most frequent side effects of digoxin are nausea, vomiting, fatigue, bradycardia, and anorexia most likely related to hypokalemia. Although weight gain **(2)** would indicate that heart failure, worsening of weight would not be reported daily. Puffy gums **(3)**, or gingival hyperplasia, is a side effect of phenytoin. Allergic reactions **(4)** are *not* common in patients taking digoxin. **EV, 6, PhI**

12. **(3)** The correct method for checking the pulse of a patient receiving an antiarrhythmic drug is to count the pulse for one full minute because the rhythm is usually irregular. A more accurate rate would be counted in one minute. Checking for an apical-radial pulse deficit **(1)** is not done routinely. Changes in pulse rate would be noted from shift to shift, *not* from week to week **(2)**. The method in option **4** is used to check the pulse in a patient not receiving an antiarrhythmic drug. **AS, 6, PhI**

13. **(2)** The next dose of digoxin should be given because the drug has not yet achieved its therapeutic effect of slowing the heart rate while also increasing cardiac contractility. If the rate slows to less than 50 beats/min, the MD should be notified **(1)**. There is no reason to hold off giving the drug **(4)** or to recheck the pulse before the next scheduled assessment of the vital signs (**3 and 4**). **EV, 6, PhI**

Hematologic Disorders

Chapter Outline

Disseminated Intravascular Coagulation (DIC)

Diffuse or widespread coagulation initially within arterioles and capillaries leading to hemorrhage.

I. Pathophysiology: activation of coagulation system resulting from tissue injury → fibrin microthrombin form in brain, kidneys, lungs → microinfarcts, tissue necrosis → red blood cells (RBCs), platelets, prothrombin, other clotting factors trapped, destroyed in process → excessive clotting → release of fibrin split products → inhibition of platelet clotting → bleeding.

II. Risk factors
- **A.** Obstetric complications.
- **B.** Neoplastic disease.
- **C.** Low perfusion states.

III. Assessment—*objective data:*
- **A.** Skin, mucous membranes: petechiae, ecchymosis.
- **B.** Extremities (fingers, toes): cyanosis.
- **C.** Bleeding: venipuncture sites, wound, oral, rectal, vaginal.
- **D.** Urine output: oliguria → anuria.
- **E.** Level of consciousness: convulsions, coma.
- **F.** Lab data: *Prolonged*—prothrombin time (PT) > 15 sec; *Decreased*—platelets, fibrinogen level.

IV. Analysis/nursing diagnosis
- **A.** *Altered tissue perfusion* related to peripheral microthrombi.
- **B.** *Risk for injury,* death, related to bleeding.
- **C.** *Risk for impaired skin integrity* related to ischemia.
- **D.** *Altered urinary elimination* related to renal tubular necrosis.

V. Nursing care plan/implementation: Goal: *prevent and detect further bleeding.*
- **A.** Carry out nursing measures designed to alleviate underlying problem (e.g., shock, birth of fetus, surgery/irradiation for cancer).
- **B.** *Medications:* heparin sodium, if ordered, to reverse abnormal clotting (controversial).
- **C.** IVs: blood to lessen shock; platelets, cryoprecipitate, fresh plasma to restore clotting factors, fibrinogen (Table 5.1).
- **D.** Observe: vital signs, *CVP* (normal, 5–15 mm Hg), *pulmonary artery pressure* (normal, 20–30 mm Hg systolic and 8–12 mm Hg diastolic), and intake and output for signs of shock or fluid overload from frequent infusions; specimens for *occult* blood (urine, stool).
- **E.** Precautions: *Avoid* IM injections if possible; pressure 5 min to venipuncture sites; *no* rectal temperatures.

VI. Evaluation/outcome criteria
- **A.** Clotting mechanism restored (increased platelets, normal PT).
- **B.** Renal function restored (urine output >30 mL/h).
- **C.** Circulation to fingers, toes; no cyanosis.
- **D.** No irreversible damage from renal, cerebral, cardiac, or adrenal hemorrhage.

Iron Deficiency Anemia
(Hypochromic Microcytic Anemia)

Inadequate production of RBCs due to lack of heme (iron); common in infants, pregnant women, and premenopausal women.

TABLE 5.1   TRANSFUSION WITH BLOOD OR BLOOD PRODUCTS

Blood or Blood Product	Indications	▶ Assessment: Side Effects	▶ Nursing Care Plan/ Implementation
Whole blood	1. Acute hemorrhage 2. Hypovolemic shock	1. Hemolytic reaction 2. Fluid overload 3. Febrile reaction 4. Pyogenic reaction 5. Allergic reaction	1. See Table 9.2, Postoperative Complications, p. 120 for complete discussion of nursing responsibilities 2. Protocol for checking blood before transfusion is begun varies with each institution; however, at least *two* people must verify that the unit of blood has been crossmatched for a specific patient
Red blood cells, packed	1. Acute anemia with hypoxia 2. Aplastic anemia 3. Bone marrow failure due to malignancy 4. Patients who need red blood cells but not volume	See Whole blood	See Whole blood
Red blood cells, frozen	1. See Red blood cells, packed 2. Patients sensitized by previous transfusions	1. Less likely to cause antigen reaction 2. Decreased possibility of transmitting hepatitis	See Whole blood
White blood cells (leukocytes)	Currently being used in severe leukopenia with infection (research still being done)	1. Elevated temperature 2. Graft-versus-host disease	1. Careful monitoring of temperature 2. *Must* be given as soon as collected
Platelet concentrate	1. Severe deficiency 2. Bleeding thrombocytopenic patients with platelet counts *below* 10,000 μL	1. Fever, chills 2. Hives 3. Development of antibodies that will destroy platelets in future transfusions *Contraindications:* 1. Idiopathic thrombocytopenic purpura 2. Disseminated intravascular coagulation (DIC)	Monitor temperature
Single-donor fresh plasma	1. Clotting deficiency or concentrates not available or deficiency not fully diagnosed 2. Shock	1. Side effects rare 2. Heart failure 3. Possible hepatitis	Use sterile, pyrogen-free filters
Plasma removed from whole blood (up to 5 d after expiration date, which is 21 d)	1. Shock due to loss of plasma 2. Burns 3. Peritoneal injury 4. Hemorrhage 5. While awaiting blood crossmatch results	See Single-donor fresh plasma	See Single-donor fresh plasma

(continued)

TABLE 5.1 **TRANSFUSION WITH BLOOD OR BLOOD PRODUCTS (*Continued*)**

Blood or Blood Product	*Indications*	✠ *Assessment: Side Effects*	✠ *Nursing Care Plan/ Implementation*
Freeze-dried plasma	See Plasma removed from whole blood	See Single-donor fresh plasma	Must be reconstituted with sterile water before use
Single-donor fresh-frozen plasma	1. See Single-donor fresh plasma 2. Inherited or acquired disorders of coagulation 3. Preoperative hemophiliac	See Single-donor fresh plasma	1. Notify blood bank to thaw about 30 min before administration 2. Give *immediately*
Cryoprecipitate concentrate (factor VIII—antihemophilic factor)	For hemophilia: 1. Prevention 2. Preoperatively 3. During bleeding episodes	Rare	0.55 mL of cryoprecipitate concentrate has same effect on serum level as 1600 mL of fresh frozen plasma
Factors II, VII, IX, and X compiled	Specific deficiencies	Hepatitis	Commercially prepared
Fibrinogen (factor I)	Fibrinogen deficiency	Increased risk of hepatitis since the hepatitis virus combines with fibrinogen during fractionation	1. Reconstitute with sterile water 2. Do *not* warm fibrinogen or use hot water to reconstitute 3. Do *not* shake 4. Must be given with a filter
Albumin or salt-poor albumin	1. Shock due to hemorrhage, trauma, infection, surgery, or burns 2. Treatment of cerebral edema 3. Low serum-protein levels	None; these are heat-treated products	Commercially prepared
Dextran	Hypovolemic shock	1. Rare allergic reaction 2. Patients with heart or kidney disease susceptible to heart failure or pulmonary edema	Commercially prepared

Source: Lagerquist, SL: *Little, Brown's NCLEX-RN Examination Review.* Boston: Little, Brown, 1996. P. 300.

I. Pathophysiology: decreased dietary intake, impaired absorption, or increased utilization of iron decreases the amount of iron bound to plasma transferrin and transported to bone marrow for hemoglobin synthesis; decreased hemoglobin in erythrocytes decreases amount of oxygen delivered to tissues.

II. Risk factors
   A. *Excessive menstruation.*
   B. *Gastrointestinal bleeding*—peptic ulcer, hookworm, tumors.
   C. *Inadequate diet*—anorexia, fad diets, cultural practices.
   D. *Poor absorption*—stomach, small intestine disease.

✠ **III. Assessment**
   A. *Subjective data:*
      1. Fatigue: increasing.
      2. Headache.
      3. Change in appetite, difficulty swallowing due to pharyngeal edema/ulceration, heartburn.
      4. Shortness of breath on exercise.
      5. Extremities: numb, tingling.
      6. Flatulence.
      7. Menorrhagia.
   B. *Objective data:*
      1. Vital signs:
         a. *BP*—increased systolic, widened pulse pressure.

   b. *Pulse*—tachycardia.
   c. *Respirations*—tachypnea.
   d. *Temperature*—normal or subnormal.
   2. Skin/mucous membranes: pale, dry.
   3. Sclera: pearly white.
   4. Nails: brittle, spoon-shaped, flattened.
   5. Lab data: *Decreased*—hemoglobin (<10 g/dL blood), serum iron (<65 µg/dL blood); *Increased*—total iron-binding capacity.

IV. Analysis/nursing diagnosis
   A. *Altered nutrition, less than body requirements,* related to inadequate iron absorption.
   B. *Altered tissue perfusion* related to reduction in RBCs.
   C. *Risk for activity intolerance* related to profound weakness.
   D. *Impaired gas exchange* related to decreased oxygen-carrying capacity.

V. Nursing care plan/implementation
   A. Goal: *promote physical and mental equilibrium.*
   1. *Position:* optimal for respiratory excursion; deep breathing; turn frequently to prevent skin breakdown.
   2. Rest: balance with activity, as tolerated; assist with ambulation.
   3. Medication (hematinics):
      a. Oral iron therapy (ferrous sulfate)—give *with* meals.
      b. Intramuscular therapy (iron dextran)—use second needle for injection after withdrawal from ampule; use **Z** *track method;* inject 0.5 cc of air before withdrawing needle to prevent tissue necrosis; use 2–3-in. needle; rotate sites; do *not* rub site or allow wearing of constricting garments after injection.
   4. Keep warm: *no* hot water bottles, heating pads, due to decreased sensitivity.
   5. *Diet:* high in protein, iron, vitamins (see Appendixes B and C); assistance with feeding, if needed.
   B. Goal: **health teaching.**
   1. Dietary regimen.
   2. Iron therapy: explain purpose, dosage, side effects (black or green stools, constipation, diarrhea); take with meals.
   3. Activity: exercise to tolerance, with planned rest periods.

VI. Evaluation/outcome criteria
   A. Hemoglobin level returns to normal range.
   B. Tolerates activity without fatigue.
   C. Selects foods appropriate for dietary regimen.

Hemolytic Anemia (Normocytic Normochromic Anemia)

Unknown factor causes antibodies to destroy the body's own erythrocytes (autoimmune); common in those over 40 yr.

I. Risk factors
   A. Malignant lymphoma.
   B. Ulcerative colitis.
   C. Lupus erythematosus.
   D. Drug therapy

II. Assessment
   A. *Subjective data:*
   1. Fatigue, physical weakness.
   2. Dizziness.
   3. Shortness of breath.
   4. Diaphoresis on slight exertion.
   B. *Objective data:*
   1. Skin: pallor, jaundice.
   2. Posture: drooping.
   3. Lab data: *Decreased* hemoglobin; *Increased* reticulocyte count; *Direct* Coombs test positive.

III. See Iron Deficiency Anemia, p. 50, for analysis, nursing care plan/implementation, and evaluation.

Pernicious Anemia (Hyperchromic Macrocytic Anemia)

Lack of intrinsic factor found in gastric mucosa, which is necessary for vitamin B_{12} (extrinsic factor) absorption; slowly developing, usually after age 50 yr; may be an autoimmune disorder.

I. Pathophysiology: atrophy or surgical removal of glandular mucosa in fundus of stomach → degenerative changes in brain, spinal cord, and peripheral nerves from lack of vitamin B_{12}.

II. Risk factors
   A. Partial or complete gastric resection.
   B. Prolonged iron deficiency.
   C. Heredity.

III. Assessment
   A. *Subjective data:*
   1. Hands, feet: tingling, numbness.
   2. Weakness, fatigue.
   3. Sore tongue, anorexia.
   4. Difficulties with memory, balance.
   5. Irritability, mild depression.
   6. Shortness of breath.
   7. Palpitations.
   B. *Objective data:*
   1. Skin: pale, flabby, jaundiced.
   2. Sclera: icterus (yellow).
   3. Tongue: smooth, glossy, red, swollen.
   4. Vital signs:
      a. *BP*—normal or elevated.
      b. *Pulse*—tachycardia.
   5. Nervous system:
      a. Decreased vibratory sense in lower extremities.
      b. Loss of coordination.
      c. *Babinski* present (flaring of toes with stimulation of sole of foot).

d. Positive *Romberg* (loses balance when eyes closed).

e. Increased or diminished reflexes.

6. Lab data:

   (a) *Increased*—hemoglobin, bilirubin;

   (b) *Decreased*—RBCs, platelets, gastric secretions, *Schilling's test* (radioactive vitamin B$_{12}$ urine test).

IV. Analysis/nursing diagnosis

A. *Altered nutrition, less than body requirements,* related to vitamin B$_{12}$ deficiency.

B. *Impaired physical mobility* related to numbness of extremities.

C. *Fatigue* related to decreased oxygen-carrying capacity.

D. *Altered oral mucous membrane* related to changes in gastric mucosa.

E. *Altered thought processes* related to progressive neurologic degeneration.

V. Nursing care plan/implementation

A. Goal: *promote physical and emotional comfort.*

1. Activity: bed rest or activity as tolerated—restrictions depend on neurologic or cardiac involvement.

2. Comfort: keep extremities warm—light blankets, loose-fitting socks.

3. Medication: vitamin B$_{12}$ therapy as ordered.

4. *Diet:*

   a. Six small feedings.

   b. Soft or pureed.

   c. Organ meats, fish, eggs.

5. Mouth care: before and after meals, to increase appetite and relieve mouth discomfort.

B. Goal: **health teaching.**

1. Medication:

   a. Lifelong therapy.

   b. Injection techniques, rotation of sites.

2. Diet.

3. Rest, exercise to tolerance.

VI. Evaluation/outcome criteria

A. No irreversible neurologic or cardiac complications.

B. Takes vitamin B$_{12}$ for the rest of life—uses safe injection technique.

C. Returns for follow-up care.

Polycythemia Vera

Abnormal increase in circulating RBCs; considered to be a form of malignancy.

I. Pathophysiology: unknown causes → massive increases of erythrocytes, myelocytes (bone marrow leukocytes), and thrombocytes → increased blood viscosity/volume and tissue/organ congestion; increased peripheral vascular resistance; intravascular thrombosis usually develops in middle age, particularly in Jewish men; in contrast, *secondary* polycythemia occurs as a compensatory response to tissue hypoxia associated with prolonged exposure to high altitude, chronic lung disease, and heart disease.

II. Assessment

A. *Subjective data:*

1. Headache; dizziness; ringing in ears.

2. Weakness; loss of interest.

3. Feelings of abdominal fullness.

4. Shortness of breath; orthopnea.

5. Pruritus, especially after bathing.

6. Pain: gouty-arthritic.

B. *Objective data:*

1. Skin: mucosal erythema, ruddy complexion (reddish purple).

2. Ecchymosis; gingival (gum) bleeding.

3. Enlarged liver, spleen.

4. Hypertension.

5. Lab data:

   (a) *Increased*—hemoglobin, hematocrit, RBCs, leukocytes, platelets, uric acid;

   (b) *Decreased*—bone marrow iron.

III. Analysis/nursing diagnosis

A. *Altered tissue perfusion* related to capillary congestion.

B. *Risk for injury* related to dizziness, weakness.

C. *Fluid volume excess* related to mass production of RBCs.

D. *Risk for impaired skin integrity* related to pruritus.

E. *Ineffective breathing pattern* related to shortness of breath, orthopnea.

III. Nursing care plan/implementation

A. Goal: *promote comfort and prevent complications.*

1. Observe for signs of bleeding, thrombosis—stools, urine, gums, skin, ecchymosis.

2. Reduce occurrence: *avoid* prolonged sitting, knee Gatch.

3. Assist with ambulation.

4. *Position:* elevate head of bed.

5. Skin care: cool-water baths to decrease pruritus; may add bicarbonate of soda to water.

6. Fluids: *force,* to reduce blood viscosity and promote urine excretion: 1500–2500 mL/24 h.

7. *Diet: avoid* foods high in iron, to reduce RBC production.

8. Assist with venesection (phlebotomy), as ordered.

B. Goal: **health teaching.**

1. *Diet:* foods to *avoid* (e.g., liver, egg yolks); fluids to be increased.

2. Signs/symptoms of complications: infections, hemorrhage.

3. *Avoid:* falls, bumps; hot baths/showers (worsens pruritus).

4. Drugs: myelosuppressive agents (busulfan [Myleran], cyclophosphamide [Cytoxan]), chlorambucil, radioactive phosphorus); purpose, side effects.

5. Procedures: venesection (phlebotomy) if ordered.

IV. Evaluation/outcome criteria

A. Acceptance of chronic disease.

B. Reports at prescribed intervals for follow-up.

C. Remission: lab data: reduction of bone marrow activity, blood volume and viscosity (RBC <6,500,000/µL; hemoglobin <18 g/dL; hematocrit <45%; white blood cell count <10,000 µL).

D. No complications (e.g., thrombi, hemorrhage, gout, heart failure, leukemia).

Leukemia (Acute and Chronic)

A neoplastic disease involving the leukopoietic tissue in either the bone marrow or lymphoid areas; acute leukemia occurs in children, young adults; chronic forms occur in later adult life.

I. Types:
  A. Acute nonlymphocytic (ANLL)—*formerly* known as *acute myelogenous leukemia* (AML); seen generally in older age (>60 yr).
  B. Acute lymphocytic (ALL)—common in children 2–10 yr.
  C. Chronic lymphocytic (CLL)—generally affects the elderly.
  D. Chronic myelogenous (CML)—also known as *chronic granulocytic leukemia* (CGL); more likely to occur between 25 and 60 yr.

II. Pathophysiology: displacement of normal marrow cells by proliferating leukemic cells (abnormal, immature leukocytes) → normochromic anemia, thrombocytopenia.

III. Risk factors
  A. Viruses.
  B. Genetic abnormalities.
  C. Exposure to chemicals.
  D. Radiation.
  E. Treatment for other types of cancer (e.g., alkylating agents).

IV. Assessment
  A. *Subjective data:*
    1. Fatigue, weakness.
    2. Anorexia, nausea.
    3. Pain: joints, bones (acute leukemia).
    4. Night sweats, weight loss, malaise.
  B. *Objective data:*
    1. Skin: pallor due to anemia, *jaundice.*
    2. Fever: frequent infections; mouth ulcers.
    3. Bleeding: petechiae, purpura, ecchymosis, epistaxis, gingiva.
    4. Organ enlargement: spleen, liver.
    5. Enlarged lymph nodes; tenderness.
    6. Bone marrow aspiration: increase in blast cells.
    7. Lab data:
      (a) WBC—15,000–500,000/mL.
      (b) RBCs—normal to severely *decreased*;
      (c) Hgb—low or normal;
      (d) Platelets—low to *elevated.*

V. Analysis/nursing diagnosis
  A. *Risk for infection* related to immature or abnormal leukocytes.
  B. *Activity intolerance* related to hypoxia and weakness.

  C. *Fatigue* related to anemia.
  D. *Altered tissue perfusion* related to anemia.
  E. *Anxiety* related to diagnosis and treatment.
  F. *Altered oral mucous membrane* related to susceptibility to infection.
  G. *Fear* related to diagnosis.
  H. *Ineffective individual or family coping* related to potentially fatal disease.

VI. Nursing care plan/implementation
  A. Goal: *prevent, control, and treat infection.*
    1. Protective isolation if indicated.
    2. Observe for early signs of infection:
      a. Inflammation at injection sites.
      b. Vital sign changes.
      c. Cough.
      d. Obtain cultures.
    3. Give antibiotics as ordered.
    4. Mouth care: clean q2h, examine for new lesions, *avoid* trauma.
  B. Goal: *assess and control bleeding, anemia.*
    1. Activity: *restrict* to prevent trauma.
    2. Observe for hemorrhage: vital signs; body orifices, stool, urine.
    3. Control localized bleeding: ice, pressure at least 3–4 min after needle sticks, positioning.
    4. Use soft-bristle or foam-rubber toothbrush to prevent gingival bleeding.
    5. Give blood/blood components as ordered (see Table 5.1); observe for transfusion reactions.
  C. Goal: *provide rest, comfort, nutrition.*
    1. Activity: 8 h sleep, daily nap.
    2. Comfort measures: flotation mattress, bed cradle, sheepskin.
    3. Analgesics: without delay.
      a. Mild pain (acetaminophen [Tylenol], propoxyphene HCl [Darvon] without aspirin).
      b. Severe pain (codeine, meperidine HCl [Demerol]).
    4. *Diet:* bland.
      a. High in protein, minerals, vitamins.
      b. Low roughage.
      c. Small, frequent feedings.
      d. Favorite foods.
    5. Fluids: 3000–4000 mL/d.
  D. Goal: *reduce side effects from therapeutic regimen.*
    1. Nausea: antiemetics, usually half hour *before* chemotherapy.
    2. Increased uric acid level: *force* fluids.
    3. Stomatitis: *antiseptic anesthetic* mouthwashes.
    4. Rectal irritation: meticulous toileting, *sitz baths*, topical relief (e.g., Tucks).
  E. Goal: *provide emotional/spiritual support.*
    1. Contact clergy if patient desires.
    2. Allow, encourage patient-initiated discussion of death (developmentally appropriate).
    3. Allow family to be involved in care.
    4. If death occurs, provide privacy, listening, sharing of grief for family.
  F. Goal: **health teaching.**
    1. Prevent infection.
    2. Limits of activity.

3. Control bleeding.
4. Reduce nausea.
5. Mouth care.
6. Chemotherapy: regimen, side effects.

VII. Evaluation/outcome criteria
   A. Alleviate symptoms; obtain remission.
   B. Prevent complications (e.g., infection).
   C. Ventilates emotions—accepts and deals with anger.
   D. Experiences peaceful death (e.g., pain free).

Idiopathic Thrombocytopenic Purpura (ITP)

Potentially fatal disorder characterized by spontaneous increase in platelet destruction; possible autoimmune response; remissions occur spontaneously or following splenectomy; in contrast, *secondary* thrombocytopenia (STP) is caused by viral infections, drug hypersensitivity (i.e., *quinidine, sulfonamides*), lupus, or bone marrow failure; treat cause.

I. Assessment
   A. *Subjective data:*
      1. Spontaneous skin hemorrhages—lower extremities.
      2. Menorrhagia.
      3. Epistaxis.
   B. *Objective data:*
      1. Bleeding: gastrointestinal, urinary, nasal; following minor trauma, dental extractions.
      2. Petechiae; ecchymosis.
      3. Lab data:
         (a) *Decreased* platelets (<100,000/mL);
         (b) *Increased* bleeding time;
         (c) Tourniquet test—positive, demonstrating increased capillary fragility.

II. Analysis/nursing diagnosis
   A. *Risk for injury* related to hemorrhage.
   B. *Altered tissue perfusion* related to fragile capillaries.
   C. *Impaired skin integrity* related to skin hemorrhages.

III. Nursing care plan/implementation
   A. Goal: *prevent complications from bleeding tendencies.*
      1. Precautions:
         a. Injections—use small-bore needles; rotate sites; apply direct pressure.
         b. *Avoid* bumping, trauma.
         c. Use swabs for mouth care.
      2. Observe for signs of bleeding, petechiae following BP reading, ecchymosis, purpura.
      3. Administer steroids (e.g., prednisone) with idiopathic thrombocytopenic purpura to increase platelet count; give platelets for count below 20,000–30,000/μL with secondary thrombocytopenic purpura.
   B. Goal: **health teaching.**
      1. *Avoid* traumatic activities:
         a. Contact sports.

b. Violent sneezing, coughing, nose blowing.
c. Straining at stool.
d. Heavy lifting.
      2. *Signs of decreased platelets*—petechiae, ecchymosis, gingival bleeding, hematuria, menorrhagia.
      3. Use MedicAlert tag/card.
      4. Precautions: self-medication; particularly *avoid* aspirin-containing drugs.
      5. Prepare for splenectomy if drug therapy unsuccessful (prednisone, cyclophosphamide, azathioprine [Imuran]).

IV. Evaluation/outcome criteria
   A. Returns for follow-up.
   B. No complications (e.g., hemorrhage).
   C. Lab data: Platelet count >200,000/μL.
   D. Skin remains intact.
   E. Resumes self-care activities.

Splenectomy

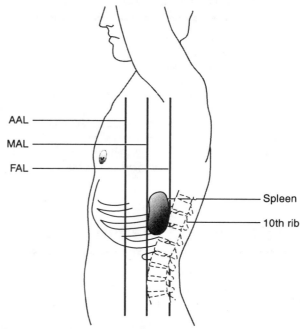

Removal of spleen following rupture due to acquired hemolytic anemia, trauma, tumor, or idiopathic thrombocytopenia purpura.

I. Assessment (see above, cause of rupture, for data)
II. Analysis/nursing diagnosis
   A. *Risk for fluid volume deficit* related to hemorrhage.
   B. *Risk for infection* related to impaired immune response.
   C. *Pain* related to abdominal distention.
III. Nursing care plan/implementation
   A. Goal: *prepare for surgery.*
      1. Give whole blood, as ordered.
      2. Insert nasogastric tube to decrease postoperative abdominal distention, as ordered.
   B. Goal: *prevent postoperative complications.*

   1. Observe for:
       a. *Hemorrhage*—bleeding tendency with thrombocytopenia due to decreased platelet count.
       b. *Gastrointestinal distention*—removal of enlarged spleen may result in distended stomach and intestines, to fill void.
   2. Recognize temperature of 101°F as normal for 10 d.
   3. Incision: splint when coughing, to prevent atelectasis (frequent complication), pneumonia with upper abdominal incision.
C. Goal: **health teaching.**
   1. Increased risk of infection after splenectomy.
   2. Report signs of infection *immediately.*
IV. **Evaluation/outcome criteria**
   A. No complications (e.g., respiratory, subphrenic abscess or hematoma, thromboemboli, infection).
   B. Complete and permanent remission—occurs in 60–80% of patients.

☞ Summary of Key Points

1. DIC occurs following low-perfusion states, such as shock. DIC should be suspected in a patient with no prior history of a bleeding tendency.
2. All types of anemia result in a decrease in oxygen-carrying capacity.
3. Fatigue, weakness, easy bruising, and bleeding gums are frequently seen in all types of leukemia.
4. If platelet count is below normal, there will be spontaneous bleeding into any part of the body.

� Study and Memory Aids

Complete Blood Count

Erythrocytes
   Hematocrit
   Hemoglobin
   Red blood cells
Leukocytes
   White blood cells
   Differential count
   Granulocytes
       Basophils
       Eosinophils
       Neutrophils
   Agranulocytes
       Lymphocytes
       Monocytes
   Thrombocytes
       Platelets

Diets

Iron Deficiency Anemia

↑ Protein, iron, vitamins

Pernicious Anemia

Small pureed feedings
Organ meat, fish, eggs

Polycythemia Vera

∅ Fe^+
↑ Fluids

Drug Review

Disseminated Intravascular Coagulation

Aminocaproic acid (Amicar) 4–5 gm IV initially, then 1–1.25 gm/h IV for 8 h. Maximum 30 gm/24 h.
Antithrombin III in fresh frozen plasma to decrease complications
Cryoprecipitate given for depletion of factors V and VIII
Fresh blood
Heparin sodium: IV, 1000 U/h adjusted according to partial thromboplastin time (PTT)
Platelets

Iron Deficiency Anemia

Ferrous sulfate (Fer-In-Sol): 300 mg 2–4 times daily; give with meals
Iron dextran (Imferon): 100–250 mg IM via Z track method. Do *not* exceed 250 mg (5 mL).

Pernicious Anemia

Vitamin derivatives to correct nutritional deficiency
Hydroxocobalamin (Vit B_{12}a): 100–200 μg monthly, given IM, SC ("Flushing" dose for Schilling's test:1000 μg/mL)

Polycythemia Vera: Drug and Other Treatment

Myelosuppressive agents to produce remission:
    radioactive phosphorus, chlorambucil, busulfan
    (Myleran), hydroxyurea (Hydrea) cyclophosphamide
    (Cytoxan)
Other treatment
    Phlebotomy
    Radiation

Leukemia

Antineoplastic drugs
    L-asparaginase
    Busulfan
    Cyclophosphamide
    Cytarabine (Ara-C) in combination with other drugs
    Daunorubicin
    Prednisone
    Vincristine
Analgesics to relieve discomfort
Antibiotics to fight infections
Antiemetics to combat nausea and vomiting

Idiopathic Thrombocytopenic Purpura: Drug and Other Treatment

Steroid therapy: prednisone, danazol (Danocrine)
Plasmapheresis until steroids take effect (Large
    volumes of the patient's plasma are removed and
    fresh plasma is administered)
Immunosuppressive therapy:
    Azathioprine (Imuran)
    Cyclophosphamide (Cytoxan)
    Vinblastine (Velban)
    Vincristine (Oncovin)

Splenectomy

Preoperative and postoperative medications, as with
    any surgical patient.
Antibiotic therapy to decrease risk of infection.

Questions

1. Which laboratory values would necessitate a nursing action?
   1. A hematocrit (Hct) value of 40%.
   2. A hemoglobin (Hgb) level of 9 g/dL.
   3. A white blood cell count (WBC) of 9,000/mm³.
   4. A potassium (K⁺) concentration of 4.8 mEq/L.
2. The nurse would record in the patient's chart the finding of large, irregular hemorrhagic areas on a patient's leg as:
   1. Ecchymoses.
   2. Hematoma.
   3. Petechiae.
   4. Hemangioma.
3. Treatment for a patient's leukemia has resulted in an apparent state of remission. The nurse explains to the patient that *remission* means that:
   1. A complete cure has occurred.
   2. The symptoms from the disease have subsided.
   3. The blood findings are normal, but the bone marrow is still affected.
   4. The leukemia will not come back because there is no evidence of disease.
4. Which group of assessment findings would be seen in a patient with acute nonlymphocytic leukemia (ANLL)?
   1. Diarrhea, nausea, and restlessness.
   2. Weakness, fever, and bleeding.
   3. Dehydration, chills, and joint pain.
   4. Tremors, lymph node tenderness, and headache.
5. As part of the preparation for a bone marrow aspiration, the nurse would:
   1. Explain the procedure to the patient and have the patient sign a consent form.
   2. Tell the patient that no anesthetic can be given because it interferes with the quality of the sample.
   3. Show the patient the location of the posterior iliac crest where the sample will be taken.
   4. Discuss the need to remain on bed rest for 6 to 8 hours after the procedure to prevent bleeding.
6. Which solution should the nurse infuse before starting a blood transfusion?
   1. 5% dextrose in water.
   2. 0.9% sodium chloride.
   3. 5% dextrose in 0.45% sodium chloride.
   4. Ringer's lactate solution.
7. The nurse finds a patient crying who is undergoing chemotherapy for leukemia. The best response for the nurse to make would be:
   1. "All of these changes in your life have been difficult."
   2. "When you're done crying I'll come back."
   3. "Fortunately there are effective treatments available."
   4. "You'll feel better when you are done crying."
8. Which nursing action is most important before starting an infusion of packed red blood cells IV?
   1. Weighing the patient as a baseline assessment.
   2. Finding out whether an 18-gauge needle is being used.
   3. Checking the Hgb and Hct levels.
   4. Clearing the existing tubing with 5% dextrose in water.
9. During the first 10 to 15 minutes of a blood transfusion, the nurse should set the rate of a transfusion to be given at 10 gtt/min at:
   1. 3–5 gtt/min.
   2. 15–20 gtt/min.
   3. 25–35 gtt/min.
   4. 40–50 gtt/min.

10. A patient receiving a blood transfusion complains of a headache and of feeling cold and a heaviness in the chest. The patient appears flushed and is shaking; blood pressure is 100/58 mm Hg. The first nursing action would be to:
1. Remove the IV immediately.
2. Clamp off the blood transfusion.
3. Continue to monitor the vital signs.
4. Call the MD.

Answers/Rationale

1. **(2)** The Hgb level for a man or woman should be 12 g/dL or higher. A level of 9 g/dL is low and may indicate the presence of anemia or blood loss. The oxygen-carrying capacity of the blood would be reduced, and as a result, the patient might be experiencing the symptoms of hypoxia, such as fatigue and shortness of breath. An Hct value of 40% **(1)** is within the normal limits of 37% or higher. The normal range of the WBC is 5000 to 10,000/mm³, so 9,000/mm³ **(3)** is normal. The normal potassium concentration ranges from 3.5 to 5.0 mEq/L, so 4.8 mEq/L **(4)** is also normal. **AN, 6, SECE**

2. **(1)** An ecchymosis is a discoloration of the skin resulting from the extravasation of blood into the subcutaneous tissues. A hematoma **(2)** is a circumscribed extravascular collection of blood, which is usually clotted. Petechiae **(3)** are pinpoint hemorrhages on a surface such as the skin or mucous membranes. A hemangioma **(4)** is a tumor composed of blood vessels. **IMP, 6, PhI**

3. **(2)** When the signs, and hence the symptoms, of a chronic condition subside, this is called a *remission*. The patient is *not* cured **(1)**. During a remission there are no symptoms **(3)**. The symptoms *often* return **(4)**, which is called an *exacerbation*. **IMP, 3, SECE**

4. **(2)** The signs and symptoms of all types of leukemia are similar. (The symptoms are also characteristic of anemia and thrombocytopenia, however.) In addition to weakness, fever, and bleeding, the patient often complains of generalized pain and headache. ANLL was formerly known as *acute myelogenous leukemia*. None of the symptoms in option **1** are those of ANLL. In option **3**, only joint pain is a symptom. Lymph node enlargement and tenderness in option **4** is a sign and headache a possible symptom, but not tremors. **AS, 6, PhI**

5. **(3)** The posterior iliac crest is the most common site for bone marrow aspiration. Other possible sites are the sternum and anterior iliac crest. Obtaining informed consent **(1)** is the responsibility of the MD, though the nurse should make sure the form is signed before the procedure. The skin and subcutaneous tissue down to the periosteum are anesthetized, and this does not interfere with the quality of the sample **(2)**. The site needs to be watched for bleeding, but bed rest **(4)** is not required. **IMP, 1, SECE**

6. **(2)** If blood is mixed with any IV solution other than normal saline outside the body, it will precipitate in the tubing. The other solutions **(1, 3, and 4)** would cause the blood to precipitate. **IMP, 6, PhI**

7. **(1)** The most therapeutic communication reflects what the patient is expressing. Such a patient needs to know the feelings are recognized and that it is okay to feel depressed and discouraged; a loss has occurred. The other responses **(2, 3, and 4)** do not recognize the patient's feelings. **IMP, 7, PsI**

8. **(2)** The needle needs to be at least an 18-gauge one to prevent lysis of the red blood cells. Vital signs, *not* weight **(1)**, are used for the baseline assessment. Hgb and Hct values **(3)** would be checked later to determine the effects of the transfusion. The line is cleared with saline, *not* dextrose **(4)**. **PL, 6, PhI**

9. **(2)** The rate of a blood transfusion during the first 15 minutes should be 1 to 2 mL/min because this is the time when transfusion reactions are most likely to occur. This would be enough blood to produce a reaction but not too much for the reaction to be easily reversed. The other rates are either too slow **(1)** to cause a reaction or too fast **(3 and 4)** and would allow too much blood to be transfused for a reaction to be easily reversed. **IMP, 6, SECE**

10. **(2)** The patient is experiencing a hemolytic transfusion reaction resulting from ABO incompatibility; the transfusion should be stopped, but the IV line left in place in case drugs need to be given in an emergency. The nurse should change the tubing immediately and infuse normal saline. If the patient goes into shock, starting a new IV may be difficult **(1)**. Vital signs would be monitored **(3)** and the MD notified **(4)** after the IV tubing has been changed. **PL, 6, PhI**

Key to Codes

Nursing process: AS, assessment; **AN,** analysis; **PL,** planning; **IMP,** implementation; **EV,** evaluation. (See Appendix M for explanation of nursing process steps.)

Category of human function: 1, protective; **2,** sensory-perceptual; **3,** comfort, rest, activity, and mobility; **4,** nutrition; **5,** growth and development; **6,** fluid-gas transport; **7,** psychosocial-cultural; **8,** elimination. (See Appendix O for explanation.)

Client need: SECE, safe, effective care environment; **PhI,** physiologic integrity; **PsI,** psychosocial integrity; **HPM,** health promotion/maintenance. (See Appendix P for explanation.)

Respiratory Disorders

Chapter Outline

Pneumonia

Acute inflammation of lungs with exudate accumulation in alveoli and other respiratory passages that interferes with ventilation.

I. Types:

  A. *Typical/classic pneumonia:* pneumococcal; related to diminished defense mechanisms, history of alcoholism, recent respiratory tract infection, viral influenza, increased age, and chronic obstructive pulmonary disease (COPD).

  B. *Atypical pneumonia:* related to contact with specific organisms.

    1. *Mycoplasma pneumoniae* or *Legionella pneumophila,* if untreated, can lead to serious complications such as disseminated intravascular coagulation (DIC), thrombocytopenic purpura, renal failure, inflammation of the heart, neurologic disorders, or possible death.

    2. *Pneumocystis carinii* in conjunction with the acquired immune deficiency syndrome (AIDS).

  C. *Aspiration pneumonia:*

    1. *Noninfectious:* aspiration of fluids (gastric secretions, foods, liquids, tube feedings) into the airways.

    2. *Bacterial aspiration pneumonia:* related to poor cough mechanisms due to anesthesia, coma (mixed flora of upper respiratory tract cause pneumonia).

  D. *Hematogenous pneumonia bacterial infections:* related to spread of bacteria from the bloodstream.

II. Pathophysiology: caused by infectious or noninfectious agents, clotting of an exudate rich in fibrogen, consolidated lung tissue.

III. Assessment

  A. *Subjective data:*

    1. Pain location: chest (affected side), referred to abdomen, shoulder, flank.

    2. Irritability, restlessness.

    3. Apprehension.

    4. Nausea, anorexia.

    5. History of exposure.

  B. *Objective data:*

    1. Cough:

      a. Productive, rust (blood) or yellowish sputum (greenish with atypical pneumonia).

      b. Splinting of affected side when coughing.

    2. Sudden increased fever, chills.

    3. Nasal flaring, circumoral cyanosis.

    4. Respiratory distress: tachypnea.

    5. Auscultation:

      a. Decreased breath sounds on *affected* side.

      b. Exaggerated breath sounds on *unaffected* side.

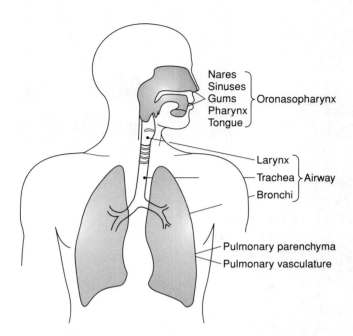

RESPIRATORY SYSTEM.
(From Judge R, Zuidema G,
Fitzgerald F. *Clinical Diagnosis.*
Boston: Little, Brown, 1989, p. 204.)

    c. Crackles, bronchial breath sounds.
    d. Dullness over consolidated area.
    e. Possible pleural friction rub.
  6. Chest retraction (air hunger in infants).
  7. Vomiting.
  8. Facial herpes simplex.
  9. *Diagnostic* studies:
    a. Chest x-ray: haziness to consolidation.
    b. Sputum culture: specific organisms, usually
      pneumococcus.
  10. Lab data:
    (1) Blood culture—organism specific except
      when viral;
    (2) White blood cell count (WBC)—leukocy-
      tosis;
    (3) Sedimentation rate—*elevated.*

IV. Analysis/nursing diagnosis
  A. *Ineffective airway clearance* related to retained se-
    cretions.
  B. *Activity intolerance* related to inflammatory pro-
    cess.
  C. *Pain* related to continued coughing.
  D. *Knowledge deficit* related to proper management
    of symptoms.
  E. *Risk for fluid volume deficit* related to tachypnea.

V. Nursing care plan/implementation
  A. Goal: *promote adequate ventilation.*
    1. Deep breathe, cough.
    2. Remove respiratory secretions, *suction* prn.
    3. High humidity with or without oxygen therapy.
    4. *Intermittent positive-pressure breathing*
      (IPPB); *incentive spirometry, chest physio-*

therapy, as ordered and needed to loosen se-
cretions.
    5. Use of expectorants, as ordered.
  B. Goal: *control infection.*
    1. Monitor vital signs; use methods to reduce ele-
      vated temperature.
    2. Administer *antibiotics,* as ordered to control
      infection—cephalexin (Keflex), cephalothin
      (Keflin), erythromycin, gentamicin sulfate
      (Garamycin), penicillin G. *Note:* need culture
      before starting on antibiotics.
  C. Goal: *provide rest and comfort.*
    1. Planned rest periods.
    2. Adequate hydration by mouth, intake and out-
      put (I&O).
    3. *Diet:* high carbohydrate, high protein to meet
      energy demands and promote healing.
  D. Goal: *prevent potential complications.*
    1. Cross-infection: use good handwashing tech-
      nique.
    2. Hyperthermia: tepid baths, hypothermia
      blanket.
    3. Respiratory insufficiency and acidosis: clear
      airway, promote expectoration of secretions.
    4. Assess cardiac and respiratory function.
  E. Goal: **health teaching.**
    1. Proper disposal of tissues, cover mouth when
      coughing.
    2. Expected side effects of prescribed medica-
      tions.
    3. Need for rest, limited interactions, increased
      caloric intake.
    4. Need to *avoid* future respiratory tract infec-
      tions.
    5. Correct dosage of antibiotics and the impor-
      tance of taking entire prescription at pre-
      scribed times (times evenly distributed
      throughout the 24-h period to maintain blood
      level of antibiotic) for increased effectiveness.

VI. Evaluation/outcome criteria
  A. Adheres to medication regimen.
  B. Has improved gas exchange, as shown by improved
    pulmonary function test results.
  C. No acid-base or fluid imbalance: normal pH.
  D. Energy level increased.
  E. Sputum production decreased, normal color.
  F. Vital signs stable.
  G. Breath sounds clear.
  H. Culture results negative.
  I. Reports comfort level increased.

Atelectasis

Collapsed alveoli in part or all of the lung.

  I. **Pathophysiology:** due to compression (tumor), airway
    obstruction, decreased surfactant production, or pro-
    gressive regional hypoventilation.
  II. **Risk factors**
    A. Shallow breathing due to pain, abdominal disten-
      tion, narcotics, or sedatives.

B. Decreased ciliary action due to anesthesia, smoking.

C. Thickened secretions due to immobility, dehydration.

D. Aspiration of foreign substances.

E. Bronchospasms.

III. Assessment

A. *Subjective data:* restlessness.

B. *Objective data:*

1. Tachypnea.
2. Tachycardia.
3. Dullness on percussion.
4. Absent bronchial breathing.
5. Tactile fremitus in affected area.
6. X-ray:
   a. Patches of consolidation.
   b. Elevated diaphragm.
   c. Mediastinal shift.

IV. Analysis/nursing diagnosis

A. *Impaired gas exchange* related to shallow breathing.

B. *Pain* related to collapse of lung.

C. *Fear* related to altered respiratory status.

V. Nursing care plan/implementation

A. Goal: *relieve hypoxia.*

1. Frequent respiratory assessment.
2. Respiratory hygiene measures, cough, deep breathe.
3. Oxygen as ordered.
4. Monitor effects of respiratory therapy, ventilators, breathing assistance measures to ensure proper gas exchange.
5. *Position* on unaffected side to allow for lung expansion.

B. Goal: *prevent complications.*

1. Antibiotics as ordered.
2. Sterile technique when tracheal bronchial suctioning to reduce risk of possible infection.
3. Turn, cough, and deep breathe.
4. *Increase fluid* intake to liquefy secretions.

C. Goal: **health teaching.**

1. Need to report signs and symptoms listed in assessment data for early recognition of problem.
2. Importance of coughing and deep breathing to improve present condition and prevent further problems.

VI. Evaluation/outcome criteria

A. Lung expanded on x-ray.

B. Acid-base balance obtained and maintained.

C. No pain on respiration.

D. Activity level increased.

Pulmonary Embolism

Undissolved mass that travels in bloodstream and occludes a blood vessel; can be thromboemboli, fat, air, or catheter. Constitutes a **critical medical emergency.**

I. Pathophysiology: obstructs blood flow to lung → increased pressure on pulmonary artery and reflex con-

striction of pulmonary blood vessels → poor pulmonary circulation → pulmonary infarction.

II. Risk factors

A. Thrombophlebitis.

B. Recent surgery.

C. Invasive procedures.

D. Immobility.

E. Obesity.

F. Myocardial infarction, heart failure.

III. Assessment

A. *Subjective data:*

1. Chest pain: substernal, localized; type—crushing, sharp, stabbing with respirations.
2. Dyspnea.
3. Restless, irritable, anxious.
4. Sense of impending doom.

B. *Objective data:*

1. Respirations: either rapid, shallow or deep, gasping.
2. Elevated temperature.
3. Auscultation: friction rub, crackles, diminished breath sounds.
4. Shock:
   a. Tachycardia.
   b. Hypotension.
   c. Skin: cold, clammy.
5. Cough: hemoptysis.
6. X-ray: area of density.
7. Lab data:
   a. *Decreased* PCO_2.
   b. *Elevated* WBC.

IV. Analysis/nursing diagnosis:

A. *Ineffective breathing pattern* related to shallow respirations.

B. *Impaired gas exchange* related to dyspnea.

C. *Pain* related to decreased tissue perfusion.

D. *Altered peripheral tissue perfusion* related to occlusion of blood vessel.

E. *Fear* related to emergency condition.

F. *Anxiety* related to sense of impending doom.

V. Nursing care plan/implementation

A. Goal: *prevent or minimize respiratory distress.*

1. Monitor blood coagulation studies, e.g., partial thromboplastin time (PTT).
2. Ambulate as tolerated and indicated.
3. Administer IVs, transfusions, and vasopressor medications.
4. Fluids, by mouth, when able.
5. Monitor signs: Homans', acidosis.
6. Prepare for surgery if peripheral embolectomy indicated.

B. Goal: **health teaching.**

1. Prevent recurrence.
2. Decrease stasis.
3. If history of thrombophlebitis, *avoid* birth control pills.
4. Need to continue medication.
5. Follow-up care.

VI. Evaluation/outcome criteria

A. No complications; no further incidence of emboli.

B. Respiratory rate returns to normal.

C. Coagulation studies within normal limits (aPTT 25–38 sec).

D. Reports comfort achieved.

Histoplasmosis

Infection found mostly in central United States. *Not transmitted from human to human but from dust and contaminated soil.* Progressive histoplasmosis, seen most frequently in middle-aged white men who have COPD, is characterized by cavity formation, fibrosis, and emphysema.

I. **Pathophysiology:** spores of *Histoplasma capsulatum* (from droppings of infected birds and bats) are inhaled, multiply, and cause fungal infections of respiratory tract. Leads to necrosis and healing by encapsulation.

II. **Assessment**
  A. *Subjective data:*
  1. Malaise.
  2. Chest pain, dyspnea.
  B. *Objective data:*
  1. Weight loss.
  2. Nonproductive cough.
  3. Fever.
  4. Positive skin test for histoplasmosis.
  5. Benign acute pneumonitis.
  6. Chest x-ray: nodular infiltrate.
  7. Sputum culture shows *H. capsulatum*.
  8. Hepatomegaly, splenomegaly.

III. **Analysis/nursing diagnosis**
  A. *Ineffective airway clearance* related to pneumonitis.
  B. *Ineffective breathing pattern* related to dyspnea.
  C. *Pain* related to infectious process.
  D. *Risk for infection* related to repeated exposure to fungal spores.
  E. *Impaired gas exchange* related to chronic pulmonary disease.
  F. *Knowledge deficit* related to prevention of disease.

IV. **Nursing care plan/implementation**
  A. Goal: *relieve symptoms of the disease:*
  1. Administer medications as ordered.
    a. Amphotericin B (IV) and ketoconazole.
    (1) Monitor for drug side effects: local phlebitis, renal toxicity, hypokalemia, anemia, anaphylaxis, bone marrow depression.
    (2) *Azotemia* (presence of nitrogen-containing compounds in blood) is monitored by biweekly with blood urea nitrogen (BUN) or creatinine levels. BUN >40 mg/dL or creatinine of 3.0 mg/dL necessitate stopping amphotericin B until values return to within normal limits.
    b. Aspirin, diphenhydramine HCl [Benadryl], promethazine HCl [Phenergan], prochlorperazine [Compazine]: used to decrease systemic toxicity of chills, fever, aching, nausea, and vomiting.
  B. Goal: **health teaching:**
  1. Desired effects and side effects of prescribed

medications; importance of taking medications for entire course of therapy (usually from 2 wk to 3 mo).

  2. Importance of follow-up laboratory tests to monitor toxic effects of drug.
  3. Identify source of contamination if possible and avoid future contact if possible.
  4. Importance of deep breathing, pursed-lip breathing, coughing (see Emphysema, p. 62, for specific care).
  5. Signs and symptoms of chronic histoplasmosis, COPD, drug toxicity, and drug side effects, as in IV.A.1 above.

V. **Evaluation/outcome criteria**
  A. Complies with treatment plan.
  B. Respiratory complications avoided.
  C. Symptoms of illness decreased.
  D. No further spread of disease.
  E. Source of contamination identified and eliminated.

Tuberculosis

Inflammatory, communicable disease that commonly attacks the lungs, although may occur in other parts of body.

I. **Pathophysiology:** exposure to causative organism (*Mycobacterium tuberculosis*) in the alveoli in susceptible person leads to inflammation. Infection spreads by lymphatics to hilus; antibodies are released, leading to fibrosis, calcification, or inflammation. Exudate formation leads to caseous necrosis, then liquefication of caseous material leads to cavitation.

II. **Risk factors**
  A. Persons who have been exposed to tubercle bacillus.
  B. Persons who have diseases or are undergoing therapies known to suppress the immune system.
  C. Immigrants from Latin America, Africa, Asia, and Oceania living in the United States for less than a year.
  D. Americans living in those regions for a prolonged time.
  E. Residents of overcrowded metropolitan cities.
  F. Men >65 yr.
  G. Women between 25–44 yr and >65 yr.
  H. Children <5 yr.

III. **Assessment**
  A. *Subjective data:*
  1. Loss of appetite, weight loss.
  2. Weakness, loss of energy.
  3. Pain: knifelike, chest.
  4. Though patient may be symptom free, the disease is found on screening.
  B. *Objective data:*
  1. Night sweats.
  2. Fever: low grade, late afternoon.
  3. Pulse: increased.
  4. *Respiratory* assessment:
    a. Productive cough, hemoptysis.
    b. Respirations: normal, increased depth.
    c. Asymmetric lung expansion.
    d. Increased tactile fremitus.

e. Dullness to percussion.

f. Crackles following short cough.

5. Diagnostic tests:

   a. *Positive tuberculin test* (*Mantoux*—reaction to test begins approximately 12 h after administration with area of redness and a central area of induration. The peak time is 48 h. Determination of positive or negative is made. A reaction is positive when it measures 10 mm. Contacts reacting from 5–10 mm may need to be treated prophylactically.)

   b. *Sputum*: positive for acid-fast bacilli (smear and culture).

   c. X-ray: infiltration, cavitation.

6. Lab data: blood: *decreased* RBCs, *increased* sedimentation rate.

---

7. **Classification of tuberculosis:**
   Class Description
   0 No TB exposure, not infected.
   1 TB exposure, no evidence of infection.
   2 TB infection, no disease.
   3 TB: current disease (persons with completed diagnostic evidence of TB—both a significant reaction to tuberculin skin test and clinical and/or x-ray evidence of disease).
   4 TB: no current disease (persons with previous history of TB or with abnormal x-ray films but no significant tuberculin skin test reaction or clinical evidence).
   5 TB: suspect (diagnosis pending) (used during diagnostic testing period of suspected persons, for no longer than a 3-mo period).

IV. Analysis/nursing diagnosis

A. *Ineffective airway clearance* related to productive cough.

B. *Impaired gas exchange* related to asymmetric lung expansion.

C. *Pain* related to unresolved disease process.

D. *Body image disturbance* related to feelings about tuberculosis.

E. *Social isolation* related to fear of spreading infection.

F. *Knowledge deficit* related to medication regimen.

V. Nursing care plan/implementation

A. Goal: *reduce spread of disease.*

1. Administer medications: isoniazid (INH), rifampin—most commonly used.

2. The following may need to take 300 mg of INH daily for 1 yr as prophylactic measure: positive skin test reactors, including contacts; persons who have diseases or are receiving therapies that affect the immune system; persons who have leukemia, lymphoma, or uncontrolled diabetes or who have had a gastrectomy.

3. *Avoid direct contact with sputum.*

   a. Use good handwashing technique after contact with patient, personal articles.

b. Have patient cover mouth and nose when coughing and sneezing, and use disposable tissues to collect sputum.

4. *Provide good circulation of fresh air* (Changes of air dilute the number of organisms. This plus chemotherapy provide protection needed to prevent spread of disease).

5. Implement respiratory isolation procedure (Table 6.1).

B. Goal: *promote nutrition.*

1. *Increase protein, calories* to aid in tissue repair and healing.

2. Small, frequent feedings.

3. *Increase* fluids, to liquefy secretions so they can be expectorated.

C. Goal: *promote increased self-esteem.*

1. Encourage patient and family to express concerns regarding long-term illness and treatment.

2. Encourage patient to maintain role in family while home treatment is ongoing and to return to work and social contacts as soon as it is determined safe for progress of treatment.

D. Goal: **health teaching.**

1. Desired effects and side effects of medications:

   a. *INH* may affect memory and ability to concentrate. May result in peripheral neuritis, hepatitis, rash, or fever.

   b. *Streptomycin* may cause eighth cranial nerve damage and vestibular ototoxicity, causing hearing loss; may cause labyrinth damage, manifested by vertigo and staggering; also may cause skin rashes, itching, and fever.

   c. Important for patient to know that medication regimen must be adhered to for entire course of treatment.

TABLE 6.1   RESPIRATORY ISOLATION

When used:
For infectious diseases that are contracted through droplet transmission (e.g., tuberculosis).
Precautions:
Isolate in private room (patients infected with same disease can be placed in same room).
Patient should wear mask if out of room for testing, etc.
Masks to be worn by personnel when working within 3 ft of patient.
Gowns *not* necessary.
Contaminated articles need to be labeled before being sent for decontamination.
Provide adequate ventilation in the patient's room.
Careful handwashing.

d. Discontinuation of therapy may allow organism to flourish and make the disease more difficult to treat.

2. Explain methods of disease prevention, encourage contacts to be tested and treated if necessary.

3. Need for follow-up, long-term care, and contact identification.

4. Importance of nutritious diet, rest, avoidance of respiratory infections.

5. Identify community agencies for support and follow-up.

6. Inform that this communicable disease must be reported.

⋈ VI. Evaluation/outcome criteria

A. Complies with medication regimen.

B. Lists desired effects and side effects of medications prescribed.

C. Gains weight, eats food high in protein and carbohydrates.

D. Sputum culture result becomes negative.

E. Retains role in family.

F. No complications (i.e., no hemorrhage, bacillus not spread to others).

Emphysema

Chronic disease with excessive inflation of the air spaces distal to the terminal bronchioles, alveolar ducts, and alveoli; characterized by increased airway resistance and decreased diffusing capacity. Emphysema, asthma, and chronic bronchitis are all examples of chronic obstructive pulmonary disease (COPD).

I. Pathophysiology: increased airway resistance during expiration results in air trapping and hyperinflation → increased residual volumes. Increased dead space → unequal ventilation → perfusion of poorly ventilated alveoli → hypoxia and carbon dioxide retention (hypercapnia). Chronic hypercapnia reduces sensitivity of respiratory center; chemoreceptors in aortic arch and carotid sinus become principal regulators of respiratory drive (respond to hypoxia).

II. Risk factors

A. Smoking.

B. Air pollution: fumes, dust.

C. Antienzymes and alpha-1/antitrypsin deficiencies.

D. Destruction of lung parenchyma.

F. Family history and increased age.

⋈ III. Assessment

A. *Subjective data:*

1. Weakness, lethargy.

2. History of repeated respiratory infections.

3. Long-term smoking.

4. Irritability.

5. Inability to accept medical diagnosis and treatment plan.

6. Refusal to stop smoking.

7. Dyspnea on exertion and at rest.

B. *Objective data:*

1. Increased blood pressure (BP).

2. Increased pulse.

3. Nostrils: flaring.

4. Cough: chronic, productive.

5. Episodes of wheezing, crackles.

6. Increased anteroposterior diameter of chest (barrel chest).

7. Use of accessory respiratory muscles, abdominal and neck.

8. Asymmetric thoracic movements, decreased diaphragmatic excursion.

9. *Position:* sits up, leans forward to compress abdomen and push up diaphragm, increasing intrathoracic pressure, producing more efficient expiration

10. Pursed lips for greater expiratory breathing phase (*"pink puffer"*).

11. Weight loss due to hypoxia.

12. Skin: ruddy color, nail clubbing; when combined with bronchitis: cyanosis (*blue bloater*).

13. Respiratory: early disease—alkalosis; late disease—acidosis, respiratory failure.

14. Spontaneous pneumothorax.

15. Cor pulmonale (emergency cardiac condition involving right ventricular failure due to increased pressure within pulmonary artery).

16. X-ray: hyperinflation of lung, flattened diaphragm.

17. *Pulmonary function tests:*

a. Prolonged, rapid, forced exhalation.

b. *Decreased:* vital capacity (<4000 mL); forced expiratory volume.

c. *Increased:* residual volume (may be 200%); total lung capacity.

18. Lab data:
(a) Po_2 <80 mm Hg; pH <7.35;
(b) Pco_2 >45 mm Hg.

Note: In patients whose compensatory mechanisms are functioning, lab values may be out of the normal range, but if a 20:1 ratio of bicarbonate to carbonic acid is maintained, then appropriate acid-base balance also will be maintained. (Carbonic acid value can be obtained by multiplying the Pco_2 value by 0.003.)

⋈ IV. Analysis/nursing diagnosis

A. *Impaired gas exchange* related to thick pulmonary secretions.

B. *Ineffective breathing pattern* related to hyperinflated alveoli.

C. *Altered nutrition, less than body requirements,* related to weight loss due to hypoxia.

D. *Activity intolerance* related to increased energy demands used for breathing.

E. *Sleep pattern disturbance* related to changes in body positions necessary for breathing.

F. *Anxiety* related to disease progression.

⋈ V. Nursing care plan/implementation

A. Goal: *promote optimal ventilation.*

1. Institute measures designed to decrease airway resistance and enhance gas exchange.

2. *Position:* Fowler's or leaning forward to encourage expiratory phase.

☞ 3. *Oxygen* with humidification, as ordered—no more than 2 L/min to prevent depression of hypoxic respiratory drive (see Oxygen Therapy, p. 71).

☞ 4. *Intermittent positive-pressure breathing* IPPB with nebulization as ordered.

5. Assisted ventilation.

☞ 6. *Postural drainage, chest physiotherapy.*

💊 7. Medications, as ordered:

    a. *Bronchodilators* to increase air flow through bronchial tree: aminophylline, theophylline, terbutaline, isoproterenol (Isuprel).

    b. *Antimicrobials* to treat infection (determined by sputum cultures and sensitivity): tetracycline and ampicillin most common (Condition deteriorates with respiratory infections).

    c. *Steroids* used when bronchodilators are ineffective or for short-term therapy in acute episodes: prednisone, methylprednisolone sodium succinate (Solu-Medrol), dexamethasone (Decadron).

    d. *Expectorants* (increase water intake to achieve desired effect): glyceryl guaiacolate (Robitussin).

    e. *Bronchial detergents*/liquefying agents (Mucomyst).

B. Goal: *employ comfort measures and support other body systems.*

☞ 1. Oral hygiene prn; frequently; patient is mouth breather.

☞ 2. Skin care: water bed, air mattress, foam pads to prevent skin breakdown.

☞ 3. Active and passive range of motion (ROM) exercises to prevent thrombus formation; antiembolic stocking or woven elastic (Ace) bandages may be applied.

4. Increase activities to tolerance.

5. Adequate rest and sleep periods to prevent mental disturbances due to sleep deprivation and to reduce metabolic rate.

🍎 **C.** Goal: *improve nutritional intake.*

1. *High-protein, high-calorie diet* to prevent negative nitrogen balance.

2. *Small, frequent* meals.

3. Supplement diet with high-calorie drinks.

4. *Push fluids* to 3000 mL/d, unless contraindicated—helps moisten secretions.

D. Goal: *provide emotional support for patient and family.*

1. Identify factors that increase anxiety:

    a. Fears related to mechanical equipment.

    b. Loss of body image.

    c. Fear of dying.

2. Assist family coping:

    a. Do not reinforce denial or encourage over-concern.

    b. Give accurate, up-to-date information on patient's condition.

    c. Be open to questioning.

    d. Encourage patient-family communication.

    e. Provide appropriate diversional activities.

🏠 **E.** Goal: **health teaching.**

☞ 1. Breathing exercises, such as pursed-lip breathing and diaphragmatic breathing.

2. Stress-management techniques.

3. Methods to stop smoking.

4. Importance of preventing respiratory infections.

5. Desired effects and side effects of prescribed medications, possible interactions with over-the-counter drugs.

6. Purposes and techniques for effective bronchial hygiene therapy.

7. Rest/activity schedule that increases activity with ability.

8. Food selection for high-protein, high-calorie diet.

9. Importance of taking 2500–3000 mL fluid per d (unless contraindicated by another medical problem).

10. Importance of medical follow-up.

⋈ VI. Evaluation/outcome criteria

A. Takes prescribed medication.

B. Participates in rest/activity schedule.

C. Improves nutritional intake, gains appropriate weight for body size.

D. No complications of respiratory failure, cor pulmonale.

E. No respiratory tract infections.

Asthma

Increased responsiveness of the trachea and bronchi to various stimuli, with difficulty breathing; caused by narrowing of the airways. *Immunologic* asthma occurs in childhood and follows other allergic disease. *Nonimmunologic* asthma occurs in adulthood and is associated with history of recurrent respiratory tract infections.

I. Pathophysiology: bronchial smooth muscle constricts, bronchial secretions increase, mucosa swells, and there is a significant narrowing of air passages. Histamine is produced by the lung. Bronchospasm, production of large amounts of thick mucus, and inflammatory response all contribute to the respiratory obstruction.

A. *Immunologic,* or allergic, asthma in persons who are atopic (hypersensitivity state that is subject to hereditary influences); immunoglobulin E usually elevated.

B. *Nonimmunologic,* or nonallergic, asthma in persons who have a history of repeated respiratory tract infections; age usually >35 yr.

C. *Mixed,* combined immunologic and nonimmunologic; any age, allergen, or nonspecific stimuli.

II. Risk factors

A. History of allergies to identified or unidentified irritants; seasonal and environmental inhalants.

B. Recurrent respiratory tract infection.

C. Decreased ability to effectively cope with emotional stress.

⋈ III. Assessment

A. *Subjective data:*
1. History: upper respiratory tract infections, rhinitis, allergies, family history of asthma.
2. Increasing tightness of the chest → dyspnea.
3. Anxiety, restlessness.
4. Attack history:
   a. *Immunologic:* contact with allergen to which person is sensitive; seen most often in children and young adults.
   b. *Nonimmunologic:* develops in adults >35 yr; aggravated by infections of the sinuses and respiratory tract.

B. *Objective data:*
1. Tachycardia, tachypnea.
2. Cough: dry, hacking, persistent.
☞ 3. Respiratory assessment: audible expiratory wheeze (also inspiratory) on auscultation; crackles, rib retraction, use of accessory muscles on inspiration.
4. General appearance: pallor, cyanosis, diaphoresis, chronic barrel chest, elevated shoulders, flattened molar bones, narrow nose, prominent upper teeth, dark circles under eyes, distended neck veins, orthopnea.
5. Expectoration of tenacious mucoid sputum.
6. *Pulmonary function* diagnostic tests:
   a. Vital capacity: *reduced.*
   b. Forced expiratory volume: *decreased.*
   c. Residual volume: *increased.*
7. Lab data: Blood gases: *elevated* PCO_2; *decreased* PO_2, pH.
   Emergency Note: Persons severely affected may suffer *status asthmaticus,* a life-threatening asthmatic attack in which symptoms of asthma persist and do not respond to usual treatment. Could lead to respiratory failure and hypoxemia.

IV. Analysis/nursing diagnosis
   A. *Ineffective airway clearance* related to tachypnea.
   B. *Impaired gas exchange* related to constricted bronchioles.
   C. *Anxiety* related to breathlessness.
   D. *Activity intolerance* related to persistent cough.
   E. *Knowledge deficit* related to causal factors.

V. Nursing care plan/implementation
   A. Goal: *promote pulmonary ventilation.*
   1. *Position:* high Fowler's for comfort.
   2. Medications as ordered:
      a. *Bronchodilators* and expectorants to improve ventilation (monitor for alterations in BP and tachycardia).
      b. *Antibiotics* to control infection.
      c. *Steroids* to reduce inflammatory response.
   ☞ 3. Oxygen therapy with increased humidity as ordered.
   4. Frequent monitoring for respiratory distress.
   5. Rest periods and gradual increase in activity.
   B. Goal: *facilitate expectoration.*
   1. High humidity.
   2. *Increase fluid* intake.
   3. Monitor for dehydration.

☞ 4. Respiratory therapy: IPPB.
C. Goal: **health teaching** *to prevent further attack.*
   1. Identify and avoid allergens.
   2. Encourage compliance with medication regimen.
   3. Medication side effects, withdrawals.
   ☞ 4. Show *postural drainage, percussion* techniques to family.
   ☞ 5. Breathing techniques to increase expiratory phase.
   6. Teach effective stress-management techniques.
   7. Recognition of precipitating factors.

VI. Evaluation/outcome criteria
   A. No complications.
   B. Has fewer attacks.
   C. Takes prescribed medications, avoids infections.
   D. Adjusts life-style.

Bronchitis

Acute or chronic inflammation of bronchus resulting as a complication from colds and flu. *Acute bronchitis* is caused by an extension of upper respiratory tract infection, such as a cold, and can be transmitted to others. It can also result from an irritation from physical or chemical agents. *Chronic bronchitis* is characterized by hypersecretion of mucus and chronic cough for 3 mo a year for 2 consecutive years.

I. Pathophysiology: bronchial walls are infiltrated with lymphocytes and macrophages; lumen becomes obstructed due to decreased ciliary action and repeated bronchospasms. Hyperventilation of alveolar sacs occurs. Long-term condition results in respiratory acidosis, recurrent pneumonitis, emphysema, or cor pulmonale.

II. Risk factors
   A. Smoking.
   B. Repeated respiratory tract infections.
   C. History of living in area where there is much air pollution.

III. Assessment:
   A. *Subjective data:*
   1. History: recurrent, chronic cough, especially when arising in the morning.
   2. Anorexia.
   B. *Objective data:*
   1. Respiratory:
      a. Shortness of breath.
      b. Use of accessory muscles.
      c. Cyanosis, dusky complexion ("blue bloater").
      d. Sputum: excessive, nonpurulent.
      e. Vesicular and bronchovesicular breath sounds, wheezing.
   2. Weight loss.
   3. Fever.
   4. *Pulmonary function* tests:
      a. Decreased forced expiratory volume.
      b. Lab data:
         PO_2 <90 mm Hg; PCO_2 >40 mm Hg.
   5. Lab data:

(a) RBC—*elevated* to compensate for hypoxia (polycythemia);

(b) WBC—*elevated* to fight infection.

◄ IV. Analysis/nursing diagnosis

  A. *Ineffective airway clearance* related to excessive sputum.

  B. *Ineffective breathing pattern* related to need to use accessory muscles for breathing.

  C. *Impaired gas exchange* related to shortness of breath.

  D. *Activity intolerance* related to increased energy used for breathing.

◄ V. Nursing care plan/implementation

  A. Goal: *assist in optimal respirations.*

    1. *Increase fluid* intake.

    ☞ 2. IPPB, chest physiotherapy.

    3. Administer medications as ordered:

      a. Bronchodilators.

      b. Antibiotics.

      c. Bronchial detergents, liquefying agents.

  B. Goal: *minimize bronchial irritation.*

    1. *Avoid* respiratory irritants—for example, smoke, dust, cold air, allergens.

    2. Environment: air-conditioned, increased humidity.

    3. Encourage nostril breathing rather than mouth breathing.

  C. Goal: *improve nutritional status.*

    1. *Diet:* soft, high calorie.

    2. *Small, frequent* feedings.

  D. Goal: *prevent secondary infections.*

    1. Administer antibiotics as ordered.

    2. *Avoid* exposure to infections, crowds.

  E. Goal: **health teaching.**

    1. *Avoid* respiratory tract infections.

    2. Medications: desired effects and side effects.

    3. Methods to stop smoking.

    4. Rest and activity balance.

    5. Stress management.

◄ VI. Evaluation/outcome criteria

  A. Stops smoking.

  B. Acid-base balance maintained.

  C. Respiratory tract infections less frequent.

Acute Adult Respiratory Distress Syndrome (ARDS)

(Formerly called by other names, including *shock lung*): noncardiogenic pulmonary infiltrations resulting in stiff, wet lungs and refractory hypoxemia in previously healthy adult. Acute hypoxemic respiratory failure without hypercapnea.

I. Pathophysiology: damage to alveolar capillary membrane, increased vascular permeability to pulmonary edema, and impaired gas exchange; decreased surfactant production and potential atelectasis; severe hypoxia → death.

II. Risk factors

  A. *Primary:*

    1. Shock, multiple trauma.

    2. Infections.

    3. Aspiration, inhalation of chemical toxins.

    4. Drug overdose.

    5. DIC.

    6. Emboli, especially fat emboli.

  B. *Secondary:*

    1. Overaggressive fluid administration.

    2. Oxygen toxicity.

◄ III. Assessment:

  A. *Subjective data:*

    1. Restlessness, anxiety.

    2. History of risk factors.

    3. Severe dyspnea.

  B. *Objective data:*

    1. Cyanosis (Table 6.2).

    2. Tachycardia.

    3. Hypotension.

    4. Hypoxemia, acidosis.

    5. Crackles.

    6. Death if untreated.

◄ IV. Analysis/nursing diagnosis

  A. *Anxiety* related to serious physical condition.

  B. *Ineffective breathing pattern* related to severe dyspnea.

  C. *Impaired gas exchange* related to alveolar damage.

  D. *Altered tissue perfusion* related to hypoxia.

◄ V. Nursing care plan/implementation

  A. Goal: *assist in respirations.*

    ☞ 1. May require mechanical ventilatory support to maintain respirations.

    2. May need to be transferred to ICU.

    ☞ 3. May need *oxygen* to combat hypoxia.

    ☞ 4. *Suction* prn.

    5. Monitor blood gas results to detect early signs of acidosis/alkalosis.

    6. If not on ventilator, assess vital signs and respiratory status every 15 min.

    7. Cough, deep breathe every hour.

    8. May need:

      ☞ a. *Chest percussion, vibration.*

      ☞ b. *Postural drainage,* suction.

      c. Bronchodilator medications.

  B. Goal: *prevent complications.*

    1. Decrease anxiety and provide psychological care:

      a. Maintain a calm atmosphere.

      b. Encourage rest to conserve energy.

      c. Emotional support.

    2. Obtain fluid balance:

      ☞ a. Slow IV flow rate.

      b. Diuretics: rapid acting, low dose.

    3. Monitor:

      a. Pulmonary artery and capillary wedge pressure.

      b. Central venous pressure, cardiac output, peripheral perfusion.

      c. I&O.

      d. Assess for bleeding tendencies, potential for DIC.

    4. Protect from infection:

      ☞ a. Strict aseptic technique.

TABLE 6.2   DIFFERENTIAL DIAGNOSIS OF DYSPNEA

◪ Assessment	Pulmonary Edema	COPD	Spontaneous Pneumothorax	Pulmonary Emboli	Asthma
Possible *history*	Symptoms of acute myocardial infarction "Water pills" *Sudden* weight gain Cough, watery sputum Orthopnea	Emphysema, bronchitis Heavy smoking Recent cold *Chronic* dyspnea "Breathing pills" or inhalers	*Sudden*, sharp chest pain *Sudden* dyspnea, brought on by strenuous exertion, coughing, air travel Patient often young, tall, thin	*Sudden*, sharp chest pain *Sudden* dyspnea Prolonged immobilization, recent surgery or trauma to lower extremities Thrombophlebitis Sickle cell anemia Birth control pills	Acute, episodic dyspnea Often younger patient Allergic history Relieved by shots in the past Cold or flu may have preceded attack
Possible *physical* findings	Distended neck veins Crackles S₃ gallop	↑ Anteroposterior diameter of chest Pursed-lip breathing Wheezing, crackles Prolonged expiratory phase of respiration Use of accessory muscles to breathe	↓ Breath sounds and ↑ resonance on side of collapsed lung Tracheal deviation	Tachypnea Tachycardia Hypotension Pleural rub Phlebitis in legs	Wheezing Hyperresonance If bronchospasm severe, chest may be silent

Source: Caroline NL. *Emergency Care in the Streets* (5th ed). Boston: Little, Brown, 1995.

⬭ **b.** Antibiotic therapy.
   5. Provide physiologic support:
      a. Maintain nutrition.
      b. Skin care.
🏠 **C.** Goal: **health teaching.**
   1. Briefly explain procedures as they are happening (emergency situation can frighten patient).
   2. Give rationale for follow-up care.
   3. Identify risk factors as appropriate for prevention of recurrence.
◪ **VI. Evaluation/outcome criteria**
   A. Patient survives and is alert.
   B. Skin warm to touch.
   C. Respiratory rate within normal limits.
   D. Lab values and pressures within normal limits.
   E. Urinary output >30 mL/h.

Chest Trauma

Flail Chest

Multiple rib fractures resulting in instability of the chest wall, with subsequent paradoxical breathing (portion of lung under injured chest wall moves in on inspiration while remaining lung expands; on expiration the injured portion of the chest wall expands while unaffected lung tissue contracts).

Sucking Chest Wound

Penetrating wound of chest wall with hemothorax and pneumothorax, resulting in lung collapse and mediastinal shift toward unaffected lung.

◪ **I. Assessment**
   A. *Subjective data:*
      1. Severe, sudden, sharp pain.
      2. Dyspnea.
      3. Anxiety, restlessness, fear, weakness.
   B. *Objective data:*
      1. Vital signs:
         a. Pulse: tachycardia, weak.
         b. BP: hypotension.
         c. Respirations: shallow, decreased expiratory force, tachypnea, stridor, accessory muscle breathing.
      2. Skin color: cyanosis, pallor.
      3. Chest:
         a. Asymmetric chest expansion (*paradoxical movement*).

b. Chest wound, rush of air through trauma site.

c. Crepitus over trauma site (from air escaping into surrounding tissues).

d. Lateral deviation of trachea, mediastinal shift.

〰 4. Pneumothorax: documented by absence of breath sounds, x-ray examination.

〰 5. Hemothorax: documented by needle aspiration by physician, x-ray examination.

6. Shock; blood and fluid loss.

7. Hemoptysis.

8. Distended neck veins.

II. Analysis/nursing diagnosis

A. *Ineffective airway clearance* related to shallow respirations.

B. *Impaired gas exchange* related to asymmetric chest expansion.

C. *Pain* related to chest trauma.

D. *Fear* related to emergency situation.

E. *Risk for trauma* related to fractured ribs.

F. *Risk for infection* related to open chest wound.

III. Nursing care plan/implementation

A. Goal: *restore adequate ventilation and prevent further air from entering pleural cavity:* **MEDICAL EMERGENCY.**

☞ 1. In emergency situation: place air-occlusive dressing or hand over open wound as patient exhales forcefully against glottis (*Valsalva maneuver* helps expand collapsed lung by creating positive intrapulmonary pressures); or place patient's weight onto *affected* side. Administer *oxygen*.

☞ 2. Assist with *endotracheal tube* insertion; patient will be placed on volume-controlled *ventilator*. (See discussion of ventilators under Oxygen Therapy, pp. 76–77.)

☞ 3. Assist with *thoracentesis* and insertion of chest tubes with connection to water-seal drainage as ordered. (See Tubes Box, p. 73.)

〰 4. Monitor vital signs to determine early shock.

5. Monitor *blood gases* to determine early acid-base imbalances.

▭ 6. Pain medications given with caution (small, frequent doses), so as not to depress respiratory center.

IV. Evaluation/outcome criteria

A. Respiratory status stabilizes, lung reexpands.

B. Shock and hemorrhage are prevented.

C. No further damage done to surrounding tissues.

D. Pain is controlled.

Pneumothorax

Presence of air within the pleural cavity; occurs spontaneously or as a result of trauma (Table 6.3).

I. Types:

A. *Closed:* rupture of a subpleural bulla, tuberculous focus, carcinoma, lung abscess, pulmonary infarction, severe coughing attack, or blunt trauma.

B. *Open:* communication between atmosphere and pleural space because of opening in chest wall.

C. *Tension:* positive pressure within chest cavity resulting from accumulated air that cannot escape during expiration. Leads to collapse of lung, mediastinal shift, and compression of the heart and great vessels.

II. Pathophysiology: pressure builds up in the pleural space, lung on the affected side collapses, and the heart and mediastinum shift toward the unaffected lung.

III. Assessment

A. *Subjective data:*

1. Pain:

a. Sharp, aggravated by activity.

b. Location—chest; may be referred to shoulder, arm on affected side.

2. Restlessness, anxiety.

3. Dyspnea.

B. *Objective data:*

1. Cough.

2. Cessation of normal movements on affected side.

3. Absence of breath sounds on affected side.

4. Pallor, cyanosis.

5. Shock.

6. Tracheal deviation to unaffected side.

〰 7. X-ray: air in pleural space.

IV. Analysis/nursing diagnosis

A. *Ineffective breathing pattern* related to collapse of lung.

B. *Impaired gas exchange* related to abnormal thoracic movement.

C. *Pain* related to trauma to chest area.

D. *Fear* related to emergency situation.

V. Nursing care plan/implementation

A. Goal: *protect against injury during thoracentesis.*

1. Provide sterile equipment.

2. Explain procedure.

3. Monitor vital signs for shock.

4. Monitor for respiratory distress, mediastinal shift.

B. Goal: *promote respirations.*

1. *Position:* Fowler's.

☞ 2. Oxygen therapy as ordered.

3. Encourage slow breathing to improve gas exchange.

▭ 4. Careful administration of narcotics to prevent respiratory depression (*avoid* morphine).

C. Goal: *prepare patient for closed-chest drainage, physically and psychologically.*

1. Explain purpose of the procedure—to provide means for evacuation of air and fluid from pleural cavity; to reestablish negative pressure in pleural space; to promote lung reexpansion.

2. Explain procedure and apparatus (see chest tubes in box, p. 73 .).

☞ 3. Cleanse skin at tube insertion site, place patient *in sitting* position, ensuring safety by having locked over-bed table for patient to lean on, or have a nurse stay with patient so appro-

TABLE 6.3   DIFFERENTIATING AMONG TENSION PNEUMOTHORAX, HEMOTHORAX, AND CARDIAC TAMPONADE

⋈ Assessment	Tension Pneumothorax	Massive Hemothorax	Cardiac Tamponade
Presenting sign or symptom	Respiratory distress	Shock	Shock
Neck veins	Distended	Flat	Distended
Trachea	Deviated	Midline	Midline
Breath sounds	Decreased or absent on side of injury	Decreased or absent on side of injury	Equal on both sides
Percussion of chest	Hyperresonant on side of injury	Dull on side of injury	Normal
Heart sounds	Normal	Normal	Muffled

Source: Caroline NL. *Emergency Care in the Streets* (5th ed). Boston: Little, Brown, 1995.

priate position is maintained throughout the procedure.

D. Goal: *prevent complications with chest tubes.*
   1. Observe for and immediately report crepitations (air under skin, also called *subcutaneous emphysema*), labored or shallow breathing, tachypnea, cyanosis, tracheal deviation, or signs of hemorrhage.
   2. Monitor for signs of infection.
   3. Ensure that tubing stays intact.
   ☞ 4. Monitor for proper tube function (*fluctuation or oscillation* of water in the tube located in the water bottle will occur with respirations; water level will *rise* in the tube when patient inhales or coughs; water level in tube will *lower* during exhalation). If *no bubbling in water*, check tubing for kinks or lack of patency. Manipulation of chest tube done only according to specific physician order.
   5. Monitor for air leaks (*continuous bubbling* of water in the bottle).
   ☞ 6. Arm and shoulder ROM.
E. Goal: **health teaching.**
   1. How to prevent recurrence by *avoiding* overexertion; *avoid* holding breath.
   2. Signs and symptoms of condition.
   3. Methods to stop smoking.
   4. Encourage follow-up care.
⋈ **VI. Evaluation/outcome criteria**
   A. No complications noted.
   B. Closed system remains intact until chest tubes are removed.
   C. Lung reexpands, breath sounds heard, pain diminished, symmetric thoracic movements.

Hemothorax

Presence of blood in pleural cavity related to trauma or ruptured aortic aneurysm. See Pneumothorax, p. 67–68, for assessment, analysis/nursing diagnosis, nursing care plan/implementation, and evaluation/outcome criteria; see also Table 6.3.

Thoracic Surgery

Performed for bronchogenic and lung carcinomas, lung abscesses, tuberculosis, bronchiectasis, emphysematous blebs, and benign tumors.

I. Types:
   A. *Thoracotomy*—incision in the chest wall, pleura is entered, lung tissue examined, biopsy specimen secured. *Chest tube is needed postoperatively.*
   B. *Lobectomy*—removal of a lobe of the lung. *Chest tube is needed postoperatively.*
   C. *Pneumonectomy*—removal of an entire lung. *No chest tube is needed postoperatively.*
⋈ **II. Analysis/nursing diagnosis**
   A. *Risk for injury* related to chest wound.
   B. *Impaired gas exchange* related to pain from surgical procedure.
   C. *Ineffective airway clearance* related to decreased willingness to cough due to pain.
   D. *Pain* related to surgical incision.
   E. *Impaired physical mobility* related to large surgical incision and chest tube drainage apparatus.
   F. *Knowledge deficit* related to importance of coughing and deep breathing to prevent complications.
⋈ **III. Nursing care plan/implementation**
   A. Preoperative care:
      1. Goal: *minimize pulmonary secretions.*
      ☞ a. *Humidify* air to moisten secretions.
      ☞ b. Use *IPPB*, as ordered, to improve ventilation.
      ⬤ c. Administer *bronchodilators, expectorants,* and *antibiotics,* as ordered.
      ☞ d. Use *postural drainage, cupping,* and *vibration* to mobilize secretions.
      2. Goal: **preoperative teaching.**
      a. Teach patient to cough against a closed glottis to increase intrapulmonary pressure for improved expiratory phase.
      ☞ b. Instruct in diaphragmatic breathing and coughing.
      c. Encourage to stop smoking.

☞ **d.** Instruct and supervise practice of postoperative arm exercises—flexion, abduction, and rotation of shoulder—to prevent ankylosis.

    e. Explain postoperative use of chest tubes, IV, and oxygen therapy.

B. Postoperative care:

  1. Goal: *maintain patent airway.*

☞ **a.** Auscultate chest for breath sounds; report diminished or absent breath sounds on unaffected side (indicates decreased ventilation → respiratory embarrassment).

    b. Turn, cough, and deep breathe, every 15 min to 1 h first 24 h and prn according to pulmonary congestion heard on auscultation.

  2. Goal: *promote gas exchange.*

☞ **a.** Splint chest during coughing—support incision to help *cough up sputum (most important activity postoperatively).*

    b. *Position:* high Fowler's.

      (1) Turn patient who has had a *pneumonectomy* to *operative* side (*avoid* extreme lateral positioning and mediastinal shift) to allow unaffected lung expansion and drainage of secretions; can also be turned onto back.

      (2) Patient who has had a *lobectomy* or *thoracotomy* can be turned on *either* side or back because chest tubes will be in place.

☞ **3.** Goal: *reduce incisional stress and discomfort*—pad area around chest tube when turning on operative side to maintain tube patency and promote comfort.

  4. Goal: *prevent complications related to respiratory function.*

☞ **a.** Maintain chest tubes to water-seal drainage system.

    b. See Chest tubes section in Tubes Box at end of chap.

    c. Observe for *mediastinal shift* (trachea should always be midline; movement toward either side indicates shift).

      (1) Move patient onto back or toward opposite side.

      (2) **MEDICAL EMERGENCY:** Notify physician immediately.

☞ **5.** Goal: *maintain fluid and electrolyte balance*—administer parenteral infusion *slowly* (risk of pulmonary edema due to decrease in pulmonary vasculature with removal of lung lobe or whole lung).

📖 **6.** Goal: **postoperative teaching.**

☞ **a.** Prevent ankylosis of shoulder—teach *passive* and *active ROM* exercises of operative arm.

    b. Importance of early ambulation, as condition permits.

    c. Importance of stopping smoking.

    d. Dietary instructions—nutritious diet to promote healing.

    e. Importance of deep breathing, coughing exercises to prevent stasis of respiratory secretions.

    f. Importance of *increased fluids* in diet to liquefy secretions.

    g. Desired effects and side effects of prescribed medications.

    h. Importance of rest, avoidance of heavy lifting and work during healing.

    i. Importance of follow-up care; give names of referral agencies where patient and family can obtain assistance.

    j. Signs and symptoms of complications.

⋈ **IV. Evaluation/outcome criteria**

  A. Patient and/or significant other will be able to:

    1. Give rationale for activity restriction and demonstrate prescribed exercises.

    2. Identify name, route, frequency, dosage, and side effects of prescribed medications.

    3. State plans for necessary modifications in lifestyle, home.

    4. Identify support systems.

  B. Wound heals without complications.

  C. Obtains ROM in affected shoulder.

  D. No complications of thoracotomy:

    1. *Respiratory*—pulmonary insufficiency, respiratory acidosis, pneumonitis, atelectasis, pulmonary edema.

    2. *Circulatory*—hemorrhage, hypovolemia, shock, myocardial infarction.

    3. *Mediastinal shift.*

    4. *Renal failure.*

    5. *Gastric distention.*

Tracheostomy

Opening into trachea, temporary or permanent. *Rationale:* airway obstruction due to foreign body, edema, tumor, excessive tracheobronchial secretions, respiratory depression, decreased gaseous diffusion at alveolar membrane, or increased dead space (e.g., severe emphysema).

⋈ **I. Analysis/nursing diagnosis**

  A. *Ineffective airway clearance* related to increased secretions and decreased ability to cough effectively.

  B. *Ineffective breathing pattern* related to physical condition that necessitated tracheostomy.

  C. *Impaired verbal communication* related to inability to speak when tracheostomy tube cuff inflated.

  D. *Fear* related to need for specialized equipment to breathe.

⋈ **II. Nursing care plan/implementation**

  A. Preoperative care:

    1. Goal: *relieve anxiety and fear.*

      a. Explain purpose of procedure and equipment.

☞   **b.** Demonstrate suctioning procedure.

      c. Establish means of postoperative communication, e.g., paper and pencil, magic slate, picture cards, and call bell. Specialized tubes such as a fenestrated tracheostomy tube or a tracheostomy button allow the patient to talk when the external opening is plugged.

    d. Remain with patient as much as possible.

B. Postoperative care:

☞ **1.** Goal: *maintain patent airway* (Table 6.4).

    2. Goal: *alleviate apprehension.*

        a. Remain with patient as much as possible.

        b. Encourage patient to communicate feelings using preestablished communication system.

🍎 **3.** Goal: *improve nutritional status.*

        a. Nutritious foods/liquids the patient can swallow.

        b. Supplemental drinks to maintain necessary calories.

TABLE 6.4   **TRACHEOSTOMY SUCTIONING PROCEDURE**

1. Suction as necessary to facilitate respirations.
2. *Position:* semi-Fowler's to prevent forward flexion of neck, facilitate respiration, promote drainage, and minimize edema.
3. Administer *mist* to tracheostomy since natural humidifying of oropharynx pathways has been eliminated.
4. Auscultate for moist, noisy respirations, as nonproductive coughing may indicate need for suctioning.
5. Prevent hypoxia by administering *100% oxygen before suctioning* (unless contraindicated).
6. Use *strict aseptic technique* and sterile suctioning catheters with each aspiration; use sterile saline to clear catheter of secretions. Keep dominant hand gloved with sterile glove, nondominant hand with nonsterile glove to control thumb control of suction. Suction tracheostomy *before* nose or mouth.
7. *Do not apply suction when inserting* suction catheter to prevent injury to respiratory tract and loss of oxygen.
8. If patient coughs during suctioning, gently remove catheter to permit ejection and suction of mucus.
9. Apply suction intermittently for *no longer* than 10 to 15 sec, as prolonged suction decreases arterial oxygen concentrations. Do *not* suction for more than 3–5 min.
10. *Cuff deflation:* if high-volume, low-pressure cuffed tube is used, deflation not necessary. If other tracheostomy cuffed tube is used, deflate for 5 min every hour to prevent damage to trachea.
11. Use caution not to dislodge tube when changing dressing or ties that secure tube.

🏠 **4.** Goal: **health teaching.**

        a. Explain all procedures.

        b. Teach alternative methods of communication (best if done before the tracheostomy if it is not an emergency situation).

☞ **c.** Teach self-care of tracheostomy as soon as possible.

⋈ **III. Evaluation/outcome criteria**

    A. Airway patent.

    B. Acid-base balance maintained.

    C. No respiratory infection/obstruction.

Laryngectomy

Radical Neck Dissection

Removal of entire larynx, lymph nodes, sternomastoid muscle, and jugular vein for cancer of the larynx that extends beyond the vocal cords. Permanent tracheostomy; new methods of speech will have to be learned.

    Partial laryngectomy: removal of lesion on larynx. Patient will be able to speak after operation, but quality of voice may be altered.

⋈ **I. Assessment**

    A. *Subjective data:*

        1. Feeling of lump in throat.

        2. Pain: Adam's apple; may radiate to ear.

        3. Dysphagia.

    B. *Objective data:*

        1. Hoarseness: persistent, progressive.

        2. Lymphadenopathy: cervical.

        3. Breath odor: foul.

⋈ **II. Analysis/nursing diagnosis**

    A. *Impaired verbal communication* related to removal of larynx.

    B. *Body image disturbance* related to radical neck dissection.

    C. *Ineffective airway clearance* related to copious amounts of mucus.

    D. *Fear* related to diagnosis of cancer.

    E. *Impaired swallowing* related to edema.

    F. *Impaired social interaction* related to altered speech.

⋈ **III. Nursing care plan/implementation**

    A. Preoperative care:

        1. Goal: *provide emotional support and optimal physical preparation.*

            a. Encourage verbalization of fears; answer all questions honestly, particularly about having no voice after surgery.

            b. Visit from person with laryngectomy (contact International Association of Laryngectomees).

        2. Goal: **health teaching.**

            a. Prepare for tracheostomy.

☞ **b.** Other means to speak (esophageal "burp" speech).

    B. Postoperative care:

        1. Goal: *maintain patent airway and prevent aspiration.*

a. *Position:* semi-Fowler's, preventing forward flexion of neck to reduce edema and keep airway open.

b. Observe for hypoxia:

(1) *Early signs:* increased respiratory and pulse rates, apprehension, restlessness.

(2) *Late signs:* dyspnea, cyanosis, swallowing difficulties—patient should chew food well and swallow with water.

c. *Laryngectomy* tube care:

(1) Observe for stridor (coarse, high-pitched inspiratory sound)—**report immediately.**

(2) Have extra laryngectomy tube at bedside.

☞ (3) Suction with sterile equipment; instill 2–3 mL of sterile saline into stoma to loosen secretions.

2. Goal: *promote optimal physical and psychological function.*

☞ **a.** Frequent mouth care.

☞ **b.** Dressings: may be pressure type; note color and amount of drainage; reinforce as ordered.

☞ **c.** *Tubes:* Hemovac (Figure 6.1); expect 80–120 mL of serosanguineous drainage first postoperative day; drainage should decrease daily; observe patency.

☞ **d.** *Post-Hemovac removal*—observe: skin flaps down, adherent to underlying tissue; may have to "roll" flaps to prevent drainage buildup.

☞ **e.** Use surgical asepsis.

f. Answer call bell *immediately;* use preestablished means of communication.

g. Reexplain all procedures while giving care.

h. Support head when lifting.

3. Goal: **health teaching.**

a. Speech rehabilitation as soon as esophageal suture is healed.

(1) Information on laryngeal speech (International Association of Laryngectomees, American Cancer Society, American Speech and Hearing Association).

(2) *Esophageal speech* best learned in speech clinic—learn to burp column of air needed for speech; new voice sounds are natural but hoarse.

☞ **b.** *Stoma* care:

(1) Cover with scarf or shirt made of a porous material (material substitutes for nasal passage—warms and filters out particles).

(2) Use source of humidification ("mister" or commercial humidifier).

(3) Caution while bathing or showering, to decrease likelihood of aspiration.

(4) Swimming and boating permitted only with snorkel device.

(5) Procedure for suctioning if cough ineffective.

☞ **c.** Simple ROM of neck; how to support head.

d. Possible *contraindications:* use of talcum powder, tissues.

IV. Evaluation/outcome criteria

A. No surgical complications (e.g., airway obstruction, infection, hemorrhage).

B. Learns alternative speech 60–90 d after surgery.

C. Demonstrates proper stoma care.

D. Resumes productive life-style (work, family).

E. Normal response to change in body image (e.g., anger, grief, denial).

Oxygen Therapy

I. Purpose—to relieve hypoxia and provide adequate tissue oxygenation.

II. Clinical indications:

A. Any patient likely to have significant *shunt* from:

1. Fluid in the alveoli:
   a. Pulmonary edema.
   b. Pneumonia.
   c. Near drowning.
   d. Chest trauma.

2. Collapsed alveoli (atelectasis).
   a. Airway obstruction:
      (1) Any unconscious patient.
      (2) Choking.
   b. Failure to take deep breaths:
      (1) Pain (rib fracture).
      (2) Paralysis of the respiratory muscles (spine injury).
      (3) Depression of the respiratory center (head injury, drug overdose).
   c. Collapse of an entire lung (pneumothorax).

3. Other gases in the alveoli:
   a. Smoke inhalation.
   b. Toxic inhalations.
   c. Carbon monoxide poisoning.

4. Respiratory arrest.

B. Cardiac arrest.

C. Shock.

D. Shortness of breath.

E. Signs of respiratory insufficiency.

F. Breathing fewer than 10 breaths/min.

G. Chest pain.

H. Stroke.

I. Anemia.

J. Fetal decelerations during labor.

III. Precautions:

A. Patients with COPD should receive oxygen at *low* flow rates, to prevent inhibition of hypoxic respiratory drive.

B. *Excessive* amounts of oxygen for prolonged periods will cause retrolental fibroplasia and blindness in premature infants.

C. Oxygen delivered *without* humidification will result in drying and irritation of respiratory mucosa, decreased ciliary action, and thickening of respiratory secretions.

FIGURE 6.1 **HEMOVAC APPARATUS FOR CONSTANT CLOSED SUCTION. IN THIS SYSTEM OF WOUND DRAINAGE, SUCTION IS MAINTAINED BY A PLASTIC CONTAINER WITH A SPRING INSIDE THAT TRIES TO FORCE APART THE LIDS AND THEREBY PRODUCES SUCTION THAT IS TRANSMITTED THROUGH THE PLASTIC TUBING. THE NECK SKIN IS PULLED DOWN TIGHT, AND NO EXTERNAL DRESSING IS REQUIRED. THE CONTAINER SERVES AS BOTH SUCTION SOURCE AND RECEPTABLE FOR BLOOD. IT IS EMPTIED AS REQUIRED, AND DRAINAGE TUBES ARE LEFT IN THE NECK FOR 3 DAYS.** (From DeWeese DD, Saunders WH. *Textbook of Otolaryngoloty* [6th ed]. St. Louis: Mosby, 1987.)

FIGURE 6.2 **CHEST DRAINAGE SYSTEM.**

REVIEW OF THE USE OF COMMON TUBES

Tube or Apparatus	Purpose	Examples of Use	▶ Key Points for Nursing Implementation
Chest tubes	1. *Anterior tube* drains mostly air from pleural space 2. *Posterior tube* drains mostly fluid from pleural space 3. Removal of fluid and air from pleural space is necessary to reestablish negative intrapleural pressure	1. *Thoracotomy* 2. *Open-heart surgery* 3. *Spontaneous pneumothorax* 4. *Traumatic pneumothorax*	1. See Key Points for each of the three entries under Drainage System, below 2. Sterile technique is used when changing dressings around the tube insertions 3. Fowler's *position* to facilitate air and fluid removal 4. Cough, deep breathe q1h; splint chest; medicate for pain 5. Manage pain carefully in order *not* to depress respirations 6. Prepare for removal when there is little or no drainage, air leak disappears, or fluctuations stop in water seal; have suture set, petrolatum gauze (or other ointment), 4 × 4s, and sturdy elastic tape ready; medicate for pain before removal; monitor breathing after removal (breath sounds, rate, chest pain)
Drainage System (see Figure 6.2, p. 72)			
#1: **drainage compartment**	Collects drainage		1. Mark level in bottle each shift to keep accurate record—*not* routinely emptied; replaced when full 2. *Never* raise container above the level of the chest; otherwise back flow will occur

(continued)

D. Oxygen supports combustion, and *fire* is a potential hazard during its administration.
  1. Ground electrical equipment.
  2. Prohibit smoking.
  3. Institute measures to decrease static electricity.
E. *High* flow rates of oxygen delivered by ventilator or cuffed tracheostomy and endotracheal tubes can produce signs of oxygen toxicity in 24–48 h.
  1. Signs and symptoms: cough, sore throat, decreased vital capacity, and substernal discomfort.
  2. Pulmonary manifestations due to:
    a. Atelectasis.
    b. Exudation of protein fluids into alveoli.
    c. Damage to pulmonary capillaries.
    d. Interstitial hemorrhage.
IV. Oxygen administration
  A. Oxygen is dispensed from cylinder or piped-in system.

B. Methods of delivering oxygen:
  1. Nasal catheter:
    a. Effective and comfortable.
    b. Delivers 30%–50% oxygen at flow rates of 6–8 L/min.
    c. Can produce excoriation of nares.
    d. Do *not* use in comatose patient.
  2. Nasal prongs/cannula:
    a. Comfortable and simple, and allows patient to move about in bed.
    b. Delivers 25%–40% oxygen at flow rates of 4–6 L/min.
    c. Difficult to keep in position unless patient is alert and cooperative.
  3. Venturi mask:
    a. Allows for accurate delivery of prescribed concentration of oxygen.
    b. Delivers 24%–40% oxygen at flow rates of 4–8 L/min.

REVIEW OF THE USE OF COMMON TUBES *(Continued)*

Tube or Apparatus	Purpose	Examples of Use	▷ Key Points for Nursing Implementation
#2: **water-seal chamber**	Water seal prevents flow of atmospheric air into pleural space; essential to prevent recollapse of the lung		1. Air bubbles from postoperative residual air *will* continue for 24–48 h 2. *Persistent* large amounts of air bubbles in this compartment indicate an *air leak* between the alveoli and the pleural space 3. Clamp tube(s) only to verify a leak; replace a broken, cracked, or full drainage unit, or verify readiness of patient for tube removal; *not* necessary to clamp when ambulating if water seal intact 4. If tube becomes disconnected, clean off tubing ends and reconnect; if dislodged from chest, seal insertion site *immediately* on expiration if possible; use sterile petrolatum gauze and adhesivetape to form *air-occlusive* dressing 5. If air leak is present, clamping the tube for very long may cause a tension pneumothorax 6. Fluctuation of the fluid level in this bottle is *expected* (when the suction is turned off) because respiration changes the pleural pressure; if there is *no fluctuation* of the fluid in the tube of this bottle (when the suction is turned off), then either the lung is fully expanded or the tube is blocked by kinking or by a clot 7. Although not routinely used, milking (gently squeezing) the tubes, if ordered, will prevent blockage from clots or debris; otherwise gravity drainage is sufficient to maintain patency 8. Drainage of >100 mL in 1 h should be *reported* to physician

(continued)

c. Useful in long-term treatment of COPD.
4. **Face mask:**
   a. Poorly tolerated—utilized for short periods; feeling of "suffocation."
   b. Delivers 50%–60% oxygen at flow rates of 8–12 L/min.

c. Significant rebreathing of carbon dioxide at low oxygen flow rates.
d. Hot—may produce pressure sores around nose and mouth.
5. **Partial rebreathing mask:**
   a. About one-third of exhaled air is rebreathed.

REVIEW OF THE USE OF COMMON TUBES (*Continued*)

Tube or Apparatus	Purpose	Examples of Use	◄ Key Points for Nursing Implementation
#3: **suction control**— connected to wall suction	Level of the column of water (i.e., 15–20 cm) is used to control the amount of suction applied to the chest tube—if the water evaporates to only *10-cm* depth, then this will be the *maximum* suction generated by the wall suction		1. Air *should continuously bubble* through this compartment when the suction is on; the bubbles are from the atmosphere—*not* the patient; when the wall suction is turned higher, the bubbling will increase, but the increased pulling of air is from the atmosphere and *not* from the pleural space 2. Since the level of H_2O determines the maximum negative pressure that can be obtained, make sure the water does *not* evaporate—keep filling the bottle to keep the ordered level; if there is *no* bubbling of air through this container, the wall suction is *too low*
Heimlich flutter valve	1. Has a one-way valve so fluids and air can drain out of the pleural space but cannot flow back 2. Eliminates the need for a water seal—no danger when tube is unclamped below the valve	Same as for other chest tubes	1. Can be connected to suction if ordered 2. Sometimes can just drain into portable bag, so patient is more mobile
Tracheostomy tube	1. Maintains patent airway and promotes better O_2-CO_2 exchange 2. Makes removal of secretions by suctioning easier 3. Cuff on tracheostomy tube is necessary if need airtight fit for an assisted ventilation	1. *Acute respiratory distress* due to poor ventilation 2. *Severe burns of head and neck* 3. *Laryngectomy* (tracheostomy is permanent)	1. Use oxygen *before* and *after* each suctioning 2. Humidify oxygen 3. Sterile technique in suctioning 4. Cleanse inner cannula as needed—only leave out *5–10 min* 5. Hemostat handy if outer cannula is expelled—have obturator taped to bed and another tracheostomy set handy 6. Cuff *must be* deflated periodically to prevent necrosis of mucosa, unless low-pressure cuff used

Note: This review focuses on care of the tubes, not on total patient care.

Source: Jane Vincent Corbett, RN, MS, EdD, Professor, School of Nursing, University of San Francisco. Used with permission.

  b. Reservoir contains mostly oxygen inspired during previous inhalation.
  c. Delivers 35%–60% oxygen at flow rates of 6–10 L/min.

6. **Nonrebreathing mask:**
  a. Reservoir bag has one-way valve preventing the patient from exhaling back into the bag.
  b. Oxygen flow rate prevents collapse of bag during inhalation.

☞ Summary of Key Points

1. Normal breath sounds over the peripheral lung fields are called *vesicular breath sounds*.
2. *Dyspnea*, difficulty breathing, is a subjective symptom and one of the most common complaints with any respiratory disorder.
3. Airways are narrowest on expiration, thus *expiratory wheezing* is heard most often.
4. *Chest pain* resulting from a respiratory disorder is frequently related to breathing and may be more localized then cardiac pain. The patient may be able to point to a specific location.
5. *Crackles*, formerly called *rales*, are usually heard on inspiration and do not clear with coughing. *Wheezing* and *rhonchi* are used interchangeably; both result from narrowing of airways. If the term *rhonchi* is used, it means fluid is the cause of the narrowing, and the sound often clears with coughing.
6. A patient who is experiencing *difficulty breathing:* will not tolerate activity, has a poor appetite, fatigues easily, speaks in broken phrases ("staccato" speech), may breathe through pursed lips (obstructive disorder), and will not be receptive to patient teaching.
7. Giving *high levels of oxygen* to a patient with *emphysema* (carbon dioxide retainer) will *interfere* with the *hypoxic drive* to breathe.
8. *Obstructive* respiratory disorders trap air, and total lung capacity is *increased;* while patients with *restrictive* disorders have a *decreased* total lung capacity and have difficulty taking in a breath.

  c. Delivers 100% oxygen at flow rates of 10–12 L/min.
  d. Ideal for severe hypoxia, but patient may complain of feelings of suffocation.
7. **T** tube:
  a. Provides humidification and enriched oxygen mixtures to tracheostomy or endotracheal tube.
  b. Delivers 40%–60% oxygen at flow rates of 4–12 L/min.

V. Ventilators
  A. *Indications:*
  1. Hypoventilation.
  2. Hypoxia.
  3. Counteract pulmonary edema by changing pressure gradient.
  4. Decrease work of breathing.
  B. *Contraindications:*
  1. Tuberculosis—may rupture tubercular bleb.
  2. Hypovolemia—increased intrathoracic pressures decrease venous return.
  3. Air trapping—increased because adequate exhalation is not allowed.
  C. *Complications:*
  1. Decreased BP; impaired venous return.
  2. Atelectasis.
  3. Infection.
  4. Oxygen toxicity.
  5. Difficulties weaning.
  6. Gastric dilatation.
  7. Pneumothorax.
  8. Hyperventilation or hypoventilation.
  9. Tracheal injury.
  D. *Types of ventilators:*
  1. **Oscillating** or **rocking bed:**
  a. Indirectly aids respirations by using weight and gravity of abdominal contents to change position of diaphragm.
  b. *Used with* paralytic disease, as an aid in weaning.
  2. **Iron lung** and **chest respirators:**
  a. Driven by motors that create negative pressure within tank or shell and thus allow air to enter patient's lungs.
  b. *Used for* neuromuscular disease.
  3. **Intermittent positive-pressure breathing** (*IPPB*):
  a. Produces greater-than-atmospheric pressures, intermittently.
  b. Improves tidal volume and minute volume and aids in overcoming respiratory insufficiency.
  c. Produces more uniform distribution of alveolar aeration and reduces work of breathing.
  d. *Used to* deliver both oxygen and medications during treatment and rehabilitative pulmonary therapy, particularly if patient has decreased tidal volume.
  e. *Contraindicated in* pneumothorax, active tuberculosis, and history of recent hemoptysis.
  4. **Pressure-constant ventilators:**
  a. *Bird*—Mark VII:
  (1) Pressure cycled, pneumatic powered.
  (2) When preset pressure is reached, valve closes, terminating inspiration.
  (3) Flow rate, sensitivity, and pressure limit are all adjustable.
  (4) Adjustable flow rate allows for increasing tidal volume.
  (5) *Disadvantage*—changes in compliance or airway resistance can affect oxygen concentration and tidal volume.
  b. *Bennett*—PR II:
  (1) Positive-pressure cycled, time cycled, flow sensitive.

(2) May be triggered by patient's inspiration or controlled by pressure or time setting.

(3) Oxygen delivery variable, so frequent monitoring is *essential.*

5. Volume-constant ventilators:

   a. *Bennett*—MA 1:

   (1) Delivers preset tidal volume.

   (2) Oxygen concentration adjusted by lighter flow being fed into machine.

   (3) Sophisticated alarms.

   (4) Has a sigh mechanism and positive end-expiratory pressure (*PEEP*), which maintains lung inflation.

   (5) *Used for* decreased compliance (stiff lungs).

   (6) Excellent humidification system.

6. Minute volume ventilators—Servo 990 C:

   a. Delivers preset inspiratory minute volume.

   b. Has PEEP, continuous positive airway pressure (*CPAP*), spontaneous intermittent mandatory ventilation (*SIMV*), and inverse ratio ventilation (*IRV*) capabilities.

   c. *Used for* patients with ARDS who have not responded to conventional treatment (PEEP, IMV) and need the advantage of IRV and prolonged inspiratory ventilation.

💡 Study and Memory Aids

Pneumonia—Signs, Sx, Tx: "FRAPPÉ"

F ever
R espiratory distress
A ntibiotics after culture
P ain, affected side
P roductive cough
E valuate effectiveness of treatment

Atelectasis—Characteristics and Tx: "COLLAPSE"

C hest tubes not necessary
O xygen
L azy breathing habits
L ung reexpansion necessary
A lveoli collapsed
P osition on unaffected side
S uction, liquefy secretions
E ncourage cough and deep breathing

Pulmonary Embolism—Signs, Dx: "SUDDEN"

S ense of doom
U ntreated → death
D yspnea
D ensity on x-ray
E mergency condition
N ew symptoms

Histoplasmosis—Characteristics: "SOIL"

S pores
O bstructive pulmonary disease
I nhaled from bird droppings
L ocation: endemic to central United States

Tuberculosis—Cause, Dx, Sx, Tx: "SPREAD"

S putum positive for acid-fast bacilli
P ositive Mantoux test
R espiratory symptoms
E xposure to *M. tuberculosis*
A ppetite decreased
D rug regimen crucial

Asthma—Sx, Cause, Dx, Tx: "WHISTLE"

W heeze
H istory of respiratory tract infections
I nflammatory response
S easonal allergies
T reat early with bronchodilators
L ab data show blood gas abnormalities
E xpectoration—facilitate

Bronchitis—Sx, Tx: "COUGH"

C yanosis
O bstructed lumen
U pper respiratory tract problem
G ive medications as ordered
H elp to stop smoking

〰 Diagnostic Studies

Pulmonary Function Studies

1. **Ventilatory studies**—utilization of a spirometer to determine how well the lung is ventilating.

a. *Vital capacity* (VC)—largest amount of air that can be expelled after maximal inspiration.
   (1) *Normally* 4000–5000 mL.
   (2) *Decreased* in restrictive lung disease.
   (3) May be normal, slightly increased, or decreased in COPD.
b. *Forced expiratory volume* (FEV)—percentage of vital capacity that can be forcibly expired in 1, 2, or 3 sec.
   (1) *Normally* 81%–83% in 1 sec, 90%–94% in 2 sec, and 95%–97% in 3 sec.
   (2) *Decreased* values indicate expiratory airway obstruction.
c. *Maximum breathing capacity* (MBC)—maximum amount of air that can be breathed in and out in 1 min with maximal rates and depths of respiration.
   (1) Best overall measurement of ventilatory ability.
   (2) *Reduced* in restrictive and chronic obstructive lung disease.

2. **Diffusion studies**—measure the rate of exchange of gases across alveolar membrane. Carbon monoxide single-breath, rebreathing, and steady-state techniques—utilized because of special affinity of hemoglobin for carbon monoxide; *decreased* when fluid is present in alveoli or when alveolar membranes are thick or fibrosed.

Sputum Studies

1. **Gross sputum evaluations**—collection of sputum samples to ascertain quantity, consistency, color, and odor.
2. **Sputum smear**—sputum is smeared thinly on a slide so that it can be studied microscopically; *used to* determine cytologic changes (malignant cell) or presence of pathogenic bacteria, e.g., tubercle bacilli.
3. **Sputum culture** —sputum samples are implanted or inoculated into special media; *used to* diagnose pulmonary infections.
4. **Gastric lavage** or **analysis**—insertion of a nasogastric tube into the stomach to siphon out swallowed pulmonary secretions; *used to* detect organisms causing pulmonary infections; especially useful for detecting tubercle bacilli in children.

Procedures to Evaluate the Respiratory System

1. **Pulmonary circulation studies**—*used to* determine regional distribution of pulmonary blood flow.
   a. *Lung scan*—injection of radioactive isotope into the body, followed by lung scintigraphy, which produces a graphic record of gamma rays emitted by the isotope in lung tissues; *used to* determine lung perfusion when space-occupying lesions or pulmonary emboli and infarct are suspected.
   b. *Pulmonary angiography*—x-ray visualization of the pulmonary vasculature after the injection of a radiopaque contrast medium; *used to* evaluate pulmonary disorders, e.g., pulmonary embolism, lung tumors, aneurysms, and changes in the pulmonary vasculature due to such conditions as emphysema or congenital defects.
2. **Bronchoscopy**—introduction of a special lighted instrument (bronchoscope) into the trachea and bronchi; *used to* inspect tracheobronchial tree for pathologic changes, remove tissue for cytologic and bacteriologic studies, remove foreign bodies or mucous plugs causing airway obstruction, assess functional residual capacity of diseased lung, and apply chemotherapeutic agents.

☞ *Prebronchoscopy nursing actions:*
   Oral hygiene.
   Postural drainage is indicated.
☞ *Postbronchoscopy nursing actions:*
   Instruct patient *not* to swallow oral secretions but to let saliva run from side of mouth.
   Save expectorated sputum for lab analysis, and observe for frank bleeding.
   NPO until gag reflex returns.
   Observe for subcutaneous emphysema and dyspnea.
   Apply ice collar to reduce throat discomfort.

3. **Thoracentesis**—needle puncture through the chest wall and into the pleura; *used to* remove fluid and, occasionally, air from the pleural space. *Nursing responsibilities before thoracentesis:*

☞ *Position:* high Fowler's position or sitting up on edge of bed, with feet supported on chair to facilitate accumulation of fluid in the base of the chest.
   If patient is unable to sit up, turn on unaffected side.
   After procedure:
   Evaluate continually for signs of shock, pain, cyanosis, increased respiratory rate, and pallor.

Roentgenologic studies (X ray)
Chest—used to determine size, contour, and position of the heart; size, location, and nature of pulmonary lesions; disorders of thoracic bones or soft tissue; diaphragmatic contour and excursion; pleural thickening or effusions; and gross changes in the caliber or distribution of pulmonary vasculature.

● Diets

Pneumonia

↑ Carbohydrate
↑ Protein

Pulmonary Tuberculosis

↑ Calories
↑ Protein

Emphysema

↑ Calories (3000/d)
↑ Fluids
↑ Protein

Bronchitis

↑ Calories
↑ Feedings
↑ Fluids

Acute Adult Respiratory Distress Syndrome

IV maintenance while patient is on ventilator

Thoracic Surgery

↑ Fluids
Nutritious diet to promote healing

☞ Drug Review

Pneumonia

Antibiotics (to control infection)
  Cephalexin (Keflex): 250–500 mg q6h
  Cephalothin (Keflin): IV, 0.5–2 g q4–6h
  Erythromycin: 250–500 mg q6–12h
  Gentamicin (Garamycin): 3–5 mg/kg/d in divided
    doses
  Penicillin G procaine (Wycillin): 1.2 million U,
    single IM dose
Antipyretics (to reduce fever): Aspirin: 325–1000 mg
  q4–6h, not to exceed 4 g/d
Expectorants: Guaifenesin (Robitussin): 100–400 mg
  q4h to clear airway

Atelectasis

Acetylcysteine (Mucomyst) 3–5 mL 3–4 times via
  nebulizer; inhalation lowers viscosity of mucus,
  allowing easier mobilization and expectoration

Pulmonary Embolism

Anticoagulants
☞ Heparin sodium: IV, 5,000 U IV to start, followed
  by 20,000–40,000 U infusion over 24 hours; SC,
  8000–10,000 U q8h, adjusted according to PTT
  Warfarin (Coumadin): 10 mg/d, adjusted according
  〰 to prothrombin time (PT)

Pain control: Morphine: IV, 2.5–15 q4h or loading
  dose of 15 mg with 0.8–10 mg/h, rate increased as
  needed; SC, 5–20 mg q4h as needed
Note: *Avoid* birth control pills after pulmonary
  embolism.

Histoplasmosis

Antiemetics: Promethazine (Phenergan): 10–25 mg
  q4h
Antifungal
  Amphotericin B: after 1 mg test dose, 0.25 mg/kg,
    increase to 0.50 mg/kg twice daily
  Ketoconazole (Nizoral): 200–400 mg/d, single dose
Antipyretics (to reduce fever): Aspirin: 325–1000 mg
  q4–6h, not to exceed 4 g/d

Pulmonary Tuberculosis

Ethambutol: 2.5 g/d
Isoniazid: 5–10 mg/kg to 300 mg with pyridoxine (10
  mg/d) to prevent neuritis
Rifampin: 600 mg/d
Streptomycin: 1 g/d (*Caution:* may cause eighth
  cranial nerve damage, nephrotoxicity)

Emphysema

Antimicrobials
  Ampicillin: 1–2 g/d q6–12h
  Tetracycline: 1–2 g/d q6–12h
Bronchodilators
  Aminophylline: loading dose, 500 mg, followed by
    250–500 mg q6–8 h. Note: monitor theophylline
    levels
  Isoproterenol (Isuprel): 1–2 inhalations 4–6 times
    daily
  Terbutaline sulfate (Bricanyl): 2 inhalations q4–6h
  Theophylline: 5 mg/kg initially then 3 mg/kg q8h
Bronchial detergents: Acetylcysteine (Mucomyst)
  inhalation 3–5 mL 3 to 4 times daily via nebulizer
Expectorants: Guaifenesin (Robitussin): 100–400 mg
  q4h to clear airway
Steroids: Should *never* be abruptly discontinued,
  gradually taper dosage to prevent complications
  Prednisone: 5–60 mg/d.
  Methylprednisolone (Medrol): 4–48 mg/d
  Dexamethasone (Decadron): 0.5–9 mg/d in single
    or divided doses

Asthma

Antibiotics
  Ampicillin: 1–2 g/d q6–12h
  Tetracycline: 1–2 g/d q6–12h

Bronchodilators
  Albuterol (Ventolin): via metered-dose inhaler, 2
    inhalations q4–6h or 2 inhalations before exercise
  Aminophylline: loading dose, 500 mg, followed by
    250–500 mg q6–8 h. Note: monitor theophylline
    levels.
  Isoproterenol (Isuprel): 1–2 inhalations 4–6 times
    daily
  Theophylline: 5 mg/kg initially then 3 mg/kg q8h

Expectorants Guaifenesin (Robitussin): 100–400 mg
  q4h to clear airway
Steroids: Should *never* be abruptly discontinued,
  gradually taper dosage to prevent complications
  Prednisone: 5–60 mg/d
  Methylprednisolone (Medrol): 4–48 mg/d
  Dexamethasone (Decadron): 0.5–9 mg/d in single
    or divided doses
  Triamcinolone (Azmacort): 2 sprays 3–4/d

Bronchitis

Antibiotics
  Ampicillin: 1–2 g/d q6–12h
  Tetracycline: 1–2 g/d q6–12h
  Cefixime (Suprox): 400 mg/d
Bronchial detergents: Acetylcysteine (Mucomyst)
  inhalation 3–5 ml 3 to 4 times daily via nebulizer
Bronchodilators
  Albuterol (Ventolin): via metered-dose inhaler, 2
    inhalations q4–6h
  Aminophylline: loading dose, 500 mg, followed by
    250–500 mg q6–8h. Note: monitor theophylline
    levels
  Isoproterenol (Isuprel): 1–2 inhalations 4–6 times
    daily
  Theophylline: 5mg/kg initially then 3 mg/kg q8h
Expectorants: Guaifenesin (Robitussin): 100–400 mg
  q4h to clear airway

Adult Respiratory Distress Syndrome

Antibiotics (to control infection)
  Cephalexin (Keflex): 250–500 mg q6h
  Cephalothin (Keflin): IV, 0.5–2 g q4–6h
  Erythromycin: 250–500 mg q6–12h
  Gentamicin (Garamycin): 3–5 mg/kg/d in divided
    doses
  Penicillin G Procaine (Wycillin): 1.2 million U
    single IM dose
Bronchodilators: Aminophylline: loading dose, 500
  mg, followed by 250–500 mg q6–8h. Note: monitor
  [ww] theophylline levels.
Diuretics: Furosemide (Lasix): 20–80 mg/d
Pharmacologic paralysis (Pancuronium bromide,
  curare) if respirations are out of phase with
  mechanical ventilation
Sedation to reduce anxiety and restlessness

Hemothorax and Pneumothorax

Pain control
  Must not depress respirations
  Small, frequent doses
Other medications according to health status

Thoracic Surgery

Antibiotics
  Cephalexin (Keflex): 250–500 mg q6h
  Cephalothin (Keflin): IV, 0.5–2 g q4–6h
  Erythromycin: 250–500 mg q6–12h
  Gentamicin (Garamycin): 3–5 mg/kg/d in divided
    doses
Bronchodilators
  Albuterol (Ventolin): via metered-dose inhaler,
    2 inhalations q4–6h
  Aminophylline: loading dose, 500 mg, followed by
    250–500 mg q6–8h. Note: monitor theophylline
    levels
  Isoproterenol (Isuprel): 1–2 inhalations 4–6 times
    daily
  Theophylline: 5 mg/kg initially then 3 mg/kg q8h
Expectorants: Guaifenesin (Robitussin): 100–400 mg
  q4h to clear airway
Pain control
  Must not depress respirations
  Small, frequent doses

Laryngectomy

Antibiotics to prevent infection
Pain control without respiratory depression
Ultrasonic nebulization to facilitate expectoration

Questions

1. The nurse would conclude that a patient with emphysema is experiencing respiratory acidosis if, on assessment, he/she observes:
   1. A change in respiratory rate from 18 to 26 breaths/min.
   2. An increasing rate and depth of respirations.
   3. A change in heart rate from 86 to 60 beats/min.
   4. A decreasing level of consciousness.
2. The breath sounds heard during a physical assessment in a patient with emphysema would be described as:
   1. Bronchovesicular.
   2. Vesicular.
   3. Bronchial.
   4. Diminished.
3. Which infection control technique is unnecessary when caring for a patient with tuberculosis (TB)?

1. Washing hands before and after contact.
2. Putting on isolation gown, mask, and gloves.
3. Avoiding face-to-face contact.
4. Careful disposal of soiled tissues.

4. The nurse would tell a patient with TB that the drug treatment for TB frequently consists of:
   1. Rifampin and ethambutol.
   2. Isoniazid and rifampin.
   3. Streptomycin and ethambutol.
   4. Isoniazid and streptomycin.

5. If a patient experiences cardiac irregularities during suctioning, the best action for the nurse to take would be to:
   1. Give an antiarrhythmic drug before suctioning.
   2. Suction no longer than 10 to 15 seconds at a time.
   3. Give additional O_2 before suctioning.
   4. Use a smaller suction catheter to reduce O_2 loss.

6. The nurse would know that an important aspect of proper tracheostomy care is to:
   1. Secure the twill ties at the back of the patient's neck.
   2. Clean the inner cannula at least once a shift.
   3. Inflate the tracheostomy cuff before tracheostomy care.
   4. Use sterile saline to clean around the stoma.

7. The nurse would know that the patient's chest tubes are functioning properly if which condition were noted?
   1. Continuous bubbling in the water seal chamber.
   2. The tubing hanging in a dependent loop to facilitate drainage.
   3. Fluid fluctuating in the water seal tube during respirations.
   4. A minimum drainage of 100 mL/h for 24 hours after insertion.

8. In what position should the nurse place a patient during thoracentesis?
   1. Supine, head elevated.
   2. Side-lying, affected lung up.
   3. Sitting up, leaning forward.
   4. Prone, affected lung down.

9. The patient with emphysema is feeling short of breath and asks the nurse to increase the oxygen flow rate. The nurse explains that if the level is increased the following may occur:
   1. More alveoli will be destroyed and breathing will become more difficult.
   2. Cilia will be destroyed and congestion will increase.
   3. Breathing will become shallow and slow and eventually stop.
   4. The serum CO_2 level will drop, causing hypocapnea.

10. A patient's pulmonary function tests show an increase in the residual volume and a reduction in vital capacity. Which nursing diagnosis would best apply to this patient?
    1. Altered health maintenance.
    2. Risk for activity intolerance.
    3. Risk for fluid volume excess.
    4. Impaired physical mobility.

11. For what expected therapeutic effect of Theo-Dur should the nurse watch a patient?

1. Dilatation of the bronchioles.
2. Improved alveolar gas exchange.
3. Increase in pulmonary compliance.
4. Decrease in pulmonary friction.

12. The patient has been receiving cefixime (Suprax) and theophylline (Theo-Vent) for the treatment of acute bronchitis. He complains of feeling nervous, anxious, and nauseated. The most appropriate action for the nurse to take would be to:
    1. Encourage the patient to use relaxation techniques.
    2. Call the MD to get an order for an antiemetic.
    3. Check the patient's most recent theophylline level.
    4. Institute a breathing treatment immediately.

13. A patient is observed using pursed-lip breathing. If the technique is working, the greatest change in the patient's pulmonary function the nurse would see would be in the:
    1. Tidal volume.
    2. Expiratory capacity.
    3. Inspiratory reserve.
    4. Vital capacity.

14. A patient with emphysema is being discharged. Discharge teaching regarding diet should include instructions to:
    1. Eat three full-size meals each day.
    2. Restrict fluid intake with meals.
    3. Increase intake of calories and carbohydrates.
    4. Limit intake of foods high in sodium.

15. Which personal factor revealed during a nursing history would be the most likely contributory cause of a patient's emphysema?
    1. Family history of diabetes.
    2. History of alcohol abuse.
    3. No regular exercise plan.
    4. Job working for highway maintenance department.

16. On assessment, the nurse should recognize which symptom as a characteristic of emphysema?
    1. Barrel chest.
    2. Dusky skin color around mouth.
    3. Vesicular breath sounds.
    4. Frequent dry cough.

17. The nurse knows that the most positive evidence of active TB is/are:
    1. A positive skin test result.
    2. A raised WBC.
    3. Positive sputum culture findings.
    4. Positive chest x-ray study findings.

18. Which assessment finding would be consistent with a pneumothorax secondary to a ruptured emphysematous bleb?
    1. Paradoxical chest motion.
    2. Chest pain on the affected side.
    3. Mediastinal shift toward the affected side.
    4. Hematemesis.

19. Patient teaching about INH therapy would include:
    1. Taking the drug on an empty stomach for best absorption.
    2. Expecting concentrated and dark urine.
    3. Avoiding the consumption of alcohol, to prevent drug toxicity.

4. Taking an antacid to relieve the gastric distress which occurs.

20. To prevent the peripheral neuropathy INH treatment can cause, the nurse should anticipate that the patient will most likely be started on a regimen of:
   1. Thiamine.
   2. Pyridoxine.
   3. Calcium.
   4. Potassium chloride.

21. After arriving at the clinic for an appointment, the patient has an asthma attack. Which event would most likely have precipitated the attack?
   1. Weeding in the yard the day before.
   2. Only 4 hours of sleep the night before.
   3. Running from the bus to the clinic for the appointment.
   4. Jogging earlier in the day.

22. For what side effect of an epinephrine inhaler should the nurse assess?
   1. Dry mouth.
   2. Tachycardia.
   3. Apnea.
   4. Hypotension.

23. Which symptom would a patient most likely complain of after an asthma attack?
   1. Dry cough.
   2. Sore chest.
   3. Restlessness.
   4. Profuse perspiration.

24. Which factor identified during a nursing history would be the most likely contributory cause of a patient's emphysema?
   1. A recent episode of pneumonia.
   2. A two–pack per day history of smoking.
   3. Patient was raised and is currently living in an industrial area.
   4. A diet high in saturated fat and cholesterol.

25. On assessment, the nurse observes that the patient with emphysema is mouth breathing and the secretions are tenacious. The first nursing action would be to:
   1. Elevate the head of the patient's bed.
   2. Increase the patient's oral fluid intake.
   3. Encourage the patient to breathe slowly and deeply.
   4. Check the breath sounds for wheezes.

26. Which breathing-enhancing strategy should the nurse teach the patient with emphysema?
   1. Diaphragmatic breathing and pursed-lip breathing during inspiration.
   2. Diaphragmatic breathing and pursed-lip breathing during exhalation.
   3. Use of upper chest and neck muscles during inhalation.
   4. Orthopnea and pursed-lip breathing during exhalation.

27. Which signs and symptoms would the nurse recognize to be side effects of aminophylline?
   1. BP 90/60 mmHg., P-120, insomnia, and headache.
   2. BP 120/70 mmHg., P-78, tremors, and lethargy.
   3. BP 140/90 mmHg., P-78, anxiety, and nausea.
   4. BP 90/50 mmHg., P-56, insomnia, and vomiting.

Answers/Rationale

1. **(4)** As the CO_2 level rises during respiratory acidosis, the patient would become more somnolent and, if breathing is not improved, would eventually lose consciousness. The patient with emphysema *normally* has a rapid respiratory rate **(1)** to compensate for the hypoxia which is present. As the CO_2 level rises, the respiratory rate would slow. Because of the disease process, the patient is unable to breathe deeply **(2)**; the patient with emphysema hypoventilates. The heart rate would most likely increase, *not* decrease **(3)**. **AS, 6, PhI**

2. **(4)** In emphysema the alveoli (the site of gas exchange) are hyperinflated or destroyed, resulting in diminished or absent breath sounds. Bronchovesicular **(1)** or bronchial **(3)** breath sounds would be abnormal if heard over the lung fields, but in emphysema there is little to no air movement to produce these sounds. Vesicular **(2)** breath sounds are *normal* sounds and would *not* be heard over the diseased lung. **AS, 6, PhI**

3. **(2)** Because TB is an airborne disease, a mask would be appropriate but the gown and gloves are *not* necessary. The mask is often put on the patient, and staff or visitors may also wear masks. It *is* necessary to use the techniques in options **1, 3,** and **4** to prevent cross-contamination. **IMP, 6, SECE**

4. **(2)** All of the drugs in the options are used in the treatment of TB, but isoniazid (INH) and rifampin are the *most commonly* used first-line drugs and are given in combination. INH is low in toxicity and a drug of choice. Rifampin is always given in combination with another agent. Ethambutol **(1** and **3)** would be the third drug of choice. Streptomycin **(3** and **4)** is used only if resistance to the other drugs occurs. **IMP, 6, PhI**

5. **(2)** Prolonged suctioning will cause hypoxia and may also produce an arrhythmia; bradycardia frequently occurs during suctioning as the result of vagal stimulation. Suctioning no longer than 10 to 15 seconds at a time decreases the likelihood of arrhythmias. Drugs **(1)** are not needed because the cause of the problem is *not* cardiac in origin. Hyperoxygenation **(3)** may be induced *if* limiting the duration of suctioning is not effective. A smaller catheter **(4)** would probably be ineffective in removing the secretions, thus necessitating more frequent suctioning. **IMP, 6, PhI**

Key to Codes

Nursing process: AS, assessment; **AN,** analysis; **PL,** planning; **IMP,** implementation; **EV,** evaluation. (See Appendix M for explanation of nursing process steps.)

Category of human function: 1, protective; **2,** sensory-perceptual; **3,** comfort, rest, activity, and mobility; **4,** nutrition; **5,** growth and development; **6,** fluid-gas transport; **7,** psychosocial-cultural; **8,** elimination. (See Appendix O for explanation.)

Client need: SECE, safe, effective care environment; **PhI,** physiologic integrity; **PsI,** psychosocial integrity; **HPM,** health promotion/maintenance. (See Appendix P for explanation.)

6. (2) The cannula must be cleaned at least once a shift to remove any mucus buildup. The ties **(1)** are secured at the *side* of the patient's neck. Although option **3** is an important aspect of tracheostomy care, not all tracheostomies have an inflatable cuff **(3)**. The correct choice must be applicable to all types of tracheostomies. Hydrogen peroxide *not* saline **(4)**, is used to clean around the stoma. **PL, 6, SECE**

7. (3) The fluid level will fluctuate with the changes in intrapleural pressure during respiration. On inspiration the fluid rises up the tube; on expiration the fluid goes down the tube. Continuous bubbling **(1)** indicates a leak in the drainage system or the pleural cavity. A dependent loop **(2)** would impair gravity drainage. Drainage of 100 mL/h **(4)** is normal only during the first 2 hours; after that, such an amount would be excessive. The total normal drainage for 24 is 500 to 1000 mL. **AS, 6, PhI**

8. (3) Having the patient sit up and lean forward with his/her arms on the lap or a bedside table exposes the area where the needle is to be inserted. The other positions **(1, 2, and 4)** would make it more difficult to get into the pleural space without puncturing the lung. **IMP, 6, SECE**

9. (3) The stimulus for the patient with emphysema to breathe is the low partial pressure of oxygen in the blood; increasing the O_2 level without the support of mechanical ventilation may actually suppress ventilation. The disease has already destroyed alveoli **(1)** and cilia **(2)**, contributing to the breathing difficulty and congestion. The CO_2 level will decrease **(4)** only if ventilation improves, but supplemental O_2 will not improve ventilation. **IMP, 6, SECE**

10. (2) The patient will experience dyspnea on exertion and activity intolerance as the result of the trapped air and reduced vital capacity. Even activities of daily living are difficult for a patient with severe respiratory disease. Health maintenance **(1)** is not specific enough. Fluid volume excess **(3)** is not causing the pulmonary function problems; the abnormalities are consistent with chronic obstructive pulmonary disease. Physical mobility **(4)** is impaired only because the patient cannot tolerate activity. The patient is able to move but tires easily as a result of the hypoxia. **AN, 6, SECE**

11. (1) Theo-Dur, an extended release theophylline, is a bronchodilator. A *secondary* effect would be an improvement in gas exchange **(2)** as a result of the improved flow of air in and out of the bronchioles. Pulmonary compliance may actually already be increased **(3)** in some patients with bronchoconstriction, such as that caused by emphysema. Anti-inflammatory agents or antibiotics would cause pulmonary friction **(4)** to be decreased. **EV, 6, PhI**

12. (3) These are the symptoms of a theophylline excess. The therapeutic level is 10 to 20 µg/mL; any level over 20 µg/mL is considered toxic. If theophylline toxicity is ruled out, the symptoms might indicate anxiety, and relaxation techniques **(1)** would help. An antiemetic **(2)** treats the symptom, not the problem. Breathing treatment **(4)** would be indicated if the symptoms were due to hypoxia. **IMP, 6, PhI**

13. (2) Pursed-lip breathing keeps the airways from collapsing on expiration, allowing more air to be exhaled; therefore the greatest change would occur in the expiratory capacity. With an increase in exhalation, there would be an improvement in inspiratory volume, which would then cause a change in all the other components of pulmonary function **(1, 3, and 4)**. However, the *greatest* effect would be on expiratory capacity. **EV, 6, SECE**

14. (3) There is more work involved in breathing, as well as hypoxemia, in a patient with a chronic obstructive pulmonary disease such as emphysema. High-calorie foods and carbohydrates provide the energy needed. It is not necessary to consume full-size meals to meet energy needs **(1)**. Fluid intake **(2)** should be increased, *not* decreased, to help liquefy secretions. There is no indication of the need to restrict sodium intake **(4)**, however, if fluid retention occurred, breathing and circulation would be further impaired. **IMP, 6, HPM**

15. (4) Constant exposure to automobile exhaust may cause lung damage. The regular inhalation of fumes, such as may occur on the job, is potentially harmful to the lungs. The conditions in the other options **(1, 2, and 3)** are *not* known to contribute to the development of lung disease. **AN, 6, PhI**

16. (1) The increase in the anteroposterior diameter of the chest, the barrel appearance, is a consequence of the alveolar hyperinflation and trapped air that occur in emphysema. These cause the patient to be unable to exhale fully and eventually to lose the elasticity of the lung. Circumoral cyanosis **(2)** may be seen with hypoxia, which is not the primary problem in emphysema. Vesicular breath sounds **(3)** are normal sounds; in emphysema the breath sounds are diminished or absent. The cough is not dry **(4)** but is often productive of thick, tenacious secretions. **AS, 6, PhI**

17. (3) A diagnosis of TB can only be established when *Mycobacterium tuberculosis* is cultured from secretions or tissue. The specimen can be from the lung or it can be gastric contents if sputum is swallowed. A skin test **(1)** may confirm the presence of TB, but false-positive results can occur. Other diseases can assume the same appearance as that of TB on an x-ray study **(4)**. An elevated WBC **(2)** indicates the presence of an infection but is not a definitive characteristic of TB. **EV, 6, SECE**

18. (2) A tension pneumothorax exerts pressure on the heart and the unaffected lung, causing the patient to experience severe pain, difficulty breathing, and a mediastinal shift toward the unaffected side. The pressure must be relieved immediately or cardiac function will be severely compromised. The mediastinal shift is *not* toward the affected side **(3)**. Paradoxical chest motion **(1)** is seen in a patient with a flail chest. Hemoptysis, *not* hematemesis **(4)**, might be present in a patient with a pneumothorax. **AS, 6, PhI**

19. (3) Regular alcohol consumption increases the risk of INH toxicity and hepatic injury or hepatitis, another drug side effect. Taking the drug on an empty stomach **(1)** is not necessary because drug absorption is not delayed when the drug is taken with food. If urine is concentrated and dark (**2**), the MD should be notified, because this would indicate liver impairment. An antacid (**4**) would delay absorption; the drug should be taken with food or milk to minimize the nausea and other forms of gastric distress that are side effects of the agent. **IMP, 6, HPM**

20. (**2**) Pyridoxine, vitamin B₆, increases neurotransmitter formation to prevent peripheral neuropathy. Thiamine (**1**), calcium (**3**), and potassium chloride (**4**) will not prevent this drug side effect. **PL, 6, PhI**

21. (**3**) There are two types of asthma—allergic and nonallergic; this attack appears to be nonallergic in origin. Precipitating factors include *recent* exercise, stress, emotion and strong odors. The nurse would look for the precipitant closest in time to the attack. The attack was immediately preceded by running. The other events (**1, 2,** and **4**) occurred several hours to a day before the attack and for this reason are unlikely causes. **AN, 6, PhI**

22. (**1**) The patient should be instructed to rinse the mouth after each use of the inhaler to prevent dryness from vasoconstriction. Other side effects of epinephrine include restlessness, insomnia, arrhythmias, bronchial irritation, and hypertension. Tachycardia (**2**), apnea (**3**), and hypotension (**4**) are *not* side effects of epinephrine. **AS, 6, HPM**

23. (**2**) There is dyspnea and use of the accessory muscles, during an asthma attack and this results in fatigue and a sore chest. During the attack the cough would be nonproductive (**1**), but after the bronchospasms are relieved, the patient will generally cough up a mucous plug. During the attack the patient is hypoxic, restless, and anxious (**3**); afterward the patient is usually calm and fatigued. Perspiration (**4**), or diaphoresis, occurs *during* the attack. **AS, 6, PhI**

24. (**2**) A major contributory cause of emphysema is smoking which destroys lung tissue. Pneumonia (**1**) would not cause emphysema but would destroy more lung tissue. Environmental irritants (**3**) may be associated with lung disease, but not as consistently so as smoking. A high fat and cholesterol diet (**4**) would contribute to the development of *heart* disease. **AN, 6, PhI**

25. (**2**) The best action for the nurse to take is to increase the patient's oral fluid intake to liquefy tenacious secretions. Mouth breathing may be pursed-lip breathing, which does not indicate the presence of respiratory distress, so the head of the bed does *not* have to be elevated (**1**). The patient will be *unable* to breathe deeply (**3**) until secretions are liquefied and mobilized. The assessment would include the checking of breath sounds (**4**). **PL, 6, PhI**

26. (**2**) Diaphragmatic (abdominal) breathing is done during both inhalation and exhalation, and pursed-lip breathing is done during exhalation only. Diaphragmatic breathing is more effective than the use of accessory muscles, such as the shoulder muscles; it can increase the tidal volume, exercise tolerance, and alveolar ventilation and decrease the respiratory rate. Pursed-lip breathing slows the flow of exhaled air, creating a back pressure, which keeps the airway open and prevents collapse; as a result, there is more complete emptying of the lungs. Pursed-lip breathing is *not* done on *inspiration* (**1**). Use of the accessory muscles (**3**) is *ineffective* and more fatiguing. Orthopnea (**4**) is dyspnea that is relieved by assuming the upright *position;* it is *not* a breathing technique. **IMP, 6, HPM**

27. (**1**) A key side effect of aminophylline is tachycardia from the chronotropic effects of the drug. If the agent is given too rapidly, hypotension will occur. In addition to complaining of insomnia and headache, the patient may appear nervous or anxious. Tremors (**2**), nausea (**3**), and vomiting (**4**) are also side effects; but in all of these options the pulse rate is normal or low, rather than rapid. **AN, 6, PhI**

Fluid and Electrolyte Imbalances

Chapter Outline

- Fluid Volume Deficits
- Fluid Volume Excess
- Common Electrolyte Imbalances
  - Sodium
  - Potassium
  - Calcium
  - Magnesium
- Acid-Base Imbalances
  - Metabolic acidosis
  - Metabolic alkalosis
  - Respiratory acidosis
  - Respiratory alkalosis
- Intravenous Therapy

- Infusion systems
- Fluid administration
- Fluid and electrolyte therapy
- Intravenous cancer therapy
- Complications of IV therapy
- Total Parenteral Nutrition
- Summary of Key Points
- Study and Memory Aids
- Diets
- Drug Review
- Questions
- Answers/Rationale

Imbalances in fluid and electrolytes may be due to changes in the total quantity of either substance (deficit or excess), protein deficiencies, and/or extracellular fluid volume shifts. Older patients and very young patients are particularly susceptible.

Fluid Volume Deficits

Decreased quantities of fluid and electrolytes may be caused by *deficient intake* (poor dietary habits, anorexia, and nausea), *excessive output* (vomiting, nasogastric suction, and prolonged diarrhea), or *failure of regulatory mechanism*.

I. Pathophysiology: water moves out of the cells to replace a significant water loss; cells eventually become unable to compensate for the lost fluid, and cellular dehydration begins, leading to circulatory collapse.

II. Risk factors
  - **A.** No fluids available.
  - **B.** Available fluids not drinkable.
  - **C.** Inability to take fluids independently.
  - **D.** No response to thirst; does not recognize the need for fluids.
  - **E.** Inability to communicate need; does not speak same language.
  - **F.** Aphasia.
  - **G.** Weakness, comatose.
  - **H.** Inability to swallow.

  I. Psychological alterations.

⋈ III. Assessment
  - **A.** *Subjective data:*
    1. Thirst.
    2. Behavioral changes: apprehension, apathy, lethargy, confusion, restlessness.
    3. Dizziness.
    4. Numbness and tingling of hands and feet.
    5. Anorexia, nausea.
    6. Abdominal cramps.
  - **B.** *Objective data:*
    1. Sudden weight loss of 5%.
    2. Vital signs:
       - **a.** *Decreased* blood pressure (BP); postural changes.
       - **b.** *Increased* temperature.
       - **c.** *Irregular,* weak, rapid pulse.
       - **d.** *Increased* rate and depth of respirations.
    3. Skin: cool and pale in absence of infection; decreased turgor.
    4. Urine: oliguria to anuria, high specific gravity.
    5. Eyes: soft, sunken.
    6. Tongue: furrows.
    7. Lab data:
       - **(1)** Blood—*increased* hematocrit and blood urea nitrogen (BUN).
       - **(2)** Urine—*decreased* 17-ketosteroids.

⋈ IV. Analysis/nursing diagnosis: *Fluid volume deficit* related to inadequate fluid intake.

V. Nursing care plan/implementation

   A. Goal: *restore fluid and electrolyte balance*—increase fluid intake to hydrate patient.

     1. IVs as ordered; small, frequent drinks by mouth.

     2. Daily weights (same time of day) to monitor progress of fluid replacement.

     3. Intake & output (I&O), hourly outputs (when in acute state).

     4. *Avoid* hypertonic solutions (may cause fluid shift when compensatory mechanisms begin to function).

   B. Goal: *promote comfort.*

     1. Frequent skin care (lack of hydration causes dry skin, which may increase risk for skin breakdown).

     2. *Position:* change every hour to relieve pressure.

     3. Medications, as ordered: *antiemetics, antidiarrheals.*

   C. Goal: *prevent physical injury.*

     1. Frequent mouth care (mucous membrane dries due to dehydration; therefore, patient is at risk for breaks in mucous membrane, halitosis).

     2. Monitor *IV* flow rate—observe for circulatory overload, pulmonary edema related to potential fluid shift when compensatory mechanisms begin, or patient's inability to tolerate rate of fluid replacement.

     3. Monitor vital signs, including *level of consciousness* (decreasing BP and level of consciousness indicate continuation of fluid loss).

     4. Prepare for surgery if hemorrhage present (internal bleeding can only be controlled by surgical intervention).

VI. Evaluation/outcome criteria

   A. Mentally alert.

   B. Moist, intact mucous membranes.

   C. Urinary output approximately equal to intake.

   D. No further weight loss.

   E. Gradual weight gain.

Fluid Volume Excess

Excessive quantities of fluid and electrolytes may be due to *increased ingestion,* tube feedings, intravenous infusions, multiple tap-water enemas, or a *failure of regulatory systems,* resulting in inability to excrete excesses.

   I. Pathophysiology: hypo-osmolar water excess in extracellular compartment leads to intracellular water excess because the concentration of solutes in the intracellular fluid is greater than that in the extracellular fluid. Water moves to equalize concentration, causing swelling of the cells.

   II. Risk factors

     A. Excessive intake of electrolyte-free fluids.

     B. Increased secretion of antidiuretic hormone in response to stress, drugs, anesthetics.

     C. Decreased or inadequate output of urine.

     D. Psychogenic polydipsia.

     E. Certain medical conditions: tuberculosis; encephalitis; meningitis; endocrine disturbances; tumors of lung, pancreas, duodenum.

     F. Inadequate kidney function or kidney failure.

III. Assessment

   A. *Subjective data:*

     1. Behavioral changes: irritability, apathy, confusion, disorientation.

     2. Headache.

     3. Anorexia, nausea, cramping.

     4. Fatigue.

     5. Dyspnea.

   B. *Objective data:*

     1. Vital signs: elevated BP.

     2. Skin: warm, moist; edema—eyelids, facial, dependent, pitting.

     3. Sudden weight gain of 5%.

     4. Pink, frothy sputum; productive.

     5. Urine: polyuria, nocturia.

     6. Lab data:

       (1) Blood—*decreasing* hematocrit, BUN;

       (2) Urine—*decreasing* specific gravity.

IV. Analysis/nursing diagnosis: *Fluid volume excess* related to excessive fluid intake or decreased fluid output.

V. Nursing care plan/implementation

   A. Goal: *maintain oxygen to all cells.*

     1. *Position:* semi-Fowler's or Fowler's to facilitate improved gas exchange.

     2. Vital signs: q4h.

     3. Fluid *restriction.*

     4. Possible *rotating tourniquets* as needed (especially for interstitial-to-plasma shift).

   B. Goal: *promote excretion of excess fluid.*

     1. Medications, as ordered: *diuretics.*

     2. If in kidney failure, may need dialysis; explain procedure.

     3. Assist patient during paracentesis, thoracentesis, phlebotomy.

       a. Monitor vital signs to detect shock.

       b. Prevent injury by monitoring sterile technique.

       c. Prevent falling by stabilizing appropriate position during procedure.

       d. Support patient psychologically.

   C. Goal: *obtain/maintain fluid balance.*

     1. Daily weights; 1 kg = 1000 mL of fluid.

     2. Measure all edematous parts, abdominal girth, I&O.

     3. *Limit:* fluids by mouth, IVs, sodium.

     4. Strict monitoring of IV fluids.

   D. Goal: *prevent tissue injury.*

     1. Skin and mouth care as needed.

     2. Evaluate feet for edema and discoloration when patient is out of bed.

     3. Observe suture line on surgical patients (potential for evisceration due to excess fluid retention).

     4. IV route preferred for parenteral medications; *Z track* if medications are to be given IM (otherwise injected liquid will escape through injection site).

🏠 **E.** Goal: **health teaching.**

🍎 1. Improve nutritional status with *low-sodium diet.*

   2. Identify cause of imbalance, methods to avoid this situation in the future.

   3. Desired effects and side effects of diuretics and other prescribed medications.

   4. Monitor urinary output, ankle edema; report to health care manager when fluid retention is noticed.

   5. Limit fluid intake when kidney/cardiac function impaired.

✉ **VI. Evaluation/outcome criteria**

   A. Fluid balance obtained.

   B. No respiratory, cardiac complications.

   C. Vital signs within normal limits.

   D. Urinary output improved, no evidence of edema.

Common Electrolyte Imbalances

Electrolytes are taken into the body in foods and fluids; normally lost through sweat and urine. May also be lost through hemorrhage, vomiting, and diarrhea. Clinically important electrolytes are:

I. Sodium (Na^+): normal 135–145 mEq/L. Most prevalent cation in extracellular fluid. Controls osmotic pressure; essential for neuromuscular functioning and intracellular chemical reactions. Aids in maintenance of acid-base balance. Necessary for glucose to be transported into cells.

   A. *Hyponatremia*—sodium *deficit,* resulting from either a sodium loss or water excess. Serum sodium level *below* 135 mEq/L; symptoms usually do not occur *until* below 120 mEq/L unless rapid drop.

   B. *Hypernatremia*—*excess* sodium in the blood, resulting from either high sodium intake, water loss, or low water intake. Serum sodium level *above* 145 mEq/L.

II. Potassium (K^+): normal 3.5–5.0 mEq/L. Direct effect on excitability of nerves and muscles. Contributes to intracellular osmotic pressure and influences acid-base balance. Major cation of the cell. Required for storage of nitrogen as muscle protein.

   A. *Hypokalemia*—potassium *deficit* related to dehydration, starvation, vomiting, diarrhea, diuretics. Serum potassium level *below* 3.5 mEq/L; symptoms may not occur *until* below 2.5 mEq/L.

   B. *Hyperkalemia*—potassium *excess* related to: severe tissue damage, renal disease, excess administration of oral or IV potassium. Serum potassium level *above* 5 mEq/L; symptoms usually occur when *above* 6.5 mEq/L.

III. Calcium (Ca^{2+}): normal 4.5–5.5 mEq/L. Essential to muscle metabolism, cardiac function, and bone

health. Controlled by parathyroid hormone; reciprocal relationship between calcium and phosphorus.

   A. *Hypocalcemia*—loss of calcium related to: inadequate intake, vitamin D deficiency, hypoparathyroidism, damage to the parathyroid gland, decreased absorption in the gastrointestinal (GI) tract, excess loss through kidneys. Serum calcium level *below* 4.5 mEq/L.

   B. *Hypercalcemia*—calcium excess related to: hyperparathyroidism, immobility, bone tumors, renal failure, excess intake of calcium or vitamin D. Serum calcium level *above* 5.5 mEq/L.

IV. Magnesium (Mg^{2+}): normal 1.5–2.5 mEq/L. Essential to cellular metabolism of carbohydrates and proteins.

   A. *Hypomagnesemia*—magnesium deficit related to: impaired absorption from GI tract, excess loss through kidneys, and prolonged periods of poor nutritional intake. Hypomagnesemia leads to neuromuscular irritability. Serum magnesium level *below* 1.5 mEq/L.

   B. *Hypermagnesemia*—magnesium excess related to: renal insufficiency, overdose during replacement therapy, severe dehydration, repeated enemas with magnesium sulfate (Epsom salts). Serum magnesium level *above* 2.5 mEq/L.

✉ **V.** Table 7.1 provides assessment, analysis, nursing care plan/implementation, and evaluation/outcome criteria information for the various electrolyte imbalances.

Acid-Base Imbalances

Concentration of hydrogen ions in extracellular fluid is determined by the ratio of bicarbonate to carbonic acid. The normal ratio is 20:1. Even when arterial blood gas values are abnormal, if the ratio remains at 20:1, no imbalance will occur. Table 7.2 shows blood gas variations with acid-base imbalances.

   I. Causes of blood gas abnormalities: Table 7.3.

   II. Types of acid-base imbalance:

   A. *Acidosis:* hydrogen ion concentration increases and pH decreases.

   B. *Alkalosis:* hydrogen ion concentration decreases and pH increases.

   C. *Metabolic imbalances: bicarbonate* is the problem. In primary conditions, the level of bicarbonate is directly *proportional* to pH.

     1. *Metabolic acidosis:* excessive acid is produced or added to the body; bicarbonate is lost or acid is retained due to poorly functioning kidneys. *Deficit* of bicarbonate.

     2. *Metabolic alkalosis:* excessive acid is lost or bicarbonate or alkali is retained. *Excess* of bicarbonate.

     3. As compensatory mechanism, PCO_2 will be *low in metabolic acidosis,* as the body attempts to eliminate excess carbonic acid and elevate pH. PCO_2 will become *elevated in metabolic alkalosis.*

TABLE 7.1   ELECTROLYTE IMBALANCES

Disorder and Related Condition	⊠ Assessment		⊠ Analysis/Nursing Diagnosis	⊠ Nursing Care Plan/ Implementation	⊠ Evaluation/ Outcome Criteria
	Subjective Data	Objective Data			
Hyponatremia Addison's disease Starvation GI suction ⊙ Thiazide diuretics Excess water intake, enemas Fever Fluid shifts Ascites Burns Small-bowel obstruction Profuse perspiration	Apathy; apprehension, mental confusion, delirium Fatigue Vertigo, headache Anorexia, nausea Abdominal and muscle cramps	*Pulse:* rapid and weak *BP:* postural hypotension Shock, coma *GI:* weight loss, diarrhea, loss through NG tubes *Muscle:* weakness	*Diarrhea* *Fluid volume deficit* *Altered nutrition, less than body requirements* *Sensory/perceptual alteration (kinesthetic)*	*Obtain normal sodium level:* identify cause of deficit, *increase sodium intake* PO (salty foods), IVs— hypertonic solutions *Prevent further sodium loss:* irrigate ☞ NG tubes with saline; hourly I&O to monitor kidney output *Prevent injury related to shock, dizziness, decreased sensorium;* dangle before ambulation *Skin care*	Na⁺ 135–145 mEq/L No complications of shock present Return of muscle strength Alert, oriented Limits intake of plain water
Hypernatremia High sodium intake Low water intake Diarrhea High fever with rapid respirations Impaired renal functions Acute tracheobronchitis	Lethargy Restlessness, agitation Confusion	*BP and temperature:* elevated *Neuromuscular:* diminished reflexes *Skin:* flushed; firm turgor *GI:* mucous membrane dry, sticky *GU:* decreased output	*Fluid volume deficit* *Fluid volume excess* *Altered nutrition: less than body requirements* *Sensory/perceptual alteration (kinesthetic)*	*Obtain normal sodium level: decrease* ⊙ *sodium intake* I&O to recognize signs and symptoms of complications, e.g., heart failure, pulmonary edema	Na⁺ 135–145 mEq/L No complaint of thirst Alert, oriented Relaxed in appearance Identifies high-sodium foods to avoid

(continued)

Hypokalemia

Causes	Signs/Symptoms	Nursing Diagnoses	Interventions	Expected Outcomes
Decreased intake: Poor potassium food intake; Excessive dieting; Nausea; Alcoholism; IV fluids without added potassium; *Increased loss:* GI suctioning, vomiting, diarrhea; Ulcerative colitis; Drainage: ostomy, fistulas; Medications: potassium-losing diuretics, digoxin, cathartics; Increased aldosterone production; Renal disorders	Apathy, lethargy, fatigue, weakness; Irritability, mental confusion; Anorexia, nausea; Leg cramps; *Muscles:* weakness, paralysis, paresthesia, hyporeflexia; *Respirations:* shallow to respiratory arrest; *Cardiac:* decreased BP; elevated, weak, irregular pulse; arrhythmias; *ECG:* low, flat T waves; prolonged ST segment; elevated U wave; potential arrest; *GI:* vomiting, flatulence, constipation; decreased motility → distention → paralytic ileus; *GU:* urine not concentrated; polyuria, nocturia; kidney damage; *Speech—slow*	*Decreased cardiac output*; *Fatigue*; *Altered cardiopulmonary tissue perfusion*; *Ineffective breathing patterns*; *Constipation*; *Bathing/hygiene self-care deficit*; *Impaired home maintenance management*; *Sensory/perceptual alteration (gustatory)*	*Replace lost potassium: increase potassium in diet (see Appendix B); liquid PO potassium medications—dilute in juice to aid taste; give potassium only if kidneys functioning; Prevent injury to tissues: prevent infiltration, pain, tissue damage; Prevent potassium loss: irrigate NG tubes with saline, not water*	K+ 3.5–5.0 mEq/L; Identifies cause of imbalance; Lists foods to include in diet; Lists signs and symptoms of imbalance; Return of muscle strength; No cardiac arrhythmias

Hyperkalemia

Causes	Signs/Symptoms	Nursing Diagnoses	Interventions	Expected Outcomes
Burns; Crushing injuries; Kidney disease; Excessive infusion or ingestion of K+; Adrenal insufficiency; Mercurial poisoning	Irritability; Weakness, muscle cramps; Nausea, intestinal cramps; *Muscles:* paresthesia, flaccid muscle paralysis (later); *Cardiac:* irregular pulse; arrhythmias; bradycardia → asystole; *ECG:* high T waves; depressed ST segment; widened QRS complex; diminished or absent P waves; ventricular fibrillation; *GI:* explosive diarrhea; hyperactive bowel sounds; *Kidney:* scanty to no urine	*Decreased cardiac output*; *Altered urinary elimination*; *Activity intolerance*; *Ineffective breathing patterns*; *Diarrhea*; *Impaired home maintenance management*	*Decrease amount of potassium in body; identify and treat cause of imbalance; give foods low in K+; avoid drugs or IV fluids containing K+; If kidney failure present, may need to prepare for dialysis*	K+ 3.5–5.0 mEq/L; No complications (e.g., arrhythmias, acidosis, respiratory failure)

(continued)

TABLE 7.1 ELECTROLYTE IMBALANCES (Continued)

Disorder and Related Condition	⊠ Assessment		⊠ Analysis/Nursing Diagnosis	⊠ Nursing Care Plan/ Implementation	⊠ Evaluation/ Outcome Criteria
	Subjective Data	Objective Data			
Hypocalcemia Acute pancreatitis Diarrhea Peritonitis Damage to parathyroid during thyroidectomy Hypothyroidism Burns Pregnancy and lactation Low vitamin D intake Multiple blood transfusions Renal disorders Massive infection	Fatigue Tingling/numbness: fingers and circumoral Abdominal cramps Palpitations Dyspnea	*Muscles:* spasms: tonic muscles, carpopedal, laryngeal; tetany → convulsions *Neuromuscular:* grimacing; hyper-irritable facial nerves *Cardiac:* arrhythmias → arrest *GI:* diarrhea *Ortho:* osteoporosis → fractures	*Pain* *Diarrhea* *Altered nutrition: less than body requirements* *Risk for injury* *Sensory/perceptual alteration (gustatory)*	💊 *Prevent tetany* (**medical emergency**): calcium gluconate IV, 2.5–5.0 mL 10% solution; repeated q10 min to maximum dose of 30 mL *Prevent tissue injury* due to hypoxia and sloughing; administer slowly; *avoid* infiltration *Prevent injury related to medication administration.* *Caution:* drug interaction with 💊 carbonate, phosphate, digitalis; *avoid* hypercalcemia *In less acute condition:* 🔴 increase calcium intake—calcium gluconate or lactate	Ca²⁺ 4.5–5.5 mEq/L No signs of tetany Absent *Trousseau's* and *Cheostek's* signs Lists foods high in vitamin D and calcium

(continued)

Hypercalcemia				
Parathyroid glands: overactive, tumor Increased immobility Decreased renal function Bone cancer Increased vitamin D and calcium intake Milk-alkali syndrome—self-administration of antacids; increased milk in diet to relieve GI symptoms	*Pain:* flank, deep bone, shin splints Muscle weakness, fatigue Anorexia, nausea Headache Thirst → polyuria	*Muscles:* relaxed *GU:* kidney stones *GI:* increased milk intake; constipation; dehydration *Neuro:* stupor → coma	Decreased cardiac output Constipation Activity intolerance Altered urinary elimination Pain	*Reduce calcium intake:* decrease foods high in *calcium;* identify cause of imbalance; give steroids, diuretics, as ordered; isotonic saline IV *Prevent injury:* prevent pathologic fractures, (e.g., advanced cancer); prevent renal calculi by increasing fluid intake	Ca²⁺ 4.5–5.5 mEq/L No pain reported No fractures/calculi seen on x-ray

Hypomagnesemia				
Impaired GI absorption Prolonged malnutrition or starvation Alcoholism Excess loss of magnesium through kidneys, related to increased aldosterone production Prolonged diarrhea Draining GI fistulas	Agitation Depression Confusion Paresthesia	*Muscles:* irritable, tremors, spasticity, tetany → convulsions *Cardiac:* arrhythmias, tachycardia	Risk for injury related to seizure activity Decreased cardiac output	*Provide safety:* prevent injury to disoriented patient; administer magnesium salts PO or IV **Health teaching:** prevention; diet—*high-magnesium* foods: fruits, green vegetables, whole grain cereals, milk, meats, nuts	Mg²⁺ 1.5–2.5 mEq/L

Hypermagnesemia				
Renal failure Diabetic ketoacidosis Severe dehydration Antacid therapy	Drowsiness, lethargy	*Neuromuscular:* loss of deep-tendon reflexes *Respiratory:* depression *Cardiac:* hypotension; cardiac arrest	Ineffective breathing pattern Decreased cardiac output Fluid volume deficit Fluid volume excess Altered cardiopulmonary tissue perfusion	*Obtain normal magnesium level.* IV calcium; fluids; possible dialysis	Mg²⁺ 1.5–2.5 mEq/L No complications (e.g., respiratory depression, arrhythmias) Identifies magnesium-based antacids (e.g., Gelusil) Deep-tendon reflexes 2+

BP = blood pressure; GI = gastrointestinal; NG = nasogastric; I&O = intake & output; GU = genitourinary; ECG = electrocardiogram.

Source: Lagerquist, SL. *Little, Brown's NCLEX-RN Examination Review.* Boston: Little, Brown, 1996. Pp. 78–80.

TABLE 7.2   BLOOD GAS VARIATIONS WITH ACID-BASE IMBALANCES

		Value with:			
Blood Gas Feature	Normal Value	Respiratory Acidosis	Respiratory Alkalosis	Metabolic Acidosis	Metabolic Alkalosis
HCO_3 (bicarbonate)	22–26 mm Hg	Normal or ↑	Normal or ↓	↓	↑
PCO_2	35–45 mm Hg	↑	↓	Normal or ↓	Normal or ↑
(carbonic acid°)	(1.05–1.35)	↑	↓	Normal or ↓	Normal or ↑
pH	7.35–7.45	↓	↑	↓	↑

↑ = increased; ↓ = decreased.

°To obtain carbonic acid level, multiply PCO_2 value by 0.03.

Source: Lagerquist, SL: *Little, Brown's NCLEX-RN Examination Review.* Boston: Little, Brown, 1996. P. 81.

D. *Respiratory imbalances: carbonic acid* is the problem. In primary conditions, PCO_2 is *inversely* proportional to the pH.
　　1. *Respiratory acidosis:* pulmonary ventilation decreases, causing an *elevation* in the level of carbon dioxide or carbonic acid. *Excess* of PCO_2.
　　2. *Respiratory alkalosis:* pulmonary ventilation increases, causing a *decrease* in the level of carbon dioxide or carbonic acid. *Deficit* of PCO_2.
　　3. As a compensatory mechanism, the level of bicarbonate will *increase in respiratory acidosis* and *decrease in respiratory alkalosis.*

▶ III. **Assessment:** Table 7.4.

▶ IV. **Analysis/nursing diagnosis**
　A. *Impaired gas exchange* related to hyperventilation.
　B. *Ineffective breathing pattern* related to decreased thoracic movements.
　C. *Ineffective airway clearance* related to retained secretions.
　D. *Risk for injury* related to poorly functioning kidneys.
　E. *Altered renal tissue perfusion* related to dehydration.
　F. *Altered urinary elimination* related to renal failure.
　G. *Fluid volume excess* related to altered kidney function.
　H. *Fluid volume deficit* related to diarrhea or dehydration.
　I. *Knowledge deficit* related to self-administration of antacid medications.

▶ V. **Nursing care plan/implementation:** see Table 7.4.

▶ VI. **Evaluation/outcome criteria:** see Table 7.4.

Intravenous Therapy

I. **Infusion systems**
　A. Plastic bag:
　　1. Contains no vacuum—needs no air to replace fluid as it flows from container.

　　2. Medication can be added with syringe and needle through a resealable latex port.
　　　a. During infusion, administration set should be completely clamped before medications are added.
　　　b. Prevents undiluted, and perhaps toxic, dose from entering administration set.
　B. Closed system:
　　1. Requires partial vacuum—however, only filtered air enters container.
　　2. Medication may be added during infusion through air vent in administration set.
　C. Administration sets:
　　1. *Standard*—deliver 10–15 gtt/mL.
　　2. *Pediatric or minidrop sets*—deliver 60 gtt/mL.
　　3. *Controlled-volume sets*—permit accurate infusion of measured volumes of fluids.
　　　a. Particularly valuable when piggybacked into primary infusion.
　　　b. Solutions containing drugs can then be administered intermittently.
　　4. *Y-type administration sets*—allow for simultaneous or alternate infusion of two fluids.
　　　a. May contain filter and pressure unit for blood transfusions.
　　　b. *Air embolism* significant hazard with this type of administration set.
　　5. *Positive-pressure sets*—designed for rapid infusion of replacement fluids.
　　　a. In emergency, built-in pressure chamber increases rate of blood administration.
　　　b. Pump chamber *must* be filled at all times to prevent air embolism.
　　　c. Application of positive pressure to infusion fluids is responsibility of *physician.*
　　6. *Infusion pumps*—utilized to deliver small volumes of fluid or doses of high-potency drugs.
　　　a. Used primarily in neonatal, pediatric, and adult intensive care units.
　　　b. Have increased the safety of parenteral therapy and reduced nursing time.

II. **Fluid administration**
　A. Factors influencing rate:

TABLE 7.3	CAUSES OF BLOOD GAS ABNORMALITIES

Blood Gas Abnormality	Cause

Elevated Pco_2 (hypercarbia, hypercapnea)	*Increased* CO_2 production:
	1. Fever
	2. Muscular exertion
	3. Anaerobic metabolism
	Decreased CO_2 elimination (hypoventilation):
	1. *Decreased* tidal volume:
	  a. Pain (rib fractures, pleurisy)
	  b. Weakness (myasthenia gravis)
	  c. Paralysis (spinal cord injury, polio)
	2. *Decreased* respiratory rate:
	  a. Head injury
	  b. Depressant drugs
	  c. Cerebrovascular accident (stroke)

Decreased Po_2 (hypoxemia, shunt)	*Fluid in the alveoli:*
	1. Pulmonary edema
	2. Pneumonia
	3. Near-drowning
	4. Chest trauma
	Collapsed alveoli (atelectasis):
	1. Airway obstruction:
	  a. By the tongue
	  b. By a foreign body
	2. Failure to take deep breaths:
	  a. Pain (rib fracture, pleurisy)
	  b. Paralysis of respiratory muscles (spinal cord injury, polio)
	  c. Depression of the respiratory center (head injury, drug overdose)
	3. Collapse of the whole lung (pneumothorax)
	Other gases in the alveoli:
	1. Smoke inhalation
	2. Inhalation of toxic chemicals
	3. Carbon monoxide poisoning
	Respiratory arrest

Source: Caroline NL. *Emergency Care in the Streets* (5th ed). Boston: Little, Brown, 1995.

1. Patient's size.
2. Patient's physical condition.
3. Patient's age.
4. Type of fluid.
5. Patient's tolerance of fluid.

B. Flow rates for parenteral infusions can be computed using the following **formula:**

$$\frac{\text{gtt/mL of given set}}{60 \text{ min/h}} \times \text{total volume/h} = \text{gtt/min}$$

Example:
If 1000 mL is to be infused in an 8-h (125 mL/h) period and the administration set delivers 15 gtt/mL, the rate is 31.2 gtt/min:

$$\frac{15}{60} \times 125 = \frac{1}{4} \times 125 = 31.2 \text{ gtt/min}$$

C. Generally the type of fluid administration set determines its rate of flow.
  1. *Fluid* administration sets—approximately 15 gtt/min.
  2. *Blood* administration sets—approximately 10 gtt/min.
  3. *Pediatric* administration sets—approximately 60 gtt/min.
  4. Always check information on the administration set box to determine the number of gtt/mL before calculating; varies with manufacturer.

D. Factors influencing flow rates:
  1. *Gravity*—a change in the height of the infusion bottle will increase or decrease the rate of flow; for example, raising the bottle will increase the rate of flow, and vice versa.
  2. *Blood clot* in needle—stopping the infusion for any reason or an increase in venous pressure may result in partial or total obstruction of needle by clot due to:
    a. *Delay* in changing infusion bottle.
    b. Blood pressure cuff on, or restraints *on* or *above* infusion needle.
    c. Patient *lying on arm* in which infusion is being made.
  3. Change in *needle position*—against or away from vein wall.
  4. *Venous spasm*—due to cold blood or irritating solution.
  5. *Plugged vent*—causes infusion to stop.

III. Fluid and electrolyte therapy
  A. Types of therapy:
    1. *Maintenance* therapy—provides water, electrolytes, glucose, vitamins, and in some instances, protein to meet daily requirements.
    2. *Restoration* of deficits—in addition to maintenance therapy, fluid and electrolytes are added to replace *previous* losses.
    3. *Replacement* therapy—infusions to replace *current* losses of fluid and electrolytes.
  B. Types of intravenous fluids (Table 7.5):
    1. **Isotonic solutions**—fluids that approximate the osmolarity (290 mOsm/L) of normal blood plasma.
      a. *Sodium chloride* (0.9%)—normal saline.
        (1) *Indications:*
          (a) Extracellular fluid replacement when Cl^- loss is equal to or greater than Na^+ loss.

TABLE 7.4   ACID-BASE IMBALANCES

Disorder and Related Conditions	Assessment		Nursing Care Plan/ Implementation	Evaluation/ Outcome Criteria
	Subjective Data	*Objective Data*		
Respiratory Acidosis Acute bronchitis Emphysema Respiratory obstruction Atelectasis Damage to respiratory center Pneumonia Asthmatic attack Drug overdose	Headache Irritability Disorientation Weakness Dyspnea on exertion Nausea	Increased respirations Cyanosis Tachycardia Diaphoresis Dehydration Coma (CO_2 narcosis) Hyperventilation to compensate if no pulmonary abnormality present HCO_3 normal, Pco_2 elevated, pH < 7.35	*Assist with normal* ☞ *breathing:* encourage coughing; *suction* airway; *postural drainage;* pursed-lip breathing; *raise* HOB ☞ *Protect from injury: oxygen* at 2 L; encourage fluids; *avoid* sedation; 💊 medications as ordered—bicarbonates, antibiotics, bronchial dilators, detergent 🏠 **Health teaching:** identify cause, prevent future episodes; increase awareness regarding risk factors and early signs of impending imbalance; encourage compliance	Normal acid-base balance obtained Respiratory rate slows, <30 breaths/min No signs of pulmonary infection (e.g., sputum colorless, breath sounds clear) Demonstrates breathing exercises (e.g., diaphragmatic breathing)
Metabolic Acidosis Diabetic ketoacidosis Hyperthyroidism Severe infections Lactic acidosis in shock Renal failure → uremia Prolonged starvation diet; low-protein diet Diarrhea, dehydration Hepatitis Burns	Headache Restlessness Apathy, weakness Disorientation Thirst Nausea, abdominal pain	*Kussmaul's* respirations: deep, rapid air hunger; ↑ temperature Vomiting, diarrhea Dehydration Stupor → convulsions → coma HCO_3 below normal Pco_2 normal, $K^+ > 5$ mEq/L; pH <7.35	*Restore normal metabolism:* correct underlying problem; sodium 💊 bicarbonate PO/IV; sodium lactate; fluid replacement, Ringer's solution; *diet:* high calorie *Prevent complica-* 💊 *tions:* regular *insulin* for ketoacidosis; hourly outputs; prepare for dialysis if in kidney failure 🏠 **Health teaching:** identify signs and symptoms of primary illness; prevent complications, cardiac arrest; diet instructions	Normal acid-base balance obtained No rebound respiratory alkalosis following therapy No tetany following return of normal pH Alert, oriented No signs of K^+ excess

(continued)

TABLE 7.4 ACID-BASE IMBALANCES (*Continued*)

Disorder and Related Conditions	▷ Assessment Subjective Data	Objective Data	▷ Nursing Care Plan/ Implementation	▷ Evaluation/ Outcome Criteria
Respiratory Alkalosis Hyperventilation— CO_2 loss Fever Metabolic acidosis Increased ICP, encephalitis ○ Salicylate poisoning After intense exercise Hypoxia, high altitudes	Circumoral paresthesia Weakness Apprehension	Increased respirations Increased neuromuscular irritability; hyperreflexia, muscle twitching, tetany, positive *Chvostek's* sign Convulsions Unconsciousness Hypokalemia HCO$_3$ normal; Pco$_2$ decreased; pH > 7.45	*Increase carbon dioxide level:* rebreathing into a paper bag; adjusting respirator for CO_2 retention and oxygen inspired *Prevent injury:* safety measures for those who are unconscious; hypothermia for elevated temperature **Health teaching:** recognize stressful events; counseling if problem is hysteria	Normal acid-base balance obtained Recognizes psychological and environmental factors causing condition Respiratory rate returns to normal limits No cardiac arrhythmias Alert, oriented
Metabolic Alkalosis Potassium deficiencies Vomiting GI suctioning Intestinal fistulas Inadequate electrolyte replacement ○ Increased use of antacids ○ Diuretic therapy, steroids ○ Increased ingestion/injection of bicarbonates	Lethargy Irritability Disorientation Nausea	Respirations: shallow; apnea, decreased thoracic movement; cyanosis Pulse: irregular → cardiac arrest *Muscle:* twitching → tetany, convulsions *GI:* vomiting, diarrhea, paralytic ileus HCO$_3$ elevated above 26; Pco$_2$ normal; K$^+$ < 3.5; pH >7.45	☞ *Obtain, maintain acid-base balance:* irrigate NG tubes with saline; monitor I&O; IV saline, potassium added; isotonic solutions PO; monitor vital signs *Prevent physical injury:* monitor for potassium loss, side effects of medications 🏠 **Health teaching:** increase sodium when loss expected; instructions regarding self-administration of medications (e.g., baking soda)	Normal acid-base balance obtained No signs of potassium deficit Respiratory rate 16– 20 breaths/min No arrhythmias— pulse regular Lists food sources high in potassium

COPD = chronic obstructive pulmonary disease; HOB = head of bed; ICP = intracranial pressure; GI = gastrointestinal; NG = nasogastric; I&O = intake & output.

Source: Lagerquist SL: *Little, Brown's NCLEX-RN Examination Review.* Boston: Little, Brown, 1996. Pp. 82–83.

TABLE 7.5   COMMONLY USED INTRAVENOUS FLUIDS

Solution	Glucose (dL)	Cations (mEq/L)			Anions (mEq/L)	
		Na⁺	K⁺	Ca²⁺	Cl⁻	Lactate
D5/W	5					
D50	50					
0.45% NaCl		77			77	
0.9% NaCl°		154			154	
Ringer's		147.5	4	4.5	156	
Ringer's lactate		130	4	3	109	28
D5/LR	5	130	4	3	109	28

°Also known as normal saline.

Source: Caroline NL. Emergency Care in the Streets (5th ed). Boston: Little, Brown, 1995.

D5/W = 5% dextrose in water; D50 = 50% dextrose; D5/LR = 5% dextrose in lactated Ringer's.

          (b) Treatment of metabolic alkalosis.
          (c) Na⁺ depletion.
          (d) Initiating and terminating blood transfusions.
      (2) Possible *side effects:*
          (a) Hypernatremia.
          (b) Acidosis.
          (c) Hypokalemia.
          (d) Circulatory overload.
   c. *5% dextrose in water (5% D/W):*
      (1) *Provides calories* for energy, *sparing body protein* and preventing ketosis resulting from fat breakdown.
          (a) 3.75 calories are provided per gram of glucose.
          (b) USP standards require use of monohydrated glucose, so only 91% is actually glucose.
          (c) 5% D/W yields 170.6 calories; 5% D/W means 5 g glucose/L.

$$50 \times 3.75 = 187.5 \text{ calories}$$
$$0.91 \times 187.5 = 170.6 \text{ calories}$$

      (2) *Indications:*
          (a) Dehydration.
          (b) Hypernatremia.
          (c) Drug administration.
      (3) Possible *side effects:*
          (a) Hypokalemia.
          (b) Osmotic diuresis—dehydration.
          (c) Transient hyperinsulinism.
          (d) Water intoxication.
   d. *5% dextrose in normal saline:*
      (1) *Prevents* ketone formation and *loss* of potassium and intracellular water.
      (2) *Indications:*

          (a) Hypovolemic shock—temporary measure.
          (b) Burns.
          (c) Acute adrenocortical insufficiency.
      (3) Same *side effects* as those of normal saline.
   d. *Isotonic multiple-electrolyte fluids*—utilized for replacement therapy; ionic composition approximates that of blood plasma.
      (1) Types—Plasmanate, Polysol, and lactated Ringer's.
      (2) *Indicated in:* vomiting, diarrhea, excessive diuresis, and burns.
      (3) Possible *side effect*—circulatory overload.
      (4) Lactated Ringer's is *contraindicated* in severe metabolic acidosis and/or alkalosis and liver disease.
      (5) Same *side effects* as those of normal saline.
2. Hypertonic solutions—fluids with an osmolarity much higher than 290 mOsm (+50 mOsm); increase osmotic pressure of blood plasma, thereby drawing fluid from the cells.
   a. *10% dextrose in normal saline.*
  ☞ (1) Administered in large vein to dilute and prevent venous trauma.
      (2) *Used for* nutrition and to replenish Na⁺ and Cl⁻.
      (3) Possible *side effects:*
          (a) Hypernatremia (excess Na⁺).
          (b) Acidosis (excess Cl⁻).
          (c) Circulatory overload.
   b. *3% and 5% sodium chloride* solutions.
      (1) Slow administration essential to prevent overload (100 mL/h).
      (2) *Indicated in* water intoxication and severe sodium depletion.
3. Hypotonic solution—fluids whose osmolarity is significantly less than that of blood plasma (−50 mOsm); these fluids lower plasma osmotic pressures, causing fluid to enter cells.
   a. *0.45% sodium chloride*—utilized for replacement when requirement for Na⁺ is questionable.
   b. 5% dextrose in 0.45% saline, and 5% dextrose in 0.2% saline—these are all hydrating fluids.
      (1) *Indications:*
          (a) Fluid replacement when some Na⁺ replacement is also necessary.
          (b) Promote diuresis in patients who are dehydrated.
          (c) Evaluate kidney status before instituting electrolyte infusions.
      (2) Possible *side effects:*
          (a) Hypernatremia.
          (b) Circulatory overload.
          (c) Use with *caution* in edematous patients with cardiac, renal, or hepatic disease.

(d) After adequate renal function is established, appropriate electrolytes should be given to prevent hypokalemia.

4. **Alkalizing agents**—fluids used in the treatment of *metabolic acidosis:*
  a. *Ringer's lactate*
    (1) Administration—rate usually not more than 300 mL/h.
    (2) *Side effects*—observe carefully for signs of alkalosis.
  b. *Sodium bicarbonate:*
    (1) *Indications:*
      (a) Replace excessive loss of bicarbonate ion.
      (b) Emergency treatment of life-threatening acidosis.
    (2) Administration:
      (a) Depends on patient's weight, condition, and carbon dioxide level.
      (b) Usual dose is 500 mL of a 1.5% solution (89 mEq).
    (3) *Side effects:*
      (a) Alkalosis.
      (b) Hypocalcemic tetany.
      (c) Rapid infusion may induce cellular acidity and death.
5. **Acidifying solutions**—fluids used in treatment of *metabolic alkalosis.*
  a. Types:
    (1) Normal saline (see *Isotonic solutions,* pp. 93, 96).
    (2) Ammonium chloride.
  b. Administration—dosage depends on patient's condition and serum lab values.
  c. *Side effects:*
    (1) Hepatic encephalopathy in presence of decreased liver function since ammonia is metabolized by liver.
    (2) Toxic effects of irregular respirations, twitching, and bradycardia.
    (3) *Contraindicated* in renal failure.
6. **Blood** *and* **blood products** (Table 5.1, pp. 48–49).
  a. *Indications:*
    (1) Maintenance of blood volume.
    (2) Supply red blood cells to maintain oxygen-carrying capacity.
    (3) Supply clotting factors to maintain coagulation properties.
    (4) Exchange transfusion.

IV. Intravenous cancer chemotherapy
  A. Usual sites: forearm, dorsum of hand, wrist, antecubital fossa.
  B. *Procedure:*
    1. Normal saline infusion usually started first, to verify vein patency, position of needle. Chemotherapy "piggybacked" into IV line that is running.
    2. Rate: usually 1 mL/min. Running slowly decreases nausea, vomiting, and the degree of vein damage.

3. Check vein patency every 3–5 min.
4. If more than one drug is to be infused, normal saline should be infused between drugs.
5. *Never* infuse against resistance.
6. Stop treatment if patient reports pain at needle site. Extravasation (infiltration of toxic drugs into tissue surrounding vessel) may be present.
7. If extravasation present, begin protocol appropriate to drug administered (e.g., flushing of line with saline, applying ice or heat, local injection of site with antidote drugs, topical application of steroid creams).
8. Once treatment is completed, remove needle, apply Bandaid, exert pressure to prevent hematoma formation.

V. Complications of IV therapy: Table 7.6.

Total Parenteral Nutrition

Provides nutrition through a central venous line to patients who are in a catabolic state; are malnourished and cannot tolerate food by mouth; are in negative nitrogen balance; or have conditions that interfere with protein ingestion, digestion, and absorption, e.g., Crohn's disease, major burns, and side effects of radiation therapy of abdomen.

I. Types of solutions
  A. Hydrolyzed proteins (Hyprotein, Amigen).
  B. Synthetic amino acids (FreAmine).
  C. Usual components:
    1. 3%–8% amino acid.
    2. 10%–25% glucose.
    3. Multivitamins.
    4. Electrolytes.
  D. Supplements that can be added:
    1. Fructose.
    2. Alcohol.
    3. Minerals: iron, copper, calcium.
    4. Trace elements: iodine, zinc, magnesium.
    5. Vitamins: A, B, C.
    6. Androgen.
    7. Insulin.

II. Administration
  A. Dosage varies with clinical condition; 1 L q5–8h; rate of flow must be constant.
  B. Solution prepared under laminar flow hood (usually in pharmacy); solution must be *refrigerated;* when refrigerated, expires in 24 h; once removed from refrigerator, expires in 12 h.
  C. Incompatible with many *antibiotics;* check with pharmacy.
  D. Route: catheter inserted in a large vein (e.g., subclavian) by physician; placement confirmed by x-ray before beginning infusion (Figure 7.1).
  E. *Side effects:*
    1. Hyperosmolar coma.
    2. Hyperglycemia >130 mg/100 mL
    3. Septicemia.
    4. Thrombosis/sclerosis of vein.

TABLE 7.6   COMPLICATIONS OF IV THERAPY

Complication	⋈ Assessment — Subjective Data	Objective Data	⋈ Nursing Care Plan/ Implementation
Infiltration—fluid infusing into surrounding tissue rather than into vessel	Pain around needle insertion	1. Infusion rate slow 2. Swelling, hardness, coolness, blanching of tissue at site of needle 3. Blood does not return into tubing when bag/bottle lowered 4. Puffiness under surface of arm	1. Stop IV 2. Apply warm towel to area 3. Restart at another side 4. Record
Thrombophlebitis—inflammatory changes in vessel; *thromboemboli*—the development of venous clots within the inflamed vessel	Pain along the vein	Redness, swelling around affected area (red line)	1. Stop IV 2. Notify physician 3. Cold compresses or warm towel, as ordered 4. Restart at another site 5. *Rest affected limb; do not rub* 6. See nursing care of thrombophlebitis, Chap. 2
Pyrogenic reaction—contaminated equipment/solution	1. Headache 2. Backache 3. Nausea 4. Anxiety	1. ↑ Temperature 2. Chills 3. Face flushed 4. Vomiting 5. ↓ BP 6. Cyanosis	1. Discontinue IV 2. Vital signs 3. Send equipment for culture/ analysis 4. Antibiotic ointment, as ordered, at injection site 5. *Prevention:* change tubing q24–48h; meticulous sterile technique; check for precipitation, expiration dates, damage to containers, tubings, etc.; refrigerate hyperalimentation fluids; discard hyperalimentation fluids that have been at room temperature 8–12 h and use new bag regardless of amount left in first bag (change, to prevent infection—excellent medium for bacterial growth)

(continued)

5. Air embolus.
6. Pneumothorax.
F. *Prolonged use:* >10 d, fat needed; intralipids piggybacked close to insertion site; do *not* give through filter; observe for hypersensitivity (e.g., tachypnea, tachycardia, nausea, urticaria).
⋈ **III. Analysis/nursing diagnosis**
    A. *Risk for fluid volume excess,* related to inability to tolerate amount and consistency of solution.
    B. *Fluid volume deficit* related to state of malnutrition.
    C. *Risk for injury* related to possible complications.

    D. *Altered nutrition, more or less than body requirements,* related to ability to tolerate parenteral nutrition.
⋈ **IV. Nursing care plan/implementation**
    A. Goal: *prevent infection.*
      1. Dressing change:
        a. Strict *aseptic* technique.
        b. Nurse and patient wear mask during dressing change.
        c. Cleanse skin with solution, as ordered:
          (1) Acetone to defat the skin, destroy the bacterial wall.

TABLE 7.6   COMPLICATIONS OF IV THERAPY (*Continued*)

| Complication | ▶ Assessment | | ▶ Nursing Care Plan/ |
	Subjective Data	Objective Data	Implementation
Fluid overload—excessive amount of fluid infused; infants/ elderly at risk	1. Headache 2. Shortness of breath 3. Syncope 4. Dyspnea	1. ↑ Pulse, venous pressure 2. Venous distention 3. Flushed skin 4. Coughing 5. ↑ Respirations 6. Cyanosis, pulmonary edema 7. Shock	1. Stop IV 2. Semi-Fowler's *position* 3. Notify physician 4. Be prepared for diuretic therapy 5. *Preventive measures:* monitor flow rate and patient's response to IV therapy (see Fluid Volume Excess, p. 86, for subjective and objective data)
Air emboli—air in circulatory system	Loss of consciousness	1. Hypotension, cyanosis 2. Tachycardia 3. ↑ Venous pressure 4. Tachypnea	1. Turn on *left* side, with head *down* 2. Administer oxygen therapy 3. **Medical emergency—call physician**
Nerve damage—improper position of limb during infusion or *tying* limb down too tight during infusion → damage to nerve	Numbness; fingers, hands	Unusual position for limb	1. Untie 2. Passive ROM exercise 3. Monitor closely for return of function 4. Record limb status
Pulmonary embolism—blood clot enters pulmonary circulation and obstructs pulmonary artery	Dyspnea	1. Orthopnea 2. Signs of circulatory and cardiac collapse	1. Slow IV to keep vein open (rate: 5–6 gtt/min) 2. Notify physician 3. **Medical emergency** 4. Be prepared for lifesaving measures and anticoagulation therapy

Source: Lagerquist SL: *Little, Brown's NCLEX-RN Examination Review.* Boston: Little, Brown, 1996. P. 302.

(2) 1% Iodine solution as antiseptic agent.
  d. Dressing changed q48–72h; transparent polyurethane dressings may be changed weekly.
  e. Mark with nurse's initials, date and time of change.
  f. Air-occlusive dressing.
2. Attach final filter on tubing setup, to prevent air embolism.
3. Solution: change q12h to prevent infection.
4. Culture wound and catheter tip if signs of infection appear.
5. Monitor temperature q4h.
6. Use lumen line for feeding only (*not* for CVP or medications).
B. Goal: *prevent fluid and electrolyte imbalance.*
  1. Daily weights.
  2. I&O.
  3. Blood glucose measured q4h using glucometer; may need insulin coverage.

4. Specific gravity q8h to determine hydration status; normal serum osmolality 275–295 mOsm, total parenteral nutrition (TPN) 600–1400 mOsm.
5. Infusion pump to maintain constant infusion rate.
C. Goal: *prevent complications.*
  1. Warm TPN solution to room temperature to prevent chills.
  2. Monitor for signs of complications (Table 7.7).
    a. Infiltration.
    b. Thrombophlebitis.
    c. Fever.
    d. Hyperglycemia.
    e. Fluid imbalance.
3. Have patient perform *Valsalva maneuver,* or apply a plastic-coated clamp when changing tubing to prevent air embolism.
4. Tape tubings together to prevent accidental separation.

FIGURE 7.1   **(A) PATIENT WITH SUBCLAVIAN HYPERALIMENTATION LINE. (B) GAUZE DRESSING. (C) TAPING HYPERALIMENTATION LINE.**

V. Evaluation/outcome criteria
1. No signs of infection.
2. Blood sugar <130 mg/100 mL.
3. Specific gravity between 1.010 and 1.020.
4. Wounds begin to heal.
5. Weight: no further loss, begins to gain.

💡 Study and Memory Aids

Acid-Base Balance: "RAMS" (Respiratory: Alternate, Metabolic: Same)

	Respiratory (alternate)		Metabolic (same)	
Acidosis	↓ pH	↑ Pco_2	↓ pH	↓ HCO_3
Alkalosis	↑ pH	↓ Pco_2	↑ pH	↑ HCO_3

Diets

Fluid Volume Deficit

Force fluids

Fluid Volume Excess

Limit fluids
Low sodium level

TABLE 7.7   COMPLICATIONS OF TOTAL PARENTERAL NUTRITION (TPN)

Complication	⋈ *Nursing Intervention*
Infection	
Local infection (pain, redness, edema)	Sterile dressings; administer ● *antibiotics* as ordered;
Generalized, systemic infection (elevated temperature, WBC)	general comfort measures
Arterial Puncture	
Artery is punctured instead of vein	Needle is withdrawn and pressure is applied
Physician aspirates bright red blood that is pulsating strongly	
Air Embolus	
Air enters venous system during catheter insertion or tubing changes; or catheter/tubing pull apart	Stat *ABGs*, chest *x-ray*, *ECG*
	☞ Connect catheter to sterile syringe and aspirate air
Chest pain, dizziness, cyanosis, confusion	Clean catheter tip, connect to new tubing
	Place patient on left side with head lowered (left Trendelenburg prevents air from going into pulmonary artery)
	☞ *Prevent: have patient perform Valsalva maneuver or use plastic-coated clamp on catheter at insertion or tubing changes*
Catheter Embolus	
Catheter must be checked for placement by *X-ray* and observed when removed to be sure it is intact	Careful observation of catheter
	Monitor for signs of distress
Pneumothorax	
If needle punctures pleura, patient reports dyspnea, chest pain	May seal off or may need chest tubes

Source: Lagerquist SL: *Little, Brown's NCLEX-RN Examination Review.* Boston: Little, Brown, 1996. P. 124.

☞ Summary of Key Points

1. Thirst is a *poor* indicator of fluid status.
2. Change in body weight is the *best* indication of hydration status.
3. An *inverse* relationship exists between calcium and potassium. Many of the signs and symptoms of an elevation in one are similar to the signs and symptoms of a decrease in the other. For example, tingling sensations and increased peristalsis are present in low-calcium or high-potassium state because each disorder causes increased excitability.
4. Fluid imbalances are *most critical* in *older* adults because the amount of body water is naturally reduced with age. Fluid reserves are decreased, and reduced heart and kidney function make rapid fluid replacement by IV difficult.
5. *Extracellular* fluid excess results primarily from increased sodium and H_2O and produces increased intravascular and interstitial fluid volumes. *Intracellular* fluid excess (water intoxication) results from increased H_2O or decreased solutes and leads to increased cerebral edema.
6. Dysrhythmias and muscle weakness occur with *both* high and low potassium levels. However, a low potassium level reduces cell excitability and a high level increases excitability initially.
7. If acid-base compensation has occurred, the pH will be in the normal range.
8. Although tissue oxygenation (PaO_2) is separate from acid-base regulation, the release of oxygen to the tissues is affected by carbon dioxide.

● **Drug Review**

Fluid Volume Deficits

Antidiarrheals
Diphenoxylate (Lomotil): 2.5 mg to 5 mg 4 times/d
Kaolin/pectin: 60–120 mL after each loose bowel movement
Loperamide (Imodium): 4 mg initially, then 2 mg after each unformed stool

Antiemetics
Prochlorperazine (Compazine): 5–10 mg, repeat once in 30 minutes as needed
Promethazine (Phenergan): 12.5–25 mg q 4–6 h
Trimethobenzamide (Tigan): 200 mg 3–4 times a day

Antipyretics (to reduce fever): Aspirin: 325–1000 mg q4–6 h *not* to exceed 4 g/d

See Intravenous Therapy, pp. 92, 93, 96–97.

Fluid Volume Excess

Diuretics
Furosemide (Lasix): 20–80 mg/d
Hydrochlorothiazide: 25–100 mg/d

Questions

1. The nurse would recognize the need for additional teaching if a patient made which statement about a low-sodium diet:
   1. "Cooking lowers the sodium content of food."
   2. "It is important to check labels for the sodium content."
   3. "Canned vegetables have more sodium than fresh vegetables."
   4. "A good rule is 'no added salt' at the table."

2. Which entree should the nurse advise a patient who is on a low-sodium diet to avoid eating?
   1. Barbecued salmon fillet.
   2. Baked chicken breast.
   3. Sliced smoked turkey.
   4. Beef tenderloin.

3. The patient has the following vital signs: pulse, 120 beats/min; respiration, 30 breaths/min; temperature, 100.4°F; blood pressure, 90/60 mm Hg. The nurse knows that these findings most likely indicate the presence of:
   1. Severe dehydration.
   2. Increased intracranial pressure.
   3. Digitalis toxicity.
   4. Cardiogenic shock.

4. Interventions to correct respiratory acidosis would first include:
   1. Administering morphine sulfate prn.
   2. Giving sodium bicarbonate in an IV push.
   3. Increasing supplemental O_2 levels.
   4. Correcting the cause of hypoventilation.

5. Which assessment finding would be expected in a patient with respiratory alkalosis?
   1. Oversedation.
   2. Heart rate of less than 60 beats/min.
   3. Intractable pain.
   4. High arterial partial pressure of O_2 (Po_2).

6. A patient has had a peripherally inserted central venous catheter in place for about 16 hours. The nurse notices erythema along the catheterized vein. What should the nurse's first action be?
   1. To apply ice to the extremity immediately.
   2. To apply warm packs, as ordered, for 24 hours.
   3. To remove the line and have it reinserted.
   4. To replace the dressing, because it is too tight.

7. Which nursing intervention will help prevent occlusion of a peripherally inserted central catheter (PICC)?
   1. Application of a proper dressing to prevent kinking of the line.
   2. Regular irrigation with streptokinase.
   3. Flushing with an equal amount of saline after drawing a blood sample.
   4. Infusion of a 1% hydrochloric acid solution prn.

8. The correct technique for removal of a peripherally inserted central catheter (PICC) from the right cephalic vein includes:
   1. Putting the patient in semi-Fowler's position with the arm placed on the over-bed table.
   2. Wearing a gown, sterile gloves, and mask.
   3. Using a hand-over-hand technique and pulling slowly without too much tension.
   4. Placing the patient flat with the arm next to his/her side to straighten the line.

9. To administer 1000 mL of IV fluid in 8 hours (15 gtt/mL), the nurse should make sure that the drops per minute will be:
   1. 25.
   2. 31.
   3. 38.
   4. 45.

10. Which arterial blood gas findings indicate the presence of acute uncompensated respiratory acidosis?
    1. Pco_2 increased, HCO_3^- normal.
    2. Pco_2 decreased, HCO_3^- normal.
    3. Pco_2 decreased, HCO_3^- decreased.
    4. Pco_2 increased, HCO_3^- increased.

11. Which of the following findings would indicate to the nurse that a patient is recovering from respiratory acidosis?
    1. Increased respiratory rate.
    2. Increased serum creatinine level.
    3. Increased heart rate.
    4. Increased HCO_3^- concentration.

12. Which arterial blood gas finding would the nurse view as a sign of metabolic acidosis?
    1. Increased Pco_2.
    2. Decreased Pco_2.
    3. Increased HCO_3^- concentration.
    4. Decreased HCO_3^- concentration.

13. The blood gas values in a patient with emphysema are as follows: Pco_2, 60 mm Hg; HCO_3^-, 30 mEq/L; pH,

7.30. The nurse would know the patient is suffering from:
1. Metabolic acidosis.
2. Metabolic alkalosis.
3. Respiratory acidosis.
4. Respiratory alkalosis.

14. A patient becomes diaphoretic, weak, and confused while she is receiving total parenteral nutrition (TPN). The initial nursing action would be to:
1. Slow the rate of the TPN infusion.
2. Increase the rate of the TPN infusion.
3. Check the patient's blood glucose level.
4. Notify the MD of the patient's symptoms.

15. A patient with diabetes mellitus is becoming lethargic. What additional change should the nurse assess for that would indicate developing metabolic acidosis?
1. Blood pressure decrease from 128/80 to 96/40 mm Hg.
2. Pulse rate change from 94 to 72 beats/min.
3. Muscle weakness.
4. Slow, shallow breathing.

16. When changing the TPN line and dressing, the nurse knows that a critical element in TPN care is to:
1. Change the dressing every shift, using a strict aseptic technique.
2. Stop the infusion briefly to prevent contamination.
3. Have the patient perform the Valsalva maneuver during the line change.
4. Use vaseline gauze as the dressing.

17. A patient is to be given 50 mL of cefazolin (Kefzol) IV over 30 minutes (10 gtt/mL). How many drops should be delivered per minute?
1. 9.
2. 12.
3. 14.
4. 17.

18. When the nurse arrives for an 8-hour shift, a patient is receiving 5% dextrose in water (D5W) at the rate of 30 gtt/min (15 gtt/mL). The IV is interrupted for 3 hours so that 650 mL of blood can be transfused. How much D5W will the patient receive during this shift?
1. 600 mL.
2. 900 mL.
3. 1250 mL.
4. 1500 mL.

19. If a patient is to receive D5W and lactated Ringer's solution at a rate of 125 mL/h, what should the rate be for a drop factor of 15 gtt/mL?
1. 28 gtt/min.
2. 29 gtt/min.
3. 30 gtt/min.
4. 31 gtt/min.

20. Which foods would the nurse recommend as the best source of calcium?
1. Spinach and mustard greens.
2. Lentils and green beans.
3. Strawberries and cantaloupe.
4. White beans and spinach.

21. The nurse would best assess the adequacy of fluid volume replacement in a patient with hypovolemia by monitoring:
1. Vital signs and daily weight.
2. Oral intake and vital signs.
3. Hemoglobin and hematocrit values.
4. Serum electrolyte levels and urinary output.

22. Muscular twitching and hyperirritability of the nervous system indicate tetany. The nurse would identify these as symptoms of which electrolyte imbalance?
1. Low sodium level.
2. High potassium level.
3. Low calcium level.
4. High magnesium level.

23. The most applicable nursing diagnosis for a patient experiencing hypercalcemia would be:
1. Risk for injury related to muscle weakness and confusion.
2. Risk for injury related to spasm or tetany.
3. Diarrhea related to decreased gastrointestinal absorption.
4. Fluid volume excess related to impaired kidney function.

24. Hyperglycemia may occur in a patient receiving TPN. How often should the blood glucose level be checked?
1. Hourly.
2. Every 6 hours.
3. Every shift.
4. Every 24 hours.

25. During insertion of a subclavian central line, the patient suddenly experiences sharp pain. Which complication of insertion would the nurse suspect?
1. Air embolism.
2. Hemothorax.
3. Pneumothorax.
4. Pleural effusion.

Answers/Rationale

1. (1) Cooking reduces the vitamin content of food, but if the food is high in sodium, the sodium content will not change significantly with cooking. Checking labels to find out the salt content **(2)**, avoiding canned and processed foods **(3)**, and not adding salt to food at the table **(4)** *are* all *effective* ways to maintain a low-sodium diet. **EV, 4, PhI**

2. (3) Smoked meats are restricted in a low-sodium diet because the preparation includes curing with salt. Fish **(1)**, chicken **(2)**, and beef **(4)**, cooked by barbecuing, baking, or broiling and carefully seasoned, would *all be included* in a low-sodium diet. **IMP, 4, HPM**

Key to Codes

Nursing process: AS, assessment; **AN,** analysis; **PL,** planning; **IMP,** implementation; **EV,** evaluation. (See Appendix M for explanation of nursing process steps.)

Category of human function: 1, protective; **2,** sensory-perceptual; **3,** comfort, rest, activity, and mobility; **4,** nutrition; **5,** growth and development; **6,** fluid-gas transport; **7,** psychosocial-cultural; **8,** elimination. (See Appendix O for explanation.)

Client need: SECE, safe, effective care environment; **PhI,** physiologic integrity; **PsI,** psychosocial integrity; **HPM,** health promotion/maintenance. (See Appendix P for explanation.)

3. (1) Tachycardia and low blood pressure are signs of low blood volume (hypovolemic shock), which could occur with severe dehydration. The fever is also a sign of dehydration. Vital signs in the presence of increased intracranial pressure (2) are the opposite of those of hypovolemic shock. The pulse would be slow in digitalis toxicity (3). Cardiogenic shock (4) is a possible choice, but if the heart is failing, the pulse rate would not likely be as high because the heart would not be able to compensate. **AN, 6, PhI**

4. (3) In respiratory acidosis, there is an increase in the CO_2 level as a result of inadequate ventilation. There is also hypoxemia in most cases. Even in a patient with emphysema who has a hypoxic drive, ventilation should be supported by giving the patient O_2 first. Giving the patient morphine sulfate (1) would only further decrease the respiratory rate and depth and would also likely cause the respiratory acidosis to worsen. Sodium bicarbonate (2) is given to correct acidosis; however, the nurse would first support the patient's ventilation by increasing the flow of O_2. It would also be important to determine the cause of the hypoventilation (4), but supplemental O_2 should be administered while diagnostic tests are being conducted. **IMP, 6, PhI**

5. (3) Patients with intractable pain will most likely breathe rapidly and excessively rid themselves of CO_2, resulting in respiratory alkalosis. Oversedation (1) will depress respirations and lead to respiratory *acidosis*. A slow heart rate (2) will result in poor perfusion and *metabolic acidosis*. Hypoxemia (low O_2 level), *not* a high O_2 level (4), is usually seen in acidosis. **AS, 6, PHi**

6. (2) Erythema along the catheterized vein does not necessarily indicate phlebitis. During the first 24 hours after insertion, the vein's epithelial lining may show irritation resulting from the insertion process. Before ordering removal of the line (3), the physician would mostly likely order the application of warm packs, *not* ice (1), for 24 hours to see whether this resolves the problem. During that time, the nurse should observe not only for a decrease in redness but also for other indicators of infection, such as a fever. As long as there is good blood return, the line flushes easily, and the patient does not feel any discomfort, the line is considered patent. The dressing, which may only be changed every 7 days, does not encircle the limb, so there would not be any tightness (4) to cause the redness. **IMP, 6, IMP**

7. (1) The most common cause of occlusion is kinked tubing, and a proper dressing technique will *prevent* such a problem. Sterile adhesive strips or sutures may be used to secure the line at the insertion site and a transparent occlusive dressing applied over the site. The PICC can be looped loosely under the dressing to prevent kinking and tugging on the line. Streptokinase (2) or urokinase are administered according to hospital policy to clear an occlusion caused by a suspected clot or fibrin plugs. After drawing a sample of blood (3), the line is flushed with 20 mL of saline regardless of the amount of blood drawn. If a drug has precipitated in the line, a 1% hydrochloric acid solution is instilled (4) to open up the line, which has *already* occluded. **IMP, 6, CECE**

8. (3) The PICC should be removed in about 30 seconds, using a gentle, slow, and a hand-over-hand technique, and without exerting too much tension. The patient should be supine with the arm placed at a 45- to 90-degree angle to the body to ensure a straight pull; the techniques named in options 1 and 4 are therefore incorrect. This prevents bending, kinking or possible breakage. Unless hospital policy states otherwise or a catheter-related infection is suspected, it is only necessary for the nurse to wear clean gloves during removal (2). **IMP, 6, SECE**

9. (2) The rate is calculated using the following formula: (mL/h $\times$ the drop factor)/60. Using this formula, the correct rate in this instance is calculated as follows: (125 mL/h $\times$ 15 gtt/mL)/60 = 31.25, or 31 gtt/min. The number of drops named in the other options (1, 3, and 4) are incorrect according to this formula. **IMP, 6, SECE**

10. (1) The P_{CO_2} is *increased* in respiratory acidosis, and the HCO_3 concentration would be normal in an uncompensated state. (The arterial P_{O_2} has no bearing on the acid-base status.) Option 2 is incorrect because the CO_2 level is decreased. Option 3 is incorrect because both the CO_2 level and the HCO_3^- concentration are decreased. Option 4 is incorrect because the HCO_3^- concentration is increased, which would be seen in the presence of *compensated* respiratory acidosis. **AN, 6, PhI**

11. (4) An increase in the HCO_3^- concentration and an increase in the CO_2 level in a patient suffering from respiratory acidosis indicate the occurrence of renal compensation. The relationship is direct: When one goes up, the other goes up. An increased respiratory rate (1) is a *symptom* of respiratory acidosis. An increased serum creatinine level (2) would be more likely to occur in metabolic acidosis resulting from renal failure. An increased heart rate (3) is a *symptom* of respiratory acidosis, and the heart rate should decrease if the patient's condition is improving. **EV, 6, PhI**

12. (4) When there is a metabolic disorder, there is a decrease in the HCO_3^- concentration. Metabolic problems (acid-base) are regulated by the kidneys which excrete or retain HCO_3, depending on the disorder. An increased P_{CO_2} (1) would be seen with respiratory acidosis. A decreased P_{CO_2} (2) occurs with respiratory alkalosis. An increased HCO_3 concentration (3) indicates metabolic alkalosis. **AN, 6, PhI**

13. (3) The CO_2 level is elevated in respiratory acidosis; the normal level is 35 to 45 mm Hg. The HCO_3^- concentration is also elevated to compensate for the raised CO_2 level; the normal concentration is 22 to 26 mEq/L. The patient's pH is below the normal range of 7.35 to 7.45, also indicating acidosis. In metabolic acidosis (1), the HCO_3^- concentration and the pH are decreased. An elevated HCO_3^- concentration and pH would occur in metabolic alkalosis (2). In respiratory alkalosis (4), the CO_2 level is decreased and the pH increased. **EV, 6, PhI**

14. (3) The patient is showing the symptoms of hypoglycemia, but additional data are needed to confirm this suspicion. Changing the rate (1 and 2) is not an independent nursing action. Transferring the decision to the

MD (**4**) is not the best choice. The best choice is a *nursing* action. **AN, 4, PhI**

15. (**3**) Metabolic acidosis in a diabetic is due to ketoacidosis and hyperglycemia. As the acidosis develops, potassium leaves the cell, resulting in hyperkalemia. The patient will experience weakness, paralysis, and paresthesia. If the metabolic acidosis goes undetected, the patient will continue to lose fluids through oliguria, leading to clinical manifestations similar to those of shock. Hypotension (**1**) would occur, but as a late sign. The pulse rate should increase, *not* decrease (**2**), as a result of shock. The breathing pattern that occurs in order to eliminate the excess CO_2 is called *Kussmaul's breathing*, and it is rapid and deep, *not* slow and shallow (**4**). **AS, 4, PhI**

16. (**3**) To prevent an air embolus from developing, the patient should hold his/her breath or bear down (the *Valsalva maneuver*) as the old tubing is disconnected and new tubing is reconnected. This prevents air from being sucked in. Although a strict aseptic technique is used, the dressing is *not* changed every shift (**1**), because the more often the dressing is changed, the greater the chance of contamination. The infusion should *not* be stopped (**2**), because this may cause the line to occlude. The dressing should be air occlusive, but vaseline is *not* used (**4**). **IMP, 4, SECE**

17. (**4**) The same formula used to calculate any IV rate is used to determine the rate in this instance: (cc or mL/h × the drop factor)/60, or (100 mL × 10 gtt/mL)/60 = 16.6, or about 17 gtt/min. The number of drops in the other options (**1, 2,** and **3**) are incorrect. **IMP, 1, SECE**

18. (**1**) At 30 gtt/min the patient will receive 2 mL/min and 120 mL/h. If the D5W is infused for only 5 hours, the patient will receive a total of 600 mL. The amounts in options **2** and **4** are mathematically incorrect. The amount in option **3** is the total of the D5W and the blood; the amount of blood transfused would be recorded separately. **IMP, 6, SECE**

19. (**4**) Using the formula mL (h × the drop factor)/60, (125 × 15)/60 = 31.25, or about 31 drops per minute. The rates in options **1, 2,** and **3** are incorrect calculations. **IMP, 6, SECE**

20. (**1**) Leafy green vegetables are the best sources of calcium, as well as of iron. Of the foods named in options **2** and **4,** only one of the foods in each, green beans and spinach, is a source of calcium. Strawberries and canta-

loupe (**3**) are high in vitamin C and potassium, respectively. **IMP, 4, HPM**

21. (**1**) Daily weight is the best indicator of volume status. Vital signs—rapid pulse and low blood pressure—can also indicate the presence of hypovolemia. Option **2** oral intake and vital signs is not the best choice; vital signs can be used to assess adequacy, but because fluid replacement is usually accomplished by the IV routes oral intake would not be an accurate indicator. The hematocrit value (**3**) is used to assess the status of volume, hemodilution, or hemoconcentration, but the hemoglobin level does not accurately reflect the status of these. The serum electrolyte levels, particularly that of sodium, and urinary output (**4**) are also affected by volume but are not the best indicators of improvement. **AS, 6, PhI**

22. (**3**) When the serum calcium level drops, nerve fibers become increasingly excitable and discharge spontaneously, causing muscles to twitch and go into spasms, or tetany. Sodium (**1**) does not interfere with the action potential of muscles. A high potassium level (**2**) causes muscle cramping, but *not* tetany. Tetany can also occur when the magnesium level is low, but *not* when it is high (**4**). **AN, 6, PhI**

23. (**1**) In the presence of high levels of calcium, smooth muscle activity decreases and there is neurologic depression, resulting in muscle weakness and confusion. The other nursing diagnoses (**2, 3,** and **4**) would be appropriate for a patient with *hypo*calcemia. **AN, 6, SECE**

24. (**2**) Every 6 hours is the best choice. Hourly (**1**) is *too often* and daily (**4**) is *not* often enough. Checking it during every shift (**3**) is *not specific* enough because shifts may be 8, 10, or 12 hours long. **PL, 4, PhI**

25. (**3**) The most common complication of insertion of a subclavian central line is pneumothorax from puncture of the lung by the needle. Breathing in this instance would be difficult, chest movements may be asymmetrical, and breath sounds would be absent. An x-ray study is needed to confirm the extent of the collapse. Air embolism (**1**) is a possible complication, but *not the most common* one and can be prevented by having the patient do the Valsalva maneuver during insertion. Hemothorax (**2**) is another possible complication but, again, *not the most common* one. Pleural effusion (**4**) is *not* a complication of subclavian insertion. **AN, 6, PhI**

Shock

Chapter Outline

- Shock
- Summary of Key Points
- Study and Memory Aids

- Drug Review
- Questions
- Answers/Rationale

Shock

A critically severe deficiency in nutrients, oxygen, and electrolytes delivered to body tissues, plus deficiency in removal of cellular wastes; results from cardiac failure, insufficient blood volume, and/or increased vascular bed size.

I. Types, pathophysiology, and risk factors:
- **A. Hypovolemic** (hemorrhagic, hematogenic)—markedly decreased **volume** of blood (hemorrhage or plasma loss from intestinal obstruction, burns, physical trauma, or dehydration) → decreased venous return, cardiac output → decreased tissue perfusion.
- **B. Cardiogenic**—failure of cardiac muscle **pump** (myocardial infarction) → generally decreased cardiac output → pulmonary congestion, hypoxia → inadequate circulation; high mortality.
- **C.** *Distributive:*
    - **1. Neurogenic**—massive **vasodilatation** from reduced vasomotor, vasoconstrictor tone (e.g., spinal shock, head injuries, anesthesia, pain); interruption of sympathetic nervous system; blood volume that is normal but inadequate for vessels → decreased venous return → tissue hypoxia.
    - **2. Vasogenic** (anaphylactic, septic, endotoxic)—severe reaction to foreign protein (insect bites; drugs; toxic substances; aerobic, gram-negative organisms) → histamine release → **vasodilatation,** venous stasis → diminished venous return.
- **II. Assessment:** varies, depending on degree of shock (Table 8.1).
    - **A.** *Subjective data:*
        - **1.** Anxiety, restlessness.
        - **2.** Dizziness, fainting.
        - **3.** Thirst.
        - **4.** Nausea.
    - **B.** *Objective data:*
        - **1.** Vital signs:
            - **a.** *Blood pressure* (BP)—hypotension (postural changes in *early* shock; systolic <70 mm Hg in *late* shock).
            - **b.** *Pulse*—tachycardia; thready, irregular (**cardiogenic shock**); could be slow if conduction system of heart damaged.
            - **c.** *Respirations*—increased depth, rate; wheezing (**anaphylactic shock**).
            - **d.** *Temperature*—decreased (elevated in **septic shock**).
        - **2.** Skin:
            - **a.** Pale (or mottled), cool, clammy (warm to touch in *septic shock*).
            - **b.** Urticaria (*anaphylactic shock*).
        - **3.** Level of consciousness: alert, oriented → unresponsive.
        - **4.** Central venous pressure (CVP):
            - **a.** *Below* 5 cm H_2O with *hypovolemic* shock.
            - **b.** *Above* 15 cm H_2O with *cardiogenic*, possibly septic shock.
        - **5.** Urine output: decreased (<30 mL/h).
        - **6.** Capillary refill: slowed (Figure 8.1).
- **III. Analysis/nursing diagnosis**
    - **A.** *Altered tissue perfusion* related to vasoconstriction or decreased myocardial contractility.
    - **B.** *Impaired gas exchange* related to ventilation-perfusion imbalance.
    - **C.** *Decreased cardiac output* related to loss of circulating blood volume or diminished cardiac contractility.
    - **D.** *Altered urinary elimination* related to decreased renal perfusion.
    - **E.** *Fluid volume deficit* related to blood loss.
    - **F.** *Anxiety* related to severity of condition.
    - **G.** *Risk for injury* related to death.
- **IV. Nursing care plan/implementation**
    - Goal: *promote venous return, circulatory perfusion.*

Clinical signs of shock—skin pale, mottled, cold, and sweaty.

A. *Position:* foot of bed *elevated* 20 degrees (12–16 in.), knees straight, trunk horizontal, head slightly elevated; *avoid* Trendelenburg position.

B. Ventilation: monitor respiratory effort, loosen restrictive clothing; *oxygen* as ordered.

C. Fluids: maintain IV infusions; give *blood, plasma expanders* as ordered (exception—*stop* blood transfusion immediately in anaphylactic shock).

D. Vital signs:
  1. *CVP* (↓ with hypovolemia) arterial line, *Swan-Ganz* (↑ pulmonary artery wedge pressure, indicating cardiac failure).
  2. Urine output (insert *catheter* for hourly output).
  3. Monitor *electrocardiogram* (↑ rate, arrhythmias).

E. Medications as ordered (depending on type of shock):
  1. *Antihypotensives*—epinephrine (Adrenalin), norepinephrine (Levophed), isoproterenol (Isuprel), dopamine (Intropin).
  2. *Antiarrhythmics.*
  3. *Cardiac glycosides.*
  4. *Adrenocorticoids.*
  5. *Antibiotics.*
  6. *Vasodilators* (nitroprusside).
  7. *Beta-blockers* (dobutamine).

F. Mechanical support: military antishock trousers (*MAST*) or pneumatic antishock garment (*PASG*); used to promote internal autotransfusion of blood from legs and abdomen to central circulation; at lower pressures may control bleeding and promote hemostasis; *do not* remove (deflate) suddenly to examine underlying areas or BP will drop precipi-

tously; *compartment syndrome* may result with prolonged use and high pressure; controversial.

V. Evaluation/outcome criteria
  A. Vital signs stable, within normal limits.
  B. Alert, oriented.
  C. Urine output >30 mL/h.

🔑 Summary of Key Points

1. All types of shock alter tissue perfusion.
2. The three basic types of shock have *different causes*—*hypovolemic shock* is due to a decrease in circulatory volume; *cardiogenic shock* occurs from pump (heart) failure; and *distributive shock* results from inadequate vascular tone.
3. Urine output is an important indicator of perfusion (circulation) through the vital organs. Normal hourly output is 60 mL. A decrease below 30 mL/h should be reported.
4. Trendelenburg positioning in shock is *contraindicated.* A head-down position actually interferes with pulmonary function and may cause cerebral edema.

TABLE 8.1	SIGNS AND SYMPTOMS OF HYPOVOLEMIC SHOCK
Blood Loss	**⋈ Assessment Parameters**
<800 mL	Usually none (equivalent to donating one unit of blood)
800–1500 mL (15%–30%)	Anxiety and restlessness Pulse >100 beats/min° Systolic pressure unchanged Diastolic pressure ↑ Urine output ↓
2000 mL (30%–40%)	Pulse >120 beats/min° Respirations >30 breaths/min Systolic pressure ↓ Mental status ↓
>2500 mL (>40%)	Pulse >120 beats/min° Respirations >30 breaths/min Narrow pulse pressure (= systolic − diastolic) Cold, clammy skin

° In some cases of abdominal trauma, there is shock without a rapid pulse.

Adapted from Caroline N. *Emergency Care in the Streets* (5th ed). Boston: Little, Brown, 1995. P 194.

FIGURE 8.1   Capillary refill test. (A) Press on the fingernail until it blanches. (B) Then release the pressure. The skin under the nail should "pink up" within 2 seconds if the patient is normally perfused. (From Caroline NL. *Emergency Care in the Streets* [5th ed]. Boston: Little, Brown, 1995.)

💡 Study and Memory Aids

💊 Drug Review

Shock:

Antiarrhythmics (some of the drugs used)
Bretylium (Bretylol): 5mg/kg bolus over 15–30 sec, not to exceed 30 mg/kg/d
Lidocaine HCl: IV, 50–100 mg (1 mg/kg) bolus; may be repeated in 5 min, then 1–4 mg/kg/min infusion (no more than 200–300 mg/h)
Procainamide (Pronestyl): 100 mg IV q 5 m until arrhythmia suppressed
Quinidine: 400–600 mg PO q2–3h, not to exceed 4 g/d

Antibiotics (to control infection)
Cephalexin (Keflex): 250–500 mg PO q6h
Cephalothin (Keflin): IV, 0.5–2 g q4–6h
Erythromycin: 250–500 mg PO q6–12h
Gentamicin (Garamycin): 3–5 mg/kg/d in divided doses
Penicillin G: 1.2 million U in single IM dose

Antihypotensives
Epinephrine (Adrenalin): 0.1–1 mg IV (1–10 ml of 1:10,000 concentration) may repeat q5–15 min
Isoproterenol (Isuprel): IV, 0.5–5 mcg/min 0.25–2.5 ml of 1:500,000 dilution
Norepinephrine (Levophed): 8–12 mcg/min IV; adjust rate of flow to maintain BP

Beta-Ac blockers agents
Atenolol (Tenorim): 25–50 mg/d
Dobutamine (Dobutrex): IV, 2.5–15 mcg/kg/min
Dopamine (Intropin): IV, 0.5–5 mcg/kg/min initially, increase at 10–30 m intervals to 50 mcg/kg/m
Metoprolol (Lopressor): 100–450 mg/d
Propranolol (Inderal): 40 mg bid

Cardiac glyosides
Digoxin (Lanoxin): digitalizing dose—IV, 0.6–1 mg over 24-h, or PO, 10–15 μg/kg over 24 h; maintenance dose, 0.125–03.75 mg/d (Take apical pulse before administering drug)

Glucocorticoids
Cortisone (Cortone): 20–300 mg/d
Dexamethasone (Decadron): 0.75–9 mg/d in single or divided doses
Methylprednisolone (Medrol): 4–48 mg/d
Prednisone (Deltasone): 5–60 mg/d

Vasodilators
Hydralazine (Apresoline): 10 mg qid for 2–4d. Increase to 25 mg q.i.d. for first week. 50 mg q.i.d. maintenance dose.
Nitroprusside (Nitropress): IV, 0.3–10 mcg/kg/min, not to exceed 10 min of therapy at 10 mcg/kg/min

Questions

1. A patient is experiencing a hemolytic transfusion reaction. Which planned nursing action should be questioned?
   1. Hanging new tubing and infusing saline.
   2. Raising the head and foot of the bed.
   3. Inserting an indwelling urinary catheter.
   4. Drawing a blood sample from the IV site.

2. What desired effects of subcutaneously administered epinephrine should the nurse watch for in a patient given this agent to manage an anaphylactic reaction?
   1. Vasodilatation and bronchodilatation.
   2. Vasodilatation and bronchoconstriction.
   3. Vasoconstriction and bronchodilatation.
   4. Vasoconstriction and bronchoconstriction.

3. Which change in a vital sign observed after surgery would require further assessment for indications of hypovolemic shock?
   1. Heart rate of 110 beats/min.
   2. Increasing diastolic pressure.
   3. Widening pulse pressure.
   4. Respiratory rate of 10 breaths/min.

4. Blood and fluid loss resulting from frequent diarrhea may cause hypovolemia. The fastest way for a nurse to assess for volume depletion is to:
   1. Measure the quantity and specific gravity of urine.
   2. Take the patient's blood pressure with the patient supine, then sitting, and noting the resultant change.
   3. Compare the patient's present weight with the weight 6 months ago.
   4. Administer the oral water test.

5. Four hours after coronary artery bypass surgery, a patient's blood pressure is 90/46 mm Hg and the central venous pressure is 6 cm H_2O; 300 mL of bloody fluid has drained from the mediastinal chest tube in the past hour. The nurse knows the patient would most likely need which measure?
   1. Milking of the mediastinal chest tube.
   2. A transfusion to replace blood loss.
   3. Premedication for a pericardiocentesis.
   4. A sodium nitroprusside (Nipride) IV push, as ordered.

Answers/Rationale

1. **(4)** A hemolytic transfusion reaction occurs as the result of the infusion of ABO incompatible blood, and any blood obtained from the IV site will be hemolyzed; that is, the red blood cells will be destroyed. The results of any laboratory test or such a blood sample would be abnormal. The extent of hemolysis will need to be determined using a sample drawn from *another* large peripheral vein with a large (19)–gauge needle. The tubing needs to be changed completely and a saline infusion *should* be started **(1)** to prevent any additional incompatible blood from being infused. Symptoms of the transfusion reaction usually include hypotension and respiratory distress, so elevation of the patient's head and feet **(2)** *will* help relieve the symptoms. A catheter *should* be in-

serted, if it is not already in place, to assess for any renal damage stemming from the reaction **(3)**. **PL, 6, PhI**

2. **(3)** Anaphylaxis causes bronchospasm and hypotension. By means of its adrenergic effects, epinephrine produces bronchodilation, which will relieve the breathing difficulty, and increases the blood pressure through vasoconstriction. Options **1, 2,** and **4** are incorrect because they include *vasodilatation* or broncho*constriction,* neither of which would be desirable in a patient in anaphylactic shock. **EV, 6, PhI**

3. **(1)** Tachycardia occurring postoperatively may indicate the development of hypovolemic shock and hypoxia, though it can also occur with pain. It would be important to look for a drop in the systolic pressure initially indicating decreased volume, followed by a decrease, not an increase, in the diastolic pressure **(2)**. The pulse pressure will initially narrow in hypovolemic shock. A widening pulse pressure **(3)** is seen in the presence of increased intracranial pressure. If the patient is experiencing hypovolemic shock and hypoxia, the respiratory rate would exceed the normal rate of 12 to 16 breaths/min. A rate of 10 breaths/min **(4)** is a slow normal one. **AN, 6, PhI**

4. **(2)** Taking a patient's vital signs supine, then sitting, will reveal the presence of postural blood pressure changes. If the patient is hypovolemic, the pressure will drop by 20 to 30 mm Hg systolic when the patient sits up. If the patient is volume depleted, the urine output **(1)** will most likely be diminished and *less frequent,* so urine output would not be a rapid way to assess volume status. Although body weight **(3)** is an excellent indicator of hydration status, it would take time to find out the prior weight. The oral water test **(4)** is a test for Addison's disease that involves the rapid intake of a large quantity of water. A normal diuresis does not occur in patient's with the disease. **AS, 6, PhI**

5. **(2)** The vital signs are indicative of hypovolemia, and the chest tube drainage is excessive for 1 hour. Judging by the large amount of fluid that has drained, the tube appears to be draining. Milking **(1)** is done if the tube is *not* draining and usually is not needed with mediastinal chest tubes. Pericardiocentesis **(3)** is done to remove blood that is collecting in the pericardium; this is not necessary in this patient because blood is draining profusely. Nipride **(4)** is a potent vasodilator and is used to treat malignant *hypertension;* this patient is hypotensive. **AN, 6, PhI**

Key to Codes

Nursing process: AS, assessment; **AN,** analysis; **PL,** planning; **IMP,** implementation; **EV,** evaluation. (See Appendix M for explanation of nursing process steps.)

Category of human function: 1, protective; **2,** sensory-perceptual; **3,** comfort, rest, activity, and mobility; **4,** nutrition; **5,** growth and development; **6,** fluid-gas transport; **7,** psychosocial-cultural; **8,** elimination. (See Appendix O for explanation.)

Client need: SECE, safe, effective care environment; **PhI,** physiologic integrity; **PsI,** psychosocial Integrity; **HPM,** health promotion/maintenance. (See Appendix P for explanation.)

Perioperative Nursing

Chapter Outline

- Preoperative Preparation
  - Teaching
  - Skin preparation
  - Gastrointestinal tract preparation
  - Day of surgery
- Intraoperative Preparation
  - Regional anesthesia
  - General anesthesia
  - Muscle relaxant
  - Hypothermia
- Postoperative Experience
  - Immediate post anesthesia nursing care
  - General postoperative nursing care
    Postoperative complications
- Review of Use of Common Tubes
- Positioning the Patient for Specific Surgical Conditions
- Summary of Key Points
- Study and Memory Aids
- Drug Review
- Questions
- Answers/Rationale

Preoperative Preparation

⋈ **I. Assessment**

  A. *Subjective data:*
  1. Understanding of proposed surgery—site, type, extent of hospitalization.
  2. Previous experiences with hospitalization.
  3. Concerns or feelings about surgery:
     a. Exaggerated ideas of surgical risk (e.g., fear of colostomy when none is being considered).
     b. Nature of anesthesia, e.g., fears of going to sleep and not waking up, saying or revealing things of a personal nature.
     c. Degree of pain, e.g., may be incapacitating.
     d. Misunderstandings regarding prognosis.
  4. Identification of significant others as a source of patient support and/or care responsibilities after discharge.

  B. *Objective data:*
  1. Speech patterns indicating anxiety—repetition, changing topics, avoiding talking about feelings.
  2. Interactions with others—withdrawn or involved.
  3. Physical signs of anxiety, i.e., increased pulse, respirations; clammy palms; restlessness.
  4. *Baseline physiologic status:* vital signs, breath sounds, peripheral circulation, weight, hydra-

〰️ tion status (hematocrit, skin turgor, urine output), degree of mobility, muscle strength.

⋈ **II. Analysis/nursing diagnosis**

  A. *Anxiety* related to proposed surgery.
  B. *Knowledge deficit* related to incomplete teaching or lack of understanding.
  C. *Fear* related to threat of death or disfigurement.
  D. *Risk for injury* related to surgical complications.
  E. *Ineffective individual coping* related to anticipatory stress.

⋈ **III. Nursing care plan/implementation**

  A. Goal: *reduce preoperative and intraoperative anxiety and prevent postoperative complications.*
  1. *Preoperative* **teaching:**
     a. Provide information about hospital and nursing routines to reduce fear of unknown.
     b. Explain purpose of diagnostic procedures to enhance ability to cooperate and tolerate procedure.
     c. What will occur and what will be expected in the postoperative period:
        (1) Will return to room, recovery room, or intensive care unit.
        (2) Special equipment—monitors, tubes, suction equipment.

  ☞ **B.** Goal: *instruct in exercises to reduce complications.*
  1. **Diaphragmatic breathing**—refers to flattening of diaphragm during inspiration, which results in enlargement of upper abdomen;

during expiration the abdominal muscles are contracted, along with the diaphragm.
  a. The patient should be in a *flat, semi-Fowler's,* or *side* position, with knees flexed and hands on the midabdomen.
  b. Have the patient take a deep breath through nose and mouth, letting the abdomen rise.
  c. Have patient exhale through nose and mouth, squeezing out all air by contracting the abdominal muscles.
  d. Repeat 10–15 times, with a short rest after each five to prevent hyperventilation.
  e. Inform patient that this exercise will be repeated 5–10 times every hour postoperatively.
2. **Coughing**—helps clear chest of secretions and, although uncomfortable, will not harm incision.
  a. Have patient lean forward slightly from a sitting position, and place patient's hands over incisional site; this acts as a splint during coughing.
  b. Have patient inhale and exhale several times.
  c. Have patient inhale deeply and cough sharply three times as exhaling—patient's mouth should be slightly open.
  d. Tell patient to inhale again and to cough deeply once or twice.
3. **Turning and leg exercises**—help prevent circulatory stasis, which may lead to thrombus formation and postoperative flatus, or "gas pains," as well as respiratory problems.
  a. Tell patient to turn on one *side* with uppermost leg flexed; use siderails to facilitate the movement.
  b. In a *supine position,* have patient bend the knee and lift the foot; this position should be held for a few seconds, then the leg should be extended and lowered; repeat five times, and do the same with the other leg.
  c. Teach patient to move each foot through full range of motion (ROM).
C. Goal: *reduce the number of bacteria on the skin to eliminate incision contamination.*
  Skin preparation:
  1. Prepare area of skin wider and longer than proposed incision in case a larger incision is necessary.
  2. Gently scrub with an antiseptic agent such as povidone-iodine (Betadine). Note possibility of allergy to iodine.
    a. Hexachlorophene should be left on the skin for 5–10 min.
    b. If benzalkonium chloride (Zephiran) solution is ordered, do *not* soap skin prior to use; soap reduces effectiveness of benzalkonium by causing it to precipitate.

3. Note any nicks, cuts, or irritations, potential infection sites.
4. Opinions differ on hair removal—may leave hair.
5. Clipping of hair or electric razor may be ordered; lower rate of infection.
6. Skin preparation may be done in surgery.
D. Goal: *reduce the risk of vomiting and aspiration during anesthesia; prevent contamination of abdominal operative sites by fecal material.*
  Gastrointestinal tract preparation:
  1. *No* food or fluid for at least 6–8 h before surgery.
  2. Remove food and water from bedside.
  3. Place NPO signs on bed or door.
  4. Inform kitchen and oncoming nursing staff that patient is NPO for surgery.
  5. Give *IV* infusions up to time of surgery if dehydrated or malnourished.
  6. *Enemas:* two or three may be given the evening prior to intestinal, colon, or pelvic surgeries; 3 d of cleansing with large-intestine procedures.
  7. Possible antibiotic therapy to reduce colonic flora with large-bowel surgery.
  8. Gastric or intestinal intubation may be done the evening prior to major abdominal surgery.
    a. **Types of tubes:**
      (1) *Levin:* single lumen; sufficient to remove fluids and gas from stomach; suction may damage mucosa.
      (2) *Salem-sump:* large lumen; prevents tissue-wall adherence.
      (3) *Miller-Abbott:* long single or double lumen; required to remove the contents of jejunum or ileum.
    b. Pressures: *low* setting with Levin and intestinal tubes, *high* setting with Salem-sump; excessive pressures will result in injury to mucosal lining of intestine or stomach.
E. Goal: *promote rest and reduce apprehension.*
  1. Medications as ordered: evening prior to surgery may give barbiturate—pentobarbital (Nembutal), secobarbital (Seconal).
  2. Quiet environment: eliminate noises, distractions.
  3. *Position:* reduce muscle tension.
  4. Back rub.
F. Goal: *protect from injury; ensure final preparation for surgery.*
  Day of surgery:
  1. Operative permit signed and on chart; physician responsible for obtaining informed consent.
  2. Shower or bathe.
    a. Dress: hospital gown.
    b. Remove: hair pins (cover hair); nail polish, to facilitate observation of peripheral circulation; jewelry (tape wedding bands securely); pierced earrings; contact lenses; dentures (store and give mouth care); if

patient objects, remove in OR; give valuable personal items to family; chart disposition of items. (See Table 9.1 for care of dentures.)

3. Proper identification—check band for secureness and legibility.
4. Vital signs—baseline data.
5. Void, to prevent distention and possible injury to bladder.
6. Give preoperative medication, to ensure smooth induction and maintenance of anesthesia:
   a. Administered 45–75 min before anesthetic induction.
   b. Siderails up (patient will begin to feel drowsy and light-headed).
   c. Expect complaint of dry mouth if atropine sulfate given.
   d. Observe for side effects—morphine sulfate and meperidine HCl (Demerol) may cause nausea and vomiting or drop in blood pressure.
   e. Quiet environment until transported to operating room.
7. Note completeness of chart:
   a. Surgical checklist completed.
   b. Vital signs recorded.
   c. Routine laboratory reports present.
   d. Preoperative medications given.
   e. Significant patient observations.
8. Assist patient's family in finding proper waiting room.
   a. Inform them that the surgeon will contact them after the procedure is over.
   b. Explain length of time patient is expected to be in post-anesthesia recovery room.
   c. Prepare family for any special equipment or devices that may be needed to care for

patient postoperatively—oxygen, monitoring equipment, ventilator, or blood transfusions.

Intraoperative Preparation

Anesthesia: blocks transmission of nerve impulses, suppresses reflexes, promotes muscle relaxation, and in some instances, achieves reversible unconsciousness.

I. **Regional anesthesia**—purpose is to block pain reception and transmission in a specified area. Commonly used drugs are lidocaine HCl, tetracaine HCl, cocaine HCl, and procaine HCl. Types of regional anesthetics:
   A. *Topical*—applied to mucous membranes or skin; drug anesthetizes the nerves immediately *below* the area. May be used for bronchoscopic or laryngoscopic examinations. *Side effects:* rare anaphylaxis.
   B. *Local infiltration*—used for minor procedures; anesthetic drug is injected directly into the area to be incised, manipulated, or sutured. *Side effects:* rare anaphylaxis.
   C. *Peripheral nerve block*—regional anesthesia is achieved by injecting drug into or around a nerve after it passes from vertebral column; procedure is named for nerve involved, such as *brachial plexus block*. Requires a high degree of anatomic knowledge. *Side effects:* may be absorbed into bloodstream. Observe for signs of excitability, twitching, changes in vital signs, or respiratory difficulties.
   D. *Field block*—a group of nerves is injected with anesthetic as the nerves branch from a major or main nerve trunk. May be used for dental procedures, plastic surgery. *Side effects:* rare.
   E. *Epidural anesthesia*—anesthetic is injected into the epidural space of vertebral canal; produces a bandlike anesthesia around body. Frequently used in obstetrics. Rare complications.
   F. *Spinal anesthesia*—anesthetic is injected into the subarachnoid space and mixes with spinal fluid; drug acts on the nerves as they emerge from the spinal cord, thereby inhibiting conduction in the autonomic, sensory, and motor systems.
      1. *Advantages:* rapid onset; produces excellent muscle relaxation.
      2. *Utilization:* surgery on lower limbs, perineum, and lower abdomen.
      3. *Disadvantages:*
         a. Loss of sensation below point of injection for 2–8 h—watch for signs of *bladder distention;* prevent injuries by maintaining alignment, keeping bedclothes straightened.
         b. Patient awake during surgical procedure—*avoid* light or upsetting conversations.
         c. Leakage of spinal fluid from puncture site—keep *flat in bed* for 8 h to prevent head-

---

TABLE 9.1   ☞ CARE OF DENTURES

Wear gloves.

If patient cannot remove own dentures, grasp upper plate at the front teeth and move up and down gently to release suction.

Lift the lower plate up one side at a time.

Use extreme care not to damage dentures while cleaning.

Use tepid, *not* hot, water to clean.

Avoid soaking for long periods.

Inspect for sharp edges.

Do oral cavity assessment.

Replace moistened dentures in patient's mouth.

Use appropriately labeled container for storage when dentures are to remain out of patient's mouth.

Source: Lagerquist SL: *Little, Brown's NCLEX-RN Examination Review.* Boston: Little, Brown, 1996. P. 310.

ache. Keep well hydrated to promote spinal fluid replacement.

  d. Depression of vasomotor responses—frequent checks of vital signs.

 G. *Intravenous regional anesthesia*—used in an extremity whose circulation has been interrupted by a tourniquet; the anesthetic is injected into vein, and blockage is presumed to be achieved from extravascular leakage of anesthetic near a major nerve trunk. Precautions: same as for peripheral nerve block.

II. General anesthesia—a reversible state in which the patient loses consciousness due to the inhibition of neuronal impulses in the brain by a variety of chemical agents; may be given intravenously, by inhalation, or rectally.

 A. *Side effects:*

  1. Respiratory depression.

  2. Nausea, vomiting.

  3. Excitement.

  4. Restlessness.

  5. Laryngospasm.

  6. Hypotension.

 B. Nursing care plan/implementation—Goal: *prevent hazardous drug interactions.*

  1. *Notify anesthesiologist* if patient is taking any of the following drugs:

   a. *Antibiotics,* such as neomycin sulfate, streptomycin sulfate, polymyxin A and B sulfate, colistin sulfate, and kanamycin sulfate—when mixed with curariform muscle relaxant, they interrupt nerve transmission and may cause *respiratory paralysis and apnea.*

   b. *Antidepressants*—particularly MAO (monoamine oxidase inhibitors), which increase *hypotensive* effects of anesthetic agents.

   c. *Diuretics*—particularly thiazide diuretics, which may induce *potassium depletion;* a potassium deficit may lead to *respiratory depression* during anesthesia.

   d. *Antihypertensives,* such as reserpine, hydralazine, and methyldopa—*potentiate* the hypotensive effects of anesthetic agents.

   e. *Anticoagulants,* such as heparin, warfarin (Coumadin)—increase bleeding times, which may result in excessive *blood loss* and/or hemorrhage.

   f. *Aspirin*—decreases platelet aggregation and may result in increased *bleeding.*

   g. *Steroids,* such as cortisone—anti-inflammatory effect may *delay* wound healing.

  2. *Stages of inhalation anesthesia and nursing goals:*

   a. *Stage I*—extends from beginning of induction to loss of consciousness. *Nursing goal: reduce external stimuli,* as all movement and noises are exaggerated for the patient and can be highly distressing.

   b. *Stage II*—extends from loss of consciousness to relaxation; stage of delirium and excitement. *Nursing goal: prevent injury* by

helping anesthesiologist *restrain* patient if necessary; maintain a quiet, nonstimulating environment.

   c. *Stage III*—extends from loss of lid reflex to cessation of voluntary respirations. *Nursing goal: reduce risk of untoward effects* by preparing the operative site, assisting with procedures, and observing for signs of complications.

   d. *Stage IV*—indicates overdose and consists of respiratory arrest and vasomotor collapse due to medullary paralysis. *Nursing goal: promote restoration of ventilation and vasomotor tone* by assisting with cardiac arrest procedures and by administering cardiac stimulants or narcotic antagonists as ordered.

III. Muscle relaxants—given to supplement general anesthetic agents, i.e., curare, succinyl-choline chloride (Anectine).

 A. *Actions:*

  1. Facilitates endotracheal intubation.

  2. Relaxes abdominal muscles.

  3. Facilitates the administration of lower doses of potent general anesthetic.

 B. Nursing care plan/implementation

  1. Goal: *observe for respiratory depression*—respiratory rate >30 breaths/min, shallow, quiet, use of accessory muscles.

  2. Goal: *document observations.*

IV. Hypothermia—a specialized procedure in which the patient's body temperature is lowered to 28°–30°C (82°–86°F).

 A. Reduces tissue metabolism and oxygen requirements.

 B. Used in heart surgery, brain surgery, and surgery on major blood vessels.

 C. Nursing care plan/implementation

  1. Goal: *prevent complications:*

   a. Monitor vital signs for shock.

   b. Note levels of consciousness.

   c. Record intake and output (I&O) accurately.

   d. Maintain good body alignment; reposition to prevent edema, pressure, or discoloration of skin.

   e. Maintain patent IV.

  2. Goal: *promote comfort.*

   a. Apply blankets to rewarm and prevent shivering.

   b. Mouth care.

V. General evaluation/outcome criteria: complete reversal of anesthetic effects (e.g., spontaneous respirations, pupils react to light).

Postoperative Experience

I. Assessment

 A. *Subjective data:*

  1. Pain: location, onset, intensity.

  2. Nausea.

B. *Objective data:*
   1. Operative summary:
      a. Type of operation performed.
      b. Pathologic findings, if known.
      c. Anesthesia and medications received.
      d. Problems during surgery that will affect recovery, (e.g., arrhythmias, bleeding [estimated blood loss]).
      e. Fluids received: type, amount.
      f. Need for drainage or suction apparatus.
   2. Observations:
      a. Patency of airway.
      b. Vital signs.
      c. Skin color and dryness.
      d. Level of consciousness.
      e. Status of reflexes.
      f. Dressings.
      g. Type and rate of IV infusion and blood transfusion.
      h. Tubes/drains: urinary, chest, Penrose, Hemovac; note color and amount of drainage.

II. Analysis/nursing diagnosis
   A. *Ineffective breathing pattern* related to general anesthesia.
   B. *Ineffective airway clearance* related to absent or weak cough.
   C. *Risk for aspiration* related to vomiting.
   D. *Pain* related to surgical incision.
   E. *Altered tissue perfusion* related to shock.
   F. *Risk for fluid volume deficit* related to blood loss.
   G. *Risk for injury* related to disorientation.
   H. *Risk for infection* related to disruption of skin integrity.
   I. *Urinary retention* related to anesthetic effects.
   J. *Constipation* related to decreased peristalsis.

III. Nursing care plan/implementation—Immediate postanesthesia nursing care: refers to time following surgery that is usually spent in the recovery room (1–2 h).
   A. Goal: *promote a safe, quiet, nonstressful environment.*
      1. Siderails up at all times.
      2. Nurse in constant attendance.
   B. Goal: *promote lung expansion and gas exchange.*
   C. Goal: *prevent aspiration and atelectasis.*
      1. *Position:* side or back, with head turned to side to prevent obstruction of airway by tongue; allows for drainage from mouth.
      2. *Airway:* leave the oropharyngeal or nasopharyngeal airway in place until patient awakens and begins to eject; gagging and vomiting may occur if not removed before pharyngeal reflex returns. Snoring is obstructed breathing.
      3. After removal of airway: turn on side in a *lateral position;* support upper arm with pillow.
      4. *Suction:* remove excessive secretions from mouth and pharynx.
      5. Encourage coughing and deep breathing: aids in upward movement of secretions.
      6. Give humidified *oxygen* as necessary: reduces respiratory irritation and keeps bronchotracheal secretions soft and moist.

   7. *Mechanical ventilation:* Bird or Bennet respirators if needed (see Ventilators in Chap. 6, pp. 76–77).
   D. Goal: *promote and maintain cardiovascular function.*
      1. Vital signs, as ordered: usually q15min until stable.
         a. Compare with preoperative vital signs.
         b. Immediately report: systolic blood pressure that *drops 20 mm Hg or more,* a pressure *below 80 mm Hg,* or a pressure that continually drops 5–10 mm Hg over several readings; pulse rates *under 60* or *over 110* beats/min, or irregularities; respirations *over* 30 breaths/min; becoming shallow, quiet, slow; use of neck and diaphragm muscles (symptoms of *respiratory depression*).
      2. Observe for other alterations in circulatory function—pallor; thready pulse; cold, moist skin; decreased urine output; restlessness.
         a. *Immediately report* to physician.
         b. Initiate *oxygen* therapy.
         c. Place patient in *shock position* unless contraindicated—feet elevated 20 degrees, legs/knees straight, head *slightly* elevated to increase venous return.
      3. *Intravenous* infusions: time, rate, orders for added medications.
      4. Monitor blood transfusions, if ordered: observe for signs of *reaction* (chills, elevated temperature, urticaria, laryngeal edema, wheezing); usually first 15–20 min. Table 9.2, p. 120, summarizes the nursing care plan/implementation.
      5. If reaction occurs, immediately stop transfusion and notify physician. Send stat urine to lab.
   E. Goal: *promote psychological equilibrium.*
      1. Reassure on awakening—orient frequently.
      2. Explain procedures even though patient does not appear alert.
      3. Answer patient's questions briefly and accurately.
      4. Maintain quiet, restful environment.
      5. Comfort measures:
         a. Good body alignment.
         b. Support dependent extremities to *avoid* pressure areas and possible nerve damage.
         c. Check for constriction: dressings, clothing, bedding.
         d. Check IV sites frequently for patency and signs of infiltration (swelling, blanching, cool to touch).
   F. Goal: *maintain proper function of tubes and apparatus.* (See Tubes Box at end of chap.).

IV. General postoperative nursing care: refers to period from admission to the general nursing unit until anticipated recovery and discharge from the hospital. See Table 9.2 for a review of postoperative complications and positioning the patient for specific surgical indications (see Positioning box at end of chapter).

TABLE 9.2   POSTOPERATIVE COMPLICATIONS

Condition and Etiology	⋈ Assessment: Signs and Symptoms	⋈ Nursing Care Plan/ Implementation
Respiratory Complications—Most Common Are Atelectasis, Pneumonias (Lobar, Bronchial, and Hypostatic), and Pleuritis; Other Complications Are Hemothorax and Pneumothorax.		
Atelectasis—undetected preoperative upper respiratory tract infections, aspiration of vomitus; irritation of the tracheobronchial tree with increased mucous secretions due to intubation and inhalation anesthesia, a history of heavy smoking, or chronic obstructive pulmonary disease; severe postoperative pain or high abdominal or thoracic surgery, which inhibits deep breathing; and debilitation or old age, which lowers the patient's resistance.	Dyspnea; ↑ temperature; absent or diminished breath sounds over affected area; asymmetric chest expansion; ↑ respirations and pulse rate; tracheal shift to affected side when severe; anxiety and restlessness.	1. *Position:* unaffected side. 2. Turn, cough, and deep breathe. ☞ 3. Postural drainage. ☞ 4. Nebulization 5. *Force* fluids, if not contraindicated.
Pneumonia—see **Atelectasis** for etiology.	Rapid, shallow, painful respirations; crackles; diminished or absent breath sounds; asymmetric lung expansion; chills and fever; productive cough, rust-colored sputum; circumoral and nailbed cyanosis.	1. *Position* of comfort—semi- to high Fowler's. 2. *Force* fluids to 3000 mL/d. ☞ 3. Humidification of air and *oxygen* therapy. ☞ 4. Oropharyngeal *suction* prn. 5. Assist during coughing. ⬤ 6. Administer antibiotics and analgesics, as ordered. ▪ 7. *Diet:* high calorie, as tolerated. 8. Cautious disposal of secretions; proper oral hygiene.
Pleuritis—see **Atelectasis** for etiology.	Knifelike chest pain on inspiration; intercostal tenderness; splinting of chest by patient; rapid, shallow respirations; pleural friction rub; ↑ temperature; malaise.	1. *Position: affected* side to splint the chest. ☞ 2. Manually splint patient's chest during cough. ☞ 3. Apply binder or adhesive strapping, as ordered. ⬤ 4. Administer analgesics, as ordered.
Hemothorax—chest surgery, gunshot or knife wounds, and multiple fractures of the chest wall.	Chest pain, increased respiratory rate, dyspnea; decreased or absent breath sounds, decreased blood pressure, tachycardia, mediastinal shift may occur (heart, trachea, esophagus, and great vessels are pushed toward unaffected side).	1. Observe vital signs closely for signs of shock and respiratory distress. 〰 2. Assist with *thoracentesis* (needle aspiration of fluid). ☞ 3. Assist with insertion of thoracotomy tube to closed-chest drainage (see care of *water-sealed drainage* system Chap. 6).

(continued)

TABLE 9.2   POSTOPERATIVE COMPLICATIONS (*Continued*)

Condition and Etiology	⋈ *Assessment: Signs and Symptoms*	⋈ *Nursing Care Plan/ Implementation*
Pneumothorax, *closed or tension* —thoracentesis (needle nicks the lung), rupture of alveoli or bronchi due to accidental injury, and chronic obstructive lung disease.	Marked dyspnea, sudden sharp chest pain, subcutaneous emphysema (air in chest wall tissue); cyanosis; tracheal shift to unaffected side; hyperresonance on percussion, decreased or absent breath sounds; increased respiratory rate, tachycardia; asymmetric chest expansion, feeling of pressure within chest; *mediastinal shift*—severe dyspnea and cyanosis, deviation of larynx and trachea toward unaffected side, deviation either medially or laterally of apex of heart, decreased blood pressure; distended neck veins; increased pulse and respirations.	1. Remain with patient—keep as calm and quiet as possible. 2. *Position:* high Fowler's (sitting). 3. Notify physician through another nurse, and have thoracentesis equipment brought to bedside. 4. Administer *oxygen* as necessary. 5. Take vital signs to evaluate respiratory and cardiac function. 6. Assist with *thoracentesis.* 7. Assist with initiation and maintenance of *closed-chest* drainage.
Circulatory Complications		
Shock—hemorrhage, sepsis, decreased cardiac contractility (myocardial infarction, cardiac failure, tamponade), drug sensitivities, transfusion reactions, pulmonary embolism, and emotional reaction to pain or deep fear.	Dizziness, fainting, restlessness, anxiety. *Blood pressure:* ↓ or falling. *Pulse:* weak, thready. *Respirations:* ↑, shallow. *Skin:* pale, cool, clammy, cyanotic. *Temperature:* ↓. *GU: oliguria* CVP < 5 cm/H_2O Thirst	1. *Position:* foot of bed raised 20 degrees, knees straight, trunk horizontal, head slightly elevated; *avoid* Trendelenburg's position. 2. Administer *blood* transfusions, plasma expanders, and intravenous infusions as ordered; medications specific to type of shock. 3. Check: vital signs, *CVP,* temperature. 4. Insert urinary *catheter* to monitor hourly urine output. 5. Administer *oxygen,* as ordered.
Thrombophlebitis—injury to vein wall by tight leg straps or leg holders during gynecologic surgery; hemoconcentration due to dehydration or fluid loss; stasis of blood in extremities due to postoperative circulatory depression.	Calf pain or cramping, redness and swelling (the left leg is affected more frequently than the right), slight fever, chills, Homans' sign and tenderness over the anteromedian surface of thigh.	1. Maintain complete bed rest, *avoiding positions* that restrict venous return. 2. Apply elastic stockings or wrap legs from toes to groin with elastic bandages to prevent swelling and pooling of venous blood. 3. Apply warm, moist soaks to area, as ordered. 4. Administer anticoagulants, as ordered. 5. Use bed cradle over affected limb. 6. Perform active and passive ROM exercises on unaffected limb.

(*continued*)

TABLE 9.2　　POSTOPERATIVE COMPLICATIONS (*Continued*)

Condition and Etiology	Assessment: Signs and Symptoms	Nursing Care Plan/ Implementation
Pulmonary embolism—obstruction of a pulmonary artery by a foreign body in bloodstream, usually a blood clot that has been dislodged from its original site.	*Sudden*, severe stabbing chest pain; *severe* dyspnea; cyanosis; *rapid* pulse; anxiety and apprehension; pupillary dilation; *profuse diaphoresis; loss* of consciousness.	1. Administer *oxygen* and *inhalants* while patient is *sitting upright*. 2. Maintain *bed rest* and frequent reassurance. 3. Administer heparin sodium, as ordered. 4. Administer analgesics, such as morphine sulfate, to reduce pain and apprehension.
Wound Complications		
Wound infection—*obesity* or *undernutrition*, particularly protein and vitamin deficiencies; *decreased* antibody production in aged; *decreased* phagocytosis in newborn; metabolic disorder, such as diabetes mellitus, Cushing's syndrome, malignancies, and shock; breakdown in aseptic technique.	Redness, tenderness, and heat in area of incision; wound drainage; ↑ temperature; ↑ pulse rate.	1. Assist in *cleansing* and irrigation of *wound* and insertion of a drain. 2. Apply hot, wet *dressings* as ordered. 3. Give antibiotics as ordered; observe responses.
Wound dehiscence and evisceration—obesity and undernutrition, particularly protein and vitamin C deficiencies; immunosuppression; metabolic disorders; cancer; liver disease; common site is midline abdominal incision, frequently about 7 d postoperatively; precipitating factors include abdominal distention, vomiting, coughing, hiccups, and uncontrolled motor activity.	Slow parting of wound edges with a gush of pinkish serous drainage or rapid parting with coils of intestines escaping onto the abdominal wall, the latter accompanied by pain and often by vomiting.	1. *Position:* bed rest, low Fowler's or horizontal position; knees flexed. 2. Notify physician stat. 3. Cover exposed coils of intestines with sterile towels or dressing and keep moist with sterile normal saline. 4. Monitor vital signs frequently. 5. Remain with patient, reassure that physician is coming. 6. Prepare for physician's arrival; set up IV, suction equipment, and NG tube; obtain sterile gown, mask, gloves, towels, and warmed normal saline. 7. Notify surgery that patient will be returning to operating room.
Urinary Complications		
Urinary retention—obstruction in bladder or urethra, neurologic disease, mechanical trauma as in childbirth or gynecologic surgery, psychological conditioning that inhibits voiding in bed, prolonged bed rest, pain with lower abdominal surgery.	Inability to void *10–18* h after surgery, despite adequate fluid replacement; palpable bladder; frequent voiding of small amounts of urine or dribbling; suprapubic pain.	1. Assist patient to stand or use bedside commode, if not contraindicated. 2. Provide privacy. 3. Reduce tension, provide support. 4. Use warm bedpan. 5. Run tap water. 6. Place patient's feet in warm water. 7. Pour warm water over perineum. 8. Catheterize if conservative measures fail.

(continued)

TABLE 9.2   POSTOPERATIVE COMPLICATIONS (*Continued*)

Condition and Etiology	▶ Assessment: Signs and Symptoms	▶ Nursing Care Plan/ Implementation
Urinary tract infections—urinary retention, bladder distention, repeated or prolonged catheterization.	*Urinary:* burning and frequency. *Pain:* low back or flank. Pyuria, hematuria; ↑ temperature, chills; anorexia; positive urine ⎍⎍⎍ *culture*.	1. *Push fluids* to 3000 mL daily, unless contraindicated. 2. *Avoid* stimulants such as caffeine. 3. Give antibiotics, sulfonamides, or acidifying agents, as ordered. 4. Give perianal care after each bowel movement.
Gastrointestinal Complications		
Gastric distention—depressed gastric motility due to sympathoadrenal stress response; idiosyncrasy to drugs; emotions, pain, shock; fluid and electrolyte imbalances.	Feeling of fullness; hiccups; overflow vomiting of dark, foul-smelling liquid; severe retention leads to decreased blood pressure (due to pressure on vagus nerve) and other symptoms of shock syndrome.	1. Report signs to physician *immediately*. 2. Insert or assist in insertion of *NG* tube; attach to intermittent suction. 3. Irrigate NG tube with *saline* (water will deplete electrolytes and result in metabolic alkalosis). 4. Administer IV infusions with electrolytes, as ordered.
Paralytic ileus—see **Gastric distention.**	Greatly decreased or absent bowel sounds; failure of either gas or feces to be passed by rectum; nausea and vomiting; abdominal tenderness, and distention; fever; dehydration.	1. Notify physician. 2. Insert or assist with insertion of *NG* tube; attach to low, intermittent suction. 3. Insert *rectal* tube. 4. Administer IV infusion with electrolytes, as ordered. 5. Irrigate NG tube with saline. 6. Assist with insertion of *Miller-Abbott* tube, if indicated. 7. Administer medications to increase peristalsis, as ordered.
Intestinal obstruction—due to poorly functioning anastomosis, hernia, adhesions, fecal impaction.	Severe, colicky abdominal pains; mild to severe abdominal distention; nausea and vomiting; anorexia and malaise; fever; lack of bowel movement; electrolyte imbalance; high-pitched tinkling bowel sounds.	1. Assist with insertion of *nasoenteric* tube and attach to intermittent *suction*. 2. Maintain IV infusions with electrolytes. 3. Encourage nasal breathing to *avoid* air swallowing. 4. Check abdomen for distention and bowel sounds every 2 h. 5. Encourage verbalization. 6. Plan rest periods for patient. 7. Administer oral hygiene frequently.

(continued)

TABLE 9.2   POSTOPERATIVE COMPLICATIONS (*Continued*)

Condition and Etiology	◣ *Assessment: Signs and Symptoms*	◣ *Nursing Care Plan/ Implementation*
Transfusions Reactions		
Allergic and febrile reactions—unidentified antigen or antigens in donor blood or transfusion equipment, previous reaction to transfusions, small thrombi, bacteria, lysed red blood cells.	Fever to 103°F, may have *sudden* onset; chills; itching; erythema; urticaria; nausea; vomiting; dyspnea and wheezing, occasionally.	1. *Stop* transfusion and notify physician. 2. Administer *antihistamines,* as ordered. 3. Send stat urine to lab for analysis. 4. Institute *cooling* measures, if indicated. 5. Maintain *strict* input and output records. 6. Send remaining blood to lab for analysis, and order recipient blood sample for analysis.
Hemolytic reaction—infusion of incompatible blood (less common, more serious).	*Early*—chills and fever; throbbing headache, feeling of burning in face; hypotension; tachycardia; chest, back, or flank pain; nausea, vomiting; feeling of doom; *later*—spontaneous and diffuse bleeding; icterus; urine: oliguria; anuria; hemoglobinuria.	1. *Stop* infusion immediately; take vital signs and notify physician. 2. Send patient blood sample and unused blood to lab for analysis. 3. Send stat urine to lab. 4. Save *all* urine for observation of discoloration. 5. Administer parenteral infusions to combat shock, as ordered. 6. Administer medications, as ordered—*diuretics, sodium bicarbonate, hydrocortisone,* and *vasopressors.*
Emotional Complications		
Emotional disturbances—grief associated with loss of body part or loss of body image; previous emotional problems; decreased sensory and perceptual input; sensory overload; fear and pain; decreased resistance to stress as a result of age, exhaustion, or debilitation.	Restlessness, insomnia, depression, hallucinations, delusions, agitation, suicidal thoughts.	1. Report symptoms to physician. 2. Encourage verbalization of feelings; give realistic assurance. 3. Orient to time and place, as necessary. 4. Provide safety measures, such as siderails. 5. Keep room lit, to reduce likelihood of visual hallucinations. 6. Administer tranquilizers, as ordered. 7. Use restraints as a *last* resort.

CVP = central venous pressure; NG = nasogastric; ROM = range of motion.

Source: Lagerquist SL: *Little, Brown's NCLEX-RN Examination Review.* Boston: Little, Brown, 1996. Pp. 108–111.

A. Goal: *promote lung expansion, gaseous exchange, and elimination of bronchotracheal secretions.*
   1. Turn, cough, and deep breathe q2h.
   2. Use *incentive spirometer* as ordered to enable patient to observe depth of ventilation.
   3. Administer nebulization as ordered to help mobilize secretions.
   4. Encourage hydration to thin mucous secretions.
   5. Assist in ambulation as soon as allowed.

B. Goal: *provide relief of pain.*
   1. Assess type, location, intensity, and duration; possible causative factors, such as poor body alignment or restrictive bandages.

2. Observe and evaluate reaction to discomfort.

☞ 3. Utilize comfort measures, such as back rubs and proper ventilation, staying with patient and encouraging verbalization.

☞ 4. Reduce incidence of pain: change position frequently; support dependent extremities with pillows, sandbags, and footboards; keep bedding dry and straight.

◙ 5. Give analgesics or tranquilizers as ordered; assure patient that they will help.

6. Observe for desired and untoward effects of medication.

C. Goal: *promote adequate nutrition and fluid and electrolyte balance.*

☞ 1. Parenteral fluids, as ordered.

2. Monitor blood pressure, I&O to assess adequate, deficient, or excessive extracellular fluid volume.

◙ 3. *Diet:* liquid when nausea and vomiting stop and bowel sounds are established; progress as ordered.

D. Goal: *assist patient with elimination.*

1. Encourage voiding within 8–10 h after surgery.

a. Allow patient to stand or use commode, if not contraindicated.

b. Run tap water or soak feet in warm water to promote micturition.

☞ **c.** Catheterization if bladder is distended and conservative treatments have failed.

2. Maintain accurate I&O records.

3. Expect bowel function to return in 2–3 d.

E. Goal: *facilitate wound healing and prevent infection.*

☞ 1. *Incision* care: *avoid* pressure to enhance venous drainage and prevent edema.

2. *Elevate* injured extremities to reduce swelling and promote venous return.

3. Support or *splint* incision when coughing.

4. Check *dressings* q2h for drainage.

☞ 5. Change dressings on draining wounds prn;
◙ *aseptic technique;* protective ointments to reduce skin irritation may be ordered.

6. Carefully observe wound suction (e.g., *Jackson-Pratt*), if applied, for kinking or twisting of the tubes.

F. Goal: *promote comfort and rest.*

1. Recognize factors that may cause restlessness—fear, anxiety, pain, oxygen lack, wet dressings.

◙ 2. Comfort measures: analgesics or barbiturates;
☞ apply *oxygen* as indicated; change positions; encourage deep breathing; massage back to reduce restlessness.

3. Allow rest periods between care-group activities.

◙ 4. Give antiemetic for relief of nausea and vomiting, as ordered.

5. Vigorous oral hygiene (brushing) to prevent "surgical mumps" or parotitis from atropine given preoperatively or general anesthesia.

G. Goal: *encourage early movement and ambulation to prevent complications of immobilization.*

1. Turn or reposition q2h.

☞ 2. ROM: passive and active exercises.

3. Encourage leg exercises.

4. Assist with standing or use of commode, if allowed.

5. Encourage resumption of personal care as soon as possible.

6. Assist with ambulation in room as soon as allowed. *Avoid* chair-sitting, as it enhances venous pooling and may predispose to thrombophlebitis.

▶ **V. Evaluation/outcome criteria**

A. Incision heals without infection.

B. No complications, (e.g., atelectasis, pneumonia, thrombophlebitis).

C. Normal bowel and bladder functions resume.

D. Carries out activities of daily living, self-care.

E. Accepts possible limitations: dietary, activity, body image (e.g., no depression, complies with treatment regimen).

⚷ Summary of Key Points

1. Assess patient carefully for factors that increase the risk of surgery associated with general anesthesia, such as hypoventilation, low perfusion, and potential for infection.

2. Document all prescribed and over-the-counter medications the patient is taking. Drugs may interact with the anesthesia, producing respiratory depression and hypotension, masking infection, or increasing bleeding.

3. Increased preoperative anxiety increases postoperative pain, nausea, and vomiting.

4. Explaining the surgical procedure and the risks to the patient is the surgeon's responsibility (informed consent).

5. Preoperative teaching is important to ensure effective postoperative coughing and use of the incentive spirometer.

6. Any noisy breathing or snoring after general anesthesia is indicative of obstructed breathing.

7. After general anesthesia, complications will most likely develop in the following order: *lung congestion* during the first 48 hours; *wound infection* or *dehiscence* and *evisceration* 3–5 d after surgery; symptoms of a *urinary tract infection* within 5–7 d; and indications of *thrombophlebitis* 7–14 d after surgery.

REVIEW OF THE USE OF COMMON TUBES

Tube or Apparatus	Purpose	Examples of Use	◄ Key Points for Nursing Implementation
Penrose drain	Soft collapsible latex rubber drain inserted to *drain serosanguineous fluid* from a surgical site; usually brought out to the skin via a stab wound.	Bowel resection.	1. Expect drainage to progress from serosanguineous to more serous. ☞ 2. *Sterile* technique when changing dressing—do often. 3. Physician will advance tube a little each day.
Nasogastric (NG) tubes			
Levin tube and small-bore feeding tubes	1. Inserted into stomach to *decompress* by removing gastric contents and air—prevents any buildup of gastric secretions, which are continuous. 2. Used when stomach needs to be washed out (*lavage*). 3. Used for feedings when patient is unable to swallow (gavage).	1. Any abdominal or other *surgery where peristalsis is absent* for a few days. 2. *Overdoses.* 3. *Gastrointestinal hemorrhage.* 4. *Cancer of the esophagus.* 5. *Early postoperative laryngectomy patient or radical neck dissection.*	☞ 1. Connect to *low* intermittent suction. ☞ 2. Irrigate prn with normal saline or puffs of air. 3. Clean, but *not* sterile, procedure. 4. Mouth care needed. 5. Report *"coffee ground"* material (digested blood). 6. For overdose: stomach is pumped out as *rapidly* as possible. 7. For hemorrhage: iced normal saline may be used to lavage. ☞ 8. Critical to make sure tube still in stomach *before* beginning feeding; listen for air passing into stomach and if possible aspirate gastric contents; small-bore tubes need placement check by ⟊ *x-ray*. 9. Follow feeding with some water to rinse out the tube. 10. Clamp tube when ambulating. ☞ 11. With larger-bore tubes, determine residuals and withhold feeding if large residuals obtained.
Miller-Abbott tube, **Cantor** tube	Longer than Levin tube—has mercury or air in bags so tube can be used to *decompress the lower intestinal tract.*	1. *Small-bowel obstructions.* 2. *Intussusception.* 3. *Volvulus.*	1. Care similar to that for Levin tube—irrigated. ☞ 2. Connected to suction, *not* sterile technique. 3. Orders will be written on how to advance the tube, gently pushing tube a few inches each hour; patient position may affect advancement of tube. ⟊ 4. X-rays determine the desired location of tube.
Salem-sump	Double-lumen tube with vent to *protect gastric mucosa* from trauma of suctioning.	Same as Levin tube.	☞ 1. Irrigate vent (blue tubing) with air *only*. 2. See Levin tube.

(continued)

REVIEW OF THE USE OF COMMON TUBES

Tube or Apparatus	Purpose	Examples of Use	► Key Points for Nursing Implementation
Gastrostomy tube	1. Inserted into stomach via abdominal wall. 2. May be used for *decompression.* 3. Used *long term for feedings.*	Conditions affecting *esophagus* where it is impossible to insert a nasogastric tube.	1. Principles of tube feedings same as with Levin nasogastric tube, *except* no danger that tube is in trachea. 2. If permanent, tube may be replaceable.
T-tube	To *drain bile* from the common bile duct *until* edema has subsided.	*Cholecystectomy* when a common duct exploration or choledochostomy was also done.	1. Bile drainage is influenced by *position* of the drainage bag. ☞2. Clamp tube as ordered to see if bile will flow into duodenum normally.
Hemovac	A type of closed-wound drainage system connected to suction—used to *drain a large amount* of serosanguineous fluid from under an incision.	1. *Mastectomy.* 2. *Total hip procedures.* 3. *Total knee procedures.*	1. May compress unit to create portable vacuum or connect to wall suction. 2. Small drainage tubes may get clogged—physician may irrigate these at times.
Jackson-Pratt	1. A method of *closed-wound suction* drainage—indicated when tissue displacement and tissue trauma may occur with rigid drain tubes (i.e., Hemovac). 2. See Hemovac.	1. *Neurosurgery.* 2. *Neck surgery.* 3. *Mastectomy.* 4. *Total knee and hip replacement.* 5. *Abdominal surgery.* 6. *Urologic procedures.*	☞1. Empty reservoir when full, to prevent loss of wound drainage and back-contamination. 2. See Hemovac.
Three-way Foley	To provide avenues for *constant irrigation and constant drainage* of the urinary bladder.	1. *Transurethral resection prostatectomy* (TURP) 2. *Bladder* infections.	1. Watch for blocking by clots—causes bladder spasms. ▬2. Irrigant solution often has antibiotic added to normal saline or sterile water. 3. *Sterile water* rather than normal saline may be used for lysis of clots.
Suprapubic catheter	To *drain bladder* via an opening through the abdominal wall above the pubic bone.	*Suprapubic* prostatectomy.	☞1. May have orders to *irrigate* prn or continuously.
Ureteral catheter	To *drain urine* from the pelvis of one kidney, or for *splinting* ureter.	1. *Cystoscopy* for diagnostic workups. 2. *Ureteral surgery.* 3. *Pyelotomy.*	1. *Never* clamp the tube—pelvis of kidney only holds 4–8 mL. ☞2. Use *only* 5 mL of sterile normal saline if ordered to irrigate.

Note: This review focuses on care of the tubes, not on total patient care.

Source: Jane Vincent Corbett, RN, MS, EdD, Professor, School of Nursing, University of San Francisco. Used with permission.

POSITIONING THE PATIENT FOR SPECIFIC SURGICAL CONDITIONS

Surgical Condition	▶ *Key Points for Nursing Implementation*	Rationale
Amputation: lower extremity	*No* pillows under stump after first 24 h. Turn patient *prone* several times a day.	Prevents flexion deformity of the limb.
Appendicitis: ruptured	Keep in *Fowler's* position—*not* flat in bed.	Keeps infection from spreading upward in the peritoneal cavity.
Burns (extensive)	Usually *flat* for first 24 h.	Potential problem is hypovolemia, which will be more symptomatic in a sitting position.
Cast, extremity	Keep extremity *elevated.*	Prevents edema.
Coronary surgery	May be ordered *flat* on back for 24 h.	Important to prevent possible hypotension, which may occur if head of bed raised.
Craniotomy	Head *elevated* with supratentorial incision; *flat* with cerebellar or brainstem incision.	Prevents collection of fluid in surgical area, which might contribute to increased intracranial pressure.
Flail chest	Position on *affected* side.	Reduces the instability of the chest wall that is causing the paradoxical respiratory movements.
Gastric resection	*Lie down after* meals.	May be useful in preventing dumping syndrome.
Hiatal hernia (*before* repaired)	Head of bed *elevated* on shock blocks.	Prevents esophageal irritation from gastric regurgitation.
Hip prosthesis	1. Keep affected leg in *abduction* (splint or pillow between legs). 2. *Avoid* adduction and flexion of the hip. 3. Use trochanter roll along outside of femur anterior joint capsule incision to keep affected leg turned slightly *inward; no* trochanter roll with posterior joint capsule incision as leg is turned slightly *outward.*	If affected leg is flexed and allowed to adduct and internally rotate, the head of the femur may be displaced from the socket.
Ileofemoral bypass; arterial insufficiency	1. Do *not* elevate legs. 2. *Avoid* hip flexion—walk or stand, but do *not* sit.	1. Arterial flow is helped by gravity. 2. Flexion of the hip compresses the vessels of the extremity.
Laminectomy; fusion	*Avoid* twisting motion when getting out of bed, ambulating.	Prevents any bending of the spine.
Liver biopsy	Place on *right* side, and position pillow for pressure.	Prevents bleeding.
Lobectomy	Do *not* put in Trendelenburg position. Position of comfort—sides, back.	Pushes abdominal contents against diaphragm; may cause respiratory embarrassment.
Mastectomy	1. Do *not* abduct arm first few days. 2. Elevate hand and arm *higher* than shoulder if lymph glands removed.	1. Puts tension on suture line. 2. Prevents lymphedema.
Pneumonectomy	Turn *only* toward *operative* side for short periods; *no* extreme lateral positioning.	1. Gives unaffected lung room for full expansion. 2. Prevents mediastinal shift. 3. In case of bleeding there will be no drainage into the unaffected bronchi.

(continued)

POSITIONING THE PATIENT FOR SPECIFIC SURGICAL CONDITIONS

Surgical Condition	⋈ *Key Points for Nursing Implementation*	*Rationale*
Radium implantation in cervix	Bedrest—usually *elevate head* to 30 degrees.	*Must* keep radium insert positioned correctly.
Respiratory distress	*Orthopnea* position usually desirable.	Allows for maximum expansion of lungs.
Retinal detachment	1. Affected area toward bed—*complete* bed rest. 2. No *sudden* movements of head—may use sand bags to prevent turning.	1. Gravity may help retina fall in place. 2. Any sudden increase in intraocular pressure may further dislodge retina. 3. Necessary to cover both eyes to reduce ocular movements.
Traction, straight	Check specific orders about how much head may be elevated.	Body is used as the countertraction—this must *not* be *less* than the pull of the traction.
Traction, balanced suspension	May give patient more freedom to move about than in straight traction.	In balanced suspension, additional weights supply countertraction.
Unconscious patient	Turn on side with head slightly *lowered*—"coma" position.	1. Important to let secretions drain out by gravity. 2. *Must* prevent aspiration.
Vein strippings; vein ligations	1. Keep legs *elevated*. 2. Do *not* stand or sit for long periods.	1. Prevents venous stasis. 2. Prevents venous pooling.

Source: Jane Vincent Corbett, RN, MS, EdD, Professor, School of Nursing, University of San Francisco. Used with permission.

💡 Study and Memory Aids

Postoperative Complications: Order "4 W's"

Wind—prevent respiratory complications
Wound—prevent infection
Water—prevent dehydration/urinary tract infection
Walk—prevent thrombophlebitis

Check for Circulation: "4 P's"

Pain
Pallor
Paresthesia
Pulse

🗩 Drug Review

Perioperative Nursing

Atropine sulfate: 0.4–0.6 mg SC 30–60 min before anesthesia
Meperidine HCl (Demerol): 50–150 mg IM or SC
Midazolam HCl (Versed): 70–80 mcg/kg 1 h before surgery to induce desired sleepiness and decrease anxiety
Morphine sulfate: 5–20 mg IM or SC q 4h
Other drugs used according to patient's medical history and anticipated health status

Questions

1. What position should the nurse place a patient in if wound evisceration occurs after abdominal surgery?
   1. Supine, with knees flexed.
   2. A semi-Fowler's position, with the feet elevated.

3. A side-lying position, with the patient's knees drawn up to the chest.
4. A position of comfort.

2. Which nursing action is the proper technique for emptying a Jackson-Pratt suction drain?
1. Opening the spout on the reservoir without gloves.
2. Disconnecting the bulb from the wound catheter.
3. Compressing the reservoir bulb with the spout open.
4. Rinsing the bulb reservoir with sterile water.

3. Which symptom would the nurse tell a patient is normal after a laparoscopy?
1. Shortness of breath.
2. Dizziness.
3. Referred shoulder pain.
4. Abdominal gas pains.

4. The effectiveness of preoperative teaching will be most negatively influenced by:
1. The presence of a significant other during the teaching session.
2. Concern regarding the amount of insurance reimbursement.
3. Prior experience with surgery in family members.
4. Abdominal pain unrelieved by medication.

5. What is the best way for the nurse to respond to a patient who refuses to remove her dentures before surgery?
1. Tell the patient that hospital policy requires that dentures must be removed.
2. Notify the operating room nurse that the dentures are still in place.
3. Leave the dentures in place and inform the anesthesiologist of this.
4. Ask the surgeon to speak to the patient.

6. A patient's comprehension of and compliance with patient teaching for same-day (out-patient) surgery will be most enhanced by:
1. Verbally giving the patient instruction during an office visit before the surgery.
2. Providing the patient with essential instructions in writing.

3. Telephoning the patient after the surgery to review instructions.
4. Showing the patient a movie regarding the procedure to reinforce verbal instructions.

Answers/Rationale

1. **(1)** A flat position with the knees bent will return the intestines to the abdominal cavity and keep them there, as well as relax the abdominal muscles. Elevating the patient's feet (**2**) may help, but having the patient sit up would *not* keep the bowel in the abdominal cavity. Side-lying (**3**) would still allow the bowel to fall forward. A position of comfort (**4**) may *not* use gravity to return the protruding bowel to the abdomen. **IMP, 1, PhI**

2. **(3)** During emptying of a Jackson-Pratt suction drain, the reservoir bulb must be compressed, but only when the spout is open, so that air is not forced into the surgical area. All of the other actions (**1, 2,** and **4**) will *increase* the likelihood of drain *contamination*. **IMP, 2, SECE**

3. **(3)** Laparoscopy involves direct visualization of the abdominal or pelvic organs using a fiberoptic light inserted into the abdomen; this causes nerve irritation that leads to shoulder pain. Shortness of breath (**1**) and dizziness (**2**) are *not* expected side effects. Although gas is used during the procedure, any abdominal gas pains (**4**) would occur as a result of bowel distention. **IMP, 1, SECE**

4. **(4)** A patient in pain will not be able to focus on teaching. In Maslow's Hierarchy of Need theory, it is hypothesized that lower-level physiologic needs, such as air, food, and comfort, must be met before a person seeks to get higher-level needs met. All of the other options (**1, 2,** and **3**) would influence a patient's receptivity to teaching, but they are related to *higher-level needs* and will have less effect. **EV, 1, PhI**

5. **(2)** The dentures can be removed after the patient is in the operating room and anesthetized. It is unnecessary to upset a patient before surgery (**1**). The best approach is for a nurse to take action, rather than calling upon the anesthesiologist (**3**) or the surgeon (**4**) to do so. **IMP, 1, PsI**

6. **(2)** Written information that the patient can refer to after the surgery is the most effective teaching tool. Patient teaching is frequently done in the MD's office (**1**), *but* the information needs to be *reinforced later* with written material. Follow-up contact (**3**) is also important, but the effects of anesthesia or pain medication may interfere with retention. A video regarding the procedure can be played for the patient while in the MD's office (**4**) but may not be available to the patient at home. **PL, 1, SECE**

Key to Codes

Nursing process: AS, assessment; **AN,** analysis; **PL,** planning; **IMP,** implementation; **EV,** evaluation. (See Appendix M for explanation of nursing process steps.)

Category of human function: 1, protective; **2,** sensory-perceptual; **3,** comfort, rest, activity, and mobility; **4,** nutrition; **5,** growth and development; **6,** fluid-gas transport; **7,** psychosocial-cultural; **8,** elimination. (See Appendix O for explanation.)

Client need: SECE, safe, effective care environment; **PhI,** physiologic integrity; **PsI,** psychosocial integrity; **HPM,** health promotion/maintenance. (See Appendix P for explanation.)

Pain

Chapter Outline

- Pain
- Summary of Key Points
- Study and Memory Aids

- Questions
- Answers/Rationale

Pain

I. Types of pain:
A. *Superficial somatic tissues*—skin, subcutaneous or fibrous tissue, and ligaments have pain receptors, and thus pain is localized.
B. *Deep somatic tissues and viscera*—pain may be diffuse and radiating because these do not have direct connection with sensory-discriminative system.
C. *Neurogenic pain*—results from damage to peripheral or central nervous system; any sensation may be perceived as pain due to abnormal processing of afferent impulses or paroxysmal activity.
D. *Psychogenic pain*—due to fantasies and psychological need for injury or punishment (called *conversion*).

II. Components of pain experience—pain related to:
A. *Stimuli*—sources: chemical, ischemic, mechanical trauma; extremes of heat/cold.
B. *Perception*—viewed with fear by children; can be altered by level of consciousness; interpreted and influenced by previous and current experience; is more severe when alone at night or immobilized.
C. *Response*—variations in physiologic, cultural, and learned responses; anxiety is created; pain seen as justified punishment; pain used as means for attention-getting.

▶ III. Assessment
A. *Subjective data:*
  1. *Site*—medial, lateral, proximal, distal.
  2. *Strength:*
    a. Certain tissues are more sensitive.
    b. Changes in intensity.
    c. Based on expectations.
    d. Affected by distraction or concentration, state of consciousness.
    e. Described as slight, medium, severe, excruciating.

3. *Quality*—aching, burning, crushing, dull, piercing, shifting, throbbing, tingling.
4. *Antecedent factors*—physical exertion, eating, extreme temperatures, physical and emotional stressors (e.g., fear).
5. *Previous experience*—influences reaction to pain.
6. *Behavioral clues*—demanding, worried, irritable, restless, difficult to distract, sleepless.
B. *Objective data:*
  1. *Verbal clues*—moaning, groaning, crying.
  2. *Nonverbal clues*—clenching teeth, grimacing, splinting of body parts, body position, knees drawn up, involuntary reflex movements, tossing/turning, rhythmic rubbing movements, voice pitch and speed, eyes shut.
  3. *Physical clues*—breathing irregularities, abdominal distention, skin color changes, skin temperature changes, excessive salivation, perspiration.
  4. *Time/duration*—onset, duration, recurrence, interval, last occurrence.

▶ IV. Analysis/nursing diagnosis
A. *Pain*, acute or chronic, related to specific patient condition.
B. *Activity intolerance* related to discomfort.
C. *Sleep pattern disturbance* related to pain.
D. *Fatigue* related to state of discomfort or emotional stress.
E. *Ineffective individual coping* related to chronic pain.

▶ V. Nursing care plan/implementation
A. Goal: *provide relief of pain.*
  1. Assess level of pain; ask patient to rate on scale of 0–10 (0 = no pain; 10 = worst pain). (Table 10.1)
  2. Determine cause:
    a. *Environmental factors:* noise, light, odors, motion.
    b. *Physiologic needs:* elimination, hunger, thirst, fatigue, circulatory impairment,

Diffuse Pain
Peritonitis
Early appendicitis
Bowel obstruction
Intestinal ischemia
Aortic aneurysm
Gastroenteritis
Pancreatitis
Diabetic ketoacidosis
Sickle cell crisis
Black widow spider bite

Right Upper
Quadrant Pain
Biliary colic
Pancreatitis
Perforated ulcer
Appendicitis
Hepatitis
Liver abscess
Right kidney stone
Right kidney infection
Herpes zoster (shingles)
Myocardial infarction
Right lower lobe
  pneumonia
Pulmonary embolism

Left Upper
Quadrant Pain
Ruptured spleen
Duodenal ulcer
Pancreatitis
Pneumonia
Gastritis
Gastric ulcer
Diverticulitis
Left kidney stone
Left kidney infection
Herpes zoster (shingles)
Myocardial infarction

Right Lower
Quadrant Pain
Appendicitis
Salpingitis
Ectopic pregnancy
Ovarian cyst
Incarcerated hernia
Diverticulitis
Regional ileitis
Psoas abscess
Kidney stone
Cecal volvulus
Cecal perforation
Pelvic inflammatory
  disease

Left Lower
Quadrant Pain
Salpingitis
Ectopic pregnancy
Ovarian cyst
Incarcerated hernia
Diverticulitis
Regional ileitis
Psoas abscess
Kidney stone
Pelvic inflammatory
  disease

POSSIBLE CAUSES OF ABDOMINAL PAIN ACCORDING TO LOCATION. (From Caroline NL. *Emergency Care in the Streets* [5th ed]. Boston: Little, Brown, 1995.)

muscle tension, ventilation, pressure on nerves.

c. *Emotional:* fear of unknown, helplessness, loneliness (especially at night).

3. Determine pain reactions; explore meaning of "pain" (how much, when, how long, where, why, what it feels like).

4. *Relieve:* anger, anxiety, boredom, loneliness.

5. Report **sudden, severe, new** pain; pain **not** relieved by medications or comfort measures; pain associated with **casts or traction.**

6. Try nursing comfort measures (non-drug):

Back rub, reassurance, reposition, relaxation techniques.

7. *Remove pain stimulus:*

a. Administer pain medication (e.g., analgesic, antispasmodic) at appropriate time intervals; do *not* withhold due to overestimated danger of addiction.

b. *Avoid* cold (to reduce immediate tissue reaction to trauma).

c. Apply heat (to relieve ischemia).

d. Change activity (e.g., restrict activity with cardiac pain).

TABLE 10.1   PQRST FORMAT FOR ASSESSING PAIN

P   What **P**rovokes the pain? Did something in particular bring it on? Does anything make it worse? Does anything make it better?

Q   What is the **Q**uality of the pain? Dull? Sharp? Cutting? Throbbing? Crushing? Squeezing?

R   Does the pain **R**adiate to any other area, or does it stay in one place?

S   What is the **S**everity of the pain? Ask the patient to grade it on a scale of 0 (no pain) to 10 (worst pain).

T   What is the **T**iming of the pain? When did it start? What has happened to it over time (gotten worse? gotten better?)? If there are associated symptoms, what is their relative timing (e.g., did the pain come on before or after the nausea?)?

Source: Caroline NL. *Emergency Care in the Streets* (5th ed). Boston: Little, Brown, 1995.

---

    e. Change, loosen dressing.
    f. Comfort (e.g., reposition, smooth wrinkled sheets, change wet dressing).
    g. Give food (e.g., for ulcer).
  8. *Reduce pain receptor reaction.*
    a. Ointment (use as coating).
    b. Local anesthetics.
    c. Padding (of bony prominences).
  9. Assist with medical/surgical procedures and interventions to *block pain impulse transmission:*
    a. Injection of local anesthetic into nerve (e.g., dental).
    b. Cordotomy—sever anterolateral spinal cord nerve tracts.
    c. Electrical stimulation—transcutaneous (skin surface), percutaneous (peripheral nerve).
    d. Peripheral nerve implant—electrode to major sensory nerve.
    e. Dorsal column stimulator—electrode to dorsal column.
  10. *Avoid causes of inadequate pain control:*
    a. Incorrect assessment.
    b. Insufficient knowledge of pharmacologic effects.
    c. Personal attitudes, e.g., concern about addiction.
    d. Fear of respiratory depression.
    e. Reluctance to accept subjective data.
  11. *Document response to pain-relief measures.*
B. Goal: *alter pain perception* by raising pain threshold.
  1. *Distraction,* e.g., TV (cerebral cortical activity blocks impulses from thalamus).

  2. *Analgesics*—give *prior* to occurrence of severe pain; give routinely for chronic/terminal pain.
  3. *Hypnosis*—assess appropriateness of use for psychogenic pain and of anesthesia; patient needs to be open to suggestion.
  4. *Acupuncture*—assess patient's emotional readiness and belief in it.
C. Goal: *alter interpretation and response to pain.*
  1. Administer narcotics—result: no longer sees pain as disturbing.
  2. Administer hypnotics—result: changes perception and decreases reaction.
  3. Help patient obtain interpersonal satisfaction from ways other than attention received when in pain.
D. Goal: *promote patient control of pain and analgesia: use patient-controlled analgesia* (PCA), an analgesic administration system designed to maintain optimal serum analgesic levels; safely delivers intermittent bolus doses of a narcotic analgesic; preset to maximum hourly dose.
  1. *Advantages:* decreased patient anxiety; improved pulmonary function; fewer side effects.
  2. *Limitations:* requires an indwelling intravenous line; analgesic targets central pain, may not relieve peripheral discomfort; cost of PCA unit.
E. Goal: **health teaching.**
  1. Explain causes of pain and how to describe pain.
  2. Explain that it is acceptable to admit existence of pain.
  3. Relaxation exercises.
  4. Biofeedback methods of pain perception and control.
  5. Proper medication administration, when necessary, for self-care.
VI. Evaluation/outcome criteria
  A. Verbalizes comfort, awareness of pain decreased.
  B. Knows source of pain, how to reduce stimulus and perception.
  C. Uses alternative measures for pain relief.
  D. Able to cope with pain, e.g., remains active, relaxed appearance; verbal and nonverbal clues to pain being absent.

Summary of Key Points

1. Pain is subjective and individualized. The patient knows best what pain is and whether a particular treatment has worked. Pain should be assessed without a preconceived idea of what the pain should or should not be.
2. Pain can be: acute, chronic, superficial, deep somatic, visceral, or referred.
3. Lack of predictable signs or expressions of pain does *not* mean lack of pain.

4. Patients should *not* have to tolerate pain for any reason.
5. Just because a patient is sleeping, it does *not* mean the patient is *not* in pain.
6. A pain assessment tool helps quantify the pain and effectiveness of treatment.
7. Anxiety *increases* pain and the need for higher doses of analgesics.
8. Pain medications should be used in combination with *nondrug interventions* such as repositioning, reassurance, a back rub, or relaxation techniques.

⚬ Study and Memory Aids

Pain: Management—"ABC's"

Assess by *asking* patient about the pain.
Believe the patient's pain is real.
Choices—let patients know their choices.
Do what you *can, when* you *said* you *would.*
Enable patients to have control over their pain.

Questions

1. Meperidine (Demerol) has been ordered for a patient for the relief of postoperative pain. Which assessment finding is a side effect of the agent?
   1. Respiratory rate of 10 breaths/min.
   2. Blood pressure of 150/90 mm Hg.
   3. Pinpoint pupils.
   4. Urine output of 20 mL/h.
2. Which nonverbal signs observed during an admitting history would indicate a patient is experiencing physical discomfort?
   1. Hesitancy in answering questions.
   2. Clenching fist and wrinkling brow.
   3. Smiling after each answer.
   4. Leaving to go to the bathroom.
3. While in the emergency room, a patient receives 4 mg of morphine sulfate IV for the relief of chest pain. Soon after admission to the unit the patient again complains of substernal chest pain. What should the nurse do first?
   1. Give the patient another dose of morphine sulfate IV.
   2. Increase the nasal oxygen flow rate to 5 L/min.
   3. Notify the physician of the resistance to pain medication.
   4. Place the patient in a high Fowler's position.
4. The patient complains of severe pain after suffering rib, arm, and leg fractures. Which pain medication would the nurse expect to provide the greatest relief?
   1. Diazepam (Valium) IV.
   2. Morphine sulfate IV.
   3. Meperidine hydrochloride (Demerol) IM.
   4. Methocarbamol (Robaxin) IM.

Answers/Rationale

1. **(1)** Demerol depresses both the rate and depth of respirations. Demerol a CNS depressant, would tend to lower blood pressure, not cause borderline hypertension **(2)**. Pinpoint pupils **(3)** can occur in patients receiving morphine. A urine output of 20 mL/h **(4)** is inadequate and would stem from decreased renal perfusion or renal failure; Demerol-induced changes in vital signs would not normally lead to such an impairment of renal function. **AS, 3, PhI**

2. **(2)** The members of some cultures and ethnic groups are reluctant to complain of pain. Nonverbal clues to tension, such as grimacing or tight fists, may be the only indication of pain. Hesitancy **(1)** may indicate fear, shyness, or lack of understanding. Smiling **(3)** after each answer may be due to uneasiness or an attempt to be cooperative. The need to go to the bathroom during the history-taking **(4)** may be prompted by urinary frequency, urgency, or nervousness. **AS, 3, PsI**

3. **(2)** The pain may be due to hypoxia, so the O_2 flow rate should be increased, unless a high O_2 flow rate is contraindicated (e.g. emphysema). The other actions listed may be appropriate, but this is a *priority* question. If ordered, the patient could be given more morphine sulfate **(1)**, but non-drug interventions should be tried *first*. Notifying the MD **(3)** would not usually be the *first* action. Positioning **(4)** is an independent nursing action that facilitates and thereby improves breathing or lowers blood pressure but is not used for *pain* management. (The patient's baseline vital signs should be assessed before positioning.) **IMP, 6, PhI**

4. **(2)** Bone pain is considered acute pain, and an opiate such as morphine should be used for the relief of moderate to severe bone pain. It is very unlikely that tolerance and dependence will develop during such short-term use as that necessitated by fractures. The opiates work by modifying the perception of the pain. Valium **(1)** and Robaxin **(4)** are not analgesics; they relieve pain by relaxing the muscles. Although an opiate, Demerol **(3)** is shorter acting than morphine sulfate and forms a toxic metabolite that stimulates the central nervous system. Demerol is not the drug of choice for the management of acute or chronic pain. **IMP, 3, PhI**

Key to Codes

Nursing process: AS, assessment; **AN,** analysis; **PL,** planning; **IMP,** implementation; **EV,** evaluation. (See Appendix M for explanation of nursing process steps.)

Category of human function: 1, protective; **2,** sensory-perceptual; **3,** comfort, rest, activity, and mobility; **4,** nutrition; **5,** growth and development; **6,** fluid-gas transport; **7,** psychosocial-cultural; **8,** elimination. (See Appendix O for explanation.)

Client need: SECE, safe, effective care environment; **PhI,** physiologic integrity; **PsI,** psychosocial integrity; **HPM,** health promotion/maintenance. (See Appendix P for explanation.)

Altered Immune System Disorders

Chapter Outline

- Acquired Immune Deficiency Syndrome (AIDS)
- Summary of Key Points
- Study and Memory Aids
  - Diet
  - Drug Review
- Questions
- Answers/Rationale

Acquired Immune Deficiency Syndrome (AIDS)

The terminal stage of the disease continuum caused by the human immunodeficiency virus (HIV), a retrovirus; typically progresses from asymptomatic seronegative status to asymptomatic seropositive status to subclinical immune deficiency to lymphadenopathy (*early* AIDS) to AIDS-related complex (*middle* stage with combination of symptoms) to AIDS; hallmarks of HIV infection include opportunistic infections: *Pneumocystis carinii* pneumonia (PCP), cytomegalovirus (CMV), *Mycobacterium tuberculosis*, hepatitis B, herpes simplex or zoster, candidiasis; may take 7–10 yr before signs and symptoms occur.

I. High-risk populations
  A. Males, homosexual or bisexual (52%).
  B. Intravenous drug users (IDU) (25%).
  C. IDU/homosexual (5%).
  D. Hemophiliacs and multiple transfusion recipients (2%).
  E. Heterosexual (9%).
  F. Undetermined/other (7%).

II. Pathophysiology: abnormal response to foreign antigen stimulation (acquired immunity) → deficiency in cell-mediated immunity—T lymphocytes, specifically helper cells (T4 cells) and hyperactivity of the humoral system (B cells).

✉ III. Assessment
  A. *Subjective data:*
    1. Fatigue: prolonged; associated with headache or light-headedness.
    2. Unexplained weight loss: >10%.
  B. *Objective data:*
    1. Fever: prolonged or night sweats >2 wk.
    2. Lymphadenopathy.
    3. Skin or mucous membrane lesions: purplish red nodules (*Kaposi's sarcoma*).
    4. Cough: persistent, heavy, dry.
    5. Diarrhea: persistent.
    6. Tongue/mouth "thrush"; oral hairy leukoplakia.
    7. Lab data. *Decreased*—CD4 (T4) lymphocytes, hematocrit, white blood cell count, platelets. Seropositive—syphilis, hepatitis B; ELISA—positive; Western blot test—positive (mean time for seroconversion is 6 wk after infection) (patient permission needed for ELISA and western blot)

✉ IV. Analysis/nursing diagnosis:
  A. *Risk for infection* related to immunocompromised state.
  B. *Fatigue* related to anemia.
  C. *Altered nutrition, less than body requirements,* related to anorexia.
  D. *Impaired skin integrity* related to nonhealing viral lesions, Kaposi's sarcoma.
  E. *Diarrhea* related to infection or parasites.
  F. *Risk for activity intolerance* related to shortness of breath.
  G. *Ineffective airway clearance* related to pneumonia.
  H. *Visual/sensory/perception alteration* related to retinitis.
  I. *Risk for altered body temperature* (fever) related to opportunistic infections.
  J. *Social isolation* related to stigma attached to AIDS.
  K. *Powerlessness* related to inability to control disease progression.
  L. *Altered thought processes* related to dementia.
  M. *Ineffective individual coping* related to poor prognosis.
  N. *Risk for violence, self-directed,* related to anger, panic, or depression.

▶ **V. Nursing care plan/implementation**
  A. Goal: *reduce risk of infection; slow disease progression.*
    1. Observe for signs of opportunistic infections: weight loss, diarrhea, skin lesions, sore throat.
    2. Monitor vital signs (including temperature).
    3. Note secretions and excretions: changes in color, consistency, or odor indicating infection.
    🍎 **4.** *Diet:* monitor fluid and electrolytes; strict measurement; encourage adequate dietary intake (high calorie, high nutrient, low bulk); 5–10 times recommended daily allowance of water-soluble vitamins (B complex, C); favorite foods from home; enteral feedings.
    ☞ **5.** *Protective isolation,* if indicated, for severe immunocompromise.
    💊 **6.** Medications, as ordered: zidovudine (Retrovir), trimethoprim-sulfamethoxazole (Septra), acyclovir (Zovirax), and/or pentamidine; do *not* give at mealtime; may need antinauseants or antiemetics to control side effects.
  B. Goal: *prevent the spread of disease.*
    ✋ **1.** Frequent handwashing, even after wearing gloves.
    ☞ **2.** *Avoid* exposure to blood, body fluids of patient; wear gloves, gowns; proper disposal of needles, IV catheters (Table 11.1).
  C. Goal: *provide physical and psychological support.*
    1. Oral care: frequent.
    ☞ **2.** Cooling bath: 1 : 10 concentration of isopropyl alcohol in tepid water; *avoid* plastic-backed pads with night sweats.
    3. Encourage verbalization of fears, concerns without condemnation; may suffer loss of job, life-style, significant other.
    4. Determine status of support network: arrange contact with support group.
    5. Observe for severe emotional symptoms (suicidal tendencies).
    6. Address issues surrounding death to ensure quality of life: designation of durable power of attorney for health care, code blue status, reassurance of comfort and pain control.
  🏠 **D.** Goal: **health teaching.**
    1. Avoidance of environmental sources of infection (kitty litter, bird cages, tub bathing).
    2. Precautions following discharge: risk-reducing behaviors—condoms (latex), limit number of sexual partners, *avoid* exposure to blood or semen during intercourse.
    3. Family counseling, availability of community resources.
    4. Information on disease progression and life span.
    ☞ **5.** Stress reduction techniques: visualization, guided imagery, meditation.
    6. Expected side effects with drug therapy, importance of compliance.
▶ **VI. Evaluation/outcome criteria**
  A. Relief of symptoms (e.g., afebrile, gains weight).
  B. Resumes self-care activities, returns to work, improved quality of life.
  C. Accepts diagnosis, participates in support group.
  D. Progression of disease slows, improved survival probability.
  E. Retains autonomy, self-worth.
  F. Permitted to die with dignity.

⚷ Summary of Key Points

1. HIV is not transmitted through casual contact but through some exposure to body fluids from an infected person.
2. Because of the compromised immune status, the AIDS patient is at greater risk for acquiring numerous opportunistic infections.
3. *Pneumocystis carinii* pneumonia is often the opportunistic infection that leads to a definitive diagnosis of AIDS.
4. *Universal precautions,* which include barrier guidelines and needle precautions, protect against exposure to blood-borne pathogens.
5. A health care worker is more likely to contract hepatitis; however, because AIDS is so devastating and not curable, there is greater fear; universal precautions must be followed.
6. Drug therapy does not cure AIDS but delays further destruction of the immune system.
7. Nursing care should focus on symptom management and dealing with the fears of isolation, loss, and death.

💡 Study and Memory Aids

🍎 Diet

AIDS

↑ Calorie
↑ Nutrient
↓ Bulk

💊 Drug Review

AIDS

Acyclovir (Zovirax): 800 mg q4h
Pentamidine: 4 mg/kg/d
Trimethoprim/sulfamethoxazole (Septra): treatment of active disease: 15–20 mg/kg/d in 3–4 divided doses q6–8h for >2 months; prevention of *Pneumocystis carinii* pneumonia 160 mg/d
Zidovudine (Retrovir) (AZT): 200 mg q4h 5 times a day

TABLE 11.1 UNIVERSAL BLOOD AND BODY FLUID PRECAUTIONS

The Centers for Disease Control (CDC) recommend universal blood and body fluid precautions (also referred to as *universal precautions*) in the care of *all* patients, especially those in emergency care settings, in which the risk of blood exposure is increased and the infection status of the patient is unknown. In other words, the nurse should treat all body substances or fluids of all patients as if they are potentially infectious.

The CDC recommend that these precautions apply to blood and to body fluids containing visible **blood,** as well as to **semen** and **vaginal** secretions, to tissues, and to the following fluids: **cerebrospinal fluid, synovial fluid, pleural fluid, peritoneal fluid, pericardial fluid,** and **amniotic fluid.** Universal precautions do *not* apply to *nasal secretions, sputum, saliva, sweat, tears, urine, feces,* and *vomitus unless* they contain visible blood. Blood is the single most important source of HIV, hepatitis B virus and other blood-borne pathogens in the health care setting.

Protective barriers—gloves, gowns, masks, and protective eyewear—reduce the risk of exposure to potentially infective materials. The following specific precautions are recommended.

- Wash your hands thoroughly and immediately after accidental contact with body substances containing blood, between patients, and immediately after gloves are removed.
- Wear gloves when touching blood and body fluids containing blood as well as when handling items or surfaces soiled with blood or body fluids.
- Change gloves between patient contacts.
- Use sterile gloves for procedures involving contact with normally sterile areas of the body.
- Use examination gloves for procedures involving contact with mucuous membranes, unless otherwise indicated, and for other patient care or diagnostic procedures that do not require the use of sterile gloves.
- Do *not* wash or disinfect surgical or examination gloves for reuse. Washing with surfactants may cause *wicking,* i.e., the enhanced penetration of liquids through undetected holes in the glove. Disinfecting agents may cause deterioration.
- Use general-purpose utility gloves (e.g., rubber household gloves) for housekeeping chores involving potential blood contact and for instrument cleaning and decontamination procedures. Utility gloves may be decontaminated and reused but should be discarded if they are peeling, cracked, or discolored or if they have punctures, tears, or other evidence of deterioration.
- Wear gloves when performing phlebotomy (venipuncture):
  - If the nurse has cuts, scratches, or other breaks in the skin.
- In situations where hand contamination with blood may occur, e.g., with an uncooperative patient.
- When the nurse is learning phlebotomy techniques.
- Wear gloves when performing finger and/or heel sticks on infants and children.
- Wear masks and protective eyewear (glasses, goggles) or face shields to protect the mucous membranes or your mouth, nose, and eyes during procedures that are likely to generate droplets of blood or other body fluids to which universal precautions apply.
- Wear a disposable plastic apron or gown during procedures that are likely to generate splatters of blood or other body fluid (e.g., peritoneal fluid) and soil your clothing.
- To prevent injuries, place used disposable needle-syringe units, scalpel blades, and other sharp items in puncture-resistant containers for disposal. Discard used needle-syringe units *uncapped* and *unbroken.* Puncture-resistant containers should be located as close as practicable to use areas.
- Place mouthpieces, resuscitation bags, or other ventilation devices in areas where the need for emergency mouth-to-mouth resuscitation is predictable—even though saliva has *not* been implicated in HIV transmission.
- If a nurse has exudative lesions or weeping dermatitis, it is necessary to refrain from all direct patient care and from handling patient-care equipment until the condition is resolved.
- Handle soiled linen as little as possible and with minimum agitation to prevent gross microbial contamination of the air and of persons handling the linen. Place and transport linen soiled with blood or body fluids in leakage-resistant bags.
- Put all specimens of blood and listed body fluids in well-constructed containers with secure lids to prevent leakage during transport. When collecting specimens, take care to *avoid* contaminating the *outside* of the container.
- Use a chemical germicide that is approved for use as a hospital disinfectant to decontaminate work surfaces after there is a spill of blood or other body fluids. In the absence of a commercial germicide, a solution of sodium hypochlorite (household bleach) in a 1:10 dilution is effective. Before decontaminating areas, first remove visible material. Wear gloves during cleaning and decontaminating procedures.
- Follow agency policies for disposal of infective waste, both when disposing of and when decontaminating contaminated materials.
- Carefully pour bulk blood, suctioned fluids, and excretions containing blood and secretions down drains that are connected to a sanitary sewer.

Source: U.S. Department of Health and Human Services, Public Health Service.

Questions

1. A hospitalized patient with AIDS has a white blood cell count (WBC) of 1500 mm³. He who is scheduled for a chest x-ray. The best response on the part of the nurse would be to:
   1. Put a mask and gown on the patient before transporting him to the x-ray department.
   2. Arrange for an x-ray to be done with a portable machine in the patient's room.
   3. Have the x-ray staff wear gowns, gloves, and masks while doing the x-ray.
   4. Have housekeeping clean the x-ray room thoroughly before the patient arrives.
2. The nurse would particularly instruct a patient with AIDS who is taking zidovudine (AZT) to avoid taking aspirin because:
   1. This would increase the chance of gastric irritation.
   2. The risk for granulocytopenia would be increased.
   3. This will cause a further reduction in the thrombocyte count.
   4. The symptoms of infection would then be masked.
3. When caring for a patient on enteric isolation, the nurse would observe which measure?
   1. Wear a gown and gloves when entering the patient's room.
   2. Wear a mask when giving direct care to the patient.
   3. Wear a gown and gloves if there is a chance of fecal contact.
   4. Wear a mask and gloves only when giving direct care.
4. Health care teaching about the most effective way to eliminate the transmission of infection through handwashing would include teaching all family members to:
   1. Rinse their hands with fingers pointing downward.
   2. Use friction when washing.
   3. Use friction and clean under fingernails.
   4. Rinse and dry hands well.
5. For which type of isolation should the nurse prepare a patient who has a WBC of 600 mm³?
   1. Respiratory.
   2. Enteric.
   3. Reverse.
   4. General.

Answers/Rationale

1. **(2)** The patient is at great risk for infection because he is in a severely immunosuppressed state. Obtaining the x-ray with a portable machine reduces the risk to the patient. Removing the patient (**1**) from protective isolation poses a risk to the patient. Protecting the x-ray staff (**3**) is not as important as protecting the patient. The safest environment for the patient is his own room; cleaning the x-ray room (**4**) may not be realistic. **IMP, 1, SECE**
2. **(2)** The co-administration of aspirin or acetaminophen with AZT causes the metabolism of AZT to be inhibited, leading to granulocytopenia. The chance of gastric irritation (**1**), although always a possible side effect of aspirin, is *not* any greater when it is taken in combination with AZT. The number of granulocytes, *not* thrombocytes (**3**), would decrease. Infection may be masked (**4**) in patients taking *steroids*. **IMP, 1, PhI**
3. **(3)** A gown and gloves should be worn any time contact with infective material is possible. It is otherwise not necessary for a nurse to wear a gown or gloves (**1**), a mask (**2**), or a mask and gloves (**4**) when entering the room of an AIDS patient casually. **IMP, 8, SECE**
4. **(3)** All of the techniques in the other options are appropriate, but the *most* effective one is to use friction to rub off pathogens and to clean under the fingernails where they can collect. The other options are less effective (**1** and **4**) or incomplete (**2**). **IMP, 1, SECE**
5. **(3)** The normal WBC is 5000 to 10000 mm³; a count of 600 mm³ is extremely low and such a patient is immunosuppressed. The risk of infection is great as a result, and the patient should be protected from infection by placing him/her in reverse or protective isolation. The other types of isolation (**1, 2,** and **4**) are designed to protect staff and visitors from the patient, *not* to protect the patient. **IMP, 1, SECE**

Key to Codes

Nursing process: AS, assessment; **AN,** analysis; **PL,** planning; **IMP,** implementation; **EV,** evaluation. (See Appendix M for explanation of nursing process steps.)

Category of human function: 1, protective; **2,** sensory-perceptual; **3,** comfort, rest, activity, and mobility; **4,** nutrition; **5,** growth and development; **6,** fluid-gas transport; **7,** psychosocial-cultural; **8,** elimination. (See Appendix O for explanation.)

Client need: SECE, safe, effective care environment; **PhI,** physiologic integrity; **PsI,** psychosocial integrity; **HPM,** health promotion/maintenance. (See Appendix P for explanation.)

Connective Tissue Disorders

Chapter Outline

- Rheumatoid Arthritis
- Systemic Lupus Erythematosus
- Lyme Disease
- Summary of Key Points
- Study and Memory Aids

- – Diet
- – Drug Review
- Questions
- Answers/Rationale

Rheumatoid Arthritis

Chronic, systemic collagen inflammatory disease; etiology unknown; may be autoimmune, viral, or genetic; affects primarily women 20–40 yr of age; present in 2%–3% of total population; follows a course of exacerbations and remissions.

I. Pathophysiology: synovitis with edema → proliferation of various blood material (formation of pannus) → destruction and fibrosis of cartilage (fibrous ankylosis); calcification of fibrous tissue (osseous ankylosis).

II. Assessment
  A. *Subjective data:*
  1. Joints: pain, stiffness, swelling.
  2. Easily fatigues, malaise.
  3. Anorexia, weight loss.
  B. *Objective data:*
  1. Subcutaneous nodules over bony prominences.
  2. Bilateral symmetric involvement of joints: crepitation, creaking, grating.
  3. Deformities: contractures, muscle atrophy.
  4. Lab data: blood: *decreased*—red blood cells (RBCs); *increased*—white blood cell count (WBCs) (12,000–15,000/mm³), sedimentation rate (>20 mm/h), rheumatoid factor.

III. Analysis/nursing diagnosis
  A. *Pain* related to joint destruction.
  B. *Impaired physical mobility* related to joint contractures.
  C. *Risk for injury* related to the inflammatory process.
  D. *Body image disturbance* related to joint deformity.
  E. *Self-care deficit* related to musculoskeletal impairment.
  F. *Risk for activity intolerance* related to fatigue and stiffness.

  G. *Altered nutrition, less than body requirements,* related to anorexia and weight loss.
  H. *Self-esteem disturbance* related to chronic illness.

IV. Nursing care plan/implementation
  A. Goal: *prevent or correct deformities.*
    1. Activity:
      a. *Bed rest* during exacerbations.
      b. Daily range of motion (ROM) exercises—active and passive exercises *even* in acute phase for 5–10-min periods; *avoid* fatigue and persistent pain.
      c. Heat and/or pain medication before exercise.
    2. Medications as ordered: *aspirin* (high dosages); *nonsteroidals; steroids; antacids* given for possible GI upset with ASA, steroids.
    3. *Fluids:* at least 1500 mL liquid daily to prevent renal calculi; milk for gastrointestinal (GI) upset.
  B. Goal: **health teaching.**
    1. Side effects of medications: tarry stools (GI bleeding), tinnitus (aspirin).
    2. Psychosocial aspects: possible need for early retirement, financial hardship, loss of libido, unsatisfactory sexual relations.
    3. Prepare for joint repair or replacement if indicated.

V. Evaluation/outcome criteria
  A. Remains as active as possible, limited loss of mobility, performs self-care activities.
  B. No side effects from drug therapy (e.g., GI bleeding).
  C. Copes with necessary life-style changes, complies with treatment.

Systemic Lupus Erythematosus (SLE)

Chronic inflammatory disease of connective tissue; may affect or involve any organ; vague etiology, but genetic factors, viruses, hormones, or drugs are being investigated; occurs *primarily in* women aged 18–35 yr.

I. Pathophysiology: possible toxic effects from immune complexes deposited in tissue—fibrinoid necrosis of collagen in connective tissue, small arterial walls (kidneys and heart particularly) → cellular death, obstructed blood flow.

II. Assessment
1. Pain: joints.
2. Anorexia, weight loss.
3. Photophobia, sensitivity to sun.
4. Weakness.
5. Nausea, vomiting.

B. *Objective data:*
1. Fever.
2. Rash: butterfly distribution across nose, cheeks.
3. Ulcerations: oral or nasopharyngeal.
4. Lab data:—blood: *increased* LE cells; *decreased* RBCs, WBCs, thrombocytes; *urine:* hematuria, proteinuria (nephritis).

III. Analysis/nursing diagnosis
A. *Risk for injury* related to possible autoimmune disorder.
B. *Pain* related to joint inflammation.
C. *Risk for activity intolerance* related to extreme fatigue, anemia.
D. *Impaired skin integrity* related to sunlight sensitivity and rashes.
E. *Altered nutrition, less than body requirements,* related to anorexia, nausea, vomiting.
F. *Altered oral mucous membrane* related to ulcerations.

IV. Nursing care plan/implementation
A. Goal: *minimize or limit immune response and complications.*
1. Activity: rest; 8–10 h sleep; unhurried environment; assist with stressful activities; *ROM* exercises to prevent joint immobility and stiffness.
2. Skin care: hygiene; topical steroid cream as ordered for inflammation, pruritus, scaling.
3. *Mouth care:* several times daily if stomatitis present; soft, bland, or liquid diet to prevent irritation.
4. *Diet:* low sodium if edematous; low protein with renal involvement.
5. Observe for signs of complications:
   a. *Cardiac/respiratory* (tachycardia, tachypnea, dyspnea, orthopnea).
   b. *GI* (diarrhea, abdominal pain, distention).
   c. *Renal* (increased weight, oliguria, decreased specific gravity).
   d. *Neurologic* (ptosis, ataxia).
   e. *Hematologic* (malaise, weakness, chills, epistaxis); report immediately.
6. Medications, as ordered:

a. *Analgesics.*
b. *Anti-inflammatory* agents (aspirin, prednisone) and *immunosuppressive drugs* (azathioprine [Imuran], cyclophosphamide [Cytoxan]) to control inflammation.
c. *Antimalarials* for skin and joint manifestations.

B. Goal: **health teaching.**
1. Disease process: diagnosis, prognosis, effects of treatment.
2. *Avoid* precipitating factors:
   a. Sun (aggravates skin lesions; thus, cover body as much as possible).
   b. Altering dosage of medications.
   c. Pregnancy (needs medical clearance).
   d. Fatigue, stress.
   e. Infections.
3. Medications: side effects of immunosuppressives and corticosteroids.
4. Regular exercise: walking, swimming; but *avoid* fatigue.
5. Wear MedicAlert bracelet.

V. Evaluation/outcome criteria
A. Attains a state of remission.
B. No organ involvement (e.g., cardiac, renal complications).
C. Keeps active within limitations.
D. Continues follow-up medical care—recognizes symptoms requiring immediate attention.

Lyme Disease

A spirochetal illness (syndrome) carried by infected ticks; incidence greatest during May through August when people are outdoors and wearing fewer clothes; only a small percentage of people hospitalized.

I. Classification
A. Stages
1. Rash at site of tick bite; *bull's-eye* or target pattern; may appear as hives or cellulitis; common in moist areas (groin, armpit, behind knees). Flulike symptoms may occur (joint pain, chills, fever).
2. If untreated, may progress to cardiac problems (10% of patients) or neurologic disturbances—Bell's palsy (10% of patients); occasionally meningitis, encephalitis, and eye damage may result.
3. From 4 wk to a year after the tick bite, "arthritis" develops in half the patients. If it goes untreated, chronic neurologic problems may develop.

II. Assessment (depends on stage)
A. *Subjective data:*
1. Malaise (I).
2. Headache (I).
3. Joint, neck, or back pain (I and III).
4. Weakness (II and III).
5. Chest pain (II).
6. Light-headedness (II).
7. Numbness, pain in arms or legs (III).

B. *Objective data:*
1. Rash—erythema migrans (I).
2. Dysrhythmias, heart block (II).

3. Facial paralysis (II).
4. Conjunctivitis, iritis, optic neuritis (II).
5. Lab data: Lyme titer—elevated (II and III).
6. Diagnostic tests: joint aspiration—fibrous exudate, WBCs, immune complexes; synovium biopsy—lymphocytic infiltrates.

III. Analysis/nursing diagnosis
  A. *Anxiety* related to diagnosis.
  B. *Pain* related to joint inflammation.
  C. *Fatigue* related to viral illness.
  D. *Impaired physical mobility* related to joint pain.
  E. *Altered thought processes* related to neurologic deficit.
  F. *Decreased cardiac output* related to dysrhythmias.
  G. *Knowledge deficit* related to treatment and course of disease.

IV. Nursing care plan/implementation
  A. Goal: *minimize irreversible tissue damage and complications.*
    1. Medications: *Stage I*—oral antibiotics for 21 d (doxycycline and penicillin V), *Stages II and III*—intravenous antibiotics for 14 d (penicillin or ceftriaxone).
    2. If hospitalized, monitor vital signs q4h for increased temperature, signs of heart failure; check level of consciousness and cranial nerve functioning.
    3. Note treatment response: worsening of symptoms during first 24 h; redder rash, higher fever, greater pain (*Jarisch-Herxheimer reaction*).
  B. Goal: *alleviate pain, promote comfort.*
    1. Medications: *salicylates, nonsteroidal anti-inflammatory agents,* or other *analgesic,* as ordered; observe for side effects (GI irritation).
    2. Rest: give instructions on relaxation techniques, create a quiet environment.
  C. Goal: *maintain physical and psychological well-being.*
    1. Activity: *ROM* exercises at regular intervals, medicate for pain prior to exercise, encourage proper posture to reduce joint stress, rest periods between activities and treatments.
    2. Referral: occupational and/or physical therapy as appropriate.
    3. Reassurance: give psychological support, encourage discussion of feelings.
  D. Goal: **health teaching.**
    1. Information on disease.
    2. Instructions for home IV antibiotics with heparin lock, if ordered.
    3. Side effects of antibiotics (drug specific), importance of completing therapy.
    4. Signs of disease recurrence (later stages of disease: less severe attacks).
    5. Preventing subsequent infections: wear proper clothing and tick repellent on clothing; conduct "tick checks" of self, children, and pets.

V. Evaluation/outcome criteria
  A. Achieves reasonable comfort.
  B. Regains normal physiologic and psychological functioning—no irreversible complications; vital signs within normal limits.
  C. Resumes previous activity level, returns to work.
  D. Adheres to follow-up care recommendations.
  E. Knows ways to minimize risk of reinfection.

🔑 Summary of Key Points

1. Disorders of connective tissue or collagen disease characteristically involve *inflammation of multiple organs.*
2. There is *no* way to *prevent* connective tissue disorders, and there is *no cure.* Treatment is symptomatic and intended to maintain optimum functioning and self-care.
3. Rheumatoid arthritis and systemic lupus erythematosus occur more frequently in *women* aged 20–40 yr, striking during the prime of life.
4. Control of *pain* is a major nursing concern in patients with rheumatoid arthritis, as is limited *mobility* and increasing loss of *joint function.*
5. The cause of death in patients with systemic lupus erythematosus is most commonly related to *renal* failure, *cardiac* involvement, or *cerebral* infarct.

💡 Study of Memory Aids

🍎 Diet

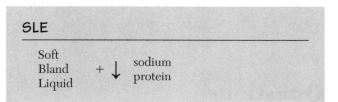

SLE

Soft
Bland   + ↓   sodium
Liquid   protein

💊 Drug Review

Rheumatoid Arthritis

Antimalarials:
  Chloroquine phosphate (Aralen phosphate) with primaquine phosphate: 300 mg of chloroquine base once weekly with evening meal
Histamine receptor antagonist: Ranitidine (Zantac): 150 mg 2 times/d
Immunosuppressive agents: Methotrexate (Mexate): 7.5 mg/wk
Nonsteroidal anti-inflammatory:
  Aspirin: 325–1000 mg q4–6h, *not* to exceed 4 g/d (enteric coated to reduce gastric irritation; antacids to relieve GI upset)
  Ibuprofen (Motrin): 300–800 mg 3–4 times a day

Naproxen (Naprosyn): 250–500 mg bid
Tolmetin (Tolectin): 400 mg tid
Steroids (should *never* be abruptly discontinued;
gradually taper dose to avoid complications)
Dexamethasone (Decadron): 0.75–9 mg/d in
single or divided doses
Methylprednisolone (Medrol): 4–48 mg/d
Prednisone (Deltasone): 5–60 mg/d.

Systemic Lupus Erythematosus

Analgesics: Aspirin: 325–1000 mg q4–6h, *not* to
exceed 4 g/d (enteric coated to reduce gastric
irritation; antacids to relieve GI upset)
Antimalarials: Chloroquine phosphate (Aralen
phosphate) with primaquine phosphate: 300 mg of
chloroquine base once weekly with evening meal.
Immunosuppressive agents:
Azathioprine (Imuran): 1 mg/kg/d for 6–8 wk,
increase to 2.5/kg/d
Cyclophosphamide (Cytoxan): 1–5 mg/kg/d
Methotrexate (Mexate): 7.5 mg/wk
Nonsteroidal anti-inflammatory:
Ibuprofen (Motrin): 200–400 mg q4–6h
Naproxen (Naprosyn): 250–500 mg bid
Tolmetin (Tolectin): 400 mg tid

Lyme Disease

Ceftriaxone (Rocephin): 1–2 g/d
Doxycycline (Vibramycin): 100–200 mg in divided
doses q12h
Penicillin V Potassium (Pen Vee K): 125–500 mg q6h
Penicillin: IV, 1–2 g/d in divided doses q4–6h

Questions

1. The nurse should encourage a patient with rheumatoid
arthritis who is suffering severe morning stiffness to:
   1. Use an electric blanket at night.
   2. Take a hot bath before going to bed and after arising
in the morning.
   3. Drink a hot herb tea upon awakening.
   4. Take aspirin or a nonsteroidal anti-inflammatory drug
(NSAID) 30 minutes before walking.
2. The nurse would conclude that the most likely cause of
fever and tachycardia in a patient with rheumatoid arthritis is:
   1. Dehydration and malnutrition.
   2. Drug toxicity resulting from ASA or NSAID.
   3. Joint pain and inflammation.
   4. GI tract bleeding resulting from excessive ASA use.
3. A patient with acute rheumatoid arthritis is being treated
with aspirin and prednisone. The nurse should monitor
for what serious side effect of both drugs?
   1. Melena stool.

   2. Headaches.
   3. Diplopia.
   4. Tinnitus.
4. A patient with rheumatoid arthritis is hesitant to move
his acutely inflamed shoulder for fear that this may
worsen his pain. The best response by the nurse would
be:
   1. "Instead of exercising, let me massage your shoulder
for relief."
   2. "Initially it may hurt more, but exercise can actually
relieve pain."
   3. "I'll give you aspirin and in 30 minutes you'll be able
to exercise vigorously."
   4. "Rest for your shoulder has been prescribed until the
inflammation subsides."

Answers/Rationale

1. **(4)**   An anti-inflammatory agent would improve mobility
by easing the joint inflammation. Aspirin (ASA) continues to be the drug of choice for the relief of joint pain.
Locally applied heat (**1** or **2**) may only work for *some*
patients. Oral heat such as that provided by a hot herb
tea drink (**3**) does *not* usually have any localized effect
on joint stiffness. **IMP, 3, HPM**
2. **(3)**   Rheumatoid arthritis is an autoimmune, systemic
inflammatory disorder of the connective tissue; the inflammation and resulting pain would cause fever and increase the heart rate. Although while dehydration (**1**)
can increase temperature and heart rate, despite their ill
appearance, patients with rheumatoid arthritis are *not*
typically dehydrated or malnourished. Fever and tachycardia are also *not* side effects of ASA or NSAID therapy
(**2**). Although GI tract bleeding is a side effect of ASA
use (**4**) and tachycardia would occur if this led to severe
blood loss, *fever* would *not* be expected. **AN, 3, PhI**
3. **(1)**   Both drugs can cause GI tract irritation and bleeding; melena stool, or black tarry stool, signifies upper GI
tract bleeding. Headaches (**2**) are a side effect of *prednisone only*. Diplopia (**3**) is *not* a side effect of either drug.
Tinnitus (**4**) only occurs in patients taking high doses of
aspirin. **EV, 4, PhI**
4. **(2)**   Exercise is done even during an acute flare-up of
rheumatoid arthritis and may help to reduce the pain.
Massage (**1**) is effective but *not as much* as exercise. Pain
medication should be given, but the exercise should *not*
be *vigorous* (**3**). Complete rest (**4**) may increase the immobility of the limb, so *some exercise* is *needed*.
IMP, 3, HPM

Key to Codes

Nursing process: AS, assessment; **AN,** analysis; **PL,** planning; **IMP,** implementation; **EV,** evaluation. (See Appendix M for explanation of nursing
process steps.)

Category of human function: 1, protective; **2,** sensory-perceptual; **3,**
comfort, rest, activity, and mobility; **4,** nutrition; **5,** growth and development; **6,** fluid-gas transport; **7,** psychosocial-cultural; **8,** elimination. (See
Appendix O for explanation.)

Client need: SECE, safe, effective care environment; **PhI,** physiologic
integrity; **PsI,** psychosocial integrity; **HPM,** health promotion/mainte-
nance. (See Appendix P for explanation.)

Biliary and Pancreatic Disorders

Chapter Outline

- Pancreatitis
- Diabetes
- Hyperglycemic Hyperosmolar Nonketotic Coma
- Cholecystitis/Cholelithiasis
- Summary of Key Points
- Diagnostic Studies
  - Glucose Testing
  - Ultrasound
    - Cholecystogram
    - Cholangiogram
- Study and Memory Aids
  - Diet
  - Drug Review
- Questions
- Answers/Rationale

Pancreatitis

Inflammatory disease of the pancreas that may result in autodigestion of the pancreas by its own enzymes.

I. Pathophysiology: proteolytic enzymes within the pancreas are activated by endotoxins, exotoxins, ischemia, anoxia, or trauma. Pancreatic enzymes begin process of autodigestion of pancreas and surrounding tissues; also activate other enzymes that digest cellular membranes. Autodigestion leads to edema, hemorrhage, vascular damage, coagulation necrosis, and fat necrosis.

II. Risk factors
   A. Obesity.
   B. Alcoholism, alcohol consumption.
   C. Biliary tract disease.
   D. Abdominal trauma.
   E. Surgery.
   F. Drugs.
   G. Metabolic diseases.
   H. Intestinal disease.
   I. Infections.
   J. Carcinoma.
   K. Adenoma.
   L. Hypercalcemia.

▶ **III. Assessment**
   A. *Subjective data:*
      1. Pain:
         a. Sudden onset; severe, widespread, constant, and incapacitating.
         b. Location—epigastrium, right and left upper quadrants of abdomen; radiates to back, flanks, and substernal area.
      2. Nausea.
      3. History of risk factors.
      4. Dyspnea.
   B. *Objective data:*
      1. *Elevated:* temperature, pulse, respirations, blood pressure (BP) (unless in shock).
      2. *Decreased* breath sounds related to atelectasis/pleural effusion.
      3. *Increased* crackles, cyanosis.
      4. Hemorrhage, shock.
      5. Vomiting.
      6. Fluid and electrolyte imbalances, dehydration.
      7. *Decreased* bowel sounds, abdominal tenderness with guarding.
      8. *Stools:* bulky, pale, foul smelling.
      9. *Skin:* pale, moist, cold; may be jaundiced.
      10. Muscle rigidity.
      11. Supine position leads to increased pain.
      12. Lab data:
         a. *Elevated:*
            (1) Amylase: serum and urine
            (2) Serum lipase, aspartate aminotransferase (AST) (serum glutamic-oxaloacetic transaminase [SGOT]).
            (3) Alkaline phosphatase.
            (4) Bilirubin, glucose: serum and urine.
            (5) Urine protein, white blood cell count (WBC).
            (6) Leukocytes
            (7) Blood urea nitrogen (BUN)
         a. *Decreased:*
            (1) Serum calcium.
            (2) Protein.

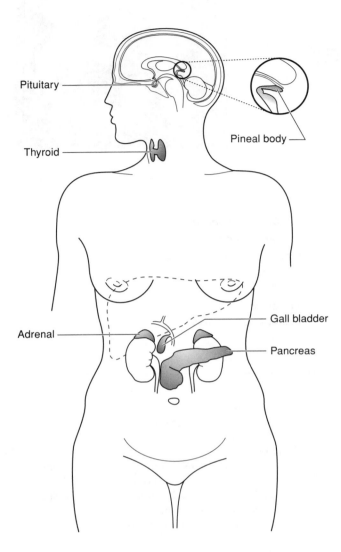

Pituitary

Pineal body

Thyroid

Gall bladder

Adrenal

Pancreas

**THE ANATOMY OF SOME OF THE
ENDOCRINE GLANDS.**

IV.   Analysis/nursing diagnosis

    A. *Altered nutrition, less than body requirements,* related to nausea and vomiting.

    B. *Pain* related to inflammatory and autodigestive processes of pancreas.

    C. *Fluid volume deficit* related to inflammation, decreased intake, and vomiting.

    D. *Ineffective breathing pattern* related to pain and pleural effusion.

    E. *Knowledge deficit* related to risk factors and disease management.

V.   Nursing care plan/implementation

    A. Goal: *control pain.*

        1. Medications: *analgesics*—meperidine (*not* morphine or codeine due to spasmodic effect).

        2. *Position:* sitting with knees flexed.

    B. Goal: *rest injured pancreas.*

        1. NPO.

        2. Nasogastric (*NG*) tube connected to low suction.

        3. Medications:

            a. *Antiulcer.*

            b. *Antiinfectives.*

            c. *Antiemetics.*

            d. *Antispasmotics.*

    C. Goal: *prevent fluid and electrolyte imbalance.*

        1. Monitor: vital signs, central venous pressure.

        2. Administer IVs: fluids, blood, albumin, plasma.

    D. Goal: *prevent respiratory and metabolic complications.*

        1. Cough, deep breathe, change position.

        2. Monitor: blood sugar level, as ordered.

        3. Monitor calcium levels: *Chvostek's* and *Trousseau's sign* positive when calcium deficit exists (see Thyroidectomy, p. 203, for description of tests).

    E. Goal: *provide adequate nutrition.*

        1. *Low-fat diet.*

        2. Bland, small, frequent meals.

        3. Vitamin supplements.

        4. *Avoid* alcohol.

    F. Goal: *prevent complications.*

        1. Monitor for signs of:

            a. Peritonitis.

            b. Bowel obstruction, perforation.

            c. Respiratory complications.

            d. Hypotension, shock.

            e. Disseminated intravascular coagulation.

            f. Hemorrhage from ulcers, varices.

            g. Anemia.

            h. Encephalopathy.

    G. Goal: **health teaching.**

        1. Food selections for low-fat, bland diet.

        2. Need for vitamin therapy.

        3. Importance of avoiding alcohol.

        4. Signs and symptoms of recurrence.

        5. Importance of rest, to prevent relapse.

        6. Desired effects and side effects of prescribed medications:

            a. *Narcotics* for pain.

            b. *Antiemetics* for nausea and vomiting.

            c. *Pancreatic hormone* and *enzymes* to replace enzymes not reaching duodenum.

VI.   Evaluation/outcome criteria

    A. Pain is relieved.

    B. No complications (e.g., peritonitis, respiratory).

    C. States dietary allowances and restrictions.

    D. Takes medications as ordered; states purposes, side effects.

Diabetes

Heterogeneous group of diseases involving disruption of the metabolism of carbohydrates, fats, and protein. If it is uncontrolled, serious vascular and neurologic changes occur.

I. **Types:**
   A. *Type I: IDDM* (insulin-dependent diabetes mellitus): formerly called *juvenile-onset diabetes.* Insulin needed to prevent ketosis; onset usually in youth but may occur in adulthood; prone to ketosis, unstable diabetes.
   B. *Type II: NIDDM* (non–insulin-dependent diabetes mellitus): formerly called *maturity-onset* or *adult-onset diabetes.* May be controlled with diet and oral hypoglycemics or insulin; patient less apt to have ketosis, except in presence of infection. May be further classified as *obese type II* or *nonobese type II.*
   C. *Type III: GDM* (gestational diabetes mellitus): glucose intolerance during pregnancy in women who were not known diabetics prior to pregnancy; will be reclassified after delivery; may need to be treated or may return to prepregnancy state and need no treatment.
   D. *Type IV:* diabetes secondary to another condition, such as pancreatic disease, other hormonal imbalances, or drug therapy such as that involving glucocorticoids.

II. **Pathophysiology:**
   A. IDDM—*absolute* deficiency of insulin due to destruction of pancreatic beta cells as the result of the interaction of genetic, immunologic, hereditary, or environmental factors.
   B. NIDDM—*relative* deficiency of insulin due to:
      1. An islet cell defect resulting in a slowed or delayed response in the release of insulin to a glucose load; or
      2. Reduction in the number of insulin receptors from continuously elevated insulin levels; or
      3. A postreceptor defect; or
      4. A major peripheral resistance to insulin induced by hyperglycemia. These factors lead to the deprivation of insulin-dependent cells → a marked decrease in the cellular rate of glucose uptake, and therefore elevated blood glucose levels.

III. **Risk factors:**
   A. Obesity.
   B. Family history of diabetes.
   C. Elderly.
   D. Women whose babies at birth weighed more than 9 lb.
   E. History of autoimmune disease.

▶ IV. **Assessment**
   A. *Subjective data:*
      1. *Eyes:* blurry vision.
      2. *Skin:* pruritus vulvae.

3. *Neuromuscular:* paresthesia, peripheral neuropathy, lethargy, weakness, fatigue, increased irritability.
      4. *Gastrointestinal (GI): polydipsia* (increased thirst).
      5. *Reproductive:* impotence.
   B. *Objective data:*
      1. *Genitourinary: polyuria,* glycosuria, nocturia (nocturnal enuresis in children).
      2. *Vital signs:*
         a. Pulse and temperature normal or elevated.
         b. BP normal or decreased, unless complications present.
         c. Respirations, increased rate and depth (*Kussmaul's* respirations).
      3. *GI:*
         a. *Polyphagia,* dehydration.
         b. Weight loss, failure to gain weight.
         c. Acetone breath.
      4. *Skin:* cuts heal slowly; frequent infections, foot ulcers, vaginitis.
      5. *Neuromuscular:* loss of strength, peripheral neuropathy.
      6. Lab data:
         a. *Elevated:*
            (1) Blood sugar > 115 mg/dL fasting or > 160 1–2 h after eating.
            (2) Glucose tolerance test.
            (3) Glycosuria (>170 mg/dL).
            (4) Potassium (>5 mEq/L) and chloride (>145 mEq/L).
            (5) Hemoglobin A_{1c} > 7%.
         b. *Decreased:*
            (1) pH (<7.4)
            (2) Pco_2 (<32 mm Hg).
      7. *Long-term pathologic* considerations:
         a. *Cataract formation and retinopathy:* thickened capillary basement membrane, changes in vascularization and hemorrhage, due to chronic hyperglycemia.
         b. *Nephropathy:* due to glomerulosclerosis, arteriosclerosis of renal artery and pyelonephritis, progressive uremia.
         c. *Neuropathy:* due to reduced tissue perfusion; affecting motor, sensory, voluntary, and autonomic functions.
         d. *Arteriosclerosis:* due to lesions of the intimal wall.
         e. *Cardiac:* angina, coronary insufficiency, myocardial infarction.
         f. *Vascular changes:* occlusions, intermittent claudication, loss of peripheral pulses, arteriosclerosis.

▶ V. **Analysis/nursing diagnosis**
   A. *Altered nutrition, less than body requirements,* related to inability to metabolize nutrients and weight loss.
   B. *Altered nutrition, more than body requirements,* related to excessive glucose intake.

C. *Risk for injury* related to complications of uncontrolled diabetes.

D. *Body image disturbance* related to long-term illness.

E. *Knowledge deficit* related to management of long-term illness.

F. *Ineffective individual coping* related to inability to follow diet/medication regimen.

G. *Sexual dysfunction* related to impotence of diabetes and treatment.

VI. Nursing care plan/implementation

  A. Goal: *obtain and maintain normal sugar balance.*

    1. Monitor: vital signs; blood glucose before meals, at bedtime, and as symptoms demand (urine testing for glucose levels is *not* as accurate as capillary blood testing).

    2. Medications: oral hypoglycemics or insulin, as ordered.

    3. *Diet,* as ordered.

      a. Carbohydrates, 50%–60%; protein, 20%; fats, 30% (saturated fats limited to 10%, unsaturated fats, 90%).

      b. Calorie reduction in obese adults; enough calories to promote normal growth and development for children or nonobese adults.

      c. Limit intake of refined sugars.

      d. Add vitamins, minerals as needed for well-balanced diet.

    4. Monitor for signs of acute or chronic complications.

  B. Goal: **health teaching.**

    1. *Diet:* foods allowed, restricted, substitutions.

    2. Medications: administration *techniques;* importance of utilizing room-temperature insulin, rotating injection sites to prevent tissue damage.

    3. Desired and side effects of prescribed insulin type; onset, peak, and duration of action of prescribed insulin.

    4. Blood glucose testing *techniques.*

    5. Signs of complications (Table 13.1).

    6. Importance of health maintenance:

      a. Infection prevention, especially foot and nail care.

      b. Routine checkups.

      c. Maintain stable balance of glucose by carefully monitoring glucose level and making necessary adjustments in diet and activity level; seek medical attention when unable to maintain balance; engage in regular exercise program.

VII. Evaluation/outcome criteria

  A. Optimal blood glucose levels achieved.

  B. Ideal weight maintained.

  C. Adequate hydration.

  D. Carries out self-care activities: blood or urine testing, foot care, exchange diets, medication administration, exercise.

  E. Recognizes and treats hyper- or hypoglycemic reactions.

  F. Seeks medical assistance appropriately.

Hyperglycemic Hyperosmolar Nonketotic Coma (HHNC)

Profound hyperglycemia and dehydration without ketosis or ketoacidosis; occurs in patients with NIDDM. The patient is *critically ill.*

  I. Pathophysiology: hyperglycemia greater than 1000 mg/100 mL causes osmotic diuresis, depletion of extracellular fluid, and hyperosmolarity, precipitated by infection or another stressor. Patient unable to replace fluid deficits with oral intake.

  II. Risk factors:

    A. Old age.

    B. History of NIDDM.

    C. Infections: pneumonia, pyelonephritis, pancreatitis, gram-negative infections.

    D. Kidney failure: uremia and peritoneal dialysis.

    E. Shock:

      1. Lactic acidosis related to bicarbonate deficit.

      2. Myocardial infarction.

    F. Hemorrhage:

      1. GI tract.

      2. Subdural.

      3. Arterial thrombosis.

    G. Medications:

      1. *Diuretics.*

      2. *Glucocorticoids.*

  III. Assessment

    A. *Subjective data:*

      1. Confusion.

      2. Lethargy.

    B. *Objective data:*

      1. Nystagmus.

      2. Dehydration.

      3. Aphasia.

      4. Nuchal rigidity.

      5. Hyperreflexia.

      6. Lab data:

        a. Blood glucose level 1000 mg/dL.

        b. Serum sodium and chloride—normal to elevated.

        c. BUN > 60 mg/dL (higher than in keto-acidosis because of more severe gluconeogenesis and dehydration).

        d. Arterial pH—slightly depressed.

  IV. Analysis/nursing diagnosis

    A. *Risk for injury* related to hyperglycemia.

    B. *Altered renal peripheral tissue perfusion* related to vascular collapse.

    C. *Ineffective airway clearance* related to coma.

  V. Nursing care plan/implementation

    A. Goal: *promote fluid and electrolyte balance.*

    1. Administer IVs: fluids and electrolytes, saline solution given initially to combat dehydration. Lab values will determine nature of fluid replacement.

TABLE 13.1   COMPARISON OF DIABETIC COMPLICATIONS

	Hypoglycemia	*Ketoacidosis*
Pathophysiology	Major metabolic complication when too little food or too large dose of insulin or hypoglycemic agents administered; interferes with oxygen consumption of nervous tissue.	Major metabolic complication in which there is insufficient insulin for metabolism of carbohydrates, fats, and proteins; seen most frequently with patients who are insulin dependent; precipitated in the known diabetic by stressors (such as infection, trauma, major illness) that increase insulin needs.
Risk factors	Too little food. Emotional or added stress. Vomiting or diarrhea. Added exercise.	Insufficient insulin or oral hypoglycemics. Noncompliance with dietary instructions. Major illness/infections. Steroid therapy. Trauma, surgery. Elevated blood sugar: >200 mg/dL.
◄ Assessment	**Behavioral change:** *Subjective data*—nervous, irritable, anxious, confused, disoriented. *Objective data*—abrupt mood changes, psychosis. **Visual:** *Subjective data*—blurred vision, diplopia. *Objective data*—dilated pupils. **Skin:** *Objective data*—diaphoresis, **pale, cool, clammy,** goose bumps (piloerection), **Vitals:** *Objective data*—tachycardia; palpitations, thready. **Gastrointestinal:** *Subjective data*—hunger, nausea. *Objective data*—diarrhea, vomiting. **Neurologic:** *Subjective data*—headache; lips/tongue: tingling, numbness. *Objective data*—fainting, yawning, speech: incoherent; convulsions; coma. **Musculoskeletal:** *Subjective data*—weakness, fatigue. *Objective data*—trembling. Blood sugar: <80 mg/dL.	**Behavioral change:** *Subjective data*—irritable, confused. *Objective data*—drowsy. **Visual:** *Objective data*—eyeballs: soft, sunken. **Skin:** *Objective data*—loss of turgor, **flushed face** **Vitals:** *Objective data*—*Kussmaul's* respiration; breath: fruity; BP: hypovolemic shock. **Gastrointestinal:** *Subjective data*—increased thirst and hunger, abdominal pain, nausea. *Objective data*—vomiting, diarrhea, dry mucous membrane; lips, tongue: red, parched. **Neurologic:** *Subjective data*—headache, irritability, confusion, lethargy, weakness. **Musculoskeletal:** *Subjective data*—fatigue, general malaise. **Renal:** *Objective data*—polyuria Blood sugar: >130 mg/dL.
◄ Analysis/nursing diagnosis	*Risk for injury* related to deficit of needed glucose. *Knowledge deficit* related to proper dietary intake or proper insulin dosage. *Altered nutrition, less than body requirements,* related to glucose deficiency.	*Risk for injury* related to glucose imbalance. *Knowledge deficit* related to proper balance of diet and insulin dosage.

(continued)

TABLE 13.1	COMPARISON OF DIABETIC COMPLICATIONS (*Continued*)	
	Hypoglycemia	*Ketoacidosis*
⬩ Nursing care plan/ implementation	Goal: *provide adequate glucose to reverse hypoglycemia:* administer simple sugar stat, PO or IV, glucose paste absorbed in mucous membrane; monitor *blood* ⬜ *sugar levels:* identify events leading to complication.	Goal: *promote normal balance of food and insulin:* ⬤ **regular** insulin as ordered; IV saline, as ordered; bicarbonate and electrolyte replacements, as ordered; potassium replacements once therapy begins and urine output is adequate.
	⬛ Goal: **health teaching:** how to prevent further episodes (see Diabetes, Health teaching, p. 142); importance of careful monitoring of balance between glucose levels and insulin dosage.	⬛ Goal: **health teaching:** diet instructions; desired effects and side effects of prescribed insulin or hypoglycemic agent (onset, peak, and duration of action); importance of recognizing signs of imbalance.
⬩ Evaluation/outcome criteria	Adheres to diet and correct insulin dosage. Adjusts dosage when activity is increased.	Serious complications avoided. Accepts prescribed diet. Takes medication (correct dose and time).
	Glucose level 80–120 mg/L.	Glucose level 80–120 mg/dL.

Source: Lagerquist SL: *Little, Brown's NCLEX-RN Examination Review.* Boston: Little, Brown, 1996. P. 127.

2. Monitor in take and output (I&O) because of the high volume of fluid replaced in the critical stage of this condition.
3. Administer nursing care for problem that precipitated this serious condition.
4. Food by mouth when patient is able.

B. Goal: *prevent complications.*

⬤ 1. Administer *regular* insulin (initial dose usually 5–15 U) and food, as ordered.
2. Uncontrolled condition leads to cardiovascular disease, renal failure, blindness, diabetic gangrene.

⬩ **VI. Evaluation/outcome criteria**

A. Blood sugar returns to normal level of 80–120 mg/dL.
B. Patient is alert to time, place, and person.
C. Primary medical problem resolves.
D. Patient recognizes and reports signs of imbalance.

Cholecystitis/Cholelithiasis

Inflammation of gallbladder due to bacterial infection, cholelithiasis (stones, cholesterol, calcium, or bile in the gallbladder), or choledocholithiasis (stone in the common bile duct) and/or obstruction. *Acute cholecystitis* is abrupt in onset, but the patient usually has a history of several attacks of fatty-food intolerance. Patient with *chronic cholecystitis* has a history of several attacks of moderate severity and has usually learned to avoid fatty foods to decrease symptoms.

I. Pathophysiology: calculi form as a result of the increased concentration of bile salts, pigments, or cholesterol due to metabolic or hemolytic disorders, biliary stasis → precipitation of salts into stones or inflammation causing bile constituents to become altered.

II. Risk factors:
  A. Women.
  B. Obesity.
  C. Pregnancy.
  D. Cirrhosis of the liver.
  E. Diabetes.

⬩ **III. Assessment**
  A. *Subjective data:*
    1. *Pain:*
      a. Type—severe colic, radiating to back under the scapula and to the right shoulder.
      ⬜ **b.** Positive *Murphy's sign*—a sign of gallbladder disease in which patient experiences pain when taking a deep breath as pressure is placed over the location of the gallbladder.
      c. Location—right upper quadrant, epigastric area, flank.
      d. Duration—spasm of duct attempting to dislodge stone lasts until dislodged or relieved by medication, or sometimes by vomiting.
    2. *GI*—anorexia, nausea, feeling of fullness, indigestion, intolerance of fatty foods.
  B. *Objective data:*
    1. *GI*—belching, vomiting, clay-colored stools.
    2. *Vital signs*—increased pulse, fever.
    3. *Skin*—chills, jaundice.
    4. *Urine*—dark amber.
    5. Lab data—*elevated:*
      a. WBC
      b. Alkaline phosphatase
      c. Serum amylase, lipase
      d. AST [SGOT]
      e. Bilirubin.

IV. Analysis/nursing diagnosis
   A. *Pain* related to obstruction of bile duct due to cholelithiasis.
   B. *Altered nutrition, more than body requirements,* related to consumption of fatty foods.
   C. *Altered nutrition, less than body requirements,* related to hesitancy to eat due to anorexia and nausea.
   D. *Risk for fluid volume deficit* related to episodes of vomiting.
   E. *Knowledge deficit* related to fat-free diet.

V. Nursing care plan/implementation
   A. **Nonsurgical interventions:**
      1. Goal: *promote comfort.*
         a. Medications as ordered: *analgesics* (meperidine), *antiinfective, antispasmodics,* electrolytes.
         b. *Avoid* morphine due to spasmodic effect.
         c. NG tube connected to low suction.
         d. *Diet:* fat free when able to tolerate food.
      2. Goal: **health teaching.**
         a. Signs, symptoms, and complications of disease.
         b. Fat-free diet.
         c. Desired effects and side effects of prescribed medications.
         d. Prepare for possible removal of gallbladder (cholecystectomy) if conservative treatment unsuccessful.
   B. **Surgical interventions:**
      1. *Preoperative*—Goal: *prevent injury:* see Preoperative Preparation, pp. 111–113.
      2. *Postoperative*—Goal: *promote comfort* (see also Postoperative Experience, pp. 114–115, 120–121).
         a. Promote tube drainage.
            (1) *NG tube* connected to low suction.
            (2) *T-tube* connected to closed-gravity drainage, to preserve patency of edematous common duct and ensure bile drainage; usual amount 500–1000 mL/24 h; dark brown drainage.
            (3) Provide enough tubing to allow turning without tension.
            (4) Empty and record bile drainage q8h.
         b. *Position:* low to semi-Fowler's to facilitate T-tube drainage.
         c. Dressing: dry to protect skin (because bile excoriates skin).
         d. Clamp T-tube as ordered.
            (1) Observe for abdominal distention, pain, nausea, chills, or fever.
            (2) Unclamp tube and notify MD if symptoms appear.
      3. Goal: *prevent complications.*
         a. *IV* fluids with vitamins.
         b. Cough, turn, and deep breathe (prone to respiratory complication because of high incision).
         c. Early ambulation to prevent vascular complications and aid in expelling flatus.
         d. Monitor for jaundice: skin, sclera, urine, stools.
         e. Monitor for signs of hemorrhage, infection.
      4. Goal: **health teaching.**
         a. *Diet:* fat free for 6 wk.
         b. Signs of complications of food intolerance, pain, infection, hemorrhage.

VI. Evaluation/outcome criteria
   A. No complications.
   B. Able to tolerate food.
   C. Plans follow-up care.
   D. Possible weight reduction.

Summary of Key Points

1. The symptoms of cholecystitis are remarkably *similar* to those of many other conditions, such as angina or myocardial infarction. An accurate assessment is therefore critical.
2. *Demerol* is the preferred analgesic in cholecystitis for pain. When pain becomes intractable (unrelieved), cholecystectomy will be done.
3. The use of laser laparoscopy for removal of the gallbladder has changed the postoperative concerns from pneumonia to *injury* to the common bile duct or other organs.
4. If the common bile duct has been explored, a *T-tube* will be inserted during surgery to ensure bile drainage. When the tube is clamped, observe the patient for jaundice or discomfort after eating.
5. The pain from pancreatitis is severe and intense; however, morphine sulfate is *contraindicated.*
6. The patient with pancreatitis is at risk for the development of *hypovolemia* and *shock* stemming from the effects of the inflammation.
7. With diabetes mellitus the kidney excretion of excess glucose and ketones *causes* diuresis (polyuria); thirst results from the loss of water (polydipsia), and hunger (polyphagia) *results* from the impaired metabolism stemming from the deficiency of insulin.
8. Despite the glucose intolerance, most of the calories in the diabetic diet come from *complex carbohydrates.*
9. Diabetics are either insulin dependent (to remember—type I has *none*) or non–insulin dependent (type II has a *few* islet cells).
10. Although exercise may increase carbohydrate metabolism and reduce the need for insulin or increase the need for food, *stored glycogen* may be released, which increases the blood sugar level.

Diagnostic Studies

Glucose Testing

To detect disorder of glucose metabolism, such as diabetes.

1. **Fasting blood sugar (FBS):** Blood sample is drawn after a 12-h fast (usually overnight). H_2O is allowed. If diabetes is present, value will be >140 mg/dL.
2. **2-h Postprandial blood sugar (PPBS):** blood is taken after a meal. For best results, patient should
   ● be on a high-*carbohydrate diet* for 2–4 d before testing. Patient fasts overnight, eats a high-carbohydrate breakfast; blood sample is drawn 2 h after eating. Patient should rest during 2-h interval. Smoking and coffee may increase glucose level.
3. **Glucose tolerance test (GTT):** done when sugar in urine or FBS or 2-h PPBS results are not conclusive. A timed test, usually 2 h. *High-carbohydrate diet* is eaten 3 d before test. Blood is drawn after overnight fast. Patient drinks a very sweet glucose liquid. All of the solution must be consumed. Blood and urine sample usually taken at 30 min, 1 h, 2 h, and sometimes 3 h after drinking solution. Blood glucose *peaks* in 30–60 min and returns to *normal*, usually *within 3 h.*

Ultrasound (sonogram)

Scanning by ultrasound is used to diagnose disorders of the thyroid, kidney, liver, uterus, gallbladder, fetus, and the intracranial structures in the neonate. It is not useful when visualization through air or bone is required (lung studies). In some hospitals the sonogram has taken the place of the oral cholecystogram in diagnosing gallbladder distention, bile duct distention, and calculi. *Patient preparation* is minimal, i.e., NPO for at least 8 h for gallbladder studies. No x-radiation. *Thirty-two ounces of water PO 30 min prior* to studies of lower abdomen or uterus.

Cholecystogram

Done if gallbladder *not* seen with ultrasound—ingestion of organic iodine contrast medium: Telepaque (iopanoic acid) or Oragrafin (preparation of calcium or sodium salt of ipodate), followed in 12 h by x-ray visualization; gallbladder disease is indicated if there is *poor* or no visualization of the bladder; accurate *only* if GI and liver function is intact; perform *before* barium enema or upper GI. *Patient preparation:* explain purpose;
● administer large amount of *water* with contrast cap-
● sules; *low-fat meal* evening *before* x-ray; *oral laxative or stool softener after meal; no food* allowed after contrast capsules; water, tea, or coffee, with no cream or sugar, usually allowed. *After completion of exam:* fluids, food, and rest; observe for any signs of allergy to contrast medium.

Cholangiogram

Intravenous injection of a radiopaque contrast medium, followed by fluoroscopic and x-ray examination of the bile ducts; failure of the contrast medium to pass certain points in the bile duct pinpoints *obstruction*.

💡 Study and Memory Aids

Diabetes—Assessment: "3 P's" (or "3 poly's")

P olydipsia (↑ thirst)
P olyphagia (↑ hunger)
P olyuria (↑ urination)

Blood Glucose (rhyme)

Symptom	Implication
Wet and **clammy** (diaphoretic)	give hard **candy** (hypoglycemia).
Hot and **dry** (dehydrated) (↑ temp, ↑ resp.)	glucose is **high** (hyperglycemia).

Source: Modified from *Memory Notebook of Nursing.* Dallas: Nursing Education Consultants, 1994.

Hypoglycemia: Signs and Symptoms—"DIRE"

D iaphoresis
I ncreased pulse
R estless
E xtra hungry

● Diet

Pancreatitis

↓ Fat
Bland, small, frequent meals
Avoid alcohol
Vitamin supplements

● Drug Review

Pancreatitis

Analgesics
  Meperidine (Demerol): 50–150 mg q3–4h as needed; IV, 15–35 mg/h as a continuous infusion
  No morphine, codeine
  Calcium carbonate (Titralac): 1–2 g with water pc and hs

Magnesium and aluminum hydroxide (Maalox suspension): 5–30 mL pc and hs
Sucralfate (Caralfate): 1 g qid
Antiinfectives—used for severe cases of pancreatitis
Cephalothin (Keflin): IV 0.5–2g q 4–6 H
Cephalexin (Keflix): 250–500 mg q 6h
Gentamicin (Garamycin): 3–5 mg/kg/d in divided doses
Penicillin G: 1.2 million U IM
Antiemetics
Prochlorperazine (Compazine): 5–30 mg qid
Promethazine (Phenergan): 10–25 mg q4h
Trimethobenzamide (Tigan): 250 mg qid
Antispasmodics: Propantheline (Pro-Banthine): 15 mg tid; 30 mg hs
Anti-ulcer: Aluminum hydroxide gel (Amphojel): 5–10 mL q2–4h or 1h pc
Replacement therapy: Exogenous pancreatic enzyme therapy includes lipase, trypsin, or histamine (H_2) receptor antagonists. Possible exogenous insulin therapy because of the destruction of islet cell tissue
Vitamin therapy according to deficiencies

Diabetes: Antihyperglycemic

Oral
Acetohexamide (Dymelor): 200–1500 mg/d
Chlorpropamide (Diabinese): 100–1,000 mg/d
Tolazamide (Tolinase): 100–500 mg/d
Tolbutamide (Orinase): 500–3,000 mg/d
Injection
Crystalline (regular) (Humulin R)—rapid acting
Lente—intermediate acting
NPH—intermediate acting
Protamine zinc insulin—slow acting
Ultralente—extended acting

See Appendix D, Review of Pharmacology.

Cholecystitis

Antiinfectives to control infection
Cephalexin (Keflex): 250–500 mg q6h
Cephalothin (Keflin): IV, 0.5–2 g q4–6h
Erythromycin: 250–500 mg q6–12h
Gentamicin (Garamycin): 3–5 mg/kg/d in divided doses
Penicillin G: 1.2 million U in single IM dose
Antispasmodics: Propantheline (Pro-Banthine): 15 mg tid, 30 mg hs
Narcotics
Meperidine (Demerol): 50–150 mg q3–4h as needed; IV 15–35 mg/h as a continuous infusion
No morphine

Questions

1. When would the nurse typically expect to hear bowel sounds after exploration of the bile duct and a cholecystectomy?
   1. 4–6 hours.
   2. 6–12 hours.
   3. 12–24 hours.
   4. 24–48 hours.
2. After the ingestion of the glucose drink used in the glucose tolerance test, the nurse would know a patient does not have diabetes mellitus if the blood glucose level returns to normal in:
   1. 2–3 hours.
   2. 4–6 hours.
   3. 7–8 hours.
   4. 10–12 hours.
3. The nurse would instruct a diabetic patient to exclude which food item from the meat exchange list?
   1. Peanut butter.
   2. Dried beans.
   3. Pasta.
   4. Cottage cheese.
4. A diabetic patient tells the nurse he drinks quite a bit of nonfat milk. The nurse's response should be:
   1. "I'm glad you are watching your fat intake."
   2. "The lactose in nonfat milk is absorbed rapidly."
   3. "Have you been craving milk more lately?"
   4. "Have you decreased the amount of another exchange food?"
5. The nurse would conclude that a patient was experiencing hypoglycemia if the assessment findings included:
   1. Diaphoresis and restlessness.
   2. Rapid, thready pulse.
   3. Vomiting and bradycardia.
   4. Rapid, bounding pulse.
6. The nurse is to give a patient 30 units of NPH and 10 units of regular insulin subcutaneously. To administer the injection the nurse would:
   1. Take the regular insulin from the refrigerator just before giving it.
   2. Draw up the regular insulin first and then the NPH.
   3. Shake the bottle to thoroughly mix the insulin.
   4. Rub the injection site slightly after the injection.
7. Which type of insulin should the nurse prepare for a direct IV push for the treatment of ketoacidosis?
   1. Regular.
   2. Semilente.
   3. NPH.
   4. Ultralente.
8. The effectiveness of insulin given through a continuous IV infusion pump would be expected to be:
   1. More rapid because of the direct vascular access afforded.
   2. Reduced because the potency is lessened by at least 20% to 80%.
   3. The same as that of the agent given subcutaneously, because of the dilution that occurs.
   4. Variable; may be either more or less potent.
9. A patient with type I diabetes (IDDM) asks if she will

still receive insulin when she is NPO before surgery. The best response by the nurse would be:
1. "No. Since you're not eating, there is no need."
2. "It depends on how stressed you feel about the surgery."
3. "Yes, because you will mostly likely receive glucose IV."
4. "Yes, but less than your regular daily amount."

10. Which plan for a snack would be appropriate for a patient receiving NPH insulin every morning at 7:00 A.M.?
1. Coffee and half a bagel an hour after the injection.
2. A piece of fruit about 4:00 P.M.
3. Cheese and crackers before bed at 10:00 P.M.
4. Hard candy every couple of hours during the day.

11. What nursing action is most important for a newly admitted patient experiencing diabetic ketoacidosis?
1. Patient teaching on self-care.
2. Insertion of a Foley catheter for urine testing.
3. Starting a peripheral IV.
4. Assessment of the patient's level of confusion.

12. Patient teaching about diabetic foot care should include the need to:
1. Rub feet with alcohol to toughen skin.
2. Use a heating pad to warm feet.
3. Inspect feet daily for cracks or cuts.
4. Disinfect scissors before removing calluses.

13. The nurse knows the patient understands the teaching about her diabetes when she says:
1. "I will need more insulin when I increase my activity."
2. "I need to eliminate sweets from my diet."
3. "I'll call with my questions after I read the brochure."
4. "Managing diabetes will be a lifetime of learning."

Answers/Rationale

1. **(4)** Bowel sounds usually return between 36 and 48 hours after abdominal surgery. Bowel sounds may return the earliest by 24 hours, due to the effects of general anesthesia, but not as early as 12 hours (**2** and **3**). Bowel sounds would never return in 4 to 6 hours in a patient receiving a general anesthetic (**1**). **AS, 8, PhI**

2. **(1)** The blood glucose level would return to normal in 2 hours in patients under 55 years of age; this may take at least 3 hours in those over 55 years. If the blood glu-

cose level stays above 200 mg/dL for more than 2 to 3 hours, the patient is likely diabetic. The timing in all the other options (**2, 3,** and **4**) is *longer* than that required for the blood glucose level of a nondiabetic patient to return to normal. **AN, 4, PhI**

3. **(3)** The meat exchange list contains only protein sources; pasta is a *carbohydrate*. All of the other foods (**1, 2,** and **4**) *are* non-meat sources of *protein*. **IMP, 4, HPM**

4. **(2)** The lack of fat in the milk actually causes the absorption of lactose, or milk sugar, to increase. If a diabetic needs to lose weight, nonfat milk is the best type of milk to be used but the amount needs to be limited to no more than one or two 8-ounce glasses daily. Reinforcing fat reduction (**1**) is not wrong, but it does not address the underlying problem in a diabetic patient. If the patient is not eating a balanced diet, there may be cravings (**3**); he/she may also not understand the limitations surrounding milk consumption. Although the diabetic diet does allow for exchanges (**4**), the overall percentage in each category needs to be consistent: 55% to 60% carbohydrates; 30% fats; and 12% to 20% protein. **AN, 4, PhI**

5. **(1)** Hypoglycemia occurs when the blood glucose level drops to 60 mg/dL or lower; diaphoresis occurs because epinephrine is released when the blood glucose level declines. The patient may act very restless and apprehensive, even drunk or psychotic. Although epinephrine would cause an increase in the pulse rate, there is no change in volume in hypoglycemia; a rapid, thready pulse (**2**) would result from *volume loss*, and a rapid, bounding pulse (**4**) would be a sign of *volume excess*. Other symptoms of hypoglycemia include weakness: headache, and lack of muscular coordination, but *not* vomiting or bradycardia (**3**). **AN, 4, PhI**

6. **(2)** The clear insulin (regular) is drawn up first, followed by the cloudy insulin (NPH). This prevents contamination of the fast-acting (regular) insulin. The current bottle of insulin does not need to be refrigerated (**1**), and in fact it is *better not* to administer *cold* insulin because this fosters lipodystrophy. The bottle should be gently rolled between the palms to mix the agent, *not shaken* (**3**). The nurse should apply gentle direct pressure and *not rub* (**4**) the injection site, because absorption may be affected. **PL, 4, SECE**

7. **(1)** Regular insulin is the *only* insulin that may be given by direct IV administration for fast action in the treatment of diabetic ketoacidosis. The other types of insulin (**2, 3,** and **4**) *cannot* be given IV. **IMP, 4, PhI**

8. **(2)** The plastic or glass container or the tubing causes the potency of the insulin to be reduced before it even reaches the venous system. The degree to which it is reduced varies, but flushing the tubing with 50 to 100 mL of IV solution minimizes the loss of potency. (Note: regular insulin is the *only* insulin that can be given IV.) Even though vascular access (**1**) is direct and insulin given in this way would take effect more rapidly, the *amount* received is *uncertain,* and the clinical effects are less predictable. The effectiveness of insulin given by IV infusion pump is not the same as that of subcutane-

Key to Codes

Nursing process: AS, assessment; **AN,** analysis; **PL,** planning; **IMP,** implementation; **EV,** evaluation. (See Appendix M for explanation of nursing process steps.)

Category of human function: 1, protective; **2,** sensory-perceptual; **3,** comfort, rest, activity, and mobility; **4,** nutrition; **5,** growth and development; **6,** fluid-gas transport; **7,** psychosocial-cultural; **8,** elimination. (See Appendix O for explanation.)

Client need: SECE, safe, effective care environment; **PhI,** physiologic integrity; **PsI,** psychosocial integrity; **HPM,** health promotion/maintenance. (See Appendix P for explanation.)

ously administered insulin (**3**), but there is a *degree of uncertainty* associated with both IV and subcutaneous administration. Insulin given by continuous IV infusion will always be *less potent,* not more (**4**). **EV, 4, PhI**

9. (**3**)   Generally an IV with dextrose in the solution is started to maintain fluid and nutrition status. Insulin is given IV according to the blood glucose determinations. Insulin is still needed even though the patient is not eating (**1**), because surgery is a stressor, which stimulates the release of glucose; the degree of stress (**2**) may affect the *amount* of insulin given, but *not whether* it will be given. Because of the IV glucose and the added stress, the amount administered may actually be increased, *not* decreased (**4**). **IMP, 4, PhI**

10. (**2**)   NPH is an intermediate-acting insulin and the action peaks in 6 to 12 hours after administration. A reaction would therefore occur between 1:00 and 7:00 P.M. A reaction in the early morning (**1**) would occur in response to *regular* insulin. A reaction later in the evening or at night (**3**) would be more likely to occur with the *long-acting* insulins. Although diabetics should carry hard candy (**4**), hypoglycemic reactions *every few hours* are *not* common. **IMP, 4, PhI**

11. (**3**)   A patient with ketoacidosis will require the IV administration of fluids to treat the severe dehydration, insulin to manage the hyperglycemia, and possibly sodium bicarbonate to treat acidosis. Teaching (**1**) should be done once the patient's condition is *stable* and *before* discharge. Urinalysis would be done to assess kidney function, but it is not needed for glucose testing; since blood is used for testing. Depending on the patient's level of consciousness and a problem with incontinence, a catheter *may or may not* be inserted (**2**). Confusion (**4**) is *not* the change in consciousness expected in a patient with ketoacidosis; the patient usually becomes comatose in the presence of severe acidosis. **PL, 4, PhI**

12. (**3**)   Peripheral circulation and wound healing are poor in diabetics, and diabetics are also more susceptible to infection. Foot care is therefore very important to prevent loss of toes or the foot. Alcohol (**1**) is drying and may foster cracking. Because the circulation and sensations are decreased, going barefoot or applying extreme heat or cold to the limbs (**2**) may only cause injury. Trimming the toenails or removing calluses (**4**) should not be done by the patient, but preferably by a podiatrist. **IMP, 4, PhI**

13. (**4**)   Diabetes is a chronic illness; although it is manageable, it is not curable. Exercise (**1**) actually *decreases* the need for insulin. Carbohydrates constitute 55% to 60% of the diabetic diet, so "sweets" (**2**) may be included but in *limited* quantities. The statement in option 3 does *not* reflect an understanding of the teaching. **EV, 4, PhI**

Hepatic Disorders

Chapter Outline

- Hepatitis: A, B, C and Delta
- Cirrhosis
- Esophageal Varices
- Summary of Key Points
- Study and Memory Aids

  - Diagnostic Studies
  - Diet
  - Drug Review
- Questions
- Answers/Rationale

Hepatitis

Inflammation of the liver.

I. Pathophysiology

  A. Infection with either hepatitis A (formerly called infectious hepatitis), hepatitis B (formerly called serum hepatitis), hepatitis C (caused by at least two unidentified viruses), or delta hepatitis (infection caused by a defective RNA virus that requires hepatitis B virus to multiply) → inflammation, necrosis, and regeneration of liver parenchyma. Hepatocellular injury impairs clearance of urobilinogen → elevated urinary urobilinogen; and, as injury increases → conjugated bilirubin not reaching the intestines → decreased urine and fecal urobilinogen → increased serum bilirubin → jaundice.

  B. Failure of liver to detoxify products → increased toxic products of protein metabolism → gastritis and duodenitis.

II. Risk factors:

  A. Exposure to virus.

  B. Exposure to carriers of virus.

  C. Exposure to hepatotoxins, such as dry cleaning agents.

  D. Nonimmunized.

⋈ III. Assessment

  A. *Subjective data:*

  1. Anorexia, nausea.
  2. Malaise, dull ache in upper right quadrant.
  3. Repugnance to food, cigarette smoke, strong odors, alcohol.
  4. Headache.
  5. Pruritus.

  B. *Objective data:*

  1. Fever.
  2. *Liver:* enlarged (hepatomegaly), tender, smooth.

  3. *Skin:* icterus in sclera of eyes, jaundice, rash, pruritus, petechiae, bruises.
  4. *Urine:* normal, dark.
  5. *Stool:* normal, clay colored, loose.
  6. Vomiting, weight loss.
  7. *Lymph nodes:* enlarged.
  8. Lab data:
      a. Blood—leukocytosis.
      b. *Increased* aspartate aminotransferase (AST), serum glutamic-oxaloacetic transaminase (SGOT), alanine aminotransferase, serum glutamic pyruvic transaminase (SGPT), bilirubin levels, alkaline phosphatase.
      c. Urine—*increased* urobilinogen.
  9. See Table 14.1.

⋈ IV. Analysis/nursing diagnosis

  A. *Pain* related to inflammation of liver.

  B. *Impaired skin integrity* related to pruritus.

  C. *Activity intolerance* related to malaise.

  D. *Risk for infection* to others related to incubation/infectious period.

  E. *Altered nutrition, less than body requirements,* related to repugnance to food.

  F. *Social isolation* related to isolation precautions.

⋈ V. Nursing care plan/implementation

  A. Goal: *promote comfort.*

  1. Bed rest to combat fatigue and reduce metabolic needs until hepatomegaly subsides; *semi-Fowler's* or *supine positioning.*
  2. Oral hygiene q1–2h to decrease nausea.
  ☞ 3. Range of motion exercises to maintain muscle strength.
  4. *Measures to reduce pruritus:*
      a. Mild, oil-based lotion to reduce itching.
      b. Nails cut short, cotton gloves, long-sleeved clothing to prevent skin injury from scratching.

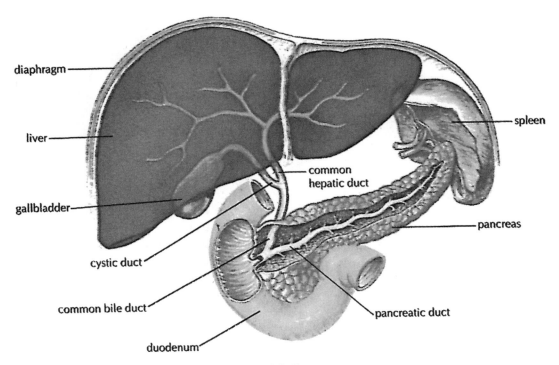

The liver and biliary system.

c. Environment: cool and dry.
☞ d. Cool wet soaks to skin.
e. Diversional activities.
💊 f. Medications as ordered:
   (1) *Emollients* to relieve dry skin.
   (2) *Topical corticosteroids* to reduce inflammation.
   (3) *Antihistamines* to reduce itch.
   (4) *Tranquilizers* and *sedatives* to allow rest and prevent exhaustion.
B. Goal: *prevent spread of infection to others.*
☞ 1. Isolation according to type:
   a. *Hepatitis A:*
      (1) Enteric precautions (Table 14.2).
      (2) Private room preferred.
      (3) Gown/gloves for direct contact with feces.
   ☞ (4) Handwashing when in direct contact with feces.
   b. *Hepatitis B:* blood and body fluid precautions.
      (1) Needle/dressing precautions.
      (2) Private room *not* necessary.
      (3) Gown: only if enteric precautions also necessary.
      🖐 (4) Handwashing; use gloves when in direct contact with blood.
   c. *Hepatitis C:* blood and body fluid precautions—Same as precautions for hepatitis B, except when in countries with fecal-oral form; then use hepatitis A precautions also.

   d. *Delta:* Same as precautions for hepatitis B.
💊 2. Passive immunity for contacts:
   a. *hepatitis A:* immune serum globulin (ISG).
   b. *Hepatitis B:* hepatitis B immune globulin (HGIB) or ISG.
   c. *Hepatitis C:* prophylaxis not as effective; immune globulin may be given.
   d. *Delta:* same as for hepatitis B.
3. Goal: *promote healing.*
   a. *Diet* as tolerated:
      (1) NPO with parenteral infusions, when in acute stage.
      (2) High protein, high carbohydrate, low fat; offered in frequent, small meals.
      (3) Push fluids, if not contraindicated; intake and output (I&O).
4. Goal: *monitor for worsening of disease process, failure to respond to treatment.*
   a. Observe urine—dark due to presence of bile and stool, clay colored.
   📈 b. Observe sclera, monitor lab test results to detect increasing jaundice.
   c. Mental confusion, unusual somnolence may indicate decreased liver function.
   d. Weigh daily—increase indicates fluid retention and possible ascites.
🏠 5. Goal: *health teaching.*
   a. Diet and fluid intake to promote liver regeneration.
   b. Importance of rest and limited activity to reduce metabolic workload of liver.

TABLE 14.1   COMPARISON OF HEPATITIS A, B, C AND DELTA HEPATITIS: ETIOLOGY, INCIDENCE, EPIDEMIOLOGY, AND CLINICAL CHARACTERISTICS

	Hepatitis A	Hepatitis B	Hepatitis C	Delta Hepatitis
Incubation	2–6 wk	4 wk–6 mo	Variable: 14–160 d; average, 50 d	4 wk–6 mo
Communicable	Until 7–9 d after jaundice occurs	Several months—as long as virus present in blood	As long as virus present in blood	As long as virus present in blood
Transmission	Fecal-oral, blood, sexual	Parenteral, sexual	Percutaneous, via contaminated blood, parenteral drug abuse; some fecal-oral forms	Parenteral, blood
Sources	Crowding; contaminated food, milk, or water	Contaminated needles, syringes, surgical instruments	Persons who have received 15 or more blood transfusions; IV drug users; persons traveling to contaminated areas	Contaminated needles, syringes
Portal of entry	GI tract; asymptomatic carriers	Integumentary: Contact with blood plasma or blood transfusion	Blood	Integumentary: blood
Hepatitis B antigen	Not present	Present	Not present	Present
Incidence	Sporadic epidemics; increased in children <15 yr	Increased in ages 15–29 yr, particularly in heroin addicts; occupational hazard for laboratory workers, nurses, physicians	All age groups; higher in adults because of exposure to risk factors	Same as for hepatitis B
⬤ Immunity	*Preexposure:* immune globulin, 0.02 mL/kg *Postexposure:* within 2 wk of exposure, as above	*Preexposure:* hepatitis B vaccine *Postexposure:* immune globulin with high amounts of anti-HBs (HBIG); hepatitis B vaccine	None; immune globulin may be given	None
Prevention	🖐 Handwashing, use of gloves	Care when handling products contaminated by blood, use of gloves	Same as for hepatitis B	Same as for hepatitis B
Severity	Mild	Mild to moderate	Mild to moderate	Moderate to severe
Fever	Common	Uncommon	Uncommon	Uncommon
Nausea/vomiting	Common	Common	Common	Common

Source: Lagerquist SL: *Little, Brown's NCLEX-RN Examination Review.* Boston: Little, Brown, 1996. P. 114.

c. Personal hygiene practices to prevent contamination.

d. *Avoid:* alcohol, blood donations, and contact with communicable infections.

e. Follow-up case referral; may take 6 mo for full recovery.

f. Teach contacts about available immunizations.

▶ **VI. Evaluation/outcome criteria**

A. Tolerates food; nausea and vomiting decreased.

B. Signs of infection/inflammation absent.

C. No complications, hemorrhage, liver damage, ascites.

D. No jaundice noted.

TABLE 14.2   ☞ ENTERIC PRECAUTIONS

1. Private room if the patient's hygiene is poor. In general, patients with the same infection *may share* a room.
2. Masks are *not* indicated.
3. Gowns are indicated if soiling is likely.
4. Gloves are indicated for touching infective material.
5. Hands must be washed *before* and *after* touching the patient or potentially contaminated articles.
6. Contaminated articles should be discarded or bagged and labeled.

Source: Lagerquist SL: *Little, Brown's NCLEX-RN Examination Review.* Boston: Little, Brown, 1996. P. 114.

Cirrhosis

Chronic inflammation and fibrosis of the liver in which some liver cells (hepatocytes) undergo necrosis and others undergo proliferative regeneration.

I. **Pathophysiology:** progressive destruction of hepatic cells → loss of normal metabolic function of the liver and formation of scar tissue. Regeneration and proliferation of fibrous tissue → obstruction of the portal vein → increased portal hypertension, ascites, liver failure, and eventual death.

II. **Risk factors**
   A. Alcohol abuse most common cause.
   B. Nutritional deficiency with decreased protein intake.
   C. Hepatotoxins.
   D. Virus.

III. **Assessment**
   A. *Subjective data:*
      1. Chronic feeling of malaise.
      2. Anorexia, nausea.
      3. Abdominal pain.
      4. Pruritus.
   B. *Objective data:*
      1. *Gastrointestinal (GI):*
         a. Malnutrition, weight loss.
         b. Vomiting.
         c. Flatulence.
         d. Ascites.
         e. Enlarged liver and spleen.
         f. Glossitis.
         g. Fetid breath (sweet, musty odor).
      2. *Blood*—coagulation defects, possible esophageal varices, portal hypertension, bleeding from gums and injection sites.
      3. *Skin and hair*—edema, jaundice, spider angioma, palmar erythema, decreased pubic and axillary hair.
      4. *Reproductive*—menstrual abnormalities, gynecomastia, testicular atrophy, impotence.

   5. *Neurologic*—memory loss, hepatic coma, decreased level of consciousness, flappy tremor, grimacing.
   6. Lab data:
      a. *Decreased:* albumin, potassium, magnesium, blood urea nitrogen;
      b. *Elevated:* prothrombin time, globulins, ammonia, AST/(SGOT), ALT/(SGPT) bromsulphalein (BSP), alkaline phosphatase, uric acid, blood sugar.

IV. **Analysis/nursing diagnosis**
   A. *Altered nutrition, less than body requirements,* related to decreased intake, nausea, and vomiting.
   B. *Risk for injury* related to decreased prothrombin production.
   C. *Activity intolerance* related to fatigue.
   D. *Fatigue* related to anorexia and nutritional deficiencies.
   E. *Self-esteem disturbance* related to physical body changes.
   F. *Risk for impaired skin integrity* related to pruritus.

V. **Nursing care plan/implementation**
   A. Goal: *provide for special safety needs.*
      1. Monitor vital signs (including neurologic) frequently for hemorrhage from esophageal varices (may have *Sengstaken-Blakemore* or *Linton* tube inserted).
      2. Prepare patient for *LeVeen shunt* surgery for portal hypertension if needed.
      3. Assist with *paracentesis* performed for ascites; monitor vital signs to prevent shock during procedure.
   B. Goal: *relieve discomfort caused by complications.*
      1. *Position:* semi-Fowler's or Fowler's to decrease pressure on diaphragm due to ascites.
      2. Deep breathing q2h to prevent respiratory complications.
      3. Skin care: topical medications to relieve pruritus, nail care to decrease possibility of further skin injury.
      4. Frequent oral hygiene necessitated by nausea, vomiting, and fetid breath.
   C. Goal: *improve fluid and electrolyte balance.*
      1. IV fluids and vitamins.
      2. I&O, hourly urine measurements during acute attacks.
      3. Daily: girths, weights to monitor fluid balance.
      4. *Diuretics* as ordered to decrease edema.
      5. May receive serum albumin to promote adequate vascular volume, prevent azotemia and encephalopathy, and promote diuresis (observe carefully, as albumin could escape quickly through cell walls and cause increase in ascites).
   D. Goal: *promote optimal nutrition within dietary restrictions.*
      1. NPO during acute episodes.
      2. Small, frequent meals when able to eat.
      3. *Low protein* (to decrease the amount of nitrogenous materials in the intestines) and *sodium* (to decrease fluid retention).

4. *Moderate carbohydrate* (to meet energy demands) and *fat* (to make diet more palatable to anorexic patients).
  E. Goal: *provide emotional support.*
    1. Quiet environment during acute episodes to decrease external stimuli.
    2. Identify community agencies for assistance for patient, e.g., Alcoholics Anonymous; for family, Alanon/Ala-teen.
  F. Goal: **health teaching.**
    1. *Avoid* alcohol, exposure to infections.
    2. Dietary allowances, restrictions (see Appendix B, Sodium-restricted diet and Purine-restricted diet, pp. 324, 325).
    3. Drugs: names, purposes.
    4. Signs, symptoms of disease and complications.
    5. Stress-management techniques.
VI. **Evaluation/outcome criteria**
  A. No complications.
  B. Nutritional status improves; lists dietary restrictions.
  C. *No* alcohol consumption.
  D. Lists signs and symptoms of disease progression and complications.
  E. Complies with discharge plan, becomes involved with an alcohol treatment program.

Esophageal Varices

Life-threatening hemorrhage from tortuous, dilated, thin-walled veins in submucosa of lower esophagus; may rupture when chemically or mechanically irritated or when pressure is increased because of sneezing, coughing, *Valsalva maneuver,* or excessive exercise.

I. **Pathophysiology:** portal hypertension related to cirrhosis of the liver → distended branches of the azygos vein and inferior vena cava where they join the smaller vessels of the esophagus.
II. **Risk factors for hemorrhage:**
  A. Exertion that increases abdominal pressure.
  B. Trauma from ingestion of coarse foods.
  C. Acid-pepsin erosion.
III. **Assessment**
  A. *Subjective data:*
    1. Fear.
    2. Dysphagia.
    3. History: alcohol ingestion, liver dysfunction.
  B. *Objective data:*
    1. Hematemesis.
    2. Hemorrhage: sudden, often fatal.
    3. Decreased blood pressure; increased pulse, respirations.
    4. Melena (occult blood in stool).
IV. **Analysis/nursing diagnosis**
  A. *Fluid volume deficit* related to blood loss.
  B. *Risk for injury* related to hemorrhage.
  C. *Fear* related to massive blood loss.
  D. *Ineffective individual coping* related to complications of cirrhosis.
V. **Nursing care plan/implementation**

A. Goal: *provide safety measures related to hemorrhage.*
    1. Recognize signs of shock; vital signs q15 min.
    2. Assist with insertion of *Sengstaken-Blakemore* (or Minnesota) or *Linton tube* (tube is large and uncomfortable for patient during insertion); explain procedure briefly to decrease fear and attempt to gain patient's cooperation.
    3. While tube in place, observe for respiratory distress; if occurs, *deflate the balloon by releasing pressure; do not cut the tube.*
    4. Deflate the balloon as ordered to prevent necrosis.
    5. NG tube connected to low gastric suction; monitor for amount of bright red blood; irrigate only as ordered using tepid, *not* iced, solutions.
    6. Vitamin K as ordered to control bleeding.
  B. Goal: *promote fluid balance.*
    1. IV fluids, expanders, blood.
    2. Fresh blood as ordered to prevent increase in ammonia; aids in coagulation.
  C. Goal: *prevent complications of hepatic coma.*
    1. Saline cathartics as ordered to remove old blood from GI tract.
    2. Antiinfectives as ordered to prevent infection.
  D. Goal: *provide emotional support.*
    1. Stay with patient.
    2. Calm atmosphere.
  E. Goal: **health teaching.**
    1. Explain use of tube to patient and family.
    2. Bland diet instructions.
    3. Recognize signs of bleeding.
    4. *Avoid* straining at stool.
    5. *Avoid* using aspirin because of increased bleeding tendency.
VI. **Evaluation/outcome criteria**
  A. Survives acute bleeding episode.
  B. Further episodes prevented by avoiding irritants, especially alcohol.
  C. Nutritional status improves.
  D. Recognizes symptoms of complications, e.g., bleeding.
  E. Demonstrates knowledge of medications by avoiding use of aspirin.

Diagnostic Studies

Celiac Angiography, Hepatoportography
Injection of a contrast medium into the portal vein or related vessel; *used to* determine patency of vessels supplying target organ or detect lesions in the organs that distort the vasculature.

Peritoneoscopy
Direct visualization of the liver and peritoneum by means of a peritoneoscope inserted through an abdominal stab wound.

Liver biopsy
Needle aspiration of tissue for the purpose of microscopic examination; *used to* determine tissue changes,

☞ Summary of Key Points

1. Before jaundice appears, the *symptoms* of a liver problem are rather vague and nonspecific.
2. Jaundice is a diagnostic *sign* indicating a problem, not a disease. Physically the skin itches, but changes in appearance may be most disturbing to the patient.
3. Even before the visible signs of jaundice occur, the patient may complain that favorite foods or drink are distasteful.
4. Check the *hard palate first* for jaundice. The sclera color is an unreliable sign in persons of color.
5. Viral hepatitis includes all of the "alphabet" types of hepatitis. They are differentiated by the *incubation* time, the *route* of transmission, and the *severity* of the clinical course.

6. Nursing interventions focus on physical and emotional rest and diet. Protein is needed for healing, but the amount consumed is adjusted according to the *blood ammonia level*. Drug therapy is used *minimally* and *cautiously* because many drugs that are normally detoxified by the liver may have toxic effects.
7. In contrast to hepatitis, which is an "itis" or inflammatory process, cirrhosis is an *"osis"* causing an *impaired flow* of blood, bile, or metabolites. Many of the signs and symptoms are the *result of pressure*, which "pushes," causing ascites, organ enlargement, and varices.
8. If hemorrhage occurs with cirrhosis, the prognosis is *poorer*.

facilitate diagnosis, and provide information regarding a disease course.

▶ *Nursing action:* place patient on *right side* and position pillow for pressure, to prevent bleeding.

Paracentesis

Needle aspiration of fluid from the peritoneal cavity; *used* to relieve excess fluid accumulation or for diagnostic studies.

▶ *Specific nursing actions* before *paracentesis*

1. Have patient void—to prevent possible injury to bladder during procedure.
2. *Position*—sitting up on side of bed, with feet supported by chair.
3. Check vital signs and peripheral circulation frequently throughout procedure.
4. Observe for signs of hypovolemic shock—may occur due to fluid shift from vascular compartment following removal of protein-rich ascitic fluid.

▶ *Specific nursing actions* after *paracentesis*

1. Apply pressure to injection site and cover with sterile dressing.
2. Measure and record amount and color of ascitic fluid; send specimens to lab for diagnostic studies.

⚲ Study and Memory Aids

Diet

Hepatitis

NPO in acute phase
High protein
High carbohydrate
Low fat
Small, frequent feeding

Cirrhosis

Small, frequent meals
Low protein
Low sodium
Moderate carbohydrate/fat

Esophageal Varices

NPO during and after bleeding episodes
Bland, soft diet when able to eat

● Drug Review

Hepatitis

Antihistamines
    Chlorpheniramine maleate (Chlor-Trimeton): 2–4 mg tid
    Diphenhydramine (Benadryl): 25–50 mg bid
Emollients: Xipamide (Aquaphor) ointment
Sedatives
    Diazepam (Valium): 2–10 mg 2–4 times a day
Topical glucocorticoids: Hydrocortisone
Tranquilizers
    Chlordiazepoxide HCl (Librium): 5–25 mg 3–4 times daily
    Phenobarbital: 30–120 mg/d in divided doses

Cirrhosis

Corticosteroids used for postnecrotic syndrome
Diuretics
    Furosemide (Lasix): 20–80 mg/d
Emollients: Xepamide (Aquaphor) ointment to
    relieve pruritus
Hydrochlorothiazide: HydroDIURIL: 25–100 mg/d
Serum albumin for acute liver failure
Vitamins: B; Fat-soluble vitamins (A, D, E, and K)

Esophageal Varices

Propranolol (Inderal) to reduce portal hypertension
Vasopressin (Pitressin) to reduce portal hypertension
Antiinfectives
Saline cathartics
    Magnesium citrate 240 ml as needed.
    Magnesium hydroxide 5–15 ml 4 times a day.
    Magnesium sulfate 10–15 G in water.
    Phosphate/biphosphate 250 mg in water 4 times
    daily.

Esophageal Varices: Restriction

Questions

1. For which possible complication should a nurse assess a
   patient with a LeVeen shunt, used to treat liver failure?
   1. Heart failure.
   2. Myocardial infarction.
   3. Respiratory distress syndrome.
   4. Acute renal failure.
2. Which physical assessment finding in a man would be a
   sign of cirrhosis?
   1. Testicular swelling.
   2. Gynecomastia.
   3. Rebound tenderness.
   4. Wheezing.
3. A patient asks why he has developed cirrhosis. Which of
   the following in the patient's history would be the most
   likely cause?
   1. Hepatitis A.
   2. Cholelithiasis.
   3. Acetaminophen use.
   4. Blunt abdominal trauma.

4. The nurse would expect which laboratory finding (5) in a
   patient with postnecrotic cirrhosis?
   1. Decreased prothrombin time and albumin level.
   2. Increased white blood cell (WBC) and thrombocyte
      counts.
   3. Increased alanine aminotransferase (ALT) and aspar-
      tate aminotransferase (AST) levels.
   4. Decreased alkaline phosphatase level.
5. The nurse can anticipate that the urine of a patient admitted for hepatitis will probably appear:
   1. Dark.
   2. Bloody.
   3. Clear.
   4. Diluted.
6. The nurse would use lactulose (Cephulac), an agent frequently used in the management of hepatic encephalopathy, in the care of a patient with which chronic
   condition?
   1. Hypoglycemia.
   2. Constipation.
   3. Colitis.
   4. Hiatal hernia.
7. Which nursing assessment is important in a patient with
   ascites?
   1. Hematest of all stools.
   2. Bowel sounds.
   3. Abdominal girth.
   4. Urine output.
8. A Minnesota (or Sengstaken–Blakemore) tube has been
   inserted in a patient to manage ruptured esophageal varices. A nursing priority in this patient would be to:
   1. Test for gastric hyperacidity.
   2. Test the gastric contents for blood (hematest).
   3. Ensure a means of communication.
   4. Maintain airway patency.
9. The nurse would recognize a worsening of hepatic encephalopathy if which sign were observed?
   1. Flapping tremor.
   2. Facial weakness.
   3. Drooling.
   4. Nystagmus.

Answers/Rationale

1. **(1)** The shunt is used to continuously reinfuse ascitic
   fluid, which accumulates as a result of liver failure, back
   into the venous system. One end of the catheter is implanted in the peritoneal cavity, and the other is chan-
   neled through the subcutaneous tissue to the superior
   vena cava. If the amount reinfused is excessive, the heart

---

Key to Codes

Nursing process: AS, assessment; **AN,** analysis; **PL,** planning; **IMP,** implementation; **EV,** evaluation. (See Appendix M for explanation of nursing
process steps.)

Category of human function: 1, protective; **2,** sensory-perceptual; **3,**
comfort, rest, activity, and mobility; **4,** nutrition; **5,** growth and development; **6,** fluid-gas transport; **7,** psychosocial-cultural; **8,** elimination. (See
Appendix O for explanation.)

Client need: SECE, safe, effective care environment; **PhI,** physiologic
integrity; **PsI,** psychosocial integrity; **HPM,** health promotion/mainte-
nance. (See Appendix P for explanation.)

may not then be able to handle the volume. A myocardial infarction (**2**), respiratory distress (**3**) and renal failure (**4**) may occur *secondary* to heart failure. **AS, 4, PhI**

2. (**2**)   Men with cirrhosis suffer breast enlargement, or gynecomastia, as well as palmar erythema, because of the increased androgen production that occurs. The testicles *atrophy* rather than swell (**1**). Rebound tenderness (**3**) is indicative of *appendicitis*. Wheezing (**4**) would be heard in the presence of *respiratory* diseases, such as bronchitis or asthma, that cause bronchospasm. If heart failure develops in a patient with cirrhosis, the patient would experience crackles. **AN, 4, PhI**

3. (**1**)   Hepatitis is the most significant infection of the liver, and the damage may be so extensive that cirrhosis results. The incidence of cirrhosis is *not* increased in patients with gallbladder or biliary (**2**) problems. The regular use of high doses of acetaminophen (**3**), such as Tylenol, has been implicated in impaired liver function, but *not consistently.* Blunt abdominal trauma (**4**) is more likely to result in *cholecystitis* or *pancreatitis*. **AN, 4, PhI**

4. (**3**)   AST (SGOT) and ALT (SGPT) are liver enzymes, and the levels would be elevated in a patient with liver disease. The *prothrombin time* (**1**) would be *increased,* even though the prothrombin and albumin levels are decreased. The number of thrombocytes (**2**), as well as red blood cells, would be *decreased.* The alkaline phosphatase (**4**) level is *elevated* in liver disease. **AS, 4, PhI**

5. (**1**)   The bile, which is not being broken down by the liver, is excreted in the urine, rendering the urine dark brown. Bloody urine (**2**), or hematuria, would occur in the presence of *bladder cancer* or *kidney* disease. Clear urine (**3**), if colorless, would be seen in *diuresis;* clearness in terms of turbidity would be a normal appearance. Diluted (**4**) urine is the same as colorless urine; it would be seen in *diuresis.* **AS, 8, PhI**

6. (**2**)   Lactulose is a cathartic and may be used if other agents for constipation are ineffective. Although lactulose does not significantly affect the serum glucose level, it is a sugar and would produce *hyperglycemia, not* hypoglycemia (**1**), if absorbed. The patient with colitis (**3**), or in-flammation of the large bowel, suffers from frequent diarrhea, so lactulose would be *contraindicated.* A hiatal hernia (**4**), which is a bulging of the esophagus where it joins the stomach, causes food to "hang up." Hot liquids, *not* lactulose, would help relieve this condition. **AN, 8, PhI**

7. (**3**)   Ascites is the accumulation of fluid in the peritoneum as a result of increased portal pressure and low serum albumin levels. Resolution of the ascites is objectively gauged by measurement of the abdominal girth. If esophageal or GI tract *bleeding* is suspected, the stools should be checked for occult blood (hematest, **1**). Bowel sounds (**2**) may be muffled in a patient with ascites, but the presence or absence of bowel sounds does *not* indicate the severity of the ascites. Urine output (**4**), if diminished, would stem from the reduced cardiac output that may occur in cirrhosis but is *unrelated* to the ascites. **AS, 4, PhI**

8. (**4**)   The Minnesota tube has inflatable balloons that are positioned in the esophagus and stomach; the tube may become dislodged and obstruct the airway. If airway obstruction is observed, the tube should not be cut, instead the balloon, or balloons, should be deflated and the tube, or tubes, removed. An acute illness will increase gastric acidity, but *routine* testing (**1**) is *not done* in a patient with the Minnesota tube. The patient should receive an antacid or H₂ blocker to prevent hyperacidity. The tube is used to stop esophageal bleeding, so a hematest (**2**) result would be positive; this finding does *not* indicate a problem with the *tube.* The tube is inserted via the nose, so communication (**3**) would *not* be impaired. **PL, 6, SECE**

9. (**1**)   Liver flap, or asterixis, which is a flapping tremor of the hand that is seen when the arm is extended, occurs with a rising ammonia level, which is a central nervous system toxin. Facial weakness (**2**) and drooling (**3**) would be seen in a patient after a *stroke* or *cranial nerve VII* (facial) damage. Nystagmus (**4**), or jerking eye movements, occurs with *cranial nerve damage* and *inner ear* disorders such as Meniere's disease. **AN, 2, PhI**

Gastric Disorders

Chapter Outline

General Nutritional Deficiencies

I. Assessment

  A. *Subjective data:*

    1. Mental irritability or confusion.

    2. History of poor dietary intake.

    3. History of lack of adequate resources to provide adequate nutrition.

    4. Lack of knowledge about proper diet, food selection, or preparation.

    5. History of eating disorders.

    6. Paresthesia (burning and tingling): hands and feet.

  B. *Objective data:*

    1. *Appearance:* listless; *posture:* sagging shoulders, sunken chest, poor gait.

    2. *Muscle:* weakness, fatigue, wasted appearance.

    3. *Gastrointestinal (GI):* indigestion; vomiting; enlarged liver, spleen.

    4. *Cardiovascular:* tachycardia on minimal exertion, bradycardia at rest, enlarged heart, elevated blood pressure.

    5. *Hair:* brittle, dry, thin, sparse; lack of natural shine; color changes; can be easily plucked out.

    6. *Skin:* dryness (*xerosis*), scaly, dyspigmentation, petechiae, lack of fat under skin.

    7. *Mouth:*

      a. *Teeth:* missing, abnormally placed, caries.

      b. *Gums:* bleed easily, receding.

      c. *Tongue:* swollen, sore.

      d. *Lips:* red, swollen, angular fissures at corners.

    8. *Eyes:* pale conjunctiva, corneal changes.

    9. *Nails:* brittle, ridged.

    10. *Nervous system:* abnormal reflexes.

    11. Lab data: blood: *decreased* albumin, iron-binding capacity, lymphocyte, hemoglobin, and hematocrit.

    12. Anthropometric measurements document nutritional deficiencies.

II. Analysis/nursing diagnosis

  A. *Altered nutrition, less than body requirements,* related to poor dietary intake.

  B. *Knowledge deficit* related to nutritional requirements.

  C. *Altered health maintenance* related to inability to provide own nutritional care.

  D. *Ineffective individual coping* related to eating disorders.

  E. *Ineffective family coping, disabling,* related to inadequate resources or knowledge to provide appropriate family nutrition.

III. Nursing care plan/implementation

  A. Goal: *prevent complications of specific deficiency.*

    1. Identify etiology of nutritional deficiency.

    2. Recognize signs of nutritional deficiencies (Table 15.1 Common Mineral Deficiencies).

    3. Identify foods high in deficient nutrient (see Appendix B).

    4. Evaluate economic resources to purchase appropriate foods.

    5. Identify community resources for assistance.

    6. Monitor progress for potential additional illnesses.

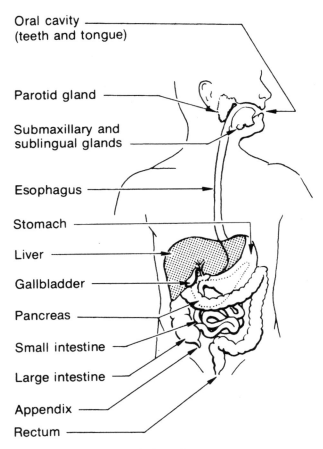

Oral cavity (teeth and tongue)

Parotid gland

Submaxillary and sublingual glands

Esophagus

Stomach

Liver

Gallbladder

Pancreas

Small intestine

Large intestine

Appendix

Rectum

Components of the digestive system.

B. Goal: **health teaching.**
   1. Effects of nutritional deficiencies on health.
   2. Foods to include in diet to avoid deficits.

IV. Evaluation/outcome criteria
   A. Complications do not occur.
   B. Patient gains weight.
   C. Patient selects appropriate foods to alleviate deficiency.

Peptic Ulcer Disease

Circumscribed loss of mucosa, submucosa, or muscle layer of the GI tract caused by decreased resistance of gastric mucosa to acid-pepsin injury. *Peptic ulcer disease* is a chronic disease and may occur in the distal esophagus, stomach, upper duodenum, or jejunum. *Gastric ulcers,* located on the lesser curvature of stomach, are larger, deeper than duodenal ulcers and tend to become *malignant. Duodenal ulcers* are located on the first part of the duodenum; they are more common than gastric ulcers. *Stress ulcers,* an acute problem, occur after a major insult to the body.

   I. **Pathophysiology:** failure of the body to regenerate mucous epithelium at a sufficient rate to counterbalance the damage to tissue during the breakdown of

protein; decrease in the quantity and quality of the mucus; poor local mucosal blood flow, along with individual susceptibility to ulceration.

II. **Risk factors**
   A. **Gastric ulcers:**
      1. Decreased resistance to acid-pepsin injury.
      2. Gastritis.
      3. Increased histamine release → inflammatory reaction.
      4. Cigarette smoking, increased caffeine/alcohol use.
      5. Family history.
      6. Difficulty coping with high-stress environment.
      7. Ulcerogenic drugs that aggravate preexisting condition.
      8. Increased hydrogen ion back-diffusion.
      9. Age: >50 yr.
   B. **Duodenal ulcers:**
      1. Elevated gastric acid secretory rate.
      2. Elevated gastric acid levels postprandially (after eating).
      3. Increased rate of gastric emptying → increased amount of acid in duodenum → irritation and breakdown of duodenal mucosa.
      4. More men than women affected; possible influence of endocrine factors such as estrogen and adrenal steroids.
      5. Seasonal influence: spring and fall.
      6. Cigarette smoking; increased caffeine/alcohol use.
      7. Family history.
      8. Difficulty coping with high-stress environment.
      9. Ulcerogenic drugs that aggravate preexisting condition.
      10. Persons with type O blood.
      11. Age 25–50 yr.
   C. **Stress ulcers:**
      1. Severe trauma or major illness.
      2. Severe burns (*Curling's ulcer*); develop in 72 h in most persons with burns over more than 35% of their body surface.
      3. Head injuries or intracranial disease (*Cushing's* ulcers).
      4. Medications in large doses: corticosteroids, salicylates, ibuprofen, indomethacin, phenylbutazone (Butazolidin).
      5. Shock.
      6. Sepsis.

III. **Assessment**
   A. *Subjective data:*
      1. **Gastric ulcers:**
         a. *Pain:*
            (1) Type: gnawing, aching, burning.
            (2) Location: epigastric, left of midline, localized.
            (3) Occurrence: periodic pain, often 2 h after eating.
            (4) Relief: antacids; may be aggravated, *not* relieved, by food.
         b. Nausea.
         c. History of risk factors, as above.

TABLE 15.1   COMMON MINERAL DEFICIENCIES

Mineral	*Function*	*Deficiency Leads to:*
Calcium	Aids in formation and maintenance of bones and teeth, permits healthy nerve functioning and normal blood clotting	↑ neuromuscular irritability, impaired blood clotting
Phosphorus	Bone building	Rickets
Magnesium	Cellular metabolism of carbohydrates and protein	↓ cellular metabolism of carbohydrates and protein, tetany
Sodium	Fluid and electrolyte balance, acid-base balance, electrochemical impulses of nerves and muscles	Fluid and electrolyte imbalance, ↓ muscle contraction
Potassium	Osmotic pressure and water balance	Fluid and electrolyte imbalance, ↓ cardiac and skeletal muscular contractility
Chloride	Fluid and electrolyte balance, acid-base balance, digestion	Fluid imbalances, alkalosis
Iron	Hemoglobin formation, cellular oxidation	Anemia
Iodine	Synthesis of thyroid hormone, overall body metabolism	Goiter
Zinc	Constituent of cell enzyme system, CO_2 carrier in red blood cell	↓ metabolism of protein and carbohydrates, delayed wound healing

2. **Duodenal ulcers:**
   a. *Pain:*
      (1) Type: gnawing, aching, burning, hungerlike, boring.
      (2) Location: right epigastric, localized; steady pain near midline of back may indicate perforation.
      (3) Occurrence: 1–3 h after eating, worse at end of day or during the night; initial attack occurs in spring or fall; history of remissions and exacerbations.
      (4) Relief: food and/or antacids.
   b. Nausea.
   c. History of risk factors (see p. 160).
3. **Stress ulcers:**
   a. *Pain:* often painless until serious complication (hemorrhage, perforation) occurs.
   b. History of risk factors (see page 160).
B. *Objective data:*
   1. **Gastric ulcer:**
      a. Vomiting.
      b. Melena (tarry stools).
      c. Weight loss.
      d. X-ray (*upper GI series*) confirms "crater" (punched-out appearance, clean base).
      e. *Endoscopy* confirms presence of ulcer; biopsy for cytologic data.
      f. Lab data—positive for *H. pylori*
      g. Monitor for blood loss: complete blood count, stool for occult blood.
   2. **Duodenal ulcer:**
      a. Eructation.
      b. Vomiting.
      c. Regurgitation of sour liquid into back of mouth.
      d. Constipation.

   e. X-ray (*upper GI series*) confirms ulcer craters and niches as well as outlet deformities: round or oval funnel-like lesion extending into musculature.
   f. Lab data—positive for *H. pylori*
   g. Common complications: hemorrhage or perforation.
3. **Stress ulcer:**
   a. GI tract bleeding.
   b. Multiple, superficial erosions affecting large area of gastric mucosa (as documented by GI series or endoscopy).
IV. **Analysis/nursing diagnosis** (all types):
   A. *Pain* related to erosion of gastric lining.
   B. *Ineffective individual coping* related to inability to change life-style.
   C. *Altered nutrition, less than body requirements,* related to inadequate intake.
   D. *Knowledge deficit* regarding preventive measures.
   E. *Risk for injury* related to possible hemorrhage or perforation.
V. **Nursing care plan/implementation** (all types):
   A. Goal: *promote comfort.*
      1. Medications as ordered to decrease pain (see Goal: **health teaching,** p. 162); sedatives to decrease anxiety.
      2. Prepare for diagnostic tests.
         a. X-rays: *upper GI series* (barium swallow), *lower GI* (barium enema).
         b. *Endoscopy.*
         c. *Gastric analysis,* to determine amount of hydrochloric acid in GI tract.
   B. Goal: *prevent/recognize signs of complications.*
      1. Monitor vital signs for shock.
      2. Check stool for occult blood/hemorrhage.

☞ **3.** Palpate abdomen for perforation (rigid, board-like), arterial bleeding.

C. Goal: *provide emotional support.*
  1. Stress-management techniques.
  2. Restful environment.
  3. Prepare for surgery, if necessary.

D. Goal: **health teaching.**
  1. Medications:
    a. *Antiulceratives: give 1–3 h after meals and at bedtime* to decrease pain by lowering acidity; monitor for:
      (1) Diarrhea (seen most often with magnesium carbonate and magnesium oxide).
      (2) Constipation (seen most often with calcium carbonate or aluminum hydroxide).
      (3) Electrolyte imbalance (seen with systemic antacid, soda bicarbonate).
      (4) Best 1–3 h *after meals.*
      (5) Liquids more effective than tablets; if taking tablets, chew slowly.
    b. *Histamine antagonists: taken with meals and at bedtime* to block the action of histamine-stimulated gastric secretions (basal and stimulated); inhibits pepsin secretion and reduces the volume of gastric secretion.
      (1) Cimetidine (Tagamet) inhibits gastrin release, can be given PO, IV, or IM; cannot be given within 1 h of antacid therapy.
      (2) Ranitidine (Zantac) causes greater reduction of acid secretion, has longer duration, requires less frequent administration (bid vs qid), and has fewer side effects than cimetidine.
    c. *Proctectant:* Sucralfate (Carafate): *given 1 h before meals and at bedtime.*
      (1) Locally active topical agent that forms a protective coat on mucosa, prevents further digestive action of both acid and pepsin.
      (2) Must *not* be given within ½ h of antacids.
    d. *Antiinfectives:* take as directed in combination with antiulcerative or H₂ antagonists. Optimal treatment regimen is under investigation.
    e. *Anticholinergic, when used, given before meals* to decrease gastric acid secretion and delay gastric emptying.
    f. Important: *avoid* aspirin use (could increase bleeding possibility).
  2. *Diet:*
    a. *Avoid:*
      (1) Stress at mealtimes.
      (2) Milk (increases gastric acid production).
      (3) Substances that provoke pain.
      (4) Coffee with or without caffeine.
      (5) Foods or liquids containing caffeine.
      (6) Alcohol.
      (7) Tobacco.
    b. *Plan:*
      (1) Small, frequent meals (to prevent exacerbation of symptoms related to an empty stomach).
      (2) Weight control.

3. Complications: signs and symptoms:
  a. Gastric ulcers may be premalignant.
  b. Perforation.
  c. Hemorrhage.
  d. Obstruction.
4. Life-style changes:
  a. *Decrease:*
    (1) Smoking.
    (2) Noise.
    (3) Rush.
    (4) Confusion.
  b. *Increase:*
    (1) Communication; verbalize concerns.
    (2) Mental/physical rest.
    (3) Compliance with medical regimen.

VI. Evaluation/outcome criteria
  A. Remains on specified diet.
  B. Takes prescribed medications.
  C. Pain decreases.
  D. No complications.
  E. States signs and symptoms of complications.
  F. Participates in stress-reduction activities.
  G. No further ulcers.

Diaphragmatic (Hiatal) Hernia

Protrusion of part of stomach through diaphragm and into thoracic cavity. *Types:* sliding (most common), paraesophageal "rolling."

I. Pathophysiology: weakening of the musculature of the diaphragm, aggravated by increased intraabdominal pressure → protrusion of the abdominal organs through the esophageal hiatus → reflux of gastric contents → esophagitis.

II. Risk factors:
  A. Congenital abnormality.
  B. Penetrating wound.
  C. Age (middle-aged or elderly).
  D. Women more affected than men.
  E. Obesity.
  F. Ascites.
  G. Pregnancy.
  H. History of constipation.

III. Assessment
  A. *Subjective data:*
    1. Pressure: substernal.
    2. Pain: epigastric, burning.
    3. Eructation, heartburn after eating.
    4. Dysphagia.
    5. Symptoms aggravated when recumbent.
  B. *Objective data:*
    1. Cough, dyspnea.
    2. Tachycardia, palpitations.
    3. Bleeding: hematemesis, melena, signs of anemia due to gastroesophageal irritation, ulceration, and bleeding.
    4. Diagnostic tests:
      a. Chest x-rays showing protrusion of abdominal organs into thoracic cavity.

b. *Barium swallow* (upper GI series) to show presence of hernia.

✖ IV. Analysis/nursing diagnosis
  A. *Pain* related to irritation of lining of GI tract.
  B. *Altered nutrition, less than body requirements,* related to dysphagia.
  C. *Sleep pattern disturbance* related to increase in symptoms when recumbent.
  D. *Risk for aspiration* related to reflux of gastric contents.
  E. *Activity intolerance* related to dyspnea.
  F. *Anxiety* related to palpitations.

✖ V. Nursing care plan/implementation
  A. *Preoperative care:*
    1. Goal: *promote relief of symptoms.*
      🍎 a. *Diet:*
        (1) Small, frequent feedings of soft, bland foods, to reduce abdominal pressure and reflux.
        (2) *Fluid* when swallowing solids; may push food into stomach; hot fluid may work best.
        (3) *Avoid* eating 2 h before bedtime.
        (4) *High-protein, low-fat* foods to decrease heartburn.
      b. *Positioning: head elevated* to increase movement of food into stomach. Symptoms may decrease if head of bed at home is elevated on 8-in. blocks.
      c. Weight reduction to decrease abdominal pressure.
      💊 d. Medications as ordered:
        (1) 30 mL of antacid 1 h after meals and at bedtime.
        (2) *Avoid* anticholinergic drugs, which decrease gastric emptying.
  B. *Postoperative care:*
    1. Goal: *provide for postoperative safety needs.*
      a. Respiratory: deep breathing, coughing; splint incision area.
      ☞ b. *Nasogastric (NG) tube:* check patency
        (1) Drainage: should be small amount.
        (2) Color: dark brown 6–12 h after surgery, changing to greenish yellow.
        (3) Do *not* disturb tube placement to *avoid* traction on suture line.
      c. *Position:* initially head of bed elevated slightly, then semi-Fowler's; turn side to side frequently to prevent pressure on diaphragm.
      ☞ d. Maintain *closed-chest drainage* if indicated (see Chap. 6 p. 73, Tubes Box).
      e. Check for return of bowel sounds.
    2. Goal: *promote comfort and maintain nutrition.*
      ☞ a. *IVs* for hydration and electrolytes.
      ☞ b. Initiate feeding through *gastrostomy* tube, if present.
        (1) Usually attached to intermittent, low *suction* after surgery.
        (2) *Aspirate* gastric contents before feeding —delay if 75 mL or more is present; report these findings to physician.

(3) Feed in *high-Fowler's* or *sitting position;* keep head elevated for 30 min *after* eating.
(4) *Warm* feeding to room temperature; *dilute* with water if too thick.
(5) Give 50 mL of water *before* feeding; 200–500 mL feeding by gravity over 10–15 min; *follow* with 50 mL of water.
(6) Give frequent mouth care.

🏠 3. Goal: **health teaching.**
  a. *Avoid* constricting clothing and activities that increase intraabdominal pressure, e.g., lifting, bending, straining at stool.
  b. Weight reduction.
  c. Dietary needs: small, frequent, soft, bland meals; chew thoroughly; *upright* position for at least *1 h after* meals.

✖ VI. Evaluation/outcome criteria
  A. Relief from symptoms, comfortable.
  B. Receiving adequate, balanced nutrition.
  C. Describes dietary changes, recommended positioning, and activity limitations to prevent recurrence.

Gastric Surgery

Performed when: medical treatment for ulcer is unsuccessful, ulcer is determined to be precancerous, or complications are present.

  I. Types:
    A. *Subtotal gastrectomy:* removal of a portion of the stomach.
    B. *Total gastrectomy:* removal of the entire stomach.
    C. *Antrectomy:* removal of entire antrum (lower) portion of the stomach.
    D. *Pyloroplasty:* repair of the pyloric opening of the stomach.
    E. *Vagotomy:* interruption of the impulses carried by the vagus nerve, which results in reduction of gastric secretions and decreased physical activity of the stomach (this procedure is now being done less often).
    F. Combination of vagotomy and gastrectomy.

✖ II. Analysis/nursing diagnosis
    A. *Pain* related to surgical incision.
    B. *Ineffective breathing pattern* related to high surgical incision.
    C. *Risk for trauma* related to possible complications after gastrectomy.
    D. *Knowledge deficit* related to inability to manage ulcer disease on medical regimen.
    E. *Fear* related to possible precancerous lesion.
    F. *Ineffective individual coping* related to risk factors for peptic ulcer disease.

✖ III. Nursing care plan/implementation
    A. Goal: *promote comfort in the postoperative period.*
      💊 1. *Analgesics:* to relieve pain and allow patient to cough, deep breathe to prevent pulmonary complications.
      2. *Position:* semi-Fowler's to aid in breathing.
    B. Goal: *promote wound healing.*

1. Keep dressing dry.

☞ **2.** *NG tube* connected to low intermittent (*Levine*) or low continuous (*Salem-sump*) suction.

    a. Check drainage from NG tube; normally bloody first 2–3 h after surgery, then brown to dark green.

    b. Excessive bright red blood drainage: take vital signs; report: vital signs, color, and volume of drainage to MD immediately.

    c. Irrigate *gently* with saline in amount ordered; do **not** irrigate against resistance; may not be done in early postoperative period.

    d. Tape securely to face, but prevent obstructed vision.

    e. Frequent mouth and nostril care.

C. Goal: *promote adequate nutrition and hydration.*

☞ **1.** Administer parenteral fluids as ordered.

    2. Accurate intake and output.

☞ **3.** Check bowel sounds, at least q4h; *NPO* 1–3 days; bowel sounds normally return after 24–36 h; *oral fluids* as ordered when bowel sounds present—usually 30 mL, then *small* feedings, then *bland* liquids to *soft* diet.

    4. Observe for nausea and vomiting due to suture line edema, food intake (too much, too fast).

D. Goal: *prevent complications.*

    1. Check dressing q4h for bleeding.

    2. Vitamin B_{12} and iron replacement as ordered to prevent pernicious or iron deficiency anemia.

    3. Prevent dumping syndrome (see below).

IV. Evaluation/outcome criteria

    A. Hemorrhage, dumping syndrome prevented.

    B. Healing begins.

    C. Adjusts life-style to prevent recurrence/marginal ulcer.

Dumping Syndrome

Hypoglycemic-type episode; occurs postoperatively after gastric resection (may also occur after vagotomy, antrectomy, or gastroenterostomy), when food and fluids that are more hyperosmolar than the jejunal secretions pass *quickly* into jejunum, producing fluid shifts from bloodstream to jejunum. This is a mild problem for about 20% of patients and disappears in a few months to a year. Symptoms are serious in about 7% of the patients. This discomfort may occur during a meal or up to 30 min after the meal and last from 20–60 min. The reaction is greatest after the ingestion of sugar.

I. Assessment

    A. *Subjective data:*

        1. Feeling of fullness, weakness, faintness.

        2. Palpitations.

        3. Nausea.

        4. Discomfort during or after eating.

    B. *Objective data:*

        1. Diaphoresis.

        2. Diarrhea.

        3. Fainting.

        4. Symptoms of hypoglycemia.

II. Analysis/nursing diagnosis

    A. *Altered nutrition, more than body requirements,* related to body's inability to properly digest high-carbohydrate, high-sodium foods.

    B. *Diarrhea* related to food passing into jejunum too quickly.

    C. *Risk for injury* related to hypoglycemia.

    D. *Knowledge deficit* related to dietary restrictions.

III. Nursing care plan/implementation

    A. Goal: **slow gastric emptying.**

        1. *Increased fat, protein* to delay emptying.

        2. Rest after meals.

        3. Eat small, frequent meals.

        4. Drink fluids *between* meals.

    B. Goal: **health teaching**

        1. Avoid foods high in *refined carbohydrates.*

        2. Practice portion control.

        3. Stress management, particularly at mealtime.

        4. Symptom management.

IV. Evaluation/outcome criteria

    A. No complications.

    B. Patient heals.

    C. Incorporates health teaching into life-style and prevents syndrome.

ᴧᴧᴧ Diagnostic Studies

Common Fluoroscopic Examinations

Upper GI—ingestion of barium sulfate or meglumine diatrizoate (Gastrografin, a white, chalky, radiopaque substance), followed by fluoroscopic and x-ray examination; *used to* determine:

    1. Patency and caliber of *esophagus;* may also detect esophageal varices.

    2. Mobility and thickness of *gastric* walls, presence of ulcer craters, filling defects due to tumors, pressures from outside the stomach, and patency of pyloric valve.

    3. Rate of passage in *small bowel* and presence of structural abnormalities.

Lower GI—rectal instillation of barium sulfate followed by fluoroscopic and x-ray examination; *used to* determine contour and mobility of colon and presence of any space-occupying tumors; perform *before* upper GI. **Patient preparation:** explain purpose; *no food after evening meal* the evening before test; *stool softeners, laxatives, enemas, and suppositories* to cleanse the bowel before the test; *NPO after midnight* prior to test; oral medications *not* permitted day of test.

After completion of exam: food, *increased liquid* intake, and rest; *laxatives for at least 2 d* or until stools are normal in color and consistency.

Examination of Gastric Contents

Gastric analysis—aspiration of the contents of the fasting stomach for analysis of free and total acid.

    1. Gastric acidity is generally *increased* in presence of duodenal ulcer.

    2. Gastric acidity is usually *decreased* in pernicious anemia, cancer of the stomach.

⌐━ Summary of Key Points

1. Gastric disorders may include problems with *ingestion* (getting the food to the stomach) or *digestion* (the process of secreting gastric juices and breaking down protein).
2. Regardless of the disorder, the patient often complains of pain (erosion or stretching), loss of appetite (impaired gastric emptying), nausea (gastric tension), bleeding (erosion or trauma), diarrhea (increased peristalsis), belching or flatus, dyspepsia (heartburn), or a combination of these.
3. Enteral (NG or gastric tube) or parenteral (TPN) feedings may be *supplemental* or *replacement*. If they are replacing oral feedings, mouth care and satisfying oral needs are important.
4. Though similar in many ways, the differences between a duodenal and gastric ulcer are distinctive. A *duodenal* ulcer is more common, the characteristic gnawing pain occurs hours after a meal or at night, and food relieves the pain.
5. Treatment is medical (rest, drugs, diet, decreased stress), unless the ulcer: becomes chronic, recurs, perforates, causes obstruction, or bleeds—then surgery is indicated.
6. Drug therapy *inhibits* acid secretion and *neutralizes* or *protects* the gastric mucosa. Patient teaching must include whether a drug is taken *before*, *with*, or how long *after* meals.
7. The dumping syndrome is controlled by regulating the *volume* and type of food—*decrease carbohydrates* and *fluids, increase protein* and *fat* to delay gastric emptying.

Stool specimens—*examined for:* amount, consistency, color, character, and melena; *used to* determine presence of: urobilinogen, fat, nitrogen, parasites, and other substances.

Esophagoscopy and gastroscopy—visualization of the esophagus, the stomach, and sometimes the duodenum by means of a lighted tube inserted through the mouth.

💡 Study and Memory Aids

Diet

Diaphragmatic Hernia

↑ Protein
↑ Feedings
↑ Soft, bland
↓ Fat
↓ Size of portions

Dumping Syndrome

↑ Fat
↑ Protein
↑ Fiber
↑ Frequency
↓ Carbohydrate
↓ Fluids at mealtime
↓ Portion size

● **Drug Review**

Peptic Ulcer Disease

Anticholinergic: Propantheline bromide (Pro-Banthine): 15 mg tid, 30 mg hs
Antiinfectives
　Amoxicillin: 250–500 mg q 8h
　Clarithromycin: (Biaxin) 250–500 mg q 12h
　Metronidazole: (Flagyl) 250 mg tid
　Tetracycline: 500 mg qid
Antiulcerative
　Aluminum hydroxide gel (Amphojel): 5–10 mL q2–4h or 1 h pc
　Calcium carbonate (Titralac): 1–2 g with water after meals and hs
　Magnesium and aluminum hydroxides (Maalox suspension): 5–30 mL pc and hs
　Omeprazole (Prilosec): 20 mg qd for 4–8 wk
Histamine antagonists
　Cimetidine (Tagamet): 300–600 mg q6h
　Ranitidine (Zantac): 150 mg bid
Protectant: Sucralfate (Carafate): 1 g ac and hs

Diaphragmatic Hernia

Antacid therapy
　Magnesium and aluminum hydroxide
　(Mylanta): 500–1000 mg 3–6 times/day
　(Maalox suspension): 5–30 ml pc and hs
　(Gaviscon): 30–60 ml pc and hs
Histamine receptor antagonist
　Ranitidine (Zantac): 150 mg b.i.d.
　Avoid anticholinergic drugs because they decrease lower esophageal sphincter function

Dumping Syndrome
Anticholinergics (e.g., propantheline): to decrease gastric activity **Vasopressor** (e.g., ephedrine): to relieve vasomotor symptoms

Questions

1. After esophagoscopy done to diagnose gastroesophageal reflux, the most important nursing action would be to:
   1. Check the patient's vital signs frequently, as ordered.
   2. Assess for cervical crepitus in the neck.
   3. Place the patient in a side-lying position to prevent aspiration.
   4. Give the patient an anesthetic lozenge for sore throat.
2. Health care counseling for a patient with a hiatal hernia should include which instruction?
   1. Restrict intake of high-carbohydrate foods, which speed emptying.
   2. Increase fluid intake with meals to facilitate food passage.
   3. Increase fat intake to delay gastric emptying.
   4. Eat three regular meals daily at least 5 hours apart.
3. When giving morphine sulfate (5 mg) in an IV push to a 65-year-old patient after a gastrectomy, the best technique would be to:
   1. Dilute it in 5 mL of normal saline and give it over 4 to 5 minutes.
   2. Dilute it in 10 mL of 5% dextrose in water and give it over 30 minutes.
   3. Give it undiluted at the injection site closest to the patient.
   4. Give it undiluted at the injection site farthest from the patient.
4. An important nursing action for a patient with a nasogastric feeding tube is to:
   1. Measure the residual contents in the stomach every morning.
   2. Clean and lubricate the external nares.
   3. Administer the feeding over 1 to 2 hours.
   4. Check the patient's blood glucose level before each feeding.
5. A patient is receiving Carafate (sucralfate) qid and Mylanta tid. The nurse explains to the patient that the best schedule for these drugs is to take:
   1. Carafate AC and HS and Mylanta PC.
   2. Carafate PC and HS and Mylanta AC.
   3. Carafate PC and HS and Mylanta PC.
   4. Carafate AC and Mylanta AC and HS.
6. A patient accidentally receives a bolus of Tagamet as the result of a faulty IV administration set. The nurse's first action would be to:
   1. Ask another nurse what problems are caused by the receipt of an overdose Tagamet.
   2. Consult a nursing textbook to find out the potential complications.
   3. Assess the patient for signs of adverse drug effects.
   4. Consult the drug formulary to find out the implications of this.
7. Which pair of drugs should the nurse plan to give at different times?
   1. Diuril (chlorothiazide) and Questran (cholestyramine) po.
   2. Atarax (hydroxyzine) and Demerol (meperidine) IM.
   3. Tylenol (acetaminophen) and Coumadin (warfarin sodium) po.
   4. Decadron (dexamethasone) and mannitol IV.
8. While being assisted to the bathroom, the patient complains of a "giving" sensation in his abdominal incision. The first nursing action would be to:
   1. Return the patient to bed and place in a supine position.
   2. Call the physician immediately.
   3. Sit the patient in a chair and check his vital signs.
   4. Culture the wound and reinforce the dressing.
9. The nurse irrigates a patient's nasogastric tube with iced saline until it is cleared of blood. What would the nurse record on the intake and output record?
   1. The amount of irrigant aspirated as output.
   2. The amount of irrigant instilled as input.
   3. The difference between the amount of the irrigant and the amount of the aspirate.
   4. Nothing about the irrigation procedure.
10. Which finding is a complication of ulcer disease and should be reported immediately?
    1. A fine rash on body.
    2. Black stool.
    3. Constipation or diarrhea.
    4. Dizziness or headache.
11. Only a small amount of fluid is draining from a patient's nasogastric tube. What is the first action the nurse should take?
    1. Irrigate the nasogastric tube.
    2. Position the patient on the right side.
    3. Determine the placement of the tube.
    4. Record the amount of drainage.
12. Which sign of bleeding would the nurse expect in a patient with a duodenal ulcer?
    1. Bright red blood in the stool.
    2. Bright red emesis.
    3. Coffee-ground emesis.
    4. Black, tarry stool.
13. Assessment of a patient with a perforated ulcer would reveal:
    1. A boardlike abdomen, tachycardia, and hypotension.
    2. A distended abdomen and hyperactive bowel sounds.
    3. A distended abdomen and belching.
    4. A boardlike abdomen, restlessness, and bradycardia.

Answers/Rationale

1. **(3)** All of the nursing actions are correct, but the *first* priority is to position the patient to prevent aspiration because a local anesthetic is sprayed on the posterior pharynx to ease the discomfort and prevent gagging when the tube is inserted, and this may impair the swallowing reflex for a while. The patient should be NPO for 2 to 4 hours afterward. Checking the vital signs (**1**) is *less important* than maintaining a clear air-

way. The finding of cervical crepitus (**2**) would indicate perforation, a *rare* complication. A sore throat (**4**) may result from the tube insertion, but it is a *less serious* concern; lozenges or a saline gargle may soothe the irritation. **IMP, 3, SECE**

2. (**2**) The main problem in a hiatal hernia is the food "hanging up" in the dilated area above the sphincter of the stomach. Hot fluids are often most effective in relaxing the sphincter. Restricting carbohydrate intake (**1**) and increasing fat intake (**3**) are appropriate measures for patients with the *dumping syndrome*. Eating three regular meals a day (**4**) is incorrect; the patients should instead eat *smaller* and *more frequent* meals.
PL, 4, HPM

3. (**1**) Morphine sulfate should be diluted when being given to an older adult to lessen potential adverse effects of IV push administration. For direct IV administration the drug should be diluted in at least 5 mL of sterile water or normal saline; 2.5 to 15 mg may be given over 4 to 5 minutes. Thirty minutes for the administration of an IV push (**2**) is *too long,* and 5% dextrose in water is used for a continuous IV, *not* an IV push. Morphine sulfate *should be* diluted to lessen the side effects (**3** and **4**). **IMP, 1, SECE**

4. (**2**) The nose may become very irritated, dried, and cracked because of the irritating effects of the tube. The residual gastric contents (**1**) should be measured *before every feeding*. The feeding should be given as prescribed (**3**); such intermittent feedings are usually administered in *less* than 1 hour. The blood glucose level (**4**) is *not* routinely tested before tube feedings.
IMP, 4, PhI

5. (**1**) Carafate is an agent used for the short-term treatment of an ulcer; it works by coating the ulcered area and should be taken 1 hour before eating and at bedtime. It does not decrease acidity or reduce H_2 (histamine) production. To effectively coat the ulcer the stomach needs to be empty, *not* full (**2** and **3**). Mylanta, an antacid, should be taken 2 to 3 hours *after* meals when acid production is greatest, *not* before meals (**2** and **4**). **PL, 4, HPM**

6. (**3**) The first priority is assessing the patient, noting any immediate effects from the excessive fluid or the large dose of the drug received. Side effects could include diarrhea, vomiting, headache, and dizziness. A colleague (**1**) and a nursing textbook (**2**) could provide inaccurate or dated data, or these actions could take time away from observation of the patient. Consulting the formulary (**4**) would be the *next* appropriate action after the patient's status has been assessed. **IMP, 4, PhI**

Key to Codes

Nursing process: AS, assessment; **AN,** analysis; **PL,** planning; **IMP,** implementation; **EV,** evaluation. (See Appendix M for explanation of nursing process steps.)

Category of human function: 1, protective; **2,** sensory-perceptual; **3,** comfort, rest, activity, and mobility; **4,** nutrition; **5,** growth and development; **6,** fluid-gas transport; **7,** psychosocial-cultural; **8,** elimination. (See Appendix O for explanation.)

Client need: SECE, safe, effective care environment; **PhI,** physiologic integrity; **PsI,** psychosocial integrity; **HPM,** health promotion/maintenance. (See Appendix P for explanation.)

7. (**1**) Questran is an antilipemic that is taken alone; administration with any other oral medication would cause the absorption of the Questran to be decreased. Atarax (**2**) or Vistaril, and Demerol *are* a common preoperative combination. Tylenol (**3**) is an analgesic that *can* be taken safely with Coumadin, an anticoagulant. Decadron and mannitol (**4**) *are* frequently administered together to head-injured patients with cerebral edema.
PL, 4, PhI

8. (**1**) The priority is to place the patient supine to keep the intestines in the abdomen if evisceration has occurred. The nurse should return the patient to bed if it is nearby; lying the patient on a gurney or a couch would also be appropriate. The MD should be called (**2**), but *not first*. Sitting (**3**) would *not* involve the use of gravity to keep the bowel in the abdomen. Wound culture (**4**) is *not* indicated in dehiscence or evisceration. **IMP, 1, PhI**

9. (**4**) The fluid used in the irrigation of a nasogastric tube in a patient suffering from gastrointestinal tract bleeding does not count as either intake or output fluid because the fluid instilled is withdrawn immediately, so there is no effect on the intake or output. The other options (**1, 2,** and **3**) are wrong because there *should be no entry* on the intake and output record for the reasons just given. **IMP, 1, SECE**

10. (**2**) Black stool, or melena, is a sign of gastrointestinal tract bleeding. Other complications are perforation, hemorrhage, shock, and peritonitis. A rash (**1**), constipation or diarrhea (**3**), and dizziness or headache (**4**) are possible side effects of one of the drugs used in the treatment of ulcers (cimetidine [Tagamet]), but they are *not potentially life-threatening* and do *not* need to be *reported immediately*. These side effects usually resolve as the body adjusts to the effects of the drug.
AS, 4, PhI

11. (**3**) The small amount of drainage could be the result of either displacement or occlusion, but to prevent possible instillation of irrigant into the lungs, tube placement must be determined before the tube is irrigated. Irrigation (**1**) would therefore *not* be the *first* action. Positioning the patient on the right side (**2**) could be tried *after* tube placement in the stomach is confirmed. This would promote gastric emptying and might cause the end of the tube to move if it is up against the stomach wall. Recording the output (**4**) is not wrong but it does *not improve* tube functioning. **IMP, 4, PhI**

12. (**4**) The digestion of blood in the duodenum results in black, tarry stools. Bright red blood in the stool (**1**) would be seen in a patient with *colitis* or *hemorrhoids*. Bright red emesis (**2**) or hemorrhage, is more common in patients with *gastric* ulcers. Acid digestion in the stomach (*gastric* ulcers) results in dark, granular emesis (**3**). **AS, 4, PhI**

13. (**1**) The abdomen becomes rigid as a consequence of the resulting chemical peritonitis, and the vital signs indicate the occurrence of hypovolemic shock. The abdomen does *not distend* (**2** and **3**) with a perforated ulcer but is tender, hard, and rigid. Peristalsis would diminish and paralytic ileus develop, so bowel sounds would be *absent* (**2**). Gas (**3**) is not a problem. There would be tachycardia, *not* bradycardia (**4**), with perforation. **AS, 4, PhI**

Intestinal Disorders

Chapter Outline

Celiac Disease (Nontropical Sprue)

Gluten-induced intestinal disease affecting adults and children, characterized by inability to digest and utilize sugars, starches, and fats.

I. Pathophysiology: intolerance to the gliadin fraction of grains, causing degeneration of the epithelial surface of the intestine, atrophy of the intestinal villi, and impaired absorption of essential nutrients.

II. Risk factors:
  A. Possible genetic or familial factors.
  B. Hypersensitivity response.
  C. History of childhood celiac disease.

III. Assessment
  A. *Subjective data:* family history.
  B. *Objective data:*
    1. Loss: weight, fat deposits, musculature.
    2. Anemia.
    3. Vitamin deficiencies.
    4. Abdomen: distended with flatus.
    5. Stools: diarrhea, foul smelling, bulky, fatty, float in commode.
    6. History of acute attacks of fluid/electrolyte imbalances.
    7. Diagnostic tests: *small-bowel biopsy, stool for fat.*
    8. *Gluten-free diet* leads to remission of symptoms.

IV. Analysis/nursing diagnosis
  A. *Altered nutrition, less than body requirements,* related to inability to digest and utilize sugars, starches, and fats.
  B. *Diarrhea* related to intestinal response to gluten in diet.
  C. *Fluid volume deficit* related to loss through excessive diarrhea.
  D. *Knowledge deficit* related to dietary restrictions to control symptoms.

V. Nursing care plan/implementation
  A. Goal: *prevent weight loss.*
    1. *Diet:* high in calories, protein, vitamins, and minerals; gluten free.
      a. *Avoid* wheat, rye, oats, barley.
      b. All other foods permitted.
    2. Daily weights to monitor changes.
  B. Goal: **health teaching.**
    1. Nature of disease.
    2. Dietary restrictions and allowances.
    3. Complications of noncompliance.
    4. Medications: *antidiarrhea* and *anticholinergic.*

VI. Evaluation/outcome criteria
  A. No further weight loss.
  B. Normal stools.
  C. Fluid/electrolyte balance obtained and maintained.

Appendicitis

Obstruction of appendiceal lumen and subsequent bacterial invasion of appendiceal wall; **acute emergency.**

I. Pathophysiology: when obstruction is partial or mild, inflammation begins in mucosa with slight appendiceal

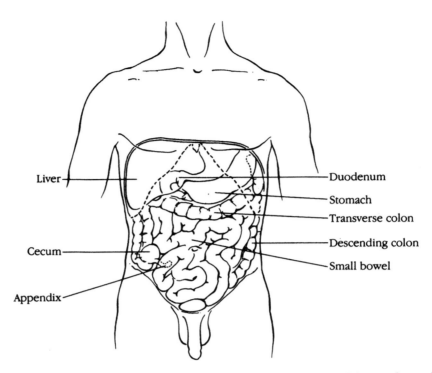

THE ABDOMINAL CONTENTS. (From Judge R, Zuidema G, Fitzgerald F. *Clinical Diagnosis.* Boston: Little, Brown, 1989, p. 331.)

swelling, accompanied by periumbilical pain. As the inflammatory process escalates and/or obstruction becomes more complete, appendix becomes more swollen, lumen fills with pus, and mucosal ulceration begins. When inflammation extends to peritoneal surface, pain is referred to right lower abdominal quadrant. *Danger:* rigidity over the entire abdomen is usually indicative of ruptured appendix; patient then prone to peritonitis.

II. Risk factors:
  A. Males affected more often than females.
  B. Most frequently seen between 10 and 30 yr old.

III. Assessment
  A. *Subjective data:*
    1. Pain: generalized, then right lower quadrant at McBurney's point, with rebound tenderness.
    2. Anorexia, nausea.
  B. *Objective data:*
    1. Vital signs: elevated temperature, shallow respirations.
    2. Either diarrhea or constipation.
    3. Vomiting, fetid breath odor.
    4. Splinting of abdominal muscles, flexion of knees onto abdomen.
    5. Lab data: elevated—white blood cell count (>10,000/mm³), neutrophil count (>75%)

IV. Analysis/nursing diagnosis
  A. *Pain* related to inflammation of appendix.
  B. *Risk for trauma* related to ruptured appendix.
  C. *Knowledge deficit* related to possible surgery.

V. Nursing care plan/implementation
  A. Goal: *promote comfort preoperatively and postoperatively.*
    1. Explain procedures; pain medications often withheld pending diagnosis.
    2. Assist with diagnostic workup.
    3. Medications as ordered: analgesics.
  B. Goal: *prevent complications.*
    1. Prevent infection: wound care, dressing technique, antiinfectives.
    2. Prevent dehydration: IVs, intake and output (I&O), fluids to solids by mouth as tolerated.
    3. Promote ambulation to prevent postoperative complications.

VI. Evaluation/outcome criteria
  A. No infection.
  B. Tolerates fluid, bowel sounds return.
  C. Heals with no complications.

Hernia

Protrusion of the intestine through a weak portion of the abdominal wall.

  I. Types:
    A. *Reducible:* visceral contents return to their normal position, either spontaneously or by manipulation.
    B. *Irreducible, or incarcerated:* contents cannot be returned to normal position.
    C. *Strangulated:* blood supply to the structure within the hernia sac becomes occluded (usually a loop of bowel).

D. Most common hernias: umbilical, femoral, inguinal, incisional, and hiatal (see Chap. 15 for hiatal hernia).

II. Pathophysiology: weakness in the wall may be either congenital or acquired. Herniation occurs when there is an increase in intraabdominal pressure from coughing, lifting, crying, straining, obesity, or pregnancy.

III. Assessment
  A. *Subjective data:*
    1. Pain, discomfort.
    2. History of feeling a lump.
  B. *Objective data:*
    1. Soft lump, especially when straining or coughing.
    2. Sometimes alteration in normal bowel pattern.
    3. Swelling.

IV. Analysis/nursing diagnosis
  A. *Activity intolerance* related to pain and discomfort.
  B. *Risk for trauma* related to lack of circulation to affected area of bowel.
  C. *Pain* related to protrusion of intestine into hernia sac.

V. Nursing care plan/implementation
  A. Goal: *prevent postoperative complications.*
    1. Monitor bowel sounds.
    2. Prevent postoperative scrotal swelling with inguinal hernia by applying ice and support to scrotum.
  B. Goal: **health teaching.**
    1. Prevent recurrence with correct body mechanics.
    2. Gradual increase in exercise.

VI. Evaluation/outcome criteria: healing occurs with no hernia recurrence.

Diverticulosis

A *diverticulum* is a small *pouch* or sac composed of mucous membrane that has protruded through the muscular wall of the intestine. *Diverticulosis* is the name for the condition in which several of these are present. *Inflammation* of the diverticula is called *diverticulitis*.

I. Pathophysiology: weakening in a localized area of muscular wall of the colon (especially the sigmoid colon), accompanied by increased intraluminal pressure.

II. Risk factors:
  A. Diverticulosis.
    1. Age: seldom before 35 yr; 60% incidence in older adults.
    2. History of constipation.
    3. Diet history: low in vegetable fiber, high in carbohydrate.
  B. Diverticulitis: highest incidence between ages 50 and 60 yr.

III. Assessment
  A. *Subjective data:* pain: cramplike left lower quadrant of abdomen.
  B. *Objective data:*
    1. Constipation or diarrhea, flatulence.
    2. Fever.

3. Rectal bleeding.
  4. Diagnostic procedures:
    a. Palpation reveals tender colonic mass.
    b. *Barium enema* (done only in absence of inflammation) reveals presence of diverticula.
    c. *Sigmoidoscopy.*

IV. Analysis/nursing diagnosis
  A. *Constipation* related to dietary intake.
  B. *Pain* related to inflammatory process in intestines.
  C. *Risk for fluid volume deficit* related to episodes of diarrhea or bleeding.
  D. *Risk for injury* related to bleeding.
  E. *Knowledge deficit* related to prevention of constipation.

V. Nursing care plan/implementation
  A. Goal: *bowel rest during acute episodes.*
    1. *Diet:* soft, liquid.
    2. Fluids, IVs if oral intake not adequate.
    3. Pain medications, as ordered.
    4. Monitor stools for signs of bleeding.
  B. Goal: *promote normal bowel elimination.*
    1. *Diet:* bland, high in vegetable fiber if no inflammation.
      a. *Include:* fruits, vegetables, whole-grain cereal, unprocessed bran.
      b. *Avoid:* foods difficult to digest (corn, nuts).
    2. Bulk-forming agents as ordered: methylcellulose, psyllium.
    3. Monitor: abdominal distention, acute bowel symptoms.
  C. Goal: **health teaching.**
    1. Methods to prevent constipation.
    2. Foods to include/avoid in diet.
    3. Relaxation techniques.
    4. Signs and symptoms of complications of chronic inflammation: abscess, obstruction, fistulas, perforation, or hemorrhage.

VI. Evaluation/outcome criteria
  A. Inflammation decreases.
  B. Bowel movements return to normal.
  C. Pain decreases.
  D. No perforation, fistulas, abscesses, obstruction, or hemorrhage noted.

Ulcerative Colitis

Inflammation of mucosa and submucosa of the distal colorectal area; inflammation leads to ulceration with bleeding; involved areas are continuous; disease is characterized by remissions and exacerbations.

I. Pathophysiology: specific physiologic response to emotional trauma. Edema and hyperemia of colonic mucous membrane → superficial bleeding with increased peristalsis, shallow ulcerations, abscesses; bowel wall thins and shortens and becomes vulnerable to perforation. Increased rate of flow of liquid ileal contents → decreased water absorption and diarrhea.

II. Risk factors:
  A. Highest occurrence in young adults (20–40 yr).
  B. Genetic predisposition: greater in whites, Jews.

   C. Autoimmune response.
   D. Infections.
   E. More common in urban areas (upper–middle incomes and higher educational levels).
   F. May be influenced by smoking.
   G. Exacerbations often related to stressful event.
III. Assessment
   A. *Subjective data:*
      1. Urgency to defecate, particularly when standing; tenesmus.
      2. Loss of appetite, nausea.
      3. Coliclike stomach pain.
      4. History of intolerance to dairy products.
      5. Emotional depression.
   B. *Objective data:*
      1. *Diarrhea:* 10–20 stools/d; can be chronic or intermittent, episodic or continual; stools contain blood, mucus, and pus.
      2. Weight loss and malnutrition, dehydration.
      3. Fever.
      4. Lab data: *decreased:* red blood cells, potassium, sodium, calcium, bicarbonate, related to excessive diarrhea.
      5. Lymphadenitis.
      6. Diagnostic tests:
         a. *Sigmoidoscopy* for visualization of lesions.
         b. *Barium* enema.
IV. Analysis/nursing diagnosis
   A. *Diarrhea* related to increased flow rate of ileal contents.
   B. *Self-esteem disturbance* related to progression of disease and increased number and odor of stools.
   C. *Pain* related to inflammatory process.
   D. *Fluid volume deficit* related to frequent episodes of diarrhea.
   E. *Knowledge deficit* related to methods to control symptoms.
   F. *Social isolation* related to continual diarrhea episodes.
V. Nursing care plan/implementation
   A. Goal: *reduce psychological stress.*
      1. Provide quiet environment.
      2. Encourage verbalization of concerns.
   B. Goal: *relieve discomfort.*
      1. Administer medications as ordered.
         a. Sedatives and tranquilizers to promote rest and comfort.
         b. Absorbents, kaolin-pectin (Kaopectate).
         c. Anticholinergics and antispasmotics to relieve cramping and diarrhea e.g., phenobarbital, atropine sulfate—diphenoxylate HCl (Lomotil).
         d. Antiinfectives to relieve bacterial overgrowth in bowel and limit secondary infection.
         e. Steroids to relieve inflammation and produce remission.
         f. Potassium supplements to relieve deficiencies.
   C. Goal: **health teaching**—*Diet:*

      1. *Avoid:* coarse-residue, high-fiber foods (e.g., raw fruits and vegetables, whole milk, cold beverages) because of inflammation.
      2. *Include:* bland, high-protein, high-vitamin, high-mineral, high-calorie foods.
      3. Parenteral hyperalimentation for severely ill.
      4. *Force fluids* by mouth.
   D. Goal: *prepare for surgery if medical regimen unsuccessful*—possible surgical procedures:
      1. Permanent ileostomy.
      2. Continent ileostomy (*Kock pouch*).
      3. Total colectomy, anastomosis with rectum.
      4. Total colectomy, anastomosis with anal sphincter.
VI. Evaluation/outcome criteria
   A. Fluid balance is obtained and maintained.
   B. Alterations in life-style managed.
   C. Stress-management techniques successful.
   D. Complications such as fistulas, obstruction, perforation, and peritonitis are prevented.
   E. Patient is prepared for surgery if medical regimen is unsuccessful or complications develop.

Crohn's Disease

A chronic, progressive inflammatory disease usually affecting the terminal ileum.

   I. Pathophysiology: *one of two conditions called "inflammatory bowel disease"* (ulcerative colitis is the other) that affect all layers of the ileum and/or the colon, causing patchy, shallow, longitudinal mucosal ulcers; possible correlation with autoimmune disease and adenocarcinoma of the bowel.
   II. Risk factors:
   A. Age: 15–20, 55–60 yr.
   B. White, especially Jewish.
   C. Familial predisposition.
   D. Possible virus involvement.
   E. Possible psychosomatic involvement.
   F. Possible hormonal or dietary influences.
III. Assessment (See Ulcerative Colitis, p. 852–6, for analysis/nursing diagnosis, nursing care plan/implementation, and evaluation/outcome criteria):
   A. *Subjective data:*
      1. Abdominal pain.
      2. Anorexia.
      3. Nausea.
      4. Malaise.
      5. History of isolated, intermittent, or recurrent attacks.
   B. *Objective data:*
      1. Diarrhea.
      2. Weight loss, vomiting.
      3. Fever, signs of infection.
      4. Fluid/electrolyte imbalances.
      5. Malnutrition, malabsorption.
      6. Occult blood in feces.

Intestinal Obstruction

Blockage of movement of intestinal contents through small or large intestine. Medical emergency because of potential for shock.

I. Pathophysiology:

A. *Mechanical causes*—physical impediments to passage of intestinal contents, e.g., adhesions, hernias, neoplasms, inflammatory bowel diseases, foreign bodies, fecal impactions, congenital or radiational strictures, intussusception, or volvulus.

B. *Paralytic causes*—passageway remains open, but peristalsis ceases, e.g., after abdominal surgery, abdominal trauma, hypokalemia, myocardial infarction, pneumonia, spinal injuries, peritonitis, or vascular insufficiency.

⋈ II. Assessment

A. *Subjective data:* pain related to:

1. *Proximal loop obstruction:* upper abdominal, sharp, cramping, intermittent pain.
2. *Distal loop obstruction:* poorly localized, cramping pain.

B. *Objective data:*

1. Bowel sounds: initially loud, high pitched; then when smooth muscle atony occurs, bowel sounds absent.
2. Increased peristalsis above level of obstruction in attempt to move intestinal contents through the obstructed area.
3. Obstipation (no passage of gas or stool through obstructed portion of bowel; no reabsorption of fluids).
4. Distention.
5. Vomiting:
   a. *Proximal loop obstruction:* profuse nonfecal vomiting.
   b. *Distal loop obstruction:* less frequent fecal-type vomiting.
6. Urinary output: decreased.
7. Elevated temperature, tachycardia, hypotension → shock if untreated.
8. Dehydration, hemoconcentration, hypovolemia.
9. Lab data:
   a. Leukocytosis.
   b. *Decreased:* sodium (<138 mEq/L), potassium (<3.5 mEq/L).
   c. *Increased:* pH (>7.45), bicarbonates (>26 mEq/L), blood urea nitrogen (BUN) (>18 mg/dL).

⋈ III. Analysis/nursing diagnosis

A. *Fluid volume deficit* related to vomiting.
B. *Pain* related to increased peristalsis above the level of obstruction.
C. *Altered nutrition, less than body requirements,* related to vomiting.
D. *Risk for trauma* related to potential perforation.

⋈ IV. Nursing care plan/implementation

A. Goal: *obtain and maintain fluid balance.*

1. Nursing care of patient with nasogastric (NG) tube (see Tubes Box in Chap. 9).
   a. *Miller-Abbott tube:* dual lumen, balloon inflated with air after insertion.
   b. *Cantor tube:* has mercury in distal sac, which helps move tube to point of obstruction.
   Caution: do *not* tape either tube to face until tube reaches point of obstruction.
2. Nothing by mouth, IV therapy, strict I&O.
3. Take daily weights (early morning), monitor central venous pressure (CVP) for hydration status.
4. Monitor abdominal girth for signs of distention and urinary output for signs of retention or shock.

B. Goal: *relieve pain and nausea.*

1. Medications, as ordered:
   a. *Analgesics, antiemetics.*
   b. If problem is paralytic: medical treatment includes neostigmine *to stimulate peristalsis.*
2. Observe for bowel sounds, flatus (tape intestinal tube to face once peristalsis begins).
3. Skin and frequent mouth care.

C. Goal: *prevent respiratory complications.*

1. Encourage coughing and deep breathing.
2. *Semi-Fowler's* or position of comfort.

D. Goal: *Postoperative nursing care* (if treated surgically): see Postoperative Experience, p. 114.

⋈ V. Evaluation/outcome criteria

A. Fluid balance obtained and maintained.
B. Shock is prevented.
C. Obstruction resolves.
D. Pain decreases.
E. Fluids tolerated by mouth.
F. Complications such as perforation and peritonitis prevented.

Fecal Diversion

Stomas: created because of disease or trauma; may be temporary or permanent.

I. Types (Table 16.1):

A. *Temporary*—fecal stream rerouted to allow GI tract to heal or to provide outlet for stool when obstructed.
B. *Permanent*—intestine cannot be reconnected. Rectum and anal sphincter removed (abdominal perineal resection). Often performed for cancer of the colon and/or rectum.

⋈ II. Analysis/nursing diagnosis

A. *Bowel incontinence* related to lack of sphincter in newly formed stoma.
B. *Altered health maintenance* related to knowledge of ostomy care.
C. *Body image disturbance* related to stoma.
D. *Fluid volume deficit* related to increased output through stoma.

⋈ III. Nursing care plan/implementation

A. Preoperative care:

TABLE 16.1   COMPARISON OF ILEOSTOMY AND COLOSTOMY

	Ileostomy	*Colostomy*
Procedure	Surgical formation of a fistula, or stoma, between the abdominal wall and *ileum;* continent ileostomy (*Kock pouch*) may be constructed.	Surgical formation of an artificial opening between the surface of the abdominal wall and *colon.* *Single barrel*—only one loop of bowel is opened to the abdominal surface. *Double barrel*—two loops of bowel, a proximal and distal portion, are open to the abdominal wall; feces is expelled from the proximal loop, mucus is expelled from the distal loop; patient may expel some excreta from rectum as well.
Reasons Performed	Unresponsive ulcerative colitis: complications of ulcerative colitis, e.g., hemorrhage, carcinoma (suspected).	*Single barrel:* colon or rectal cancer. *Double barrel:* relieve obstruction.
Results	Permanent stoma.	*Single barrel:* permanent stoma. *Double barrel:* temporary stoma.
Discharge	Green liquid, nonodorous.	Consistency of feces dependent on diet and portion of the bowel used as the stoma; from brown odorous liquid to normal stool consistency.
Nursing Care	See Fecal Diversion, p. 173.	See Tables 16.2 to 16.4 and Fecal Diversion p. 173.

Source: Lagerquist SL: *Little, Brown's NCLEX-RN Examination Review.* Boston: Little, Brown, 1996. P. 134.

1. Goal: *prepare bowel for surgery.*
   - a. Administer neomycin as ordered to reduce colonic bacteria.
   - b. Administer cathartics, *enemas* as ordered to cleanse the bowel of feces.
   - c. Administer *low-residue or liquid diet* as ordered.
2. Goal: *relieve anxiety and assist in adjustment to surgery.*
   - a. Provide accurate, brief, and reassuring explanations of procedures; allow time for questions.
   - b. Have enterostomal nurse visit to discuss ostomy management and placement of stoma appliance.
   - c. Offer opportunity for a visit with an Ostomy Association Visitor.
3. Goal: **health teaching.**
   - a. Determine knowledge of surgery and potential impact.
   - b. Begin teaching regarding ostomy.
B. **Postoperative care:**
   1. Goal: *maintain fluid balance.*
      - a. Monitor I&O, as large volume of fluid is lost through stoma.
      - b. Administer IV fluids as ordered.
      - c. Monitor losses through *NG tube.*
   2. Goal: *prevent other postoperative complications.*
      - a. Monitor for signs of intestinal obstruction.
      - b. Maintain sterility when changing dressings; *avoid* fecal contamination of incision.
      - c. Observe appearance of stoma: rosy pink, raised.
   3. Goal: *initiate ostomy care.*
      - a. Protect skin around stoma: use commercial preparation to toughen skin and use protective barrier wafer (Stomahesive) or paste (karaya or substitute) to keep drainage (which can cause excoriation) off the skin.
      - b. Keep skin around stoma clean and dry; empty appliance frequently. Check for drainage in appliance at least twice during each shift. If drainage (diarrhea-type stool) is present, empty colostomy appliance (Table 16.2).

TABLE 16.2 ☞ **EMPTYING COLOSTOMY APPLIANCE**

Check for drainage in appliance at least twice during each shift. If drainage present (diarrhea-type stool):

Do	**Do Not**
1. Unclip the bottom of bag.	1. Remove appliance each time it needs emptying.
2. Drain into bedpan.	2. Use any materials that could irritate bowel.
3. Use a squeeze-type bottle filled with warm water to rinse inside of appliance.	3. Ignore patient's needs.
4. Clean off clamp if soiled.	
5. Put a few drops of deodorant in appliance if not odorproof.	
6. Fasten bottom of appliance securely (fold bag over clamp 2–3 times before closing).	
7. Check for leakage under appliance every 2–4 h.	
8. Communicate with patient while attending to appliance.	

Source: Lagerquist SL: *Little, Brown's NCLEX-RN Examination Review.* Boston: Little, Brown, 1996. P. 309.

    c. Change appliance when drainage leaks around seal, or approximately every 2–3 d. Initially, stoma will be large due to edema. Pouch opening should be slightly larger than stoma, so it will not constrict. Stoma will need to be measured for each change until swelling subsides to ensure appropriate fit. (See Table 16.3).

    ✋ **d.** Use deodorizing drops in appliance and provide adequate room ventilation to decrease odors. *Caution:* deodorizing drops must be safe for mucous membranes. *No* pinholes in pouch.

    e. If a continent ileostomy, a *Kock pouch,* has been constructed, the patient does not have to wear an external pouch. The stool is stored intraabdominally. The patient drains the pouch several times daily, when there is a feeling of fullness, using a catheter. The stoma is flat and on the right side of the abdomen.

    4. Goal: *promote psychological comfort.*
      a. Support patient and family—accept feelings and behavior.
      b. Recognize that such a procedure may initiate the grieving process.

🏠 **5.** Goal: **health teaching.**
      a. Self-management skills related to ostomy appliance, skin care, and irrigation, if indicated (Table 16.4).
      ● **b.** *Diet:* adjustments to control character of feces; *avoid* foods that increase flatulence.
      c. Signs of complications of infection, obstruction, or electrolyte imbalance.
      d. Community referral for follow-up care.

⋈ **IV. Evaluation/outcome criteria**
    A. Demonstrates self-care skill for independent living.
    B. Makes dietary adjustments.
    C. Ostomy functions well.
    D. Adjusts to alteration in bowel elimination pattern.

Hemorrhoids

Enlarged vein in mucous membrane of rectum.

    I. Pathophysiology: venous congestion and interference with venous return from hemorrhoidal veins → increase in pelvic pressure, swelling, and distortion.

II. Risk factors:
    A. Straining to expel constipated stool.
    B. Pregnancy.
    C. Intraabdominal or pelvic masses.
    D. Interference with portal circulation.
    E. Prolonged standing or sitting.
    F. History of low-fiber, high-carbohydrate diet, which contributes to constipation.
    G. Family history of hemorrhoids.
    H. Enlarged prostate.

⋈ **III. Assessment**
    A. *Subjective data:* discomfort, anal pruritus, pain.
    B. *Objective data:*
      1. Bleeding, especially on defecation.
      2. Narrowing of stool.
      3. Grapelike clusters around anus (pink, red, or blue).
      4. Diagnosis:
        a. Visualization for *external* hemorrhoids.
      〰️ **b.** *Digital exam* or *proctoscopy* for *internal* hemorrhoids.

⋈ **IV. Analysis/nursing diagnosis**
    A. *Pain* related to defecation.
    B. *Constipation* related to dietary habits and pain at time of defecation.
    C. *Knowledge deficit* related to foods to prevent constipation.

⋈ **V. Nursing care plan/implementation**
    A. Goal: *reduce anal discomfort.*
    ☞ **1.** Sitz baths, as ordered; perineal care to prevent infection.
    ☞ **2.** Hot or cold compresses, as ordered, to reduce inflammation and pruritus.

TABLE 16.3   ☞ CHANGING COLOSTOMY APPLIANCE

Gather equipment: gloves, skin prep packet, colostomy appliance measured to fit stoma properly (if new surgical stoma, it will continue to shrink with healing; use stoma measuring guide), skin barrier, warm water and soap, face cloth/ towel, plastic bag for disposal of old equipment. Remember that bowel is very fragile; also, working near bowel increases peristalsis, and feces and flatulence may be expelled.

Do

1. Remove old appliance carefully, pulling from area with least drainage to area with most drainage.
2. Wash skin area with soap and water.
3. Observe skin area for potential breakdown.
4. Use packet of skin prep on the skin around the stoma; allow skin prep solution to dry on skin before applying colostomy appliance.
5. Apply skin barrier you have measured and cut to size.
6. Put appliance on so that the bottom of the appliance is easily accessible for emptying (e.g., if patient is *out* of bed most of the time, put the bottom facing the feet; if patient is *in* bed most of the time, have bottom face the side); picture-frame the adhesive portion of the appliance with 1-in. (2.5-cm) tape.
7. Put a few drops of deodorant in appliance if not odor-proof.
8. Use clamp to fasten bottom of appliance.
9. Talk to patient (or communicate in best way possible for patient) during and after procedure. This is a very difficult alteration in body image.
10. Use good handwashing technique.

Do Not

1. Tear appliance quickly from skin.
2. Wash stoma with soap; put anything dry onto stoma.
3. Irritate skin or stoma.
4. Put skin prep solution onto stoma; it will cause irritation.
5. Make opening too large (increases risk of leakage).
6. Have appliance attached so patient can't be involved in own care.
7. Use any materials that would irritate bowel.
8. Avoid conversation/eye contact.
9. Contaminate other incisions.

Source: Lagerquist SL: *Little, Brown's NCLEX-RN Examination Review.* Boston: Little, Brown, 1996. P. 310.

---

    3. Topical medications as ordered.
       a. *Anti-inflammatory:* hydrocortisone cream.
       b. *Astringents:* witch hazel–impregnated pads.
       c. *Topical anesthetics:* dibucaine (Nupercaine).
   B. Goal: *prevent complications related to surgery.*
     1. Encourage postoperative ambulation.
     2. Pain relief until packing removed.
     3. Monitor for: bleeding, infection, pulmonary emboli, phlebitis.
     4. Facilitate bowel evacuation: stool softeners, laxatives, suppositories, oil enemas, as ordered.
     5. Monitor for syncope/vertigo during first postoperative bowel movement.
     6. *Diet:*
       a. Low residue (postoperative)—*until* healing has begun.
       b. High fiber to prevent constipation *after* healing.
       7. *Increase* fluid intake.
   C. Goal: **health teaching**—methods to avoid constipation.
VI. Evaluation/outcome criteria
   A. No complications.
   B. Patient has bowel movement.
   C. Incorporates knowledge of correct foods into lifestyle.

TABLE 16.4   COLOSTOMY IRRIGATION

1. Assemble all equipment for irrigation and appliance change.
2. Remove and discard old pouch.
3. Clean the peristomal skin.
4. Apply the irrigating sleeve; place in toilet or bedpan.
5. Fill container with 500–1000 mL of warm water, *never* more than 1000 mL. Clear air from tubing. Insert lubricated tubing 2–4 in. (5–10 cm) into stoma. Do *not* force. Hold container about 18 in. (45 cm) above stoma. Infuse gently over 7–10 min.
6. Allow stool to empty into toilet. Evacuation usually occurs in 20–25 min.
7. If no return after irrigation, ambulate, gently massage abdomen, or give patient a warm drink.
8. Once complete, remove the sleeve and follow guidelines for applying appliance.

Source: Lagerquist SL: *Little, Brown's NCLEX-RN Examination Review.* Boston: Little, Brown, 1996. P. 135.

☞ Summary of Key Points

1. *Auscultation* of bowel sounds is done *after* inspection because palpation or percussion done before auscultation will change the bowel sounds.
2. Only an intestinal obstruction is more of an emergency than appendicitis. The chance of a ruptured appendix places the patient at risk for *peritonitis* leading to sepsis.
3. Instruct a patient with a hernia to seek assistance if the hernia cannot be reduced or pain occurs that could be indicative of *strangulation*.
4. If the patient has an inflammatory bowel condition (an "itis"), the diet should be *low fiber or low residue*.
5. Patients with ulcerative colitis may have more that 20 diarrhea stools per day. Assess for *fluid* and *electrolyte* imbalance.
6. Surgical removal of the entire inflamed colon is the common treatment for ulcerative colitis, but only sections of the diseased bowel are removed in patients with Crohn's disease. Surgical options include a *per*

manent ileostomy with a stoma and an external appliance; a *Kock's pouch*, a *continent* ileostomy (a stoma but no appliance), or a *restorative* procedure (anastomosis or J pouch reservoir), which allows for rectal evacuation.
7. A colostomy is indicated after *removal* of the rectum or part of the colon (*permanent*) or when the colon is being allowed to rest (*temporary*).
8. For all types of fecal diversion, a sufficient oral intake of fluid is essential; high-fiber foods may cause obstruction of an ileostomy but are needed to manage constipation in a colostomy patient.
9. An intestinal obstruction is an *emergency* situation because fluid and electrolyte absorption is seriously impaired and mortality is high if it goes untreated.
10. With a *mechanical* obstruction, bowel sounds (peristalsis) will be *increased* initially in an attempt to move the obstruction. Bowel sounds are *absent* from the beginning of a paralytic ileus (*functional* obstruction).

💡 Study and Memory Aids

⌇⌇⌇ Diagnostic Studies

Proctoscopy
Visualization of rectum and colon by means of a lighted tube inserted through the anus.

Small-bowel Biopsy
A specimen is obtained by passing a tube through the oral cavity and is microscopically examined for changes in cellular morphology.
☞ *Nursing responsibilities:* *no* food or fluids 8 h before procedure. Obtain written consent. Remove dentures if present. Monitor vital signs before, during, and after procedure for indications of hemorrhage. Procedure takes about an hour.

🍎 Diet

Celiac Disease

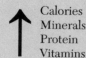
↑ Calories
  Minerals
  Protein
  Vitamins

Diverticulosis

Bowel rest:
  NPO initially
  Liquid to soft food
  Increase fluids
Bowel cleansing:
  Bland food

  High-fiber food (fruits, vegetables, whole-grain cereal, unprocessed bran)
Avoid foods that are difficult to digest (corn, nuts)

Hemorrhoids

Postoperative: ↓ residue
After healing: ↑ fiber
             ↑ fluids

Ulcerative Colitis: Diet

  Bland
  Calories
  Minerals
  Protein
AVOID:
  Coarse residue, high-fiber foods
  Raw fruits and vegetables
  Whole milk
  Cold beverages

● Drug Review

Celiac Disorders

Anticholinergic (Belladonna alkaloid: 0.25–0.5 mg
3 times a day oral or sublingual) to inhibit gastric
motility
Antidiarrheals
Diphenoxylate HCl with atropine sulfate (Lomotil):
2.5–5 mg 4 times a day
Kaolin with pectin (Kaopectate): 60–120 ml after
each loose bowel movement

Appendicitis

Analgesics
Meperidine HCl (Demerol): IM or SC, 50–150 mg
Morphine sulfate: IM or SC, 5–20 mg
Other drugs used according to patient's medical
history and postoperative health status
Antibiotics
Ampicillin 1–2 g/day q 6–12 h

Hernia

Analgesics
Meperedine HCL (Demerol): 50–150 mg
Morphine sulfate: IM or SC 5–50 mg. (may use
patient controlled analgesia—PCA)
Oxycodone (Roxicodone) with acetaminophen
(Percocet): 5 mg q 6h as needed

Diverticulosis

Analgesics
Morphine sulfate: 5–20 mg IM, SC
Oxycodone (Roxicodone) with acetaminophen
(Percocet) 5 mg q 6h as needed.
Antiinfectives
Cephalothin sodium (Keflin): 0.5–1 g q6h IV

Ulcerative Colitis

Antiinfectives
Ampicillin: 1–2 g/d q6–12h
Cephalexin (Keflex): 250–500 mg q6h
Cephalothin (Keflin): IV, 0.5–2 g q4–6h
Erythromycin: 250–500 mg q6–12h
Gentamicin (Garamycin): 3–5 mg/kg/d in divided
doses
Penicillin G: 1.2 million U in single IM dose
Tetracycline: 1–2 g/d q6–12h

Anticholinergics/antispasmodics
Atropine: 0.3–1.2 mg q 4–6h
Phenobarbital: 30–120 mg/d in divided doses
Antidiarrheals
Diphenoxylate HCl and atropine sulfate (Lomotil):
2.5–5 mg 4 times/d
Kaolin with pectin (Kaopectate): 60–120 ml after
each loose bowel movement
Loperamide hydrochloride (Imodium): 4 mg
initially, then 2 mg after each loose bowel
movement.
Potassium supplements: Potassium chloride: 16–24
mEq/d in divided doses
Sedatives/tranquilizers
Chlordiazepoxide HCl (Librium): 5–25 mg 3–4
times daily
Diazepam (Valium): 2–10 mg 2–4 times daily
Steroids: (should *never* be discontinued abruptly;
gradually taper dose to prevent complications)
Dexamethasone (Decadron): 0.5–9 mg/d in single
or divided doses
Methylprednisolone (Medrol): 4–48 mg/d
Prednisone: 5–60 mg/d

Crohn's Disease

Anticholinergic: Propantheline (Pro-Banthine): 15
mg tid, 30 mg hs
Antidiarrheals
Loperamide hydrochloride (Imodium) 4 mg initially
then 2 mg after each loose stool.
No opiate preparations
Antiinfectives: inflammatory
Sulfasalazine (Azulfidine): 500 mg 4/d
Antispasmodics (to reduce postprandial pain)
Belladonna Alkaloid: 0.25–0.5 mg 3 times/d
Glycopyrrolate (Robinol): 11 mg t.i.d.
Propantheline bromide (Pro-Banthine): 15 mg tid,
30 mg hs
Antiulceratives
Aluminum hydroxide gel (Amphojel): 5–10 mL q2–
4h or 1 h pc
Calcium carbonate (Titralac): 1–2 g with *water pc*
and *hs*
Magnesium and aluminum hydroxide (Maalox
suspension): 5–30 mL pc and hs
Sucralfate (Carafate): 1 g qid
Histamine antagonists
Cimetidine (Tagamet): 300–600 mg q6h
Ranitidine (Zantac): 150 mg bid
Hydrophilic mucilloids—psyllium (Metamucil):
1 rounded tsp in water 1–3 times/d; methyl-
cellulose (Citrucel): 15 ml in water 1–3 times/d (for
stool consistency)
Immunosuppressive agents: 6-Mercaptopurine
Steroids (should *never* be abruptly discontinued;
gradually taper dose to prevent complications)
Dexamethasone (Decadron): 0.5–9 mg/d in single
or divided doses
Methylprednisolone (Medrol): 4–48 mg/d
Prednisone: 5–60 mg/d

Intestinal Obstruction

Analgesics
    Meperidine HCl (Demerol): IM or SC, 50–150 mg
    Morphine sulfate: IM or SC, 5–20 mg
Antiemetics
    Prochlorperazine (Compazine): 5–10 mg IM; repeat
        once as needed
    Promethazine (Phenergan): 12.5–25 mg q 4–6 h as
        needed
    Trimethobenzamide (Tigan): 200 mg IM; 3–4
        times/day
Cholinergics
    Neostigmine (Prostigmin): used for paralytic ileus
        0.5–1 mg SC or IM

Fecal Diversion

Neomycin: 1 g/h for 4 h, then 1 g q4h for 24 h
    preoperatively

Hemorrhoids

Anti-inflammatory: Hydrocortisone cream
Astringents: Witch hazel–impregnated pads
Topical anesthetics: dibucaine (Nupercaine)

Questions

1. The dietary instructions the nurse gives a patient with ulcerative colitis would include a recommendation to eat foods that are low in:
   1. Residue.
   2. Carbohydrate.
   3. Fat.
   4. Calories.
2. The nursing priority in a patient who 2 days before has undergone an uncomplicated abdominoperineal resection and a colostomy would be to:
   1. Give instructions regarding colostomy irrigation.
   2. Record the patient's vital signs and intake and output.
   3. Check stomal drainage and the condition of the incision.
   4. Institute dietary restrictions and plan menus because patient is ready to start eating.
3. Which patient complaint should the nurse recognize as a symptom or sign of colorectal cancer?
   1. Nausea and vomiting.
   2. Left lower quadrant pain.
   3. Increased flatulence.
   4. Change in stool color.
4. Which statement that a patient makes about a scheduled colonoscopy would indicate to the nurse a need for further teaching?
   1. "A flexible tube will be inserted into my rectum."
   2. "I will be conscious, but sedated."
   3. "A scope will be inserted through my belly button."
   4. "I will need to have several enemas before the test."
5. Before the surgical removal of a rectal mass and a sigmoid colostomy, a patient will be receiving neomycin PO. The nurse knows that the purpose of this medication is to:
   1. Sterilize the bowel before surgery.
   2. Treat the infection caused by the tumor.
   3. Provide prophylactic anti-infective therapy.
   4. Decrease intestinal motility.
6. Which food should the nurse remove from the tray of a patient on a low-residue diet?
   1. Cottage cheese.
   2. Chicken breast.
   3. Mashed potatoes.
   4. Green beans.
7. The nurse explains to a colleague that the purpose of keeping a Foley catheter in place for several days after an abdominal perineal resection with a colostomy is to:
   1. Prevent a urinary tract infection.
   2. Prevent urine retention and resulting perineal wound pressure.
   3. Minimize the chance of wound contamination from urine.
   4. Determine whether the surgery caused bladder trauma.
8. Which nursing diagnosis would be a priority during the first 72 hours after surgery in a patient who has undergone a sigmoid colostomy?
   1. Knowledge deficit.
   2. Risk for infection.
   3. Body image disturbance.
   4. Self-care deficit.
9. The most important nursing action in a patient experiencing an acute episode of ulcerative colitis would be to:
   1. Replace the fluid and sodium lost as a result of the diarrhea.
   2. Monitor regularly for an increased serum glucose level from steroid therapy.
   3. Restrict dietary intake of high-potassium foods.
   4. Note change in color and consistency of stool.
10. Which side effects of propantheline (Pro-Banthine), given for the control of gastrointestinal tract spasms, would the nurse educate a patient about?
    1. Pupillary constriction and photophobia.
    2. Urinary frequency and urgency.
    3. Bradycardia and dizziness.
    4. Dry mouth and constipation.
11. The greatest concern in a 74-year-old patient who has been given midazolam (Versed) and fentanyl (Sublimaze) to produce conscious sedation during colonoscopy would be:
    1. An increased risk of postural hypotension.
    2. Management of abdominal discomfort resulting from constipation.
    3. Decreased bowel function stemming from reduced peristalsis.
    4. Assessment for return of motor function.

12. After self-irrigation of a sigmoid colostomy, there is no return. What should the nurse tell the patient to do?
    1. Massage the abdomen gently.
    2. Instill another 150 mL of water.
    3. Lie down, supine, until there is a return.
    4. Wait 45 minutes for initial emptying to occur.
13. When performing a physical assessment in a patient complaining of abdominal pain, the nurse would first:
    1. Auscultate to determine whether there are changes in bowel sounds.
    2. Observe the contour of the abdomen.
    3. Palpate the abdomen for a mass.
    4. Percuss the abdomen to determine whether fluid is present.
14. To assess the function of a colostomy 3 days after the procedure, the nurse would assess for:
    1. An appliance filled with flatus (gas).
    2. Semiformed stool.
    3. Continuous liquid drainage.
    4. A flat, pale-pink stoma.

Answers/Rationale

1. **(1)** It is important for a patient with col*itis*, an inflammation, to consume a low-residue, low-fiber diet. (A high-fiber diet is called for in patients with divertic*ulosis*.) The carbohydrate (**2**), fat (**3**), and calorie (**4**) content of foods is *not* a concern in inflammatory bowel disease. **IMP, 8, HPM**

2. **(3)** Around 36 hours the wound should be assessed for signs of infection, and the character of any drainage should be noted. Instruction on irrigation (**1**) should be done *before discharge.* Vital signs and I&O (**2**) would be the priority during the *first 24 hours* after surgery. Dietary planning (**4**) would also be an emphasis around this time, but this is a priority question and diet would be a *lesser* concern. **IMP, 8, PhI**

3. **(1)** Nausea and vomiting, as well as rectal bleeding, a change in bowel habits, abdominal pain, weight loss, and anorexia, may occur in colorectal cancer. Tumors of the small bowel and ascending (right) colon are usually associated with nausea and vomiting. Rectal bleeding is the usual finding that alerts a patient to a problem. Left lower quadrant pain (**2**) is more consistent with *ulcerative colitis.* Flatulence (**3**) is seen with *gallbladder* problems and *dietary* intolerance. A change in stool color (**4**) would more likely be due to a problem in the *biliary* system, such as gallstones. **AS, 8, PhI**

4. **(3)** In a colonoscopy the lining of the large intestine is

Key to Codes

Nursing process: **AS,** assessment; **AN,** analysis; **PL,** planning; **IMP,** implementation; **EV,** evaluation. (See Appendix M for explanation of nursing process steps.)

Category of human function: 1, protective; 2, sensory-perceptual; 3, comfort, rest, activity, and mobility; 4, nutrition; 5, growth and development; 6, fluid-gas transport; 7, psychosocial-cultural, 8, elimination. (See Appendix O for explanation.)

Client need: **SECE,** safe, effective care environment; **PhI,** physiologic integrity; **PsI,** psychosocial integrity; **HPM,** health promotion/maintenance. (See Appendix P for explanation.)

visualized by means of a flexible endoscope that is inserted rectally. (A *laparoscope* is inserted through the navel.) The statement in option **1** is therefore accurate, and requires *no* further teaching. Conscious sedation (**2**) *is* used, often a combination of midazolam (Versed) and fentanyl (Sublimaze). Bowel preparation *does* include enemas (**4**) to clean the bowel and ensure visualization. **EV, 8, SECE**

5. **(1)** It is important to minimize the bacterial growth in the bowel, because otherwise, when the bowel is incised, bacteria from the bowel could contaminate the peritoneum. Sterilizing the bowel before surgery minimizes the chance of postoperative infection. Infection (**2**) is *not* a common characteristic of colorectal cancer. General anti-infective therapy (**3**) is a plausible choice, but bowel sterilization is a *more specific* answer. Antiinfectives frequently cause diarrhea, which stems from an increase, *not* decrease (**4**), in motility. **PL, 8, PhI**

6. **(4)** Green beans are high in fiber, or residue, and such foods are usually eliminated from the diet of a patient with a bowel inflammation to reduce fecal bulk and mechanical irritation. The other foods (**1, 2,** and **3**) *are* low in residue and would be easily tolerated. **IMP, 4, PhI**

7. **(2)** Because general anesthesia and abdominal pain may make voiding difficult, the Foley catheter would be placed to prevent urine retention and the resultant bladder distention, which would then exert pressure on the surgical area. Catheters actually *increase* the risk of a urinary tract infection; they *do not prevent* such infections (**1**). There has been no intentional surgical incision into the urinary tract, so urine should *not* be leaking into the surgical wound (**3**). Bladder trauma (**4**) is always a possibility, and the appearance of the urine draining from the catheter would alert the nurse to blood in the urine or inadequate output; however, this is *not* the *initial* purpose of the catheter. **PL, 8, SECE**

8. **(2)** All of the diagnoses could apply in a patient who has undergone a sigmoid colostomy, but the diagnosis of postoperative complications is a *priority* during the first few days after surgery. The bowel sterilization procedure carried out preoperatively should minimize the risk for infection, however. Other complications to observe for include hemorrhage, wound disruption, thrombophlebitis, and abnormal stomal function. Knowledge about stoma care (**1**) would need to be assessed *before discharge. Once* the risk of postoperative complications is reduced, body image (**3**) becomes a major concern. The patient's ability to care for the stoma (**4**) would also need to be determined *before discharge.* **AN, 8, SECE**

9. **(1)** If a patient is suffering an acute episode of ulcerative colitis, there will be a minimum of 20 diarrhea stools per day, with a resultant fluid loss of as much as 17,000 mL in 24 hours. Steroid therapy will be ordered and will reduce the inflammation, but it is not curative. Steroids will increase the serum glucose level over a long term, but hyperglycemia (**2**) is *not* a priority concern during treatment for an acute episode. Steroids cause a loss of potassium; if the patient were eating, the dietary intake of potassium would therefore be increased, *not* restricted (**3**). The frequency of the stools, *not* the color (**4**), is important. **IMP, 8, PhI**

10. **(4)** Propantheline is an anticholinergic drug that causes dry mouth and constipation. It also causes pupillary dilatation, *not* constriction, and photophobia **(1)**; urinary retention, *not* frequency and urgency **(2)**; and tachycardia *not* bradycardia, and dizziness **(3)**. **IMP, 8, PhI**

11. **(1)** Both drugs cause hypotension, and this risk is greater in the elderly. Position changes should therefore be made slowly and with assistance to prevent fainting and falls. The drugs do *not* cause constipation. Air is used during the colonoscopy to increase visualization, thus cramping may occur during the procedure, but there is little subsequent discomfort resulting from the gas distention or the drugs **(2)**. These drugs have *no* effect on peristalsis **(3)**. The drugs do *not* have an effect on motor function **(4)** (e.g. no paralysis) per se. Any problems with ambulation would be related to fainting. **PL, 1, SECE**

12. **(1)** Usually 300 to 500 mL of fluid, and up to 1000 mL, is instilled over 3 to 5 minutes. If there is no return, the nurse should tell the patient to massage the abdomen gently. Additional fluid **(2)** would *only* be indicated if the fluid was returning as it was being instilled. If unable to sit up, the patient should lie on the left side to facilitate drainage, *not* on the *back* **(3)**. The whole procedure may take an hour, but the bowel is usually stimulated soon after the fluid is instilled; it should *not* take 45 minutes for initial emptying to occur **(4)**. **IMP, 8, HPM**

13. **(2)** The nurse should always observe or inspect before proceeding with the next step in the physical assessment. Auscultation **(1)** should be done after inspection and before palpation **(3)** and percussion **(4)**. **AS, 8, PhI**

14. **(1)** Initially there would be gas or mucus in the appliance. Stool is *not* present until 4 to 5 days postoperatively, and the expected *consistency cannot be determined* in this question because the location of the colostomy is not specified. Semiformed stool **(2)** would be expected with a *transverse* colostomy; continuous liquid **(3)** would be expected with an *ascending* (right) colostomy. Option **4** describes the stoma and is *unrelated to functioning*. **AS, 8, PhI**

Renal Disorders

Chapter Outline

Pyelonephritis

Acute or chronic inflammation due to bacterial infection of the parenchyma and pelvis of the kidney; 95% of cases caused by gram-negative enteric bacilli (*Escherichia coli*); occurs more frequently in young women and older men.

I. **Pathophysiology:** inflammation of renal medulla or lining of the renal pelvis → nephron destruction; hypertrophy of nephrons needed to maintain urine output → impaired sodium reabsorption (salt wasting), inability to concentrate urine, progressive renal failure, hypertension (two-thirds of all cases).

II. **Risk factors:**
   A. Obstruction.
   B. Hypertension.
   C. Hypokalemia.
   D. Diabetes mellitus.
   E. Pregnancy.
   F. Catheterization.

III. **Assessment**
   A. *Subjective data:*
      1. *Pain:* flank—one or both sides, back, dysuria; headache.
      2. *Loss of appetite,* weight loss.
      3. *Night sweats,* chills.
      4. *Urination:* frequency, urgency.
   B. *Objective data:*
      1. Fever.

   2. Lab data:
      a. *Blood*—polymorphonuclear leukocytosis >11,000/mm³.
      b. *Urine*—leukocytosis, hematuria, white blood cell casts, proteinuria (<3 g in 24 h), positive cultures, specific gravity—normal or *increased* with acute pyelonephritis; *decreased* with chronic pyelonephritis; cloudy, foul smelling.
      3. *Intravenous pyelogram (IVP)*—may show structural changes; see p. 195.

IV. **Analysis/nursing diagnosis**
   A. *Altered urinary elimination* related to kidney disease.
   B. *Pain* related to dysuria and kidney damage.
   C. *Altered nutrition, less than body requirements,* related to impaired sodium reabsorption and protein loss.
   D. *Risk for fluid volume* excess related to renal failure.

V. **Nursing care plan/implementation**
   A. Goal: *combat infection, prevent recurrence, alleviate symptoms.*
      1. Medications:
         a. *Antiinfectives, urinary antiseptics,* and/or sulfonamides appropriate for causative organism; also reduces pain.
         b. *Analgesics* for pain—phenazopyridine (Pyridium); stronger if calculi present.
         c. *Antipyretics* for fever—acetaminophen (Tylenol).

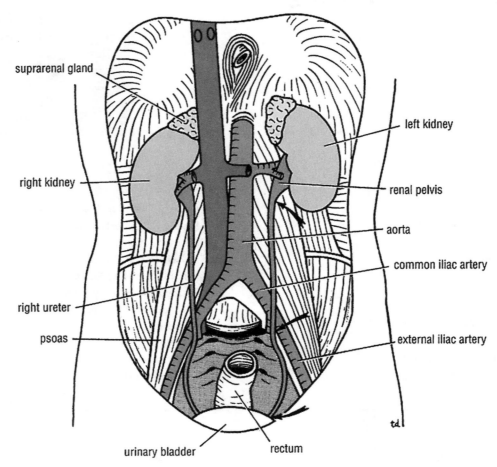

suprarenal gland

right kidney

right ureter

psoas

urinary bladder   rectum

left kidney

renal pelvis

aorta

common iliac artery

external iliac artery

td

POSTERIOR ABDOMINAL WALL, SHOWING KIDNEYS AND URETERS IN SITU. ARROWS INDICATE THREE SITES WHERE URETER IS NARROWED.

2. *Fluids:* 1500–2000 mL/d to flush kidneys, relieve dysuria, reduce fever, prevent dehydration.

☞ 3. Observe hydration status: intake and output (I&O) (output minimum, 1500 mL/24 h); daily weight; urine—check each voiding for *protein,* blood, *specific gravity;* vital signs q4h to monitor for hypertension, tachycardia; skin turgor.

◐☞ 4. Hygiene: meticulous *perineal* care, cleanse with soap and water, antiinfective ointment may be used around urinary meatus with retention catheter.

☞ 5. Cooling measures: tepid sponging.

◑ 6. *Diet:* sufficient calories and protein to prevent malnutrition, sodium supplement as ordered.

B. Goal: *promote physical and emotional rest.*

1. Activity: bed rest or as tolerated—depends on whether anemia or fever is present; encourage activities of daily living as tolerated.

2. Emotional support: encourage expression of fears (possible renal failure, dialysis); provide diversional activities; include family in care; answer questions.

🏠 C. Goal: **health teaching.**

1. Medications: take regularly to maintain blood level; side effects.

2. Personal care: perineal hygiene, *avoid* urethral contamination, *avoid* tub baths.

3. Possible recurrence with pregnancy.

4. Monitoring daily weight.

◪ VI. **Evaluation/outcome criteria**

A. Normal renal function (minimum 1500 mL of urine/24 h).

B. Blood pressure (BP) within normal range.

C. No recurrence of symptoms.

Acute Glomerulonephritis*

Acute glomerulonephritis (AGN) is a bilateral inflammation of the glomeruli of the kidneys. It is twice as common in men as in women. Like rheumatic fever, AGN is thought to result from an antigen-antibody reaction to a *Streptococcus* infection; however, unlike rheumatic fever, it does *not* tend to recur, since specific immunity is conferred after the first episode

*From Colombraro GC. Nursing Care of Children and Families. In *Little, Brown's NCLEX-RN Examination Review,* SL Lagerquist (ed). Boston: Little, Brown, 1996. p 529.

of AGN. Postinfectious AGN is primarily a disease of children occurring about 21 d after infection. AGN from other bacterial, viral, or parasitic infections occurs within a few days after illness.

I. Pathophysiology: Immunologic disorder often associated with an infection; circulating antigen–antibody complexes are trapped within glomerulus → inflammation → ↓ glomerular function, ↑ glomerular porosity → proteinuria and hematuria.

II. Risk factors
   A. Beta-hemolytic streptococcal infection of skin or upper respiratory system
   B. Systemic lupus erythematosus
   C. Vascular injury (e.g., hypertension)
   D. Diabetes
   E. Disseminated intravascular coagulation

III. Assessment
   A. Typical concerns from family about urine: change in color/appearance of urine (thick, reddish brown; decreased amounts).
   B. Acute edematous phase—usually lasts 4–10 d.
      1. Lab examination of urine:
         a. Severe **hematuria.**
         b. Mild proteinuria.
         c. Increased specific gravity.
      2. Hypertension
         a. Headache.
         b. Potential hypertensive encephalopathy → seizures, increased intracranial pressure.
      3. Mild–moderate edema: chiefly periorbital; increased weight due to fluid retention.
      4. General:
         a. Abdominal pain.
         b. Malaise.
         c. Anorexia.
         d. Vomiting.
         e. Pallor.
         f. Irritability.
         g. Lethargy.
         h. Fever.
   C. Diuresis phase:
      1. Copious diuresis.
      2. Decreased body weight.
      3. Marked clinical improvement.
      4. Decrease in gross hematuria, but microscopic hematuria may persist for weeks/months.

IV. Analysis/nursing diagnosis
      1. *Fluid volume excess* related to decreased urine output.
      2. *Pain* related to fluid retention.
      3. *Altered nutrition, less than body requirements,* related to anorexia and vomiting.
      4. *Impaired skin integrity* related to immobility.
      5. *Activity intolerance* related to fatigue.
      6. *Knowledge deficit* related to disease process, treatment, and follow-up care.

V. Nursing care plan/implementation
   A. Goal: *monitor fluid balance, observing carefully for complications.*
      1. Check and record BP at least every 4 h to monitor hypertension.
      2. Monitor daily weights.
      3. Urine: strict I&O; specific gravity and dipstick for blood every void.
      4. Note edema: extent, location, progression.
      5. Adhere to fluid restrictions if ordered.
      6. Bed rest, chiefly necessitated by hypertension: monitor for possible development of hyperten-

sive encephalopathy (seizures, increased intracranial pressure); report any changes stat to physician.
      7. Administer medications as ordered:
         a. *Antiinfectives*—eradicate any lingering *Streptococcus* infection.
         b. *Antihypertensives,* e.g., hydralazine HCl (Apresoline).
         c. Rarely use diuretics—limited value.
         d. *If heart failure develops*—may use digoxin.
         e. Refer to Appendix D for additional information on medications.
   B. Goal: *provide adequate nutrition.*
      1. *Diet: low sodium, low potassium*—to prevent fluid retention and hyperkalemia; *high protein* to replace protein being lost in the urine. Refer to Appendix B for additional information on diets.
      2. Stimulate appetite: offer small portions, attractively prepared; meals with family or others; offer preferred foods, if possible; encourage family to bring in special foods, e.g., culturally related preferences.
   C. Goal: *provide reasonable measure of comfort.*
      1. Encourage visiting by family.
      2. Provide for positional changes, give good skin care.
      3. Provide appropriate diversion, as tolerated.
   D. Goal: *prevent further infection.*
      1. Use good handwashing technique.
      2. Screen staff, other patients, visitors to limit contact with infectious persons.
      3. Administer *antiinfectives* if ordered (usually only for patients with positive cultures).
      4. Keep warm and dry, stress good hygiene.
      5. Note possible sites of infection: increased skin breakdown secondary to edema.
   E. Goal: *health teaching.*
      1. Teach how to check urine at home: dipstick for protein and blood. (*Note:* occult hematuria may persist for months.)
      2. Teach activity restriction: *no strenuous activity* until hematuria is completely resolved.
      3. Teach family how to prepare low-sodium, low-potassium diet.
      4. Arrange for follow-up care: physician, home health nurse.
      5. *Stress:* subsequent recurrences are *rare* because specific immunity is conferred.

VI. Evaluation/outcome criteria
   A. No permanent renal damage occurs.
   B. Normal fluid balance is maintained/restored.
   C. Adequate nutrition is maintained.
   D. No secondary infections occur.
   E. Verbalizes understanding of the disease, its treatment, and its prognosis.

Acute Renal Failure

Broadly defined as the rapid onset of oliguria accompanied by a rising blood urea nitrogen (BUN) and serum creatinine; usually reversible.

I. **Pathophysiology:** acute renal ischemia → tubular necrosis → decreased urine output. *Oliguric phase* (<400 mL/24 h)—waste products are retained → metabolic acidosis → water and electrolyte imbalances → anemia. *Recovery phase*—diuresis → dilute urine → rapid depletion of sodium, chloride, and water → dehydration.

II. **Types and risk factors:**
   A. *Prerenal*—due to factors outside of kidney; usually circulatory collapse—hemorrhage, severe dehydration, myocardial infarction, shock, vascular obstruction.
   B. *Intrinsic renal*—parenchymal disease resulting from ischemia or nephrotoxic damage; nephrotoxic agents—poisons, (such as carbon tetrachloride); heavy metals (arsenic, mercury); antiinfectives (kanamycin sulfate, neomycin sulfate); incompatible blood transfusion; alcohol myopathies; acute renal disease—AGN, acute pyelonephritis.
   C. *Postrenal*—obstruction in collecting system: renal or bladder calculi, tumors of bladder, prostate, or renal pelvis; gynecologic or urologic surgery in which ureters are accidentally ligated.

▶ III. **Assessment**
   A. *Subjective data:*
      1. Sudden decrease or cessation of urine output (<400 mL/24 h).
      2. Anorexia, nausea, vomiting resulting from azotemia.
      3. Sudden weight gain resulting from fluid accumulation.
      4. Headache.
   B. *Objective data:*
      1. Vital signs (vary according to cause and severity):
         a. *BP*—usually elevated.
         b. *Pulse*—tachycardia, irregularities.
         c. *Respirations*—increased rate, depth, crackles.
      2. *Neurologic:* decreasing mentation, unresponsive to verbal or painful stimuli, psychoses, convulsions.
      3. Mouth/oral: halitosis, cracked mucous membranes.
      4. *Skin:* dry, rashes, purpura, itchy, pale.
      5. Lab data:
         a. Blood: *increased*—potassium BUN; creatinine, white blood cell count (WBC); *decreased*—pH, bicarbonate, hematocrit, hemoglobin.
         b. Urine: *decreased*—volume, specific gravity (↓ 1,010); *increased*—protein, casts, red and white blood cells, sodium.

▶ IV. **Analysis/nursing diagnosis**
   A. *Altered urinary elimination* related to kidney malfunction.
   B. *Fluid volume excess* related to decreased urine output.
   C. *Altered nutrition, less than body requirements,* related to anorexia.
   D. *Altered oral mucous membrane* related to stomatitis.
   E. *Altered thought processes* related to uremia.

▶ V. **Nursing care plan/implementation**

   A. Goal: *maintain fluid and electrolyte balance and nutrition.*
      1. Monitor: daily weight (should not vary more than ± 1 lb); vital signs—include central venous pressure (*CVP*). Blood chemistries: BUN 6–20 mg/dl; creatinine 0.6–1.5 mg/dl
   ☞ 2. *Fluids:* IV as ordered; blood: plasma, packed cells, electrolyte solutions to replace losses; restricted to 400 mL/24 h if hypertension present or during oliguric phase to prevent fluid overload.
   ● 3. *Diet:* as tolerated: *high* carbohydrate, low protein, may be *low* potassium and *low* sodium; ☞ hypertonic glucose (total parenteral nutrition) if oral feedings not tolerated; intravenous L-amino acids and glucose.
   ● ☞ 4. Control hyperkalemia: infusions of hypertonic glucose and insulin to force potassium into cells; calcium gluconate (IV) to reduce myocardial irritability from potassium; sodium bicarbonate (IV) to correct acidosis; sodium polystyrene sulfonate (Kayexalate) or other exchange resins, orally or rectally (*enema*), to remove excess potassium (K⁺); *peritoneal dialysis or hemodialysis.*
   ● 5. Medications—*diuretics* (mannitol, furosemide [Lasix]).
   B. Goal: *use assessment and comfort measures to reduce occurrence of complications.*
   〰 ☞ 1. Respiratory: monitor rate, depth, breath sounds, *arterial blood gases;* encourage deep breathing, coughing, turning; use *incentive spirometer* or *nebulizer* as indicated.
      2. Frequent oral care to prevent stomatitis.
      3. Observe for signs of:
         a. *Infection*—elevated temperature, localized redness, swelling, heat, or drainage.
         b. *Bleeding*—stools, gums, venipuncture sites.
   C. Goal: *maintain continual emotional support.*
      1. Same caregivers, consistency in procedures.
      2. Give opportunities to express concerns, fears.
      3. Allow family interactions.
   D. Goal: *health teaching.*
      1. Preparation for dialysis (indications: uremia, uncontrolled hyperkalemia, or acidosis).
      2. *Dietary restrictions:* low sodium, fluid restriction.
      3. Disease process; treatment.

▶ VI. **Evaluation/outcome criteria**
   A. Return of kidney *function*—normal creatinine level (<1.5 mg/dl) urine output.
   B. Resumes normal life pattern (about 3 mo after onset).

Chronic Renal Failure

Because of progressive destruction of kidney tissue, the kidneys are no longer able to maintain their homeostatic functions; considered irreversible.

I. **Pathophysiology:** destruction of glomeruli → reduced glomerular filtration rate → retention of metabolic waste products; decreased urine output; severe fluid, electrolyte, acid-base imbalances → uremia. Clinical picture includes:
  A. Ammonia in skin and alimentary tract resulting from bacterial interaction with urea → inflammation of mucous membranes.
  B. Retention of phosphate → decreased serum calcium → muscle spasms, tetany, and increased parathormone release → demineralization of bone.
  C. Failure of tubular mechanisms to regulate blood bicarbonate → metabolic acidosis → hyperventilation.
  D. Urea osmotic diuresis → flushing effect on tubules → decreased reabsorption of sodium → sodium depletion.
  E. Waste product retention → depressed bone marrow function → decreased circulating red blood cells (RBCs) → renal tissue hypoxia → decreased erythropoietin production → further depression of bone marrow functioning → anemia.

II. **Risk factors:**
  A. Polycystic kidney disease.
  B. Chronic glomerulonephritis.
  C. Chronic urinary obstruction, ureteral stricture, calculi, neoplasms.
  D. Chronic pyelonephritis.
  E. Severe hypertension.
  F. Congenital or acquired renal artery stenosis.
  G. Systemic lupus erythematosus.

III. **Assessment**
  A. *Subjective data:* excessive fatigue, weakness.
  B. *Objective data*
    1. Skin: bronze-colored, uremic frost.
    2. Ammonia breath.
    3. See also Acute Renal Failure, p. 186; symptoms gradual in onset.

IV. **Analysis/nursing diagnosis**
  A. In addition to the following, see Acute Renal Failure, p. 186.
  B. *Fatigue* related to severe anemia.
  C. *Risk for impaired skin integrity* related to pruritus.
  D. *Ineffective individual coping* related to chronic illness.
  E. *Body image disturbance* related to need for dialysis.
  F. *Noncompliance* related to denial of illness.

V. **Nursing care plan/implementation**
  A. Goal: *maintain fluid/electrolyte balance and nutrition.* (See also Acute Renal Failure, p. 186.)
    1. *Diet: low* sodium; foods *high* in calcium, vitamin B complex, vitamins C and D, and iron (to reduce edema, replace deficits, and promote absorption of nutrients).
    2. Administer medications: calcium carbonate; supplemental vitamins if deficient; electrolyte modifier (aluminum hydroxide [Alu-Cap., Amphojel]).
    3. I&O; intake should be limited to no more than 600–800 mL more than previous day's output to prevent fluid retention.
  B. Goal: *employ comfort measures that reduce distress and support physical function.*
    1. Activity: bed rest; facilitate ventilation; turn, cough, deep breathe q2h; range of motion exercises—active and passive, to prevent thrombi.
    2. Hygiene: *mouth care* to prevent stomatitis and reduce discomfort from mouth ulcers; *perineal* care.
    3. Skin care: soothing lotions to reduce pruritus.
    4. Encourage communication of concerns.
  C. Goal: **health teaching.**
    1. Dietary restrictions: *no* added salt when cooking; change cooking water in vegetables during process to decrease potassium; read food labels to *avoid* sodium and potassium intake.
    2. Importance of daily weight: same scale, time, clothing.
    3. Prepare for dialysis, transplantation.

VI. **Evaluation/outcome criteria**
  A. Acceptance of chronic illness (no indication of indiscretions, destructive behavior, suicidal tendency).
  B. Compliance with dietary restriction—no signs of protein excess (e.g., nausea, vomiting) or fluid/sodium excess (e.g., edema, weight gain).

Dialysis

Diffusion of solute through a semipermeable membrane that separates two solutions; direction of diffusion depends on concentration of solute in each solution; rate and efficiency depend on concentration gradient, temperature of solution, pore size of membrane, and molecular size; two methods available (Table 17.1).

I. Indications: acute poisonings, acute or chronic renal failure, hepatic coma, metabolic acidosis, extensive burns with azotemia.

II. Goals:
  A. *Reduce level of nitrogenous waste.*
  B. *Correct acidosis, reverse electrolyte imbalances, remove excess fluid.*

III. **Hemodialysis:** circulation of patient's blood through a compartment formed of a semipermeable membrane (cellophane or cuprophane) surrounded by dialysate fluid.
  A. Types of dialyzers:
    1. Coil type.
    2. Parallel plate.
    3. Capillary.
  B. Types of venous access for hemodialysis:
    1. *External shunt* (Figure 17.1).
      a. Cannula is placed in a large vein and a large artery that are approximate.
      b. External shunts, which provide easy and painless access to bloodstream, are prone to infection and clotting and cause erosion of the skin around the insertion area.
        (1) Daily cleansing and application of a sterile dressing.

TABLE 17.1   COMPARISON OF HEMODIALYSIS AND PERITONEAL DIALYSIS

	Hemodialysis	Peritoneal Dialysis
Process	*Rapid*—uses either external AV shunt (acute renal failure) or internal AV fistula (chronic renal failure); typical treatment is 3–4 h 3 d/wk; also used for barbiturate overdoses to remove toxic agent quickly.	*Intermittent*—up to 24–72 h for hospitalized patients; outpatients 10–14 h 3–4 times a week; *dwell time* 30–45 min for manual dialysis or 10–20 min for automatic cycler; either rigid stylet catheter or surgically inserted soft catheter; advantage for patients who cannot tolerate rapid fluid and electrolyte changes. *Continuous*—four cycles in 24 h; *dwell time* is 4–5 h during the day and 8 h overnight; no need for machinery, electricity, or water source; surgically inserted soft catheter; closely resembles normal renal function.
Vascular access	Required.	Not necessary; therefore suitable for patients with vascular problems.
⬤ Heparinization	Required; systemic or regional.	Little or no heparin necessary; therefore suitable for patients with bleeding problems.
Complications (other than fluid and electrolyte imbalances, which are common to all)	Dialysis dysequilibrium syndrome (preventable) Mechanical dysfunctions of dialyzer	Peritonitis Hypoalbuminemia Bowel or bladder perforation Plugged or dislodged catheter.

AV = arteriovenous.

Source: Lagerquist SL: *Little, Brown's NCLEX-RN Examination Review.* Boston: Little, Brown, 1996. P. 139.

(2) Prevention of physical trauma and *avoidance* of some activities, such as swimming.
2. *Arteriovenous fistulas* (Figure 17.2).
   a. Large artery and vein are sewn together (anastomosed) below the surface of the skin.
   b. Purpose is to create one blood vessel for withdrawing and returning blood.
   c. *Advantages:* greater activity range than arteriovenous shunt and no protective asepsis.
   d. *Disadvantage:* need for two venipunctures with each dialysis.
C. **Complications** during hemodialysis:
   1. *Dysequilibrium syndrome*—rapid removal of urea from blood → reverse osmosis, with water moving into brain cells → cerebral edema → possible headache, nausea, vomiting, confusion, and convulsions; usually occurs with initial dialysis treatments; shorter dialysis time and slower rate minimizes.
   2. *Hypotension*—results from excessive ultrafiltration or excessive antihypertensive medications.
   3. *Hypertension*—results from volume overload (water and/or sodium), causing dysequilibrium syndrome or anxiety.
   4. *Transfusion reactions* (see Chap. 5).
   5. *Arrhythmias*—due to hypotension, fluid overload, or rapid removal of potassium.
   6. *Psychological problems:*

   a. Patients react in varying ways to dependence on hemodialysis.
   b. Nurse needs to identify patient reactions and defense mechanisms and to employ supportive behaviors, i.e., include patient in care; continual repetition and reinforcement; do *not* interpret patient's behavior—for example, do not say, "You're being hostile" or "You're acting like a child"; answer questions honestly regarding quality and length of life with dialysis and/or transplantation; encourage independence as much as possible.
IV. **Intermittent peritoneal dialysis:** involves introduction of a dialysate solution into the abdomen, where the peritoneum acts as the semipermeable membrane between the solution and blood in abdominal vessels. *Procedures:*
   ⬤ A. Area around umbilicus is prepared, anesthetized with local anesthetic, and a catheter is inserted into the peritoneal cavity through a trocar; the catheter is then sutured into place to prevent displacement.
   B. Warmed dialysate is then allowed to flow into the peritoneal cavity. Inflow time: 5–10 min; 2 liters of solution are used in each cycle in the adult; solutions contain glucose, Na^+, Ca^{2+}, Mg^{2+}, K^+, Cl^-, and lactate or acetate.
   C. When solution bottle is empty, dwell time (exchange time) begins. *Dwell time:* 10–20 min with automatic, 30–45 min with manual; processes of diffusion, osmosis, and filtration begin to move

A On Dialyzer

B Off Dialyzer (before bandaging)

Cannula clamps

FIGURE 17.1 **ARTERIOVENOUS SHUNT (CANNULAS).**
(Adapted and used by permission of Ann Holmes, RN, West Contra Costa Dialysis Clinic, San Pablo, CA.)

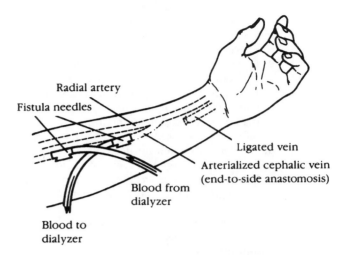

FIGURE 17.2 **ARTERIOVENOUS FISTULA.**
(Adapted and used by permission of Ann Holmes, RN, West Contra Costa Dialysis Clinic, San Pablo, CA.)

waste products from bloodstream into peritoneal cavity.
   D. Draining of the dialysate begins with the unclamping of the outflow clamp. *Outflow time:* usually 20 min; return of <2 liters usually results from incomplete peritoneal emptying; turn side to side to increase return; 30 cycles in 24 h is ideal.
V. **Continuous ambulatory peritoneal dialysis (CAPD)** Functions on the same principles as peritoneal dialysis, yet allows greater freedom and independence for patient. *Procedure:*
   A. Dialysis solution is infused into peritoneum three times daily and once before bedtime.
   B. *Dwell time*—5 h for each daily exchange, overnight for the fourth (8 h).
   C. Indwelling peritoneal catheter is connected to solution bag at all times—serves to fill and drain peritoneum; concealed in cloth pouch, strapped to the body during dwell time; patient can move about doing usual activities.

Kidney Transplantation

Placement of a donor kidney (from sibling, parent, cadaver) into the iliac fossa of a recipient and the anastomosis of its ureter to the bladder of the recipient; indicated in end-stage renal disease.

   I. *Criteria for recipient:* irreversible kidney function; under 70 yr of age; patent and functional lower urinary tract; and good surgical risk, free of serious cardiovascular complications. *Contraindicated* in metastatic carcinoma and oxalosis (excessive oxalate in urine).
  II. *Donor selection:*
   A. Sibling or parent—survival rate of kidney is greater; preferred for transplantation.
   B. Cadaver—greater rate of rejection after transplantation, although cadaver kidneys are used for most transplantations.
 III. *Bilateral nephrectomy:* necessary for patients with rapidly progressive glomerulonephritis, malignant hypertension, or chronic kidney infections; prevents complications in transplanted kidney (see Nephrectomy for nursing care, p. 191).
 IV. **Analysis/nursing diagnosis**
   A. *Altered urinary elimination* related to kidney failure.
   B. *Fear* related to potential transplant rejection.
   C. *Risk for infection* related to immunosuppression.
   D. *Body image disturbance* related to immunosuppression.
  V. **Nursing care plan/implementation**
   A. **Preoperative care:**
     1. Goal: *promote physical and emotional adjustment.*
      a. Informed consent.

b. Lab work completed—histocompatibility, complete blood count, urinalysis, blood type and cross-match.

c. Skin preparation.

2. Goal: *encourage expression of feelings:* origin of donor, fear of complications, rejection.

3. Goal: *minimize risk of organ rejection:* give medications: begin *immunosuppression* (azathioprine, corticosteroids, cyclosporine); anti-infectives if ordered.

4. Goal: **health teaching.**

   a. Nature of surgery, placement of kidney.

   b. Postoperative expectations: deep breathing, coughing, turning, early ambulation, reverse isolation.

   c. Medications: immunosuppressive therapy: purpose, effect.

B. Postoperative care:

1. Goal: *promote uncomplicated recovery of recipient.*

   a. Vital signs; *CVP;* I&O—may see large amounts urine (3–20 L) in early postoperative period from sodium diuresis, or kidney may not work for a week or more and dialysis will be needed within 24–48 h.

   b. *Isolation:* strict reverse isolation with immunosuppression, wear face mask when out of room.

   c. *Position:* back to nonoperated sides, semi-Fowler's to promote gas exchange.

   d. Indwelling catheter care: characteristics of urine—report gross hematuria, heavy sediment; clots; perineal care (see p. 194).

   e. Activity: ambulate 24 h after surgery, *avoid* prolonged sitting.

   f. *Weigh daily.*

   g. Medications: *immunosuppressives, analgesics* as ordered.

   h. Drains: irrigate *only* on physician's order, *meticulous* catheter care.

   i. *Diet:* regular; liberal amounts of protein; *restrict* fluids, sodium, potassium *only if* oliguric.

2. Goal: *observe for signs of rejection*—most dangerous complication. Three classifications:

   a. *Hyperacute*—occurs within 5–10 min up to 48 h after transplantation (RARE).

   b. *Acute*—signs and symptoms are evident at approximately 6 weeks after transplantation. Rejection is most common at 3 mos. after transplantation.

   c. *Chronic*—occurs several months to years after transplantation.

   d. Assessment

     (1) *Subjective data:*

       (a) Lethargy, anorexia.

       (b) Tenderness over graft site.

     (2) *Objective data:*

       (a) Lab data: urine: *decreased*—output creatinine clearance, sodium;

increased—protein; Blood, *increased*—BUN, creatinine.

       (b) Rapid weight gain.

       (c) Vital signs: BP, temperature—elevated.

3. Goal: *maintain immunosuppressive therapy.*

   a. Azathioprine (Imuran)—an antimetabolite that interferes with cellular division. *Side effects:*

     (1) Gastrointestinal (GI) bleeding (give PO form *with food*).

     (2) Bone marrow depression, *leukopenia, anemia.*

     (3) Development of malignant neoplasms.

     (4) Infection.

     (5) Liver damage.

   b. Prednisone—believed to affect lymphocyte production by inhibiting nucleic acid synthesis, anti-inflammatory action helps prevent tissue damage if rejection occurs. *Side effects:*

     (1) Stress ulcer with bleeding (give with food).

     (2) Decreased glucose tolerance (hyperglycemia).

     (3) Muscle weakness.

     (4) Osteoporosis.

     (5) Moon facies.

     (6) Acne and striae.

     (7) Depression and hallucinations.

   c. Cyclosporine (Cyclosporin A)—a polypeptide antibiotic used to prevent rejection of kidney, liver, or heart allografts; PO dose given *with* room temperature chocolate milk or orange juice in a glass dispenser. *Side effects:*

     (1) Nephrotoxicity (increased *BUN, creatinine*).

     (2) Hypertension.

     (3) Tremor.

     (4) Hirsutism, gingival hyperplasia.

     (5) *GI*—nausea, vomiting, anorexia, diarrhea, abdominal pain.

     (6) *Infections*—pneumonia, septicemia, abscesses, wound.

   d. Additional drugs may include cyclophosphamide (Cytoxan), methylprednisolone, antithymocyte (ATGAM), antilymphocyte globulin, and anti–T-lymphocyte monoclonal antibody.

4. Goal: **health teaching.**

   a. Signs of rejection (see goal 2).

   b. Drugs: side effects of immunosuppression (see goal 3. above).

   c. Self-care activities: temperature, BP, I&O, urine specimen collection.

   d. Prevention of infection.

   e. See also goals of care, Postoperative Experience, pp. 114–115.

VI. Evaluation/outcome criteria

A. No signs of rejection (e.g., weight gain, oliguria).

B. No depression.

C. Resumes role responsibilities.

Nephrectomy

Removal of kidney through flank, retroperitoneal, abdominal, thoracic, or thoracic-abdominal approach; indicated with malignant tumors, severe trauma, or under certain conditions before renal transplantation (see Kidney Transplantation, pp. 189–190).

I. Analysis/nursing diagnosis

   A. *Pain* related to surgical incision.

   B. *Risk for infection* related to wound contamination.

   C. *Risk for aspiration* related to vomiting.

   D. *Constipation* related to paralytic ileus.

   E. *Anxiety* related to possible loss of function in remaining kidney.

   F. *Dysfunctional grieving* related to perceived loss.

II. Nursing care plan/implementation:

   A. Preoperative care: Goal: *optimize physical and psychological functioning* (see Preoperative Preparation, pp. 111–113).

   B. Postoperative care: Goal: *promote comfort and prevent complications.*

      1. Observe for signs of:

         a. *Paralytic ileus*—abdominal distention, absent bowel sounds, vomiting (common complication following renal surgery).

         b. *Hemorrhage.*

      2. Fluid balance: daily weight—maintain within 2% of preoperative level.

III. Evaluation/outcome criteria

   A. No complications (e.g., hemorrhage, paralytic ileus, wound infection).

   B. Acceptance of loss of kidney.

Renal Calculi (Urolithiasis)

Formation of calculi (stones) in renal calyces or pelvis that pass to lower regions of urinary tract—ureters, bladder, or urethra; occurs after age 30 yr, with greatest incidence in *men,* particularly over age 50 yr.

   I. Pathophysiology: organic crystals form (75% of stones contain calcium) → obstruction, infection; increased backward pressure in kidney → hydronephrosis → atrophy, fibrosis of renal tubules.

   II. Risk factors:

   A. Changes in urine pH and concentration from readily precipitable, crystalline materials—sulfonamides, uric acid, calcium salts.

   B. Urinary tract infection.

   C. Indwelling Foley catheter.

   D. Vitamin A deficiency.

III. Assessment (depends on size, shape, location of stone):

   A. *Subjective data:*

      1. Pain: occasional, dull, in loin or back when stones are in calyces or renal pelvis; *excruciating* in flank area (renal colic), radiating to groin when stones are ureteral.

      2. Nausea associated with pain.

   B. *Objective data:*

      1. Pallor, sweating, syncope, shock, and vomiting due to pain.

      2. Palpable kidney mass with hydronephrosis.

      3. Fever and pyuria with infection.

      4. Lab data:

         a. Urinalysis: abnormal—pH (acidic or alkaline), RBCs (injury), WBCs (infection); *increased*—specific gravity, casts, crystals, other organic substances, depending on type of stone (i.e., uric acid, calcium); positive culture.

         b. Blood: *increased*—calcium phosphorus, total protein, alkaline phosphatase, creatinine, uric acid, BUN.

      5. Diagnostic tests:

         a. *IVP:* reveals nonopaque stones, degree of obstruction. See p. 195.

         b. X-ray: radiopaque stones seen.

         c. Ultrasound may also be used.

IV. Analysis/nursing diagnosis

   A. *Pain* related to passage of stone.

   B. *Altered urinary elimination* related to potential obstruction.

   c. *Urinary retention* related to obstruction of urethra.

V. Nursing care plan/implementation

   A. Goal: *reduce pain and prevent complications.*

      1. Medication: *narcotics, antiemetics, antiinfectives.*

      2. *Fluids:* 3–4 L/d; *IVs* if nauseated, vomiting.

      2. Activity: ambulate to promote passage of stone, except bed rest during acute attack (colic).

      3. Reduce spasms: warm soaks to affected flank.

      4. Observe for signs of:

         a. *Obstruction*—decreased urinary output, increased flank pain.

         b. *Passage of stone*—cessation of pain; filter urine with gauze.

      5. Monitor: hydration status—I&O, daily weight; vital signs—particularly temperature for sign of infection; urine—color, odor.

   B. Goal: **health teaching.**

      1. Importance of *fluids:* minimum 3000 mL/d; 2 glasses during night.

      2. *Diet:* modify according to stone type and amount of urinary excretion of organic substance (i.e., calcium).

         a. *Uric acid stones*—low purine.

         b. *Calcium oxalate and calcium phosphate stones*—low calcium phosphorus, and oxalate (e.g., *avoid* tea, cocoa, cola, beans, spinach, acidic fruits). Low calcium diet may be contraindicated, as it may cause bone demineralization, particularly in postmenopausal women.

         c. *Cystine stones*—low protein.

      3. *Acid-ash diet* with: calcium oxalate and calcium phosphate stones, magnesium and ammonium phosphate stones.

      4. *Alkaline-ash diet* with: Uric acid, and cystine stones (see Review of Nutrition in Appendix B).

      5. Signs of urinary tract infection: dysuria, frequency, hematuria; seek immediate treatment.

☞ **6.** Prepare for removal if indicated; 60%–80% of patients will have lithotripsy done (see below); cystoscopy (see p. 195) or ureterolithotomy may also be ordered; nephrectomy in *extreme cases.*

⋈ VI. Evaluation/outcome criteria
   A. Relief from pain.
   B. No signs of urinary obstruction (e.g., increased flank pain, decreased urine output).
   C. No recurrence of lithiasis (adheres to diet and fluid regimen).

Extracorporeal Lithotripsy

A noninvasive mechanical procedure used to break up renal calculi so they can pass spontaneously, in most cases. The trunk of the patient is submerged in water. In addition to being strapped to a frame, the patient may also be sedated, as the procedure takes 30–45 min and remaining still is important. An underwater electrode generates shock waves that fragment the stone, so it can be excreted in the urine a few days after the procedure. A degree of renal colic may occur, necessitating treatment with *antispasmodics.*

   ⋈ *Nursing measures:* encourage ambulation and promote diuresis through *forcing fluids.*

Urinary Diversion (Ileal Conduit)

Implantation of ureters into a portion of the terminal ileum, with formation of a stoma; common method for urinary diversion; also known as *Bricker's procedure.*

   I. Indications:
      A. Congenital anomalies of bladder.
      B. Neurogenic bladder.
      C. Mechanical obstruction to urine flow (e.g., bladder cancer).
      D. Severe cystitis.
      E. Trauma to lower urinary tract.
   ⋈ II. Analysis/nursing diagnosis
      A. *Altered urinary elimination* related to surgical diversion.
      B. *Risk for impaired skin integrity* related to leakage of urine.
      C. *Risk for infection* related to contamination of stoma.
      D. *Constipation* related to absence of peristalsis.
      E. *Body image disturbance* related to stoma.
   ⋈ III. Nursing care plan/implementation
      A. Preoperative care: optimal bowel and stoma site preparation.
         1. *Diet:* nonresidue several days before surgery.
         2. Medications:
            a. Neomycin.
         3. Bowel cleansing activities
            a. cathartics
            ☞ **b.** enemas

4. Site selection: appliance faceplate must bond securely; *avoid* areas where there would be pressure from clothing (waistline); usual site is right or left lower abdominal quadrant.
5. See also Preoperative Preparation, p. 111.
B. Postoperative care:
   1. Goal: *prevent complications and promote comfort.*
      a. Observe for signs of:
         ☞ **(1)** *Paralytic ileus* (common complication) —keep *nasogastric tube* patent.
         (2) *Stoma necrosis*—dusky or cyanotic color (**emergency** situation).
      ☞ **b.** Skin care: check for leakage around ostomy bag.
      c. See Postoperative Experience, p. 114.
   ⌂ **2.** Goal: **health teaching.**
      a. Self-care activities:
         ☞ **(1)** *Peristomal skin care*—prevent irritation, breakdown; proper cleansing— soap and water; adhesive remover, if needed.
         ☞ **(2)** *Appliance application and emptying*— do not remove each day, change appliance every 4–5 d or when leaking.
         (3) *Odor control*—dilute urine; *acid-ash diet;* hygiene; *avoid* asparagus, tomatoes; an increase in mucus is normal.
         (4) *Use of night drainage system* if necessary for uninterrupted sleep.
      b. Signs of *complications:* change in urine color, clarity, quantity, smell; stomal color change.
⋈ IV. Evaluation/outcome criteria
   A. Acceptance of new body image.
   B. Regains independence.
   C. Demonstrates confidence in management of self-care activities.

Prostatic Hypertrophy (Prostatism)

Malfunction of the urinary tract resulting from a lesion (benign or malignant) of the prostate gland.

   I. Pathophysiology: prostate enlarges, bulges upward, blocks flow of urine from bladder into urethra → obstruction → hydroureter, hydronephrosis.
   II. Risk factors:
      A. *Benign:*
         1. Changes in estrogen and androgen levels.
         2. Men >50 yr.
      B. *Malignant:*
         1. Genetic tendency.
         2. Hormonal factors (e.g., late puberty, greater sperm count).
         3. Diet (high fat).
         4. Exposure to chemical carcinogens (fertilizer, rubber, cadmium batteries).

▶ III. **Assessment**
  A. *Subjective data—urination:*
    1. Difficulty starting stream.
    2. Smaller, less forceful.
    3. Dribbling.
    4. Frequency.
    5. Urgency.
    6. Nocturia.
    7. Retention (incomplete emptying).
    8. Inability to void after ingestion of alcohol or exposure to cold.
  B. *Objective data:*
    1. Catheterization for residual urine: 25–50 mL after voiding.
    2. Enlarged prostate on digital rectal exam (DRE).
    3. Lab data:
      a. Urine—*increased* RBC, WBC.
      b. Blood—*increased* creatinine. Prostate Specific Antigen (PSA)—*elevated* with cancer.

▶ IV. **Analysis/nursing diagnosis:**
  A. *Urinary retention* related to incomplete emptying.
  B. *Altered urinary elimination* related to obstruction.
  C. *Urinary incontinence* related to urgency, pressure.
  D. *Anxiety* related to potential surgery.
  E. *Body image disturbance* related to threat to male identity.

▶ V. **Nursing care plan/implementation**
  A. Goal: *relieve urinary retention.*
    1. Catheterization: release maximum of 1000 mL initially; *avoid* bladder decompression, which results in hypotension, bladder spasms, ruptured blood vessels in bladder; empty 200 mL every 5 min.
    2. Patency: irrigate intermittently or continually, as ordered.
    3. *Fluids:* minimum of 2000 mL/24 h.
  B. Goal: **health teaching.**
    1. Preparation for surgery (cystostomy, prostatectomy):
      a. Expectations—indwelling catheter (will feel urge to void).
      b. *Avoid* pulling on catheter (this increases bleeding and clots).
      c. Bladder spasms common 24–48 h after surgery, particularly with transurethral resection (TUR) and suprapubic approaches.
      d. Threatening nature of procedure (possibility of impotence and/or incontinence).
    2. See also Preoperative Preparation, pp. 111–113.

Prostatectomy

Surgical procedure to relieve urinary retention and frequency caused by benign prostatic hypertrophy or cancer of the prostate.

  I. Types
  A. *Transurethral resection (TUR)*—removal of obstructive prostatic tissue surrounding urethra by an electric wire (resectoscope) introduced through the urethra; hypertrophy may recur, and TUR may need to be repeated.
  B. *Suprapubic*—low midline incision is made directly over the bladder; bladder is opened and large mass of prostatic tissue is removed through incision in urethral mucosa.
  C. *Retropubic*—removal of hypertrophied prostatic tissue high in pelvic area through a low abdominal incision; bladder is not opened.
  D. *Perineal*—removal of prostatic tissue low in pelvic area is accomplished through an incision made between the scrotum and the rectum; usually results in impotency because procedures involves nerve transection.

▶ II. **Nursing care plan/implementation**
  A. *Preoperative care:* see Prostatic Hypertrophy, pp. 192–193.
  B. *Postoperative care:*
    1. Goal: *promote optimal bladder function and comfort.*
      a. *Urinary drainage:* sterile closed-gravity system—maintain external traction as ordered.
      b. Reinforce purposes, sensations to expect.
      c. *Bladder irrigation* to control bleeding, keep clots from forming (see Three-way Foley, p. 194).
      d. *Suprapubic catheter* care (suprapubic prostatectomy)—closed-gravity drainage system; observe character, amount, flow of drainage see p. 194.
      e. *After removal:*
        (1) Observe for urinary drainage q4h for 24 h.
        (2) Skin care.
        (3) Report excessive drainage to physician.
      f. *Dressings:* keep dry, clean; reinforce if necessary (may need to change suprapubic dressing if urinary drainage); notify physician of *excessive bleeding.*
      g. Observe for signs of:
        (1) *Bladder distention*—distinct mound over pubis, slow drop in collecting bottle; irrigate catheter as ordered.
        (2) *Increased bleeding*—bright red drainage and clots; cool, clammy, pale skin; increased pulse rate.
    2. Goal: *assist in rehabilitation.* Emotional support: *fears* of incontinence, loss of male identity, impotence.
    3. Goal: **health teaching.**
      a. Expectations: mild incontinence, dribbling for a while (several months) after surgery; need to void as soon as urge is felt; *push fluids.*
      b. Exercises: perineal 1–2 d after surgery—buttocks are tightened for a count of ten, 20–50 times daily.
      c. *Avoid:*

REVIEW OF THE USE OF COMMON TUBES

Tube or Apparatus	Purpose	Examples of Use	☞ Key Points
Three-way Foley	To provide avenues for *constant irrigation and constant drainage* of the urinary bladder.	1. Transurethral resection. 2. *Bladder* infections.	1. Watch for blocking by clots—causes bladder spasms 2. Irrigant solution often has antiinfective added to normal saline or sterile water 3. Sterile water rather than normal saline may be used for lysis of clots
Suprapubic catheter	To *drain bladder* via an opening through the abdominal wall above the pubic bone.	*Suprapubic* prostatectomy.	May have orders to irrigate prn or continuously
Ureteral catheter	To *drain urine* from the pelvis of one kidney, or for *splinting* ureter.	1. *Cystoscopy* for diagnostic workups. 2. *Ureteral surgery*. 3. *Pyelotomy*.	1. *Never* clamp the tube—pelvis of kidney only holds 4–8 mL. 2. Use *only* 5 mL of sterile normal saline if ordered to irrigate.

Note: This review focuses on care of the tubes, not on total patient care.

Source: Jane Vincent Corbett, RN, MS, EdD, Professor, School of Nursing, University of San Francisco. Used with permission.

⚷ Summary of Key Points

1. Kidney infections such as pyelonephritis and glomerular nephritis, may result in kidney failure. It is therefore important to recognize patients at high risk, such as those with an untreated streptococcal infection, bowel incontinence, or history of urinary reflux.
2. A classic symptom of a kidney infection is *flank pain*.
3. *Acute* renal failure is considered *reversible. Chronic* renal failure is *irreversible*.
4. Frequently the *specific gravity* of the scanty urine output in renal failure is *low* because the kidney is unable to concentrate water. Reduced urine output resulting from dehydration will lead to an elevated urine output, indicating concentration of particles from water loss.
5. The best indicator of the status of glomerular function is the serum *creatinine* level. BUN is *increased* in renal failure, dehydration, and malnutrition.
6. Dialysis may be: permanent or temporary; stationary or ambulatory; fast or slow; intermittent or continuous;

and the access external or internal. Patient needs will be varied.
7. The effectiveness of dialysis is measured by both a *decrease* in serum creatinine and BUN, but also the *reduction in fluid retention* (1 kg = 1000 mL).
8. After a kidney transplantation the greatest concern is *rejection*, which may be immediate or take months or a year or more to develop.
9. *Pain* is usually greater after a nephrectomy than after a kidney transplantation. The pain from renal colic (renal calculi) is excruciating, requiring pain management and rest until the pain is relieved.
10. Expect *mucus* in the urine after the construction of an ileal conduit.
11. *Impotence* is expected after a perineal prostatectomy because the procedure involves nerve transection. If present after the other approaches, the cause may be psychological.

(1) Long auto trips, vigorous exercise, heavy lifting, and sexual intercourse until medical permission given, as this may increase tendency to bleed.
(2) Alcoholic beverages for 1 mo, as this may cause burning on urination.

(3) Tub baths, as this increases chance of infection.
   d. Medications: stool softeners or mild cathartics to decrease straining.
◀ **III. Evaluation/outcome criteria**
    A. Relief of symptoms.
    B. No complications (e.g., hemorrhage, impotence).

Study and Memory Aids

⟪⟫ Diagnostic Studies— Renal System

Kidney, Ureter, and Bladder X-ray
Used to determine size, shape, and position of kidneys, ureters, and bladder.

Cystogram
Installation of radiopaque medium through a catheter into the bladder; *used to* visualize bladder wall and evaluate ureterovesical valves for reflux.

Intravenous Urography (IVU) or Pyelography (IVP)
Injection of a radiopaque contrast substance, followed by fluoroscopic and x-ray films of kidneys and urinary tract; *used to* identify lesions in kidneys and ureters and provide a rough estimate of kidney function.

24-h Urine Collection
A true and accurate evaluation of kidney function, primarily glomerular filtration. Substances excreted by the kidney are excreted at different rates, amounts, and times of day or night. Timed urine collection is done for *protein, creatinine, electrolytes, urinary steroids,* etc. A large container is used, with or without preservative. Label with patient name, type of test, and exact time test starts and ends. Not usually necessary to measure urine. Have patient void, discard urine; test starts at this time. Have patient void as close to the end of the 24-h period as possible. If refrigeration is required, urine may be stored in iced container.

Renal Angiogram
Small catheter is inserted into the femoral artery and passed into the aorta or renal artery, radiopaque fluid is instilled, and serial films are taken.
1. *Used to* diagnose renal hypertension and pheochromocytoma and differentiate renal cysts from renal tumors.
2. *Postangiogram nursing actions:* check pedal pulse for signs of decreased circulation.

Cystoscopy
Visualization of bladder, urethra, and prostatic urethra by insertion of a tubular, lighted, telescopic lens (cystoscope) through the urinary meatus.
1. *Used to:* directly inspect the bladder, collect urine from the renal pelvis, obtain biopsy specimens from bladder and urethra, remove calculi, and treat lesions in the bladder, urethra, and prostate.
2. *Nursing actions following* procedure:
   a. Observe for urinary retention.
   b. Warm sitz baths to relieve discomfort.

Renal biopsy
Needle aspiration of tissue from the kidney for the purpose of microscopic examination.

Diet

Acute Renal Failure

↑ carbohydrate
↓ protein
↓ sodium
Fluid restriction

Chronic Renal Failure

Low sodium
High calcium, vitamin B complex, vitamins C and D
High iron
Avoid: foods high in potassium

Kidney Transplantation

↓ Sodium, potassium, fluids if oliguric

Drug Review

Pyelonephritis: Medications

Analgesics: Phenazopyridine (Pyridium): 200 mg tid
Antiinfectives (to control infection)
   Cephalexin (Keflex): 250–500 mg q6h
   Cephalothin (Keflin): IV, 0.5–2 g q4–6h
   Erythromycin: 250–500 mg: q6–12h
   Gentamicin (Garamycin): 3–5 mg/kg/d in divided doses q 8h
   Penicillin G: 1.2 million U in single IM dose
   Sulfamethoxazole (Gantanol DS): 1 g q8–12h; with trimethoprim (Septra)
Antipyretics
   Acetaminophen (Tylenol): 325–1000 mg q6h
   Aspirin: 325–1000 mg q4–6h, *not to exceed* 4 g/d
Urinary antiseptics

Acute Renal Failure

Sodium polystyrene sulfonate (Kayexalate): 15 g qid
Diuretics:
   Furosemide (Lasix): 20–80 mg/d
   Mannitol (Osmitrol): IV, 50–100 g as 5–10% solution

👄 Chronic Renal Failure

Electrolyte Modifiers
   Calcium carbonate
   Vitamin supplements (dose varies with symptoms):
      Water soluble: folic acid 0.4 mg to 1 mg/day;
      pyridoxine 2.5–10 mg/day ascorbic acid 45–60
      mg/day; Vitamin D supplements 0.25 mcg/day
      (if deficient)
   Aluminum hydroxide (Amphojel): 1.9–4.8 g 3–4
      times daily

Kidney Transplantation

Analgesics
   Meperidine (Demerol): 50–150 mg q 3–4 h as
      needed; IV 15–35 mg/h as a continuous infusion
   Morphine: IV 2.5–15 mg q 4h or loading dose of 15
      mg with 0.8–10 mg/h rate increased as needed;
      SC 5–20 mg q4h as needed
Corticosteroids
   Dexamethasone (Decadron): 0.5–9 mg daily in
      single on divided doses
   Prednisone (Deltasone): 5–60 mg/d
   Methylprednisolone (Medrol): 4–48 mg/d
Immunosuppresive Therapy
   Antithymocyte (ATGAM) (antilymphocyte
      globulin): 10–30 mg/kg for 14 days, then
      alternate days for total of 21 doses in 4 weeks
   Anti-T-lymphocyte monoclonal antibody (OKT$_3$): 5
      mg/day for 14 days
   Aza thioprine (Imuran): 3–5 mg/kg/day
   Cyclophosphamide (Cytoxan): 1–5 mg/kg/day
   Cyclosporine (Sandimmune): 15 mg/kg/day

Renal Calculi

Antiinfectives (to control infection)
   Cephalexin (Keflex): 250–500 mg q6h
   Cephalothin (Keflin): IV, 0.5–2 g q4–6h
   Erythromycin: 250–500 mg q6–12h
   Gentamicin (Garamycin): 3–5 mg/kg/d in divided
      doses
   Penicillin G: 1.2 million U in single IM dose
Antiemetics
   Prochlorperazine (Compazine): 5–10 mg IM—
      repeat once as needed
   Promethazine (Phenergan): 12.5–25 mg IM q4–6h
      as needed
   Trimethobenzamide (Tigan): 200 mg IM 3–4 times/d
Narcotics: Meperidine (Demerol): 50–150 mg q3–4h
   as needed; IV, 15–35 mg/h as a continuous infusion

Urinary Diversion

Neomycin (Mycifradin): 1 g q/h for 4h, then 1 gm
   q4h for 24h preoperatively to decrease incidence of
   infection.

Questions

1. During the immediate postoperative period after a
   transurethral resection of the prostate (TURP), what
   common physical problem should the nurse observe
   for?
   1. Sexual impotence.
   2. Thrombophlebitis.
   3. Venous bleeding.
   4. Atelectasis.
2. Three days after renal transplantation, a patient's urine
   output decreases to 720 mL in 24 hours. The nurse
   would respond to this by:
   1. Calling the patient's physician.
   2. Increasing the intravenous infusion rate.
   3. Checking the urine specific gravity.
   4. Checking the output hourly for 8 hours.
3. To minimize bleeding after a TURP, the most important nursing action would be to maintain:
   1. Traction on the in-dwelling catheter.
   2. Continuous irrigation of the bladder.
   3. The patient on bedrest until bleeding diminishes.
   4. The patency of the catheter drainage system.
4. The nurse would recognize which of the following as a
   complication of peritoneal dialysis?
   1. Oliguria.
   2. Pink-tinged urine.
   3. Cloudy dialysate return.
   4. Yellow dialysate drainage.
5. What characteristic urinalysis findings would the nurse
   note in a patient with glomerulonephritis?
   1. Decreased specific gravity and hematuria.
   2. Decreased specific gravity and proteinuria.
   3. Increased specific gravity and glycosuria.
   4. Increased specific gravity and proteinuria.
6. After a cystectomy and construction of an ileal conduit,
   which complication should the nurse advise the patient
   to take special precautions against?
   1. Paralytic ileus.
   2. Urinary calculi.
   3. Pyelonephritis.
   4. Mucus in the urine.
7. When the amount of peritoneal dialysate returned is
   less than that infused, the nurse should:
   1. Turn the patient from side to side gently.
   2. Apply suction to the abdominal catheter.
   3. Reduce the amount of dialysate infused during the
      next exchange.
   4. Apply gentle pressure to the abdomen to move the
      catheter tip.

8. The nurse should advise a middle-aged man that it is recommended that the prostate be examined:
   1. Once a month, when showering, after age 40.
   2. Every 3 months after age 50.
   3. During an annual physical examination after age 40.
   4. Every other year after age 50.

9. Which nursing diagnosis is a priority concern in a patient in acute renal failure?
   1. Risk for impaired skin integrity.
   2. Altered nutrition: less than body requirements.
   3. Fluid volume excess.
   4. Anxiety.

10. The nursing care plan for a patient suffering from acute renal failure should include a diet that is:
    1. High in protein and calories.
    2. Low in protein and high in calories.
    3. High in protein and low in calories.
    4. Low in protein and calories.

11. Which fruit should the nurse suggest as a snack for a patient in acute renal failure?
    1. Apricots.
    2. Apples.
    3. Nectarines.
    4. Oranges.

12. Patient teaching on the way in which continuous ambulatory peritoneal dialysis works would include the fact that:
    1. The dialysate solution is absorbed intravascularly, and waste products are excreted by the kidneys.
    2. Urine is drawn into the dialysate solution and eliminated with each exchange.
    3. Waste products move out of the blood into the dialysate solution and are drained out.
    4. The instillation of fluid into the abdomen stimulates the kidneys to concentrate waste products.

13. The nurse tells a patient undergoing continuous ambulatory peritoneal dialysis that a common side effect of the treatment is:
    1. Diarrhea.
    2. Bloody effluent.
    3. Back pain.
    4. Nausea.

14. The nurse should anticipate that, during an attack of ureteral colic stemming from a kidney stone, a patient will most likely show what change in his urine?
    1. Ketonuria.
    2. Glycosuria.
    3. Hematuria.
    4. Proteinuria.

15. Intravenous pyelography has been ordered to search for kidney stones. In preparation, the nurse must first:
    1. Weigh the patient.
    2. Determine whether the patient has any allergy to iodine.
    3. Note the last bowel movement.
    4. Record the baseline vital signs.

16. Which nursing measure is a priority for a patient with renal calculi?
    1. Monitoring for extreme variations in blood pressure.
    2. Straining the urine to obtain sediment or stone particles.
    3. Encouraging the patient to drink 3 to 4 liters of fluids daily.
    4. Record the urine output to assess kidney function.

17. Which assessment finding would be an early indication of a postoperative complication that frequently occurs after the construction of an ileal conduit?
    1. Mucus in the urinary drainage.
    2. Absent bowel sounds.
    3. Boardlike abdomen.
    4. Diminished breath sounds.

18. Which discharge teaching should the nurse question in a patient with calcium renal calculi?
    1. Limit amount of protein in the diet.
    2. Drink 3 to 4 liters of fluid daily.
    3. Void every 2 to 3 hours.
    4. Take vitamin C daily.

19. The nurse should anticipate that an infection in the kidney would most likely produce which complaint?
    1. Burning on urination.
    2. Flank or abdominal pain.
    3. Blood in the stool.
    4. Difficulty starting urinary stream.

20. Which statement regarding the usual postoperative urinary elimination would guide the nursing actions?
    1. A well-hydrated patient usually voids within 6 to 8 hours after surgery.
    2. The amount of fluids administered IV after abdominal surgery is restricted to prevent diuresis.
    3. The amount of the first voiding after surgery is usually 800 to 1000 mL.
    4. The total urinary output the day of surgery usually exceeds 3000 mL.

Answers/Rationale

1. **(3)** Venous bleeding is common for several days after a TURP. The blood is dark red, and it is also less viscous than arterial blood. Sexual dysfunction (**1**) is not an expected complication of the transurethral approach, because there would be *no physiologic* cause for impotence. The patient ambulates early after a TURP to prevent problems stemming from immobility (**2**). Atelectasis (**4**) would be more likely in a patient who receives a general anesthetic, *not* spinal anesthesia, which is used for a TURP. **AS, 8, PhI**

2. **(3)** The 24-hour volume equals 30 mL/h, the minimum hourly output, so additional data are needed to determine whether this change is due to dehydration or rejection. Calling the physician (**1**) turns the decision-

Key to Codes

Nursing process: AS, assessment; **AN,** analysis; **PL,** planning; **IMP,** implementation; **EV,** evaluation. (See Appendix M for explanation of nursing process steps.)

Category of human function: 1, protective; **2,** sensory-perceptual; **3,** comfort, rest, activity, and mobility; **4,** nutrition; **5,** growth and development; **6,** fluid-gas transport; **7,** psychosocial-cultural; **8,** elimination. (See Appendix O for explanation.)

Client need: SECE, safe, effective care environment; **PhI,** physiologic integrity; **PsI,** psychosocial integrity; **HPM,** health promotion/maintenance. (See Appendix P for explanation.)

making process over to the MD. Increasing the infusion rate (2) is *not* an *independent nursing action*. Waiting another 8 hours (4) would not be in the patient's best interests, because intervention may be needed in the meantime. **EV, 8, PhI**

3. (1) Venous bleeding is often controlled by the pressure exerted by the fluid-filled balloon of the urethral catheter. Irrigation (2) would prevent clogging of the drainage system with clots but would *not stop* the bleeding. Lengthy bedrest (3) would lead to problems stemming from immobility. Keeping the catheter drainage system patent (4) would also *not stop* the bleeding. **IMP, 8, PhI**

4. (3) Cloudy dialysate would indicate the presence of peritonitis caused by organisms that have entered the peritoneum after insertion of the dialysis catheter. Small urine volume, or oliguria (1), would indicate that renal function is compromised and is *not* a complication of the treatment. Blood in the urine (2) would indicate the existence of bladder or kidney problems. If blood were in the dialysate, this would indicate that trauma occurred during insertion of the trocar. Protein would color the dialysate yellow (4), but this is *not* a complication of peritoneal dialysis. **AS, 8, PhI**

5. (4) The urinalysis findings would reflect damage to the glomeruli with the resultant leaking of protein and red blood cells into the urine, but the kidney would still have the ability to concentrate wastes, so specific gravity would be increased. Hematuria (1) and proteinuria (2) would be found, but the specific gravity is *increased* in glomerulonephritis. Sugar in the urine, or glycosuria (3), would *not* occur in glomerulonephritis. **EV, 8, SECE**

6. (3) This urinary diversion procedure increases the risk of infection because the bladder has been removed which normally reduces the chance of organisms reaching the kidneys. There is *nothing* the patient can do *to prevent* ileus (1), which is a complication of surgery. The likelihood of kidney stones (2) forming is not greater in patients who undergo this procedure, and this is *not necessarily preventable*. The mucus in the urine (4) is *normal* and expected after the surgery. **IMP, 8, HPM**

7. (1) The tip of the catheter may lodge up against the bowel. By turning the patient, the tip of the catheter may shift and the dialysate return increase. Suction is *not* applied (2); return of the dialysate is achieved by gravity. Reducing the amount of the next exchange (3) is *not an independent nursing decision*. The use of even gentle pressure (4) may cause trauma to the bowel if the trocar is rigid. **IMP, 8, PhI**

8. (3) The prostate is examined annually during a rectal examination performed by a physician. The prostate is not examined while showering (1), and self-examination is *not possible*. Examination every 3 months (2) is *more often* than necessary. Examination every other year (4) after age 50 is *not often enough*. **IMP, 8, HPM**

9. (3) Acute renal failure is a reversible dysfunction of the kidneys; if the kidneys are not working, elimination of water, electrolytes and waste products is impaired and there would be a fluid excess. Skin problems (1)

occur in *chronic* renal failure. As electrolytes (K^+, Na^+) accumulate, there would be more, *not* less, nutrition to meet body requirements (2). Anxiety (4) is *not* specific to acute renal failure but may be due to many other patient circumstances. Changes in the patient's psychological status are seen in *chronic* renal failure as the level of metabolic wastes increases in the serum. **AN, 8, SECE**

10. (2) During the acute phase of renal failure the kidney cannot eliminate the nitrogenous waste products given off during protein metabolism, so protein intake is restricted to those proteins consisting of essential amino acids. A high-calorie intake is necessary to prevent catabolism, and the source is carbohydrates, not protein. Options 1 and 3 are incorrect because the diet should be *low* in protein. Option 4 is incorrect because the diet should be *high* in calories. The diet may also be low in sodium and potassium. **PL, 4, PhI**

11. (2) Apples are acceptable for a snack in patients in acute renal failure because they are low in potassium which is restricted in renal failure. All of the other fruits (1, 3, and 4) are high in potassium, which is restricted in renal failure. **IMP, 4, PhI**

12. (3) The peritoneal membrane acts as a semipermeable membrane. When the dialysate comes in contact with the peritoneal blood vessels, the waste substances in the blood are exchanged for the bicarbonate and acetate in the dialysate. In continuous ambulatory dialysis there is continuous exchange and better clearance of certain elements during the prolonged 4 to 8-hour dwell time. The concentration gradient between the serum and dialysate causes wastes to move *out of the serum, not* into the vascular space (1). In renal failure, the kidneys are *not* producing sufficient amounts of urine to eliminate waste (2) and to concentrate waste products.(4). **IMP, 8, SECE**

13. (3) Low back pain may develop because of the added abdominal weight from the fluid which affects posture. Appropriate exercises may help relieve the discomfort. Diarrhea (1) is a symptom of *bowel perforation*. Bloody effluent (2), although usually insignificant initially, may also be an indication of *bowel perforation*. Nausea (4) is a symptom of *peritonitis*. **IMP, 8, PhI**

14. (3) As the stone moves through the ureter, there is trauma to the ureter, with the result that the ureter becomes infected and blood appears in the urine. Ketonuria (1) and glycosuria (2) would occur in *diabetes*. Proteinuria (4) is a sign of *renal disease*. **AN, 8, PhI**

15. (2) The contrast dye used for pyelography is an iodine-based agent, and severe, even fatal, allergic reactions can occur in a patient allergic to iodine or seafood. Weight (1) is the best indicator of *fluid status;* it would be important to determine this *if* the patient had hydronephrosis stemming from obstruction. It is important to know the status of the bowel (3), but the presence of stool would *not be life-threatening;* if the bowel were full of fecal matter, visualization of the kidneys would be partially or totally obscured. Cathartics, enemas, or suppositories are used to clear the bowel and ensure good visualization. Vital signs (4) are impor-

tant, but the first action is to determine whether the patient is at any risk for anaphylaxis. **IMP, 8, SECE**

16. **(2)** It is important to collect the stone so that its composition can be determined. Dietary changes can be made on the basis of the stone's composition to minimize the formation of more stones. Blood pressure changes **(1)** are *not* expected in patients with calculi unless the obstruction leads to renal failure. Fluid intake **(3)** is very important, and 3 to 4 liters per day may be needed to produce sufficient urine to flush out the stone; however, knowing the composition of the stone is *more* important clinically. Keeping track of the urine output **(4)** is also important, but collecting the stone is *more* important from the standpoint of long-term treatment. **IMP, 8, PhI**

17. **(2)** Paralytic ileus is a frequent complication of ileal conduit construction. Resection of the bowel segment and general anesthesia inhibit peristalsis, causing bowel sounds to be absent. Mucus in the urine **(1)** is *normal,* because the urine irritates the bowel mucosa of the ileal pouch. A boardlike abdomen **(3)** would *not* be expected unless there was gastrointestinal tract bleeding. Diminished breath sounds **(4)** are a possible complication of general anesthesia and hypoventilation but are *not* directly related to the surgical procedure. **AS, 8, PhI**

18. **(4)** Vitamin C supplements increase oxalate, not calcium, excretion. If calcium phosphate stones are present, protein intake *should* be restricted **(1)**; otherwise a high-protein diet promotes calcium excretion and stone formation. Fluid intake *should be* increased regardless of the type of stone **(2)**. The patient *should,* and will need to, void every 2 to 3 hours **(3)**. An acid-ash diet is also indicated for patients with calcium stones. Such food includes meat, fish, poultry, grains, corn, cranberries, prunes, and plums. **EV, 8, SECE**

19. **(2)** Infection in the kidney causes edema and swelling, and the symptom of this is flank pain. The pain often radiates down the ureter or toward the epigastric area, causing the abdominal pain. Burning **(1)** is a symptom of a *bladder* infection. Blood in the stool **(3)** would be seen in *hemorrhoids* or *colorectal* problems; a kidney infection would most likely cause blood to be excreted in the *urine*. Difficulty starting urine flow **(4)** is a characteristic problem associated with an enlarged *prostate*. **AS, 6, PhI**

20. **(1)** Before surgery a patient is NPO; however, IV solutions administered during surgery should maintain hydration unless the patient hemorrhages during surgery. If a catheter is not inserted during the surgery, the patient should need to void within 6 to 8 hours. It is important to check for bladder distention. In addition, abdominal pain may affect the patient's ability to relax the sphincter muscles. The amount of fluids administered IV is increased, *not* decreased **(2)**, after surgery because PO intake is generally restricted. The bladder is palpable when it contains 250 mL of urine; if the patient voids 800 to 1000 mL **(3)** initially there would have been bladder distention, which should be avoided. Retention of sodium and water is common, but, diuresis does not occur until 5 to 7 days after surgery, *not* the *day* of surgery **(4)**. **AN, 1, PhI**

Endocrine Disorders

Chapter Outline

Thyroid and Parathyroid Disorders

Hyperthyroidism

(Also called *Thyrotoxicosis, Graves' disease*): spectrum of symptoms of accelerated metabolism caused by excessive amounts of circulating thyroid hormone.

I. Pathophysiology: diffuse hyperplasia of thyroid gland → overproduction of thyroid hormone and increased blood serum levels. Hormone stimulates mitochondria to increase energy for cellular activities and heat production. As metabolic rate increases, fat reserves are utilized, despite increased appetite and food intake. Cardiac output is increased to meet increased tissue metabolic needs, and peripheral vasodilation occurs in response to increased heat production. Neuromuscular hyperactivity → accentuation of reflexes, anxiety, and increased alimentary tract mobility. *Graves' disease* is caused by stimulation of the gland by immunoglobulins of the G class.

II. Risk factors:
- **A.** Possible autoimmune response resulting in increase of a gamma globulin called *long-acting thyroid stimulator* (LATS).
- **B.** Occurs in third and fourth decades.
- **C.** Affects women more than men.
- **D.** Emotional trauma, infection, increased stress.
- **E.** Overdose of medications used to treat hypothyroidism.
- **F.** Use of certain weight-loss products.

III. Assessment
- **A.** *Subjective data:*
  1. Nervousness, mood swings.
  2. Palpitations.
  3. Heat intolerance.
  4. Dyspnea.
  5. Weakness.
- **B.** *Objective data:*
  1. *Eyes:* exophthalmos, characteristic stare, lid lag.
  2. *Skin:*
     - **a.** Warm, moist, velvety.
     - **b.** Increased sweating, melanin pigmentation.
     - **c.** Pretibial edema with thickened skin and hyperpigmentation.
  3. *Weight:* loss *despite* increased appetite.
  4. *Muscle:* weakness, tremors, hyperkinesia.
  5. *Vital signs:* blood pressure (BP)—increased systolic pressure, widened pulse pressure; tachycardia.
  6. Goiter: thyroid gland noticeable and palpable.
  7. GYN: abnormal menstruation.
  8. GI: frequent bowel movements.
  9. *Activity* pattern: overactivity leads to fatigue, which leads to depression, which stimulates patient to overactivity, and pattern continues. *Danger:* total exhaustion.
  10. Lab data:
      - **a.** *Elevated:* serum thyroxine (T_4) (>11 μg/dL), free T_4 or free T_4 index, triiodothyronine (T_3) level ($>35\%$) and free T_3 level.
      - **b.** *Elevated:* thyroid uptake of radioiodine (see Diagnostic Studies Box).

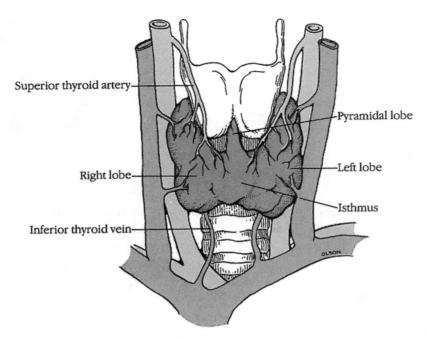

ANATOMY OF THE THYROID GLAND. (From Judge R, Zuidema G, Fitzgerald F. *Clinical Diagnosis.* Boston: Little, Brown, 1989, P. 186.)

c. *Elevated:* basal metabolic rate (BMR).
d. *Decreased:* white blood cell count (WBC) caused by decreased granulocytosis (<4500 mm³).

IV. Analysis/nursing diagnosis
A. *Altered nutrition, less than body requirements,* related to elevated BMR.
B. *Risk for injury* related to exophthalmos and tremors.
C. *Activity intolerance* related to fatigue from overactivity.
D. *Fatigue* related to overactivity.
E. *Anxiety* related to tachycardia.
F. *Sleep pattern disturbance* related to excessive amounts of circulating thyroid hormone.

V. Nursing care plan/implementation
A. Goal: *protect from stress:* private room, restrict visitors, quiet environment.
B. Goal: *promote physical and emotional equilibrium.*
   1. Environment: quiet, cool, well ventilated.
   2. Eye care:
      a. Sunglasses to protect from photophobia, dust, wind.
      b. Protective drops (methylcellulose) to soothe exposed cornea.
   3. *Diet:*
      a. High: calorie, protein, vitamin B.
      b. 6 meals/d, as needed.
      c. Weigh daily.
      d. *Avoid* stimulants (coffee, tea, colas, tobacco).
C. Goal: *prevent complications.*
   1. Medications as ordered:
      a. Propylthiouracil to *block thyroid synthesis;* hyperthyroidism returns when therapy is stopped.

b. Methimazole (Tapazole) to inhibit synthesis of thyroid hormone.
c. Iodine preparations: used in combination with above medications when hyperthyroidism not well controlled; saturated solution of potassium iodide (SSKI) or Lugol's solution; more palatable if *diluted* with water, milk, or juice; give through a *straw* to prevent staining teeth. Takes 2–4 wk before results are evident.
d. Propranolol to *relieve tachycardia, tremors, and anxiety.*

2. Monitor for *thyroid storm (crisis)*—**medical emergency:** acute episode of thyroid overactivity caused when increased amounts of thyroid hormone are released into the bloodstream and metabolism is markedly increased.

a. **Risk factors**—*thyroid storm:* patient with uncontrolled hyperthyroidism (usually *Graves' disease*) subjected to severe, sudden stress, such as:
   (1) Infection.
   (2) Surgery.
   (3) Beginning of labor.
   (4) Taking inadequate antithyroid medications before thyroidectomy.
b. **Assessment**
Subjective data
   (1) Apprehension.
   (2) Restlessness.
Objective data
   (1) Vital signs: elevated temperature (106° F), hypotension, extreme tachycardia.

(2) Marked respiratory distress, pulmonary edema.

(3) Weakness and delirium.

(4) **If untreated, patient could die of heart failure.**

c. Medications—*thyroid storm:*

(1) Propylthiouracil or methimazole (Tapazole) to decrease synthesis of thyroid hormone.

(2) Sodium iodide IV, Lugol's solution orally to *facilitate thyroid hormone synthesis.*

(3) Propranolol (Inderal) to *slow heart rate.*

(4) Aspirin to *decrease temperature.*

(5) *Steroids* to *combat crisis.*

(6) *Diuretics,* digitalis to *treat heart failure.*

D. Goal: **health teaching.**

1. Stress-reduction techniques.

2. Importance of medications, their desired and side effects.

3. Methods to protect eyes from environmental damage.

4. Signs and symptoms of thyroid storm (see p. 202).

E. Goal: *prepare for additional treatment as needed.*

1. *Radioactive iodine therapy:* ^{131}I, a radioactive isotope of iodine to decrease thyroid activity.

a. ^{131}I dissolved in water and given by mouth.

b. Hospitalization necessary only when large dose is administered.

c. Minimal precautions needed for usual dose:

(1) Sleep alone for several nights.

(2) Flush toilet several times after use.

d. Effectiveness of therapy seen in 2–3 wk; single dose controls 90% of patients.

e. Monitor for signs of hypothyroidism.

2. Surgery: see Thyroidectomy, below.

VI. Evaluation/outcome criteria

A. Complications avoided.

B. Compliance with medical regimen.

C. No further weight loss.

D. Able to obtain adequate sleep.

Thyroidectomy

Partial removal of thyroid gland (for hyperthyroidism) or total removal (for malignancy of thyroid).

I. Risk factor: unsuccessful medical treatment of hyperthyroidism.

II. Analysis/nursing diagnosis

A. *Risk for injury* related to possible trauma to parathyroid gland during surgery.

B. *Ineffective breathing pattern* related to neck incision.

C. *Pain* related to surgical incision.

D. *Altered nutrition, less than body requirements,* related to difficulty in swallowing because of neck incision.

E. *Impaired verbal communication* related to possible trauma to nerve during surgery.

F. *Risk for altered body temperature* related to thyroid storm.

III. Nursing care plan/implementation: *prepare for surgery* (see Preoperative Preparation, p. 111). *Postoperative Care:*

A. Goal: *promote physical and emotional equilibrium.*

1. *Position:* semi-Fowler's to reduce edema.

2. Immobilize head with pillows/sandbags.

3. Support head during position changes to prevent stress on sutures, flexion or hyperextension of neck.

B. Goal: *prevent complications of hypocalcemia and tetany,* due to accidental trauma to parathyroid gland during surgery; signs of tetany indicate need for *calcium gluconate IV.*

1. Check *Chvostek's sign*—tapping face in front of ear produces spasm of facial muscles.

2. Check *Trousseau's* sign—compression of upper arm (usually with BP cuff) elicits carpal (wrist) spasm.

3. Monitor for *respiratory distress* (due to laryngeal nerve injury, edema, bleeding); keep tracheostomy set/suction equipment at bedside.

4. Monitor for elevated temperature, indicative of *thyroid storm* (see objective assessment data for thyroid storm, p. 202).

5. Monitor vital signs, check dressing and beneath head, shoulders for bleeding q1h and prn for 24 h; *hemorrhage* is possible complication; if swallowing is difficult, loosen dressing. If patient still complains of tightness when dressing is loosened, look for further signs of hemorrhage.

6. Check voice postoperatively as soon as patient responsive after anesthesia and every hour (assessing for possible *laryngeal nerve damage*); crowing voice sound indicates laryngeal nerves on both sides have been injured, making *respiratory distress possible due to swelling.*

a. *Avoid* unnecessary talking to lessen hoarseness.

b. Provide alternative means of communication.

C. Goal: *promote comfort measures.*

1. *Narcotics,* as ordered.

2. Offer *iced fluids.*

3. Ambulation and *soft diet,* as tolerated.

D. Goal: **health teaching.**

1. How to support neck to prevent pressure on suture line: place both hands behind neck when moving head or coughing.

2. Signs of hypothyroidism; needs supplemental thyroid hormone if total thyroidectomy.

3. Signs and symptoms of hemorrhage and respiratory distress.

4. Importance of adequate rest and nutritious diet.

5. Importance of voice rest in early recuperative period.

IV. Evaluation/outcome criteria

A. No respiratory distress, hemorrhage, laryngeal damage, tetany.

B. Preoperative symptoms relieved.

C. Normal range of neck motion obtained.
D. States signs and symptoms of possible complications.

Hypothyroidism (*Myxedema*)

Deficiency of circulating thyroid hormone; often a final consequence of *Hashimoto's thyroiditis* and *Graves' disease*.

I. Pathophysiology: atrophy, destruction of gland by endogenous antibodies or inadequate pituitary thyrotropin production → insidious slowing of body processes, personality changes, and generalized, interstitial nonpitting (mucinous) edema—myxedema; pronounced involvement in systems with high protein turnover (e.g., cardiac, gastrointestinal [GI], reproductive, hematopoietic).

II. Risk factors:
  A. Total thyroidectomy, inadequate replacement therapy.
  B. Inheritance of autosomal recessive genes coding for disorder.
  C. Hypophyseal failure.
  D. Dietary iodine deficiencies.
  E. Irradiation of thyroid gland.
  F. Overtreatment of hyperthyroidism.

III. Assessment
  A. *Subjective data:*
    1. Weakness, fatigue, lethargy.
    2. Headache.
    3. Slowed memory, psychotic behavior.
    4. Loss of interest in sexual activity.
  B. *Objective data:*
    1. Depressed BMR.
    2. Cardiomegaly, bradycardia, hypotension, anemia.
    3. Menorrhagia, amenorrhea, infertility.
    4. Dry skin, brittle nails, coarse hair, hair loss.
    5. Slowed speech, hoarseness, thickened tongue.
    6. Weight gain: edema, generalized interstitial; peripheral nonpitting; periorbital puffiness.
    7. Intolerance to cold.
    8. Hypersensitivity to narcotics and barbiturates.
    9. Radioactive iodine uptake test: low uptake (see Diagnostic Studies at end of chapter).
    10. Lab data:
      a. *Elevated:* thyroid releasing hormone (TRH), thyroid stimulating hormone (TSH), cholesterol (>200 mg/dL), lipids (>850 mg/dL), protein (>8 g/dL).
      b. Normal—low: serum thyroxine (T_4), serum triiodothyronine (T_3).
      c. *Decreased:* radioactive iodine uptake (RAIU) (see Diagnostic Studies box).

IV. Analysis/nursing diagnosis
  A. *Risk for injury* related to hypersensitivity to drugs.
  B. *Altered nutrition, more than body requirements,* related to decreased BMR.
  C. *Activity intolerance* related to fatigue.
  D. *Constipation* related to decreased peristalsis.
  E. *Decreased cardiac output* related to hypotension and bradycardia.

F. *Risk for impaired skin integrity* related to dry skin and edema.
G. *Social isolation* related to lethargy.

V. Nursing care plan/implementation
  A. Goal: *provide for comfort and safety.*
    1. Monitor for infection or trauma; may precipitate *myxedema coma,* which is manifested by unresponsiveness, bradycardia, hypoventilation, hypothermia, hypotension.
    2. Provide warmth, prevent heat loss and vascular collapse.
    3. Administer thyroid medications as ordered: levothyroxine (Synthroid)—most common drug used; liothyronine sodium (Cytomel); dosage adjusted according to symptoms.
  B. Goal: **health teaching.**
    1. *Diet:* low calorie, high protein.
    2. Signs and symptoms of hypothyroidism and hyperthyroidism.
    3. Life-long medications, dosage, desired and side effects.
    4. Medication dosage adjustment: take ⅓–½ usual dose of narcotics and barbiturates.
    5. Stress-management techniques.
    6. Exercise program.

VI. Evaluation/outcome criteria
  A. No complications noted. Most common complications: atherosclerotic coronary heart disease, acute organic psychosis, and myxedema coma.
  B. Dietary instructions followed.
  C. Medication regimen followed.
  D. Thyroid hormone balance obtained and maintained.

Adrenal Disorders
Cushing's Disease

Overactivity of adrenal gland, leading to prolonged elevated plasma concentration of adrenal steroids.

I. Pathophysiology
  A. Excess glucocorticoid production, leading to:
    1. *Increased* gluconeogenesis → raised serum glucose levels → glucose in urine, increased fat deposits in face and trunk.
    2. *Decreased* amino acids → protein deficiencies, muscle wasting, poor antibody response, lack of collagen.

II. Risk factors
  A. Adrenal hyperplasia.
  B. Excessive hypothalamic stimulation.
  C. Tumors: adrenal, hypophyseal, pituitary, bronchogenic, gallbladder.
  D. Excessive steroid therapy.

III. Assessment
  A. *Subjective data:*
    1. Headache, backache.
    2. Weakness, decreased work capacity.
    3. Mood swings.

B. *Objective data:*
   1. Hypertension, weight gain, pitting edema.
   2. Characteristic supraclavicular fat deposits (*buffalo hump*).
   3. Pendulous abdomen, purple striae, easy bruising.
   4. Moon face, acne.
   5. Hirsutism: face, arms, legs.
   6. Hyperpigmentation.
   7. Menstrual changes.
   8. Impotence.
   9. Lab data:
      a. Urine: *elevated* 17-ketosteroids (>12 mg/24 h), glucose (>120 mg/dL).
      b. Plasma: *elevated* 17-hydroxycorticosteroids, cortisol (>10 µg/dL). Cortisol level does not decrease during the day as it should.
      c. Serum: *elevated*—glucose, red blood cells, WBC; *diminished*—potassium, chlorides, eosinophils, lymphocytes.
   10. X-rays and scans to determine tumors/metastasis (see also 8 h IV ACTH test in Diagnostic Studies Box).

IV. Analysis/nursing diagnosis
   A. *Body image disturbance* related to changes in physical appearance.
   B. *Activity intolerance* related to backache and weakness.
   C. *Risk for injury* related to infection and bleeding.
   D. *Knowledge deficit* related to management of disease.
   E. *Pain* related to headache.

V. Nursing care plan/implementation
   A. Goal: *promote comfort.*
      1. Assist with preparation for diagnostic workup.
      2. Explain procedures.
      3. Protect from trauma.
   B. Goal: *prevent complications;* monitor for:
      1. Fluid balance—intake and output (I&O), daily weights.
      2. Glucose metabolism—blood, urine for sugar and acetone.
      3. Hypertension—vital signs.
      4. Infection—skin, urinary tract; check temperature.
      5. Mood swings—observe behavior.
   C. Goal: **health teaching.**
      1. *Diet: increased* protein, potassium; *decreased* calories, sodium.
      2. Medications:
         a. *Cytotoxic* agents: aminoglutethimide (Cytadren), trilostane (*Modrastane*), mitotane (Lysodren)—decrease cortisol production.
         b. *Replacement hormones* as needed.
      3. Signs and symptoms of increased disease as noted in assessment.
      4. Preparation for adrenalectomy if medical regimen unsuccessful.

VI. Evaluation/outcome criteria
   A. Symptoms controlled by medication.
   B. No complications—adrenal steroids within normal limits.
   C. If adrenalectomy necessary, see following section.

Adrenalectomy

Surgical removal of adrenal glands because of tumors or uncontrolled overactivity; also, bilateral adrenalectomy may be performed to control metastatic breast or prostate cancer.

I. Risk factors:
   A. Pheochromocytoma.
   B. Adrenal hyperplasia.
   C. Cushing's syndrome.
   D. Metastasis of prostate or breast cancer.
   E. Adrenal cortex or medulla tumors.

II. Assessment
   A. *Objective data:* validated evidence of:
      1. Benign lesion (unilateral adrenalectomy) or malignant tumor (bilateral adrenalectomy).
      2. Adrenal hyperfunction that cannot be managed medically.
      3. Metastasis of breast.
      4. Metastasis of prostate carcinoma.

III. Analysis/nursing diagnosis
   A. *Knowledge deficit* related to planned surgery.
   B. *Risk for physical injury* related to hormone imbalance.
   C. *Risk for decreased cardiac output* related to possible hypotensive state resulting from surgery.
   D. *Risk for infection* related to decreased normal resistance.
   E. *Altered health maintenance* related to need for self-administration of steroid medications, orally or by injection.

IV. Nursing care plan/implementation
   A. Goal: **preoperative:** *reduce risk of postoperative complications.*
      1. Prescribed *steroid* therapy, given 1 wk before surgery, is gradually decreased; will be given again postoperatively.
      2. *Antihypertensive* drugs are discontinued, as surgery may result in severe hypotension.
      3. *Sedation* as ordered.
      4. General preoperative measures (see p. 111).
   B. Goal: **postoperative:** *promote hormonal balance.*
      1. Administer hydrocortisone parenteral therapy, as ordered; rate determined by fluid and electrolyte balance, blood sugar level, and blood pressure.
      2. Monitor for signs of adrenal crisis (see p. 206).
   C. Goal: *prevent postoperative complications.*
      1. Monitor vital signs until stability is regained; if on *vasopressor* drugs such as metaraminol (Aramine):
         a. Maintain flow rate as ordered.
         b. Monitor BP q5–15min, notify physician of significant elevations in BP (dose needs to be decreased) or drop in BP (dose needs to be increased). *Note:* readings that are nor-

motensive for some may be hypotensive for patients who have been hypertensive.

☞ **2.** NPO—attach nasogastric (*NG*) tube to intermittent suction; abdominal distention is common side effect of this surgery.

3. Respiratory care:

   a. Turn, cough, deep breathe.

   b. Splint flank incision when coughing.

💊 **c.** Administer *narcotics* to reduce pain and allow patient to cough; flank incision is close to diaphragm, making coughing very painful.

☞ **d.** Auscultate breath sounds q2h; decreased or absent sounds could indicate *pneumothorax.*

   e. Sudden chest pain and dyspnea should be reported *immediately,* as spontaneous pneumothorax can occur.

4. *Position:* flat or semi-Fowler's.

5. Mouth care.

☞ **6.** Monitor dressings for bleeding; reinforce prn.

7. Ambulation, as ordered.

   a. Check BP q15min when ambulation is first attempted.

☞ **b.** Place elastic stockings on lower extremities to enhance stability of vascular system.

8. Diet—as tolerated, once NG tube removed.

🏠 **D.** Goal: **health teaching.**

1. *Signs and symptoms of* **adrenal crisis:**

   a. Pulse: rapid, weak, or thready.

   b. Temperature: elevated.

   c. Severe weakness and hypotension.

   d. Headache.

   e. Convulsions, coma.

💊 **2.** Importance of adhering to *steroid* therapy schedule to ensure therapeutic serum level.

3. Weigh daily.

📟 **4.** Monitor blood glucose levels daily.

5. Report undesirable side effects of steroid therapy or adrenal crisis to physician.

6. *Avoid* persons with infections, due to decreased resistance.

7. Daily schedule: include adequate rest, moderate exercise, good nutrition.

📧 **V.** **Evaluation/outcome criteria**

A. Adrenal crisis avoided.

1. Vital signs within normal limits.

2. No neurologic deficits noted.

B. Healing progresses: no signs of infection or wound complications.

C. Adjusts to alterations in physical status.

1. Complies with medication regimen.

2. Avoids infections.

3. Incorporates good nutrition, periods of rest and activity into daily schedule.

Addison's Disease

Chronic primary adrenocorticotropic hormone (ACTH) insufficiency.

   I. Pathophysiology

A. Atrophy of adrenal gland is most common cause of adrenal insufficiency; manifested by *decreased* adrenocortical secretions.

1. Deficiency in mineralocorticoid secretion (*aldosterone*) → increased sodium excretion → dehydration → hypotension → decreased cardiac output and resulting decrease in heart size.

2. Deficiency in glucocorticoid secretion (*cortisol*) → decrease in gluconeogenesis → hypoglycemia and liver glycogen deficiency, emotional disturbances, diminished resistance to stress. Cortisol deficiency → failure to inhibit anterior pituitary secretion of ACTH and melanocyte-stimulating hormone → increased levels of ACTH and hyperpigmentation.

3. Deficiency in androgen hormone → less axillary and pubic hair in women (testes supply adequate sex hormone in men, so no symptoms are produced).

   II. Risk factors:

A. Autoimmune processes.

B. Infection.

C. Malignancy.

D. Vascular obstruction.

E. Bleeding.

F. Environmental hazards.

G. Congenital defects.

H. Bilateral adrenalectomy.

📧 **III.** **Assessment**

A. *Subjective data:*

1. Muscle weakness, fatigue, lethargy.

2. Dizziness, fainting.

3. Nausea, food idiosyncrasies, anorexia.

4. Abdominal pain, cramps.

B. *Objective data:*

1. *Vital signs:* decreased BP, orthostatic hypotension, widened pulse pressure.

2. *Pulse*—increased, collapsing, irregular.

3. *Temperature*—subnormal.

4. *GI:* vomiting, diarrhea.

5. Tremors.

6. Skin: poor turgor, excessive pigmentation (bronze tone).

7. Lab data:

   a. Blood: *decreased:* sodium (<135 mEq/L); glucose (<60 mg/dL), chloride (<98 mEq/L), bicarbonate (<23 mEq/L). *Increased:* hematocrit, potassium (>5 mEq/L).

   b. Urine: *decreased* (or absent) 17-ketosteroids (<5 mg/24 h), 17-hydroxycorticosteroids (<2 mg/24 h).

8. See also Diagnostic Studies Box, p. 207.

📧 **IV.** **Analysis/nursing diagnosis**

A. *Fluid volume deficit* related to decreased sodium level.

B. *Altered renal tissue perfusion* related to hypotension.

C. *Decreased cardiac output* related to aldosterone deficiency.

D. *Risk for infection* related to cortisol deficiency.

E. *Activity intolerance* related to muscle weakness and fatigue.

F. *Altered nutrition, less than body requirements,* related to nausea, anorexia, and vomiting.

V. Nursing care plan/implementation

   A. Goal: *decrease stress.*

      1. Environment: quiet, nondemanding schedule.

      2. Anticipate events where extra resources will be necessary.

   B. Goal: *promote adequate nutrition.*

      1. *Diet: acute phase*—high sodium, low potassium; *nonacute phase*—increased carbohydrates and protein.

      2. *Fluids:* force, to balance fluid losses; monitor I&O, daily weights.

      3. Administer life-long exogenous replacement therapy as ordered.

         a. *Glucocorticoids*—prednisone, hydrocortisone.

         b. *Mineralocorticoids*—fludrocortisone (Florinef).

   C. Goal: **health teaching.**

      1. Take medications *with* food or milk.

      2. May need *antacid* therapy to prevent GI disturbances.

      3. Side effects of steroid therapy.

      4. *Avoid* stress, may need adjustment in medication dosage when stress is increased.

      5. Signs and symptoms of *adrenal (addisonian) crisis:* very serious condition characterized by: severe hypotension, shock, coma, and vasomotor collapse related to strenuous activity, infection, stress, omission of prescribed medications. **If untreated, could quickly lead to death.**

   D. Goal: *prevent serious complications if addisonian crisis evident.*

      1. Complete bed rest, *avoid* stimuli.

      2. High dose of hydrocortisone IV or cortisone IM.

   3. Treat shock—IV saline.

   4. I&O, vital signs q15min to 1 h or prn until crisis passes.

VI. Evaluation/outcome criteria

   A. No complications occur.

   B. Medication regimen followed, is adequate for patient's needs.

   C. Adequate nutrition and fluid balance obtained.

Diagnostic Studies

Radioactive Iodine Uptake Test (^{131}I Uptake)—ingestion of a tracer dose of ^{131}I, followed in 24 h by a scan of the thyroid for amount of radioactivity emitted.

   1. *High* uptake indicates hyperthyroidism.

   2. *Low* uptake indicates hypothyroidism.

Eight-hour Intravenous ACTH Test—administration of 25 U of ACTH in 500 mL of saline over an 8-h period.

   1. *Used to* determine function of adrenal cortex.

   2. 24-h urine specimens are collected, before and after administration, for measurement of 17-ketosteroids and 17-hydroxycorticosteroids.

   3. In *Addison's disease,* urinary output of steroids does *not increase* after administration of ACTH; *normally* steroid excretion *increases three- to fivefold* after ACTH stimulation.

   4. In *Cushing's syndrome,* hyperactivity of the adrenal cortex *increases* the urine output of steroids tenfold in the second urine specimen.

Summary of Key Points

1. In hyperthyroidism the body responses and systems are *accelerated,* resulting in: tachycardia, agitation, muscle tremors, diarrhea, and fever. In hypothyroidism the same responses and systems are *depressed,* resulting in: bradycardia, sluggishness, and sensitivity to cold.

2. Drug doses may need to be *increased* in hyperthyroidism and *reduced* in hypothyroidism.

3. After complete or partial removal of the thyroid gland, observing for *airway obstruction* is a priority.

4. Note signs of *tetany (carpopedal spasm),* indicating injury to or accidental removal of the parathyroid glands.

5. Cushing's disease involves an excess of sugar (increased glucose), salt (increased sodium), and sex hormones (increased androgens). These changes adversely affect body image, with weight gain and abnormal hair distribution resulting.

6. The signs and symptoms of Cushing's disease are the *same* regardless of whether it is caused by *hyperadrenalism* or *steroid therapy.*

7. The greatest concern in a patient with Addison's disease is the occurrence of a *crisis,* causing severe *hypovolemic shock* and *vascular collapse.*

💡 Study and Memory Aids

Diet

Cushing's Syndrome: Signs—"3 S's"

Sugar (hyperglycemia)
Salt (hypernatremia)
Sex (excess androgens)

Addison's Disease

Acute: ↑ sodium
↓ potassium
Non acute: ↑ carbohydrate
↓ protein

Hyperthyroidism

↑ Calorie
  Protein
  Vitamin B
Avoid stimulants: no coffee, tea, chocolate, cola; no
  tobacco

Drug Review

Hyperthyroidism

Methimazole (Tapazole): 15–60 mg/d for 6–8 wk;
  maintenance dose, 15–30 mg/d in single or divided
  doses
Potassium iodide (SSKI): 250 mg (5 drops) tid. **Mix
  with fruit juice.** Used for 10 days before
  thyroidectomy.
Propylthiouracil: 50–600 mg/d in single or divided
  doses
Strong iodine solution (Lugol's solution): 0.1–0.3 mL
  tid. Used for 10 days before thyroidectomy.

Thyroid Storm Crisis

Antipyretic:
  Aspirin: 325–1000 mg q4–6h, *not* to exceed 4 g/d
Antiarrhythmic:
  Digoxin (Lanoxin): 0.6–1 mg IV in divided doses
    over 24 hours; maintenance dose, Rapid loading
    dose, 150 μg/d.
  Propranolol (Inderal): 1–3 mg; IV repeat in 2 min if
    needed
Diuretics:
  Furosemide (Lasix): 20–80 mg/d
  Mannitol (Osmitrol): IV, 50–100 g as 5%–25%
    solution

Antithyroid:

Methimazole (Tapazole): 15–60 mg/d for 6–8 wk;
  maintenance dose, 15–30 mg/d in single or divided
  doses
Propylthiouracil: 50–600 mg/d in single or divided
  doses
Strong iodine solution (Lugol's solution): 0.1–0.3 mL
  tid. Used for 10 days before thyroidectomy
Steroids (should never be abruptly discontinued;
  gradually taper dose to prevent complications)
  Dexamethasone (Decadron): 0.5–9 mg/d in single
    or divided doses
  Prednisone: 5–60 mg/d
  Methylprednisolone (Medrol): 4–48 mg/d

Thyroidectomy

Potassium iodide (SSKI): 250 mg (5 drops) tid. **Mix
  with fruit juice.** Used for 10 days before
  thyroidectomy.
Strong iodine solution (Lugol's solution): 0.1–0.3 mL
  tid. Used for 10 days before thyroidectomy

Hypothyroidism

Levothyroxine (Synthroid): 0.05 mg/d. Increase by
  0.025 mg q 2–3 weeks; maintenance dose 0.1–0.2
  mg/d
Liothyronine (Cytomel): 25 μg/d; increase by 12.5–25
  μg/d at 1 to 2-wk intervals; usual maintenance dose,
  25–50 μg/d

Cushing's Disease

Aminoglutethimide (Cytadren): 250 mg q6h increased
  by 250 mg/d at 1- to 2-wk intervals up to daily total
  of 2 g
Mitotane (o, p'-DDD, Lysodren): 3–6 g/d in 3–4
  divided doses, decreased to maintenance dose of
  500 mg twice weekly (half-life, 18–159 d)

Adrenalectomy

Steroids (should *never* be abruptly discontinued;
  gradually taper dose to prevent complications)
  Dexamethasone (Decadron): 0.5–9 mg/d in single
    or divided doses
  Hydrocortisone: Solu-Cortef—10–320 mg/d in
    divided doses; IM, IV, 100–500 mg
    q2–6 h (succinate)
  Methylprednisolone (Medrol): 4–48 mg/d
  Prednisone: 5–60 mg/d
Tranquilizers
  Chlordiazepoxide HCl (Librium): 5–25 mg 3–4
    times daily
  Diazepam (Valium): 2–10 mg 2–4 times daily
  Phenobarbital: 30–120 mg/d in divided doses

Addison's Disease

Antiulcer therapy
    Aluminum hydroxide gel (Amphojel): 5–10 mL
       q2–4h or 1 h pc
    Calcium carbonate (Titralac): 1–2 g with water pc
       and hs
    Magnesium and aluminum hydroxides (Maalox
       suspension): 5–30 mL pc and hs
    Sucralfate (Carafate): 1 g qid
Glucocorticoids
    Short acting
       Cortisone (Cortone): 20–300 mg/d
       Hydrocortisone (Solu-Cortef): 10–320 mg/d in
         divided doses; succinate—IM, IV, 100–500
         mg q2–6h (succinate)
    Intermediate acting
       Prednisolone (Deltasone): 5–60 mg in single or
         divided doses
       Methylprednisolone (Medrol): 4–48 mg/d in
         single or divided doses
    Long acting
       Betamethasone (Valisone): 0.6–7.2 mg/d
       Dexamethasone (Decadron): 0.5–9 mg/d in
         single or divided doses
Mineralocorticoids: Fludrocortisone (Florinef):
    100 μg/d (range, 100 μg 3 times weekly to 200
    μg/d)
Note: **Steroids** should *never* be abruptly
discontinued; gradually taper dose to prevent
complications.

Questions

1. The nurse would counsel a patient taking cortisone to observe a diet:
   1. High in protein, calcium, and potassium.
   2. High in carbohydrates and low in sodium.
   3. Low in sodium, calcium, and carbohydrates.
   4. Low in protein, potassium, and sodium.
2. Which of the following are signs and symptoms of hyperthyroidism?
   1. Nervousness and weight loss.
   2. Lethargy and slow pulse.
   3. Weight gain and diaphoresis.
   4. Slow pulse and increased appetite.
3. The nurse tells a patient that the most appropriate diet to follow the week before surgery to remove a suspected thyroid tumor is one that is:
   1. Increased in carbohydrates and protein.
   2. Decreased in carbohydrates and increased in protein.
   3. Decreased in fat and protein.
   4. Increased in fat and decreased in protein.
4. To assess for laryngeal nerve damage after a thyroidectomy, the nurse would observe the patient for:
   1. Dyspnea, intercostal muscle retraction, and stridor.
   2. Difficulty swallowing, deviated uvula, and hoarseness.
   3. Stridor, difficulty swallowing, and cough.
   4. Dysphagia, weakened voice, and wheezing.

Answers/Rationale

1. **(1)** Corticosteroids, such as cortisone, have a catabolic effect on protein, resulting in a negative nitrogen balance, so protein is needed to compensate for this loss. Aldosterone secretion is also stimulated, leading to sodium retention and potassium loss, and thus making added potassium intake important. Cortisone also decreases the intestinal transport of calcium and promotes calcium loss through the kidneys, and so extra calcium is needed in the diet to make up for the loss. The diet should be *low* in carbohydrates **(2).** As already noted, calcium **(3)** as well as protein and potassium **(4)** intake should be *increased.* The sodium intake, however, should be *decreased* to compensate for the sodium retained. **PL, 4, PhI**
2. **(1)** Hyperthyroidism, or Graves' disease, results from an overproduction of thyroid-stimulating hormone. This causes the metabolic rate of the patient to be accelerated, leading to: agitation, weight loss, heat intolerance, tachycardia, exophthalmos, goiter, diaphoresis, increased appetite, and diarrhea. Lethargy **(2)** and slow pulse **(2 and 4)** would be seen in *hypothy*roidism. Weight gain **(3)** is also a symptom of *hypo*thyroidism. **AS, 3, PhI**
3. **(1)** Because of the increased metabolism in such a patient, the caloric and protein intake would need to be high to prevent catabolism (a negative nitrogen balance) before surgery. The carbohydrate **(2)** and protein **(3 and 4)** intake should both be *increased.* **PL, 4, PhI**
4. **(4)** Thyroidectomy is the most common cause of laryngeal nerve damage because of the proximity of the gland and the nerve. The primary symptom is hoarseness or a weakened voice. There may also be temporary dysphagia, or difficulty swallowing, and if both vocal cords are involved, there would be airway compromise (wheezing). The problems listed in option **(1)** may occur if the person is active but would *not* be seen in the *early* postoperative period. A deviated uvula **(2)** would be seen in a patient with *glossopharyngeal* nerve damage. A cough **(3)** is *not* characteristic. **AS, 3, PhI**

Key to Codes

Nursing process: AS, assessment; **AN,** analysis; **PL,** planning; **IMP,** implementation; **EV,** evaluation. (See Appendix M for explanation of nursing process steps.)

Category of human function: 1, protective; **2,** sensory-perceptual; **3,** comfort, rest, activity, and mobility; **4,** nutrition; **5,** growth and development; **6,** fluid-gas transport; **7,** psychosocial-cultural; **8,** elimination. (See Appendix O for explanation.)

Client need: SECE, safe, effective care environment; **PhI,** physiologic integrity; **PsI,** psychosocial integrity; **HPM,** health promotion/maintenance. (See Appendix P for explanation.)

Sensory Disorders

Chapter Outline

- Ear Disorders
  - Meniere's Disease
  - Otosclerosis
  - Stapedectomy
  - Deafness
- Eye Disorders
  - Glaucoma (acute and chronic)
    - Acute (closed angle)
    - Chronic (open angle)
  - Cataract

- Cataract removal
  - Retinal Detachment
  - Blindness
- Diagnostic Studies
- Summary of Key Points
- Study and Memory Aids
  - Diets
  - Drug Review
- Questions
- Answers/Rationale

Ear Disorders

Meniere's Disease

Chronic, recurrent disorder of inner ear; attacks of vertigo, tinnitus, and vestibular dysfunction; lasts 30 min to full day; usually no pain or loss of consciousness.

I. Pathophysiology: associated with excessive dilatation of cochlear duct (unilateral) resulting from overproduction or decreased absorption of endolymph → progressive sensorineural hearing loss.

II. Risk factors:
  A. Emotional or endocrine disturbance (diabetes mellitus).
  B. Spasms of internal auditory artery.
  C. Head trauma.
  D. Allergic reaction.
  E. High salt intake.
  F. Smoking.
  G. Ear infections.

III. Assessment
  A. *Subjective data:*
    1. Tinnitus.
    2. Headache.
    3. True vertigo: sudden attacks, room appears to spin.
    4. Depression, irritability, withdrawal.
    5. Nausea on sudden head motion.
  B. *Objective data:*
    1. Impaired hearing, especially *low* tones.
    2. Change in gait, lack of coordination.

3. Vomiting with sudden head motion.
    4. Nystagmus—during attacks.
    5. Diagnostic test: *caloric* (cold water in ear canal)—may precipitate attack; audiometry—loss of hearing (See Diagnostic Studies box).

IV. Analysis/nursing diagnosis
  A. *Risk for injury* related to vertigo, lack of coordination.
  B. *Auditory sensory/perceptual alteration* related to progressive hearing loss.
  C. *Anxiety* related to uncertainty about treatment.
  D. *Risk for activity intolerance* related to sudden onset of vertigo.
  E. *Sleep pattern disturbance* related to tinnitus.
  F. *Ineffective individual coping* related to chronic disorder.

V. Nursing care plan/implementation
  A. Goal: *provide safety and comfort during attacks.*
    1. Activity: *bed rest* during attack, siderails up; lower to chair or floor if attack occurs while standing; assist with ambulation (sudden dizziness common).
    2. *Position:* recumbent, affected ear uppermost usually.
    3. Identify prodromal symptoms (aura, ear pressure, increased tinnitus).
    4. Call bell within reach.
  B. Goal: *minimize occurrence of attacks.*
    1. Give medications as ordered:
      a. *Diuretics* (chlorothiazide [Diuril], acetazolamide [Diamox]) to decrease endolymphatic fluids.

211

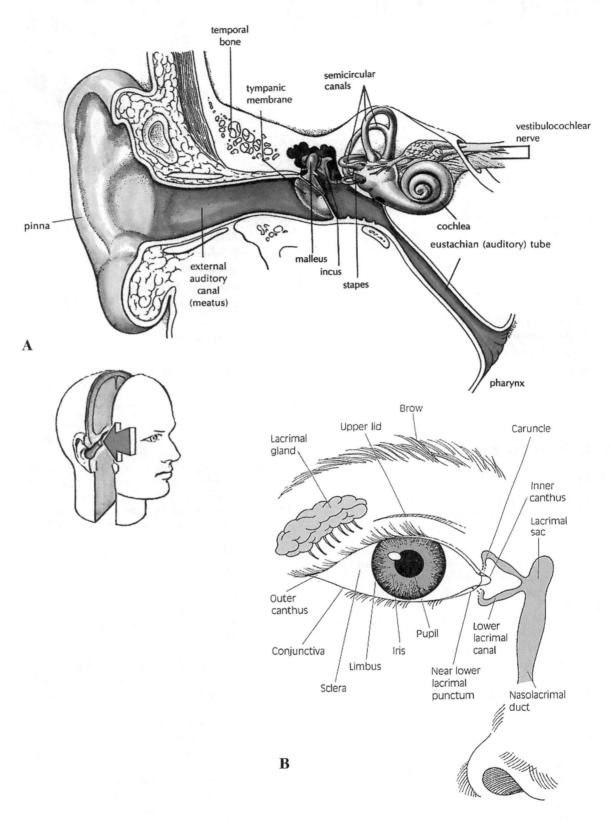

(A) THE EAR, SHOWING THE EXTERNAL, MIDDLE, AND INTERNAL SUBDIVISIONS.
(Adapted from Chaffee EE, Lytle IM: Basic Physiology and Anatomy, 4th ed, p. 227.
Philadelphia, JB Lippincott, 1980.) **(B) STRUCTURES OF THE EXTERNAL EYE AND
POSITION OF THE INTERNAL LACRIMAL STRUCTURES.**

b. *Antihistamines* (dimenhydrinate [Drama-mine], diphenhydramine HCl [Benadryl]) to inhibit tissue edema.

c. *Vasodilators* (nicotinic acid) to control vasospasms.

d. *Antiemetics and antivertigo agents* (diazepam [Valium], meclizine HCl [Antivert]).

2. *Diet:* low sodium, limited fluids to reduce endolymphatic pressure.

3. *Avoid* precipitating stimuli: bright, glaring lights; noise; sudden jarring; turning head or eyes (stand in front of patient when talking).

C. Goal: *health teaching.*

1. No smoking (causes vasospasm) or alcoholic beverages (fluid retention, contraindicated with medications).

2. Management of symptoms: play radio to mask tinnitus, particularly at night.

3. Keep medication available at all times.

4. Prepare for surgery if indicated (*labyrinthectomy* if hearing is gone or *endolymphatic sac decompression* to preserve hearing).

VI. Evaluation/outcome criteria

A. Decreased frequency of attacks.

B. Complies with treatment regimen and restrictions (e.g., low-sodium diet, no smoking).

C. Hearing preserved.

Otosclerosis

Insidious, progressive deafness; most common cause of conductive deafness; cause unknown.

I. Pathophysiology: formation of new spongy bone in labyrinth → fixation of stapes → prevention of sound transmission through ossicles to inner ear fluids.

II. Risk factors:

A. Heredity.

B. Females, puberty to 45 yr.

III. Assessment

A. *Subjective data:*

1. Tinnitus.

2. Difficulty hearing—gradual loss in both ears.

B. *Objective data*—diagnostic tests:

1. *Rinne* (tuning fork placed over mastoid bone)—reduced sound conduction by air and intensified by bone.

2. *Weber* (tuning fork placed on top of head)—increased sound conduction to affected ear.

3. *Audiometry*—diminished hearing.

IV. Analysis/nursing diagnosis

A. *Auditory sensory/perceptual alteration* related to hearing loss.

B. *Body image disturbance* related to hearing aid.

C. *Ineffective individual coping* related to grief reaction to loss.

D. *Impaired social interaction* related to hearing loss.

V. Nursing care plan/implementation, evaluation/ outcome criteria: see Stapedectomy, following.

Stapedectomy

Removal of the stapes and replacement with a prosthesis (steel wire, Teflon piston, or polyethylene); treatment for deafness due to otosclerosis, which fixes the stapes, preventing it from oscillating and transmitting vibrations to the fluids in the inner ear.

I. Analysis/nursing diagnosis

A. *Sensory/perceptual alteration* related to edema and ear packing.

B. See Perioperative Experience, p. 111, for diagnoses relating to surgery.

II. Nursing care plan/implementation

A. Preoperative care: health teaching.

1. Important postoperatively to keep head in position ordered by physician.

2. *Avoid:* sneezing, blowing nose, vomiting, coughing—all of which increase pressure in eustachian tubes.

3. Breathing exercises.

B. Postoperative care:

1. Goal: *promote physical and psychological equilibrium.*

a. *Position:* as ordered by physician—varies according to preference; side-rails up, as vertigo is common.

b. Activity: assist with ambulation; *avoid* rapid turning, which might increase vertigo.

c. Dressings: check frequently; may change cotton pledget in outer ear.

d. Give medications as ordered:

(1) *Antiemetics.*

(2) *Analgesics.*

(3) *Antibiotics.*

e. Reassurance: reduction in hearing is normal, hearing may *not* immediately improve after surgery.

2. Goal: **health teaching.**

a. Ear care: keep covered outdoors; keep outer ear plug clean, dry, and changed.

b. *Avoid:*

(1) Washing hair for 2 wk.

(2) Swimming for 6 wk.

(3) Air travel for 6 mo.

(4) People with upper respiratory tract infections.

(5) Heavy lifting or straining.

III. Evaluation/outcome criteria

A. Hearing improves—evaluate 1 mo postoperatively (may require hearing aid).

B. Returns to work (usually 2 wk after surgery).

C. Continues medical supervision.

Deafness

(1) *Hard of hearing*—slight or moderate hearing loss that is serviceable for performing activities of daily living. (2) *Deaf*—hearing is nonfunctional for carrying out activities of daily living.

I. Risk factors:

A. *Conductive* hearing losses (transmission deafness):
   1. Impacted cerumen (wax).
   2. Foreign body in external auditory canal.
   3. Defects (thickening, scarring) of eardrum.
   4. Otosclerosis of ossicles.

B. *Sensorineural* hearing losses (perceptive or nerve deafness):
   1. Arteriosclerosis.
   2. Infectious diseases (mumps, measles, meningitis).
   3. Drug toxicities (quinine, streptomycin, neomycin sulfate).
   4. Tumors.
   5. Head trauma.
   6. High-intensity noises.

II. Assessment—*objective data:*
   A. Inattentive or strained facial expression.
   B. Excessive loudness or softness of speech.
   C. Frequent need to clarify content of conversation or inappropriate responses.
   D. Tilting of head while listening.
   E. Lack of response when others speak.

III. Analysis/nursing diagnosis
   A. *Auditory sensory/perceptual alteration* related to loss of hearing.
   B. *Impaired social interaction* related to deafness.

IV. Nursing care plan/implementation
   A. Goal: *maximize hearing ability and provide emotional support.*
      1. Gain person's attention before speaking, *avoid* startling.
      2. Provide adequate lighting so person can see you when you are speaking.
      3. Look at the person when speaking.
      4. Use nonverbal cues to enhance communication, e.g., writing, hand gestures, pointing.
      5. Speak slowly, distinctly; do *not* shout (excessive loudness distorts voice).
      6. If person does not understand, use different words; write it down.
      7. Use alternative communication system:
         a. Speech (lip) reading.
         b. Sign language.
         c. Hearing aid.
         d. Paper and pencil.
         e. Flash cards.
      8. Supportive, nonstressful environment.
   B. Goal: **health teaching.**
      1. Prepare for evaluative studies—audiogram.
      2. Appropriate community resources: National Association of Hearing and Speech Agencies for *counseling* services; National Association for the Deaf to assist with *employment, education, legislation;* Alexander Graham Bell Association for the Deaf, Inc., serves as *information* center for those working with the deaf; American Hearing Society provides educational information, employment services, *social clubs.*
      3. Use of hearing aid: care, testing, carry spare battery at all times. (See Table 19.1 for care of hearing aid.)

TABLE 19.1   ☞ CARE OF A HEARING AID

Clean earmold as often as needed. Warm water and mild soap may be used, or wipe nightly with alcohol. Use a pipe cleaner to remove wax. Dry earmold completely before connecting to hearing aid.

Keep the hearing aid dry. Do *not* wear in the shower or at the hairdresser. Aid may not work as well in hot, humid climate because of moisture in ear or hearing aid.

Turn hearing aid off at night or when not in use. Keep spare batteries. Batteries may be removed completely at night.

Store away from pets. Dogs and cats like the smell of ear wax and will chew or roll on hearing aid.

Leave the aid in the same place every night.

If the aid does not work: check on-off switch, inspect for wax, examine battery for correct insertion, replace batteries (may only last a few days or a few weeks), check for correct placement of earmold.

---

      4. Safety precautions: when crossing street, driving.

V. Evaluation/outcome criteria
   A. Method of communication established.
   B. Achieves independence (use of Dogs for Deaf, special telephones, visual signals).
   C. Copes with life-style changes (minimal depression, anger, hostility).

Eye Disorders

Glaucoma (Acute and Chronic)

Increased intraocular pressure; affects 2% of population >40 yr.

I. Pathophysiology
   A. *Acute (closed-angle)*—impaired passage of aqueous humor into the circular canal of Schlemm due to closure of the angle between the cornea and the iris. **Medical emergency;** *requires surgery.*
   B. *Chronic (open-angle)*—local obstruction of aqueous humor between the anterior chamber and the canal. *Most common; treated with medication* (miotics, carbonic anhydrase inhibitors).
   C. Untreated: imbalance between rate of secretion of intraocular fluids and rate of absorption of aqueous humor → increased intraocular pressures → decreased peripheral vision → corneal edema → halos and blurring of vision → blindness.

II. Risk factors—unknown, but associated with:
   A. Emotional disturbances.
   B. Hereditary factors.
   C. Allergies.
   D. Vasomotor disturbances.

III. Assessment

    A. *Subjective data:*

        1. *Acute* (closed-angle):

            a. Pain: severe, in and around eyes.

            b. Headache.

            c. Rainbow halos around lights.

            d. Blurring of vision.

            e. Nausea, vomiting.

        2. *Chronic* (open-angle):

            a. Eyes tire easily.

            b. Loss of peripheral vision.

    B. *Objective data:*

        1. Corneal edema.

        2. Decreased peripheral vision.

        3. Increased cupping of optic disc.

        4. Tonometry—pressures >22 mm Hg.

        5. Pupils: dilated.

        6. Redness of eye.

IV. Analysis/nursing diagnosis

    A. *Visual sensory/perceptual alterations* related to increased intraocular pressure.

    B. *Pain* related to sudden increase in intraocular pressure.

    C. *Risk for injury* related to blindness.

    D. *Impaired physical mobility* related to impaired vision.

V. Nursing care plan/implementation

    A. Goal: *reduce intraocular pressure.*

        1. Activity: bed rest.

        2. *Position:* semi-Fowler's.

        3. Medications as ordered:

            a. *Miotics* (pilocarpine, carbachol).

            b. *Carbonic anhydrase inhibitors* (acetazolamide [Diamox]).

            c. *Anticholinesterase* (demecarium bromide [Humorsol]) to facilitate outflow of aqueous humor.

            d. *Ophthalmic* (timolol) to decrease intraocular pressure.

    B. Goal: *provide emotional support.*

        1. Place personal objects within field of vision.

        2. Assist with activities.

        3. Encourage verbalization of concerns, fears of blindness, loss of independence.

    C. Goal: **health teaching.**

        1. *Prevent* increased intraocular pressure by *avoiding:*

            a. Anger, excitement, worry.

            b. Constrictive clothing.

            c. Heavy lifting.

            d. Excessive *fluid* intake.

            e. Atropine or other mydriatics, which cause dilation.

            f. Straining at stool.

            g. Eye strain.

        2. Relaxation techniques; stress-management techniques, if indicated.

        3. Prepare for surgical intervention, if ordered: *laser trabeculoplasty, trabeculectomy* (filtering).

        4. Medications: purpose, dosage, frequency; eyedrop installation; have extra bottle in case of breakage or loss.

        5. Activity: moderate exercise—walking.

        6. Safety measures: eye protection (shield or glasses); MedicAlert band or tag; *avoid* driving 1–2 h after instilling miotics.

        7. Community resources as necessary.

VI. Evaluation/outcome criteria

    A. Eyesight preserved if possible.

    B. Intraocular pressure lowered (<22 mm Hg).

    C. Continues medical supervision for life—reports reappearance of symptoms immediately.

Cataract

Developmental or degenerative opacification of the crystalline lens.

    I. General

        A. **Risk factors:**

            1. Aging (most common).

            2. Trauma.

            3. Toxins.

            4. Congenital defect.

         B. **Assessment**

            1. *Subjective data*—vision: blurring, loss of acuity (see best in low-lit conditions); distortion; diplopia; photophobia.

            2. *Objective data:*

                 a. Blindness: unilateral or bilateral (particularly in congenital cataracts).

                 b. Loss of red reflex, gray opacity of lens.

        C. **Analysis/nursing diagnosis**

            1. *Visual sensory/perceptual alterations* related to opacity of lens.

            2. *Risk for injury* related to accidents.

            3. *Social isolation* related to impaired vision.

    II. **Cataract removal:** removal of opacified lens because of loss of vision; extracapsular cataract extraction followed by intraocular lens (IOL) insertion is procedure of choice.

        A. **Nursing care plan/implementation**

            1. **Preoperative care:**

                 a. Goal: *prepare for surgery. Antibiotic* drops or ointment, *mydriatic* eyedrops as ordered; note dilatation of pupils; *avoid* glaring lights; usually done under local anesthesia with sedation.

                 b. Goal: **health teaching.** Postoperative expectations: do *not* rub, touch, or squeeze eyes shut after surgery; eye patches will be on; assistance will be given for needs; overnight hospitalization not required unless complications occur; mild iritis usually occurs.

            2. **Postoperative care:**

                 a. Goal: *reduce stress on the sutures and prevent hemorrhage.*

                    (1) Activity: ambulate as ordered, usually soon after surgery; generally discharged 5–6 h after surgery.

                    (2) *Position:* flat or low Fowler's; on back or turn to *nonoperative* side, as turning to operative side increases pressure.

(3) *Avoid* activities that increase intraocular pressure: straining at stool, vomiting, coughing, brushing teeth, brushing hair, shaving, lifting objects over 20 lb, *bending,* or *stooping;* wear glasses or shaded lens during day, eyeshield at night.

(4) Provide: mouthwash, hair care, personal items within easy reach, "step-in" slippers.

b. Goal: *promote psychological well-being.* With elderly, frequent contacts to prevent sensory deprivation.

c. Goal: **health teaching.**

(1) If prescriptive glasses are used (*aphakic glasses*), explain about magnification, perceptual distortion, blind areas in peripheral vision; guide through activities with glasses; need to look through central portion of lens and turn head to side when looking to the side to decrease distortion.

(2) Eye care: *instillation of eyedrops* (mydriatics and carbonic anhydrase inhibitors to prevent glaucoma and adhesions if IOL not inserted; with IOL steroid-antibiotic used); eye shield at night to prevent injury for 1 mo.

(3) Signs/symptoms of: *infection* (redness, pain, edema, drainage); *iris prolapse* (bulging or pear-shaped pupil); *hemorrhage* (sharp eye pain, half-moon of blood).

(4) *Avoid:* heavy lifting, potential eye trauma.

B. Evaluation/outcome criteria
1. Vision restored.
2. No complications (e.g., severe eye pain, hemorrhage).
3. Performs self-care activities (e.g., instills eyedrops).
4. Returns for follow-up ophthalmology care—recognizes symptoms requiring immediate attention.

Retinal Detachment

Separation of retina from choroid.

I. Risk factors
   A. Trauma.
   B. Degeneration.
II. Assessment
   A. *Subjective data:*
      1. Flashes of light before eyes.
      2. Vision: blurred, sooty (sudden onset); sensation of floating particles; blank areas of vision.
   B. *Objective data*—ophthalmic exam: retina is grayish in area of tear; bright red, horseshoe-shaped tear.
III. Analysis/nursing diagnosis
   A. *Visual sensory/perceptual alteration* related to blurred vision.
   B. *Anxiety* related to potential loss of vision.

C. *Risk for injury* related to blindness.
IV. Nursing care plan/implementation
   A. Preoperative care:
      1. Goal: *reduce anxiety and prevent further detachment.*
         a. Encourage verbalization of feelings, answer all questions, reinforce physician's explanation of surgical procedures.
         b. Activity: *bed rest,* eyes usually covered to promote rest and maintain normal position of retina, siderails up.
         c. *Position:* according to location of retinal tear: involved area of eye should be in a *dependent* position.
         d. Give medications as ordered: *cycloplegic* or *mydriatics* to dilate pupils widely and decrease intraocular movement.
         e. Relaxing diversion: conversation, music.
      2. Goal: **health teaching.** Prepare for surgical intervention:
         a. *Cryotherapy*—supercooled probe is applied to the sclera, causing a scar, which pulls the choroid and retina together.
         b. *Laser photocoagulation*—a beam of intense light from a carbon arc is directed through the dilated pupil onto the retina; seals hole if retina not detached.
         c. *Scleral buckling*—the sclera is resected or shortened to enhance the contact between the choroid and retina.
         d. *Banding or encirclement*—silicone band or strap is placed under the extraocular muscles around the globe.
   B. Postoperative care:
      1. Goal: *reduce intraocular stress and prevent hemorrhage.*
         a. *Position:* flat or low Fowler's; sandbags may be used to position head; turn to *nonoperative side* if allowed, retinal tear dependent; special positions may be prone, side-lying, or sitting with face down on table.
         b. Activity: *bed rest;* decrease intraocular pressure by *not* stooping, bending, or assuming prone position.
         c. Give medications as ordered:
            (1) *Mydriatics.*
            (2) *Antiinfectives.*
            (3) *Corticosteroids* to reduce eye movements, inflammation, and prevent infection.
         d. Range of motion exercises—isometric, passive; elastic stockings to prevent thrombus related to immobility.
      2. Goal: *support coping mechanisms.*
         a. Plan all care with patient.
         b. Encourage verbalization of feelings, fears.
         c. Encourage family interaction.
         d. Diversional activities.
      3. Goal: **health teaching.**
         a. Eye care: eye patch or shield at night to prevent touching of the eye while asleep; dark glasses; *avoid* rubbing, squeezing eyes.

b. Limitations: *no* reading for 3 wk, no physical exertion for 6 wk.

c. Medications: dosage, frequency, purpose, side effects; *avoid* nonprescription medications.

d. *Signs of redetachment:* flashes of light, increase in "floaters," blurred vision.

◄ **V. Evaluation/outcome criteria**

  A. Vision restored.

  B. No further detachment—recognizes signs and symptoms.

  C. No injury occurs—accepts limitations.

Blindness

Legally defined as vision less than 20/200 with the use of corrective lenses, or a visual field of no greater than 20 degrees; greatest incidence after 65 yr.

I. Risk factors:

  A. Glaucoma.

  B. Cataracts.

  C. Diabetic retinopathy.

  D. Atherosclerosis.

  E. Trauma.

◄ **II. Analysis/nursing diagnosis**

  A. *Visual sensory/perceptual alteration* related to blindness.

  B. *Impaired social interaction* related to loss of sight.

  C. *Risk for injury* related to visual impairment.

  D. *Self-care deficit* related to visual loss.

◄ **III. Nursing care plan/implementation**

   A. Goal: *promote independence and provide emotional support.*

   1. Familiarize with surroundings, encourage use of touch.

   2. Establish communication lines, answer questions.

   3. Deal with feelings of loss, overprotectiveness by family members.

   4. Provide diversional activities: radio, records, talking books, tapes.

   5. Encourage self-care activities; allow voicing of frustrations when activity is not done to satisfaction (spilling or misplacing something), to decrease anger and discouragement.

  B. Goal: *facilitate activities of daily living.*

   1. *Eating:*

    a. Establish routine placement for tableware, (e.g., plate, glass).

    b. Help person mentally visualize the plate as a clock or compass (e.g., "3 o'clock" or "east").

    c. Take person's hand and guide the fingertips to establish spatial relationship.

   2. *Walking:*

    a. Have person hold your *forearm:* walk a half step in front.

    b. Tell the person when approaching stairs, curb, incline.

   3. *Talking:*

    a. Speak when approaching person; tell them *before* you touch them.

    b. Tell them who you are and what you will be doing.

    c. Do *not avoid* using words such as "see" or discussing the appearance of things.

  C. Goal: **health teaching.**

   1. Accident prevention in the home.

   2. Community resources:

    a. Voluntary agencies:

     (1) American Foundation for the Blind—provides catalogs of devices for visually handicapped.

     (2) National Society for the Prevention of Blindness—comprehensive educational programs and research.

     (3) Recording for the Blind, Inc.—provides recorded educational books on free loan.

     (4) Lion's Club.

     (5) Catholic Charities.

     (6) Salvation Army.

    b. Government agencies;

     (1) Social and Rehabilitation Service—counseling and placement services.

     (2) Veterans Administration—screening and pensions.

     (3) State Welfare Department, Division for the Blind—vocational.

   3. Care of artificial eye—see Table 19.2.

◄ **IV. Evaluation/outcome criteria**

  A. Acceptance of disability—participates in self-care activities, remains socially involved.

  B. Regains independence with rehabilitation.

〰 Diagnostic Studies

Caloric Stimulation Test

Used to evaluate the vestibular portion of the eighth cranial nerve, identify the impairment or loss of thermally induced nystagmus. Reflex eye movements (nystagmus) result in response to cold or warm irrigations of the external auditory canal if the nerve is intact. A *diminished or absent* response occurs in Meniere's disease or acoustic neuroma. Nausea, vomiting, or dizziness can be precipitated by the test.

💡 Study and Memory Aids

● Diet

Meniere's Disease

Low sodium
No alcohol

☞ Summary of Key Points

1. Regardless of the type of sensory disorder, concern for patient safety is a priority because of the accompanying *dizziness* (vertigo), impaired vision, or *altered depth perception*.
2. Meniere's disease is a relatively common disorder of *balance*. Medical treatment is instituted first; hospitalization is necessary only if surgery is needed to preserve hearing or manage symptoms.
3. Ringing in the ears (tinnitus) is *not* normal and usually indicates a problem.
4. The patient should be told that hearing will not immediately improve after surgery for otosclerosis.
5. Hearing losses are either *conductive or sensorineural*. A conductive loss involves the *external, middle,* or *inner* ear. Sensorineural loss means there is *nerve damage*.
6. When talking to a patient with an inner ear problem, stand *in front* of the patient to avoid causing head movement and prevent dizziness.
7. Talking *louder* does *not* improve communication with a blind person.
8. The patient with glaucoma must *avoid* using drugs that dilate the pupil and impair the outflow of aqueous humor. *Miotics* are used to constrict the pupil.
9. A rule of thumb—unless otherwise stated, the patient should *not lie on* the *operative* side after eye surgery.
10. The most common cause of cataract is *aging*. An intraocular *lens* will most likely be inserted after cataract removal. Postoperative complications are less with such a lens implant, and depth perception is not altered; therefore accidents are less likely. Contact lenses are less desirable for older adults with decreased manual dexterity.
11. If a gas or air bubble is injected to seal a retinal tear, postoperative *positioning is key* to maximizing the gravitational force. The patient may need to assume a *head-down* position while sitting and lie *prone* while sleeping.

TABLE 19.2 ☞ CARING FOR AN ARTIFICIAL EYE

With gloved hand pull lower eyelid down over the infraorbital bone and exert pressure below the eyelid.
Pressure will make the eye pop out.
Handle eye prosthesis carefully.
Using aseptic techniques, cleanse socket with saline-moistened gauze, stroking from the inner to outer canthus.
Wash the prosthesis in warm normal saline.
To reinsert, gently pull the patient's lower lid down, raise the upper lid if necessary, slip the saline-moistened eye prosthesis gently into the socket, and release the lids.

Source: Lagerquist SL: *Little, Brown's NCLEX-RN Examination Review.* Boston: Little, Brown, 1996. P. 310.

Drug Review

Meniere's Disease

Antiemetics
   Prochlorperazine (Compazine): 5–10 mg qid
   Promethazine (Phenergan): 10–25 mg q4h
   Trimethobenzamide (Tigan): 250 mg qid
Antihistamines
   Dimenhydrinate (Dramamine): 5–200 mg q4–6h, not to exceed 400 mg/d

   Diphenhydramine HCl (Benadryl): 25–50 mg q4–6h
Antivertigo
   Diazepam (Valium): 2–10 mg 3–4 times daily
   Meclizine (Antivert): 25–100 mg/d in divided doses
Diuretics
   Acetazolamide (Diamox): 250 mg 2–4 times daily
   Hydrochlorothiazide (Diuril, HydroDIURIL): 25–100 mg/d in 1–2 doses
Vasodilators: Niacin (nicotinic acid): 500 mg/d in divided doses

Stapedectomy

Analgesics
   Acetaminophen/codeine (Tylenol #1, #2, #3): 1–2 tablets q3–4h, as needed
   Meperidine HCl (Demerol): IM or SC, 50–150 mg
   Morphine sulfate: IM or SC, 5–20 mg
   Oxycodone/acetaminophen (Tylox, Percocet): 5 mg q3–6h, as needed
Antiinfectives
   Cephalexin (Keflex): 250–500 mg q6h
   Cephalothin (Keflin): IV, 0.5–2 g q4–6h
   Erythromycin: 250–500 mg q6–12h
   Gentamicin (Garamycin): 3–5 mg/kg/d in divided doses
   Penicillin G: 1.2 million U in single IM dose
Antiemetics
   Prochlorperazine (Compazine): 5–10 mg qid
   Promethazine (Phenergan): 10–25 mg q4h
   Trimethobenzamide (Tigan): 250 mg qid

Eye Medications

My**d**riatic = **d**ilated (big) pupils
Mio**t**ic = **t**iny (constricted) pupils

Source: Modified from Zerwekh J, et al. *Memory Notebook of Nursing.* Dallas: Nursing Education Consultants, 1994, p. 44.

Glaucoma

Anticholinesterase: Demecarium bromide
(Humorsol): 1–2 drops twice a week up to 1–2
drops twice a day
Carbonic anhydrase inhibitors: Acetazolamide
(Diamox): 250 mg 2–4 times daily
Miotics (pupil will constrict)
Carbachol (Miostat Intraocular): 1–2 drops 4 times
a day
Pilocarpine (Ocuset): 1–2 drops up to 6 times daily
Ophthalmic: Timolol (Timoptic) 1 drop 1–2 times
daily

Cataract Removal: Restriction

Cataract

Mydriatics (pupil will dilate)
Cyclopentolate (Cyclogyl): 1 drop daily
Homatropine (Homatrine): 1–2 drops daily

Questions

1. The nurse would question a patient's understanding of the discharge instructions after removal of a cataract if he says:
   1. "I'll protect my eye with glasses or a shield."
   2. "I'll remember to drink plenty of fluids."
   3. "I'll wash around my eye with warm water."
   4. "I'll take a laxative every night."
2. Patient teaching about the things to expect after cataract surgery would include the fact that:
   1. Nausea and vomiting may result from general anesthesia.
   2. Narcotics will be available to manage surgical pain.
   3. The patient will be tested for increased intraocular pressure.
   4. The patient will need to significantly restrict activities after surgery.
3. The nurse would know that a patient understands the possible precipitating causes of Meniere's disease if she states that she:
   1. Will increase her fluid intake.
   2. Plans to quit smoking.
   3. Must begin to do vigorous exercises regularly.
   4. Likes wine with her dinner.
4. The nurse knows that the vertigo in Meniere's disease may be relieved if the patient lies:
   1. On the side with the affected ear uppermost.
   2. On the side with the unaffected ear uppermost.
   3. Supine with the head of the bed elevated 30 degrees.
   4. Supine with the head of the bed flat.
5. The best technique the nurse can use to improve communication with a patient with hearing impairment is to:
   1. Speak loudly and accentuate the words.
   2. Tap the patient's shoulder before talking.
   3. Stand with a light on his/her face while talking.
   4. Give one-word answers to the patient's questions.
6. Besides frontal headaches, the nurse would expect a patient with open-angle glaucoma to:
   1. Experience a decrease in peripheral vision.
   2. See colored halos around lights.
   3. Have dilated pupils, even in light.
   4. Have cloudy corneas.
7. Routine discharge teaching in a patient who has undergone removal of a cataract from the right eye would include the need to:
   1. Avoid sexual activity for a month.
   2. Report immediately any eye aching.
   3. Sleep supine or lying on the nonoperated side.
   4. Remove the eye patch at night only.
8. Which aspect of a physical assessment of the eyes would be unaffected in a patient with a cataract?
   1. Red reflex testing.
   2. Funduscopy.
   3. Visual acuity.
   4. Pupillary reaction.
9. Which nursing action would be inappropriate in a patient with Meniere's disease suffering an attack of vertigo?
   1. Supporting each side of the patient's head with a pillow.
   2. Speaking into the patient's unaffected ear to facilitate hearing.
   3. Keeping the patient on bedrest with side rails up.
   4. Having the patient ask for assistance when turning.
10. A patient is preparing to go home after surgery for glaucoma. Which instruction would not be included in the discharge teaching?
    1. Washing hands well before instilling eye drops.
    2. Refraining from smoking for 1 week postoperatively.
    3. Avoiding driving at night for 6 weeks.
    4. Wearing a protective eyeshield during sleep for several weeks.

11. Which instruction is part of the proper care of a hearing aid?
    1. Cleaning off the ear mold weekly.
    2. Storing the hearing aid in a warm, dry place.
    3. Removing accumulated lint from the casing monthly.
    4. Replacing the batteries every month.
12. Which action to determine the cause of hearing aid failure should the nurse take first?
    1. Replacing the existing batteries.
    2. Checking for proper fit in the ear.
    3. Examining the ear for cerumen.
    4. Checking to see if the hearing aid is "on."

Answers/Rationale

1. **(2)** The intake of plenty of fluids, although an important measure in most patients, is *not* going to promote recovery after cataract surgery. Protecting the eye (1), careful cleaning (3), and preventing straining at stool (4) *are* all important and *appropriate* measures. **EV, 2, SECE**

2. **(3)** Secondary glaucoma is one of the major complications of cataract extraction. Usually this resolves within 24 to 72 hours, however. *Local* anesthesia, *not* general anesthesia, is used for the procedure, so nausea and vomiting (1) are *not* expected. Acetaminophen (Tylenol) is usually effective enough to relieve the postoperative discomfort (2). Restrictions are *minimal* (4). Normally, patients should avoid lifting and straining but they may resume other usual activities within 24 hours. **IMP, 2, SECE**

3. **(2)** Quitting smoking eliminates one source of vasospasm and vasoconstriction, which may inhibit the absorption of endolymph and cause ear pressure to increase. If fluid intake is increased (1), fluid retention may result and the symptoms will be aggravated. Vigorous, sudden movement (3) may precipitate an attack, so vigorous exercise should be *avoided*. Alcohol (4), like smoking, may cause vasoconstriction and hence increased endolymph accumulation. **EV, 2, PhI**

4. **(1)** Some patients have experienced relief if they lie on their side with the affected ear uppermost. This may reduce inner ear pressure. Lying with the unaffected ear up (2), with the head elevated (3), or supine (4) has *not* been found to produce any *relief.* **IMP, 2, PhI**

5. **(3)** Standing with a light on the nurse's face helps the patient speech read. It is best to speak slowly in a *normal* tone and *not* to overaccentuate (1). To get the patient's attention, the nurse should raise an arm or hand; tapping the patient on the shoulder (2) may startle the patient. It is also best *not* to use one-word answers (4), but to use phrases, which convey more meaning. In general, the nurse should not avoid conversation with a hearing-impaired patient. **IMP, 2, HPM**

6. **(1)** A patient with open-angle glaucoma suffers a gradual loss of peripheral vision, but central vision remains good. A patient with *closed*-angle glaucoma sees colored halos around lights (2). *Cranial nerve III* (oculomotor) damage or drugs cause pupillary dilatation (3). Patients with *cataracts* have cloudy corneas (4). **AS, 2, PhI**

7. **(3)** Discharge teaching should emphasize the need to avoid activities that place strain on the eye. Unless otherwise stated, sleeping on the back or the nonoperated side is recommended. Sexual activity (1) is *not* routinely restricted, but this varies with each patient and MD. *Mild* pain and aching (2) are *expected* and relieved with mild analgesia. Sudden, sharp pain should be reported. A patch *is* worn at night (4) to protect the eye from rubbing against the bedclothes and keep the patient from rubbing the eye during sleep. **IMP, 2, SECE**

8. **(4)** The pupillary response, which is controlled by cranial nerve III, would still be intact, because this is elicited by light, which can still penetrate the cornea. Cataract *would interfere* with the red reflex (1), which is the bright red-orange glow seen through the pupil. The opacity of the lens caused by a cataract *would* make it difficult for the examiner to see through the lens into the posterior portion of the eye (2) and the central vision acuity (3) of the patient *would be impaired.* **AS, 2, PhI**

9. **(2)** It is inappropriate to make the patient turn the head or move the eyes to look at the nurse, because this may worsen dizziness. Head support (1) and assistance in turning (4) *can* minimize sudden movements or jerking, which could increase discomfort and aggravate the symptoms. The side rails (3) *would* be up to prevent falls during dizzy spells. **IMP, 2, PhI**

10. **(3)** There are usually no driving restrictions unless visual impairment has resulted. The instructions in options 1, 2, and 4 *are* appropriate for patients who have undergone glaucoma surgery. **IMP, 2, SECE**

11. **(4)** Replacing the batteries every month will prevent battery failure as a source of a patient's inability to hear. The instructions in options 1 and 3 specify exact times for cleaning, whereas cleaning is actually done only as needed when wax or lint buildup warrant. The ear mold is cleaned off daily with soap and warm water, and with a pipe cleaner if necessary. The hearing aid is usually *not stored* (2) when not in use; when it is not in the ear, it is kept on the patient's bedside stand. **IMP, 2, SECE**

12. **(4)** The nurse should start with the obvious: checking to see if the hearing aid is on. Next check to see if the ear mold is clean. After this the battery should be checked to make sure it is correctly inserted. The other actions would *follow* these steps: replacing the battery if necessary (1), then checking the position of the hearing aid in the ear (2), and finally checking to see if there has been a buildup of cerumen (3). **IMP, 2, SECE**

Key to Codes

Nursing process: AS, assessment; **AN,** analysis; **PL,** planning; **IMP,** implementation; **EV,** evaluation. (See Appendix M for explanation of nursing process steps.)

Category of human function: 1, protective; **2,** sensory-perceptual; **3,** comfort, rest, activity, and mobility; **4,** nutrition; **5,** growth and development; **6,** fluid-gas transport; **7,** psychosocial-cultural; **8,** elimination. (See Appendix O for explanation.)

Client need: SECE, safe, effective care environment; **PhI,** physiologic integrity; **PsI,** psychosocial integrity; **HPM,** health promotion/maintenance. (See Appendix P for explanation.)

Musculoskeletal Disorders

Chapter Outline

Fractures

Disruptions in the continuity of bone as the result of trauma or various disease processes, such as Cushing's syndrome, that weaken the bone structure.

I. Types:

  A. *Open or compound*—fractured bone extends *through skin* and mucous membranes; increased potential for infection.

  B. *Closed or simple*—fractured bone *does not* protrude through skin.

  C. *Complete*—fracture extends through *entire bone,* disrupting the periosteum on both sides of the bone, producing two or more fragments.

  D. *Incomplete*—fracture extends *only part way* through bone; bone continuity is not totally interrupted.

  E. *Greenstick* or *willow-hickory stick*—fracture of *one* side of bone; *other side merely bends;* usually seen only in children.

  F. *Impacted or telescoped*—fracture in which bone fragments are *forcibly driven into* other or adjacent bone structures.

  G. *Comminuted*—fracture having *more than one* fracture line and with bone fragment broken into *several pieces.*

  H. *Depressed*—fracture in which bone or bone fragments are driven *inward,* as in skull or facial fractures.

II. Methods used to reduce/immobilize fractures: reduction or setting of the bone—restores bone alignment as nearly as possible.

  A. *Closed reduction*—manual traction or manipulation. Usually done under general anesthesia to reduce pain and muscle spasm. Maintenance of reduction and immobilization is accomplished by casting (fiberglass or plaster of Paris).

  B. *Open reduction*—operative procedure utilized to achieve bone alignment; pins, wire, nails, or rods may be used to secure bone fragments in position; prosthetic implants may also be used.

  C. *Traction reduction*—force is applied in two directions, to obtain alignment and to reduce or eliminate muscle spasm. Used for fractures of long bones. May be:

    1. *Continuous*—used with fractures or dislocations of bones or joints.

    2. *Intermittent*—used to reduce flexion contractures or lessen pain and muscle spasm.

    3. Applied as follows:

      a. *Skin*—traction applied to skin using a commercial foam-rubber *Buck's* traction splint or an adhesive, plastic, or moleskin strip bound to the extremity by elastic bandage; exerts indirect traction on bone or muscles (e.g., *Buck's* extension, *Bryant's, Russell's,* pelvic). (Figure 20.1A to 20.1D.)

      b. *Skeletal*—direct traction applied to bone using pins (*Steinman*), wires (*Kirschner*). Pin is inserted through the bone in or close

FIGURE 20.1   **TYPES OF TRACTION. (A) Buck's extension.** Skin traction applied to the medial and lateral aspects of an extremity with adhesive foam, moleskin, or use of "Buck's boot." **(B) Bryant's traction.** Vertical suspension skin traction in which pelvis is elevated from the bed. **(C) Russell's traction.** Skin traction composed of Buck's extension on the foreleg, three pulleys at the bottom, and a sling under the knee. Affords more freedom of movement than Buck's. **(D) Pelvic traction.** Skin traction applied to the lumbosacral region by means of a pelvic belt. **(E) Head halter.** Cervical traction applied to the head by means of a halter under the chin. **(F) Crutchfield tongs.** Cervical traction using tongs into the skull. **(G) Thomas' splint.** Full-leg splint that keeps the leg fully extended and the long bones in alignment. Pressure is on the ischium and perineal area. May be used with skin or skeletal traction. **(H) Halo vest assembly.** Applied in operating room. Patient will usually be ambulatory 24 hours after application. (From Saxton DF. The Addison-Wesley Manual of Nursing Practice. Menlo Park, CA. Addison-Wesley, 1983.)

to the involved area and usually protrudes through skin on both sides of the extremity. Skeletal traction for fractured vertebrae accomplished with tongs (*Crutchfield tongs, Gardner-Wells tongs*).

4. Specific types of traction:

a. *Cervical*—direct traction applied to cervical vertebrae using a head halter or *Crutchfield, Gardner-Wells,* or *Vinke* tongs that are inserted into the skull (see Figure 20.1E and 20.1F). Traction is increased with weights until vertebrae move into position and alignment is regained. After reduction is obtained, weights are decreased to the amount needed to maintain reduction. *Weight amount is prescribed by physician.*

b. *Balanced suspension*—countertraction produced by a force other than patient's body weight; additional weights supply countertraction. Extremity is suspended in a traction apparatus that maintains the line of traction despite changes in the patient's position (e.g., *Russell's* leg traction, *Thomas'* splint with *Pearson's* attachment). (See Figure 20.1C and 20.1G.) Patient has more freedom to move about than in straight or running traction.

c. *Running*—traction that exerts a pull in one plane; countertraction is supplied by the weight of the patient's body (this must not be less than the pull of the traction) or can be increased through use of weights and pulleys in the opposite direction (e.g., *Buck's* extension, *Russell's* traction). Check specifics orders to determine how much the head may be elevated (See Figure 20.1A and 20.1C).

d. *Halo*—an apparatus that employs both a plastic and metal frame; molded frame extends from the axilla to iliac crest and houses a metal frame. The struts of the frame extend to skull and attach to round metal (halo) device. The halo is attached to skull by four pins—two located anterolaterally and two located posterolaterally. They are inserted into external cortex of the cranium. (See Figure 20.1H.) Used to immobilize the cervical spine after spinal fusion, somewhat corrects scoliosis before spinal fusion, immobilizes nondisplaced fracture of spine.

D. *Immobilization*—maintains reduction and promotes healing of bone fragments. Achieved by:

1. *External fixation:*

a. *Casts*—types:

(1) *Spica*—applied to immobilize hip or shoulder joints.

(2) *Body cast*—applied to trunk.

(3) *Arm or leg cast*—joints above and below site included in cast.

b. *Splints*—continuous traction.

c. External fixation devices (*Charnley* pillow)—multiple pins/rods through limb above and below fracture site, attached to external metal supports; patient able to become ambulatory.

2. *Internal fixation*—pins, wires, nails, rods. See Total Hip Replacement, p. 239, and Total Knee Replacement, p. 241.

III. Assessment

A. *Subjective data:*

1. Pain, tenderness.
2. Tingling, numbness.
3. Nausea.
4. History of trauma.
5. Muscle spasm.

B. *Objective data:*

1. Function: abnormal or lost.
2. Deformities.
3. Ecchymosis, increased heat over injured part.
4. Localized edema.
5. Crepitation (grating sensations heard or felt as bone fragments rub against each other).
6. Signs of shock.
7. Indicators of anxiety.
8. X-ray: *fracture*—positive interruption of bone; *dislocation*—abnormal position of bone.

IV. Analysis/nursing diagnosis

A. *Pain* related to interruption in bone.

B. *Impaired physical mobility* related to fracture/treatment.

C. *Risk for injury* related to complications of fractures.

D. *Knowledge deficit* regarding cast care, crutch walking, traction.

E. *Constipation* related to immobilization.

F. *Risk for impaired skin integrity* related to immobility or friction from materials used to immobilize the fracture during healing.

V. Nursing care plan/implementation

A. Goal: *promote healing and prevent complications of fractures* (Table 20.1).

1. *Diet:* high protein, iron, vitamins, *to improve tissue repair;* moderate carbohydrates, to *prevent weight* gain; *no* increase in calcium, to *prevent kidney stones* (decalcification and demineralization occur when patient is immobilized).

2. Encourage *increased fluid intake, to prevent kidney stones.*

3. *Prevent* or alleviate *constipation* by *increasing bulk foods, fruits, and fruit juices* or by administering prescribed *stool softeners, laxatives,* or *cathartics,* as necessary.

4. Provide activities to reduce perceptual deprivation—reading, handicrafts, music, special interests/hobbies that can be done while maintaining correct position for healing.

B. Goal: *prevent injury or trauma in relation to:*

1. *Fracture care:*

a. Maintain affected part in optimal alignment.

TABLE 20.1   COMPLICATIONS OF FRACTURES

Complication	⊠ Assessment	⊠ Analysis/Nursing Diagnosis	⊠ Nursing Care Plan/ Implementation	⊠ Evaluation/Outcome Criteria
Shock (see Chap. 8).				
Thrombophlebitis (see p. 14).				
Fat emboli: serious, potentially life-threatening complication in which pressure changes in interior of fracture force molecules of fat from marrow into systemic circulation; may cause problems in respiratory or nervous system; seen most frequently on third day after multiple fractures, fractures of long bones, or comminuted fracture.	*Subjective data:* dyspnea, severe chest pain; confusion, agitation; decrease in level of consciousness; numbness; feeling faint; history of diabetes, obesity.	*Risk for injury* related to fat emboli.	1. *Position:* high Fowler's to relieve respiratory symptoms.	Alert, oriented. Pain relieved.
	Objective data: cyanosis; pupillary changes; muscle twitching; petechiae—chest, buccal cavity, axilla, conjunctiva, soft palate; extremities—pallor, cold; shock, vomiting.	*Altered tissue perfusion* related to fat emboli.	2. Administer *oxygen stat,* to relieve anoxia and reduce surface tension of fat globules.	Respiratory, cardiac, and neurologic problems cause no permanent damage.
			3. Institute respiratory support measures, as ordered—intermittent positive-pressure breathing, respiratory assistive devices: **be prepared for cardiopulmonary resuscitation** in event of respiratory failure.	
			4. Monitor vital signs, cardiac monitor, q15min during acute episode and prn (shock/cardiac failure possible).	
			5. Obtain baseline data and monitor *level of consciousness, neurologic signs* q15min during acute episode and prn (neurologic involvement possible).	
			6. Administer *parenteral fluids,* as ordered: IV alcohol, blood and fluid replacements.	
			7. Administer medications as ordered: corticosteroids, digitalis, aminophylline, heparin sodium.	
			8. **DO NOT RUB ANY LEG CRAMPS, BUT REPORT IMMEDIATELY.**	

(continued)

Assessment	Nursing Diagnosis	Nursing Plan/Implementation	Evaluation/Expected Outcomes
Nerve compression: pressure on nerve in affected area from edema, dislocation of bone, or immobilization apparatus; if pressure not relieved, permanent paralysis can result.	*Subjective data:* discomfort, pain, referred pain, burning, tingling, "stinging sensation," numbness, altered sensation, inability to distinguish touch. *Objective data:* limited movement; muscle weakness; paralysis; reflexes—diminished, irritable, or absent; color changes related to impaired circulation.	*Pain* related to pressure on nerve. *Risk for physical injury* related to pressure on nerve. *Impaired tissue perfusion* related to impaired circulation. *Impaired physical mobility* related to joint contracture, numbness.	1. Monitor for potential signs q1h for first 48 h; neurovascular assessment q12h and prn as condition indicates CSM (*circulation, sensation, motion*). 2. *Position: elevate* affected limb; flex hand or foot of affected extremity; passive and active ROM exercises. 3. **Be prepared to cut cast or remove constrictions if signs of impairment present.** 4. Begin active ROM exercises to unaffected extremities. 5. Use footboard to prevent footdrop. 6. Encourage use of trapeze if applicable. 7. Isometric exercises, as ordered. 8. Ambulation, weight bearing as ordered; support casts.	Sensation, motor function are normal. No complications noted.
Avascular necrosis/ circulatory impairment: interference with normal circulation to affected area due to interruption of blood vessel, pressure on the vessel from dislocation, edema, or immobilization devices; impaired circulation leads to discomfort and, if not eliminated, to necrosis of tissue and bone due to lack of oxygen supply.	*Subjective data:* tenderness; pain, especially on passive motion. *Objective data:* edema, swelling in affected area; decreased color, temperature, mobility; bleeding from wound.	*Risk for altered peripheral tissue perfusion,* related to vessel damage.	1. Monitor for potential signs q1h for first 48 h: blanching, coolness, edema; palpate pulse above and below injury; report absent or major discrepancies stat. 2. *Position: elevate* affected limb to decrease edema. 3. Report to physician if signs persist. 4. Be prepared to assist with bivalving of casts, or cut cast to relieve pressure. 5. Monitor size of drainage stains on casts; measure accurately and report if they enlarge.	Circulation adequate to limb, to prevent tissue damage.

(continued)

TABLE 20.1   COMPLICATIONS OF FRACTURES (Continued)

Complication	☒ Assessment	☒ Analysis/Nursing Diagnosis	☒ Nursing Care Plan/ Implementation	☒ Evaluation/Outcome Criteria
Infection	*Subjective data:* pain. *Objective data:* elevated temperature and pulse; erythema—discoloration of surrounding skin; edema—sudden, local in-duration; drainage—thin, watery, foul-smelling exu-date; crepitation (may be indicative of gas gan-grene); with cast—warm area, foul smell.	*Risk for injury* related to tis-sue destruction. *Altered peripheral tissue perfusion* related to swell-ing.	1. Monitor vital signs, drainage. 2. Ensure patient has had prophylac-tic tetanus toxoid. 3. May have prophylactic antiinfec-tives ordered if wound was con-taminated at time of injury. 4. Instruct patient *not to* touch open wound, pin sites or put anything inside cast (could interrupt skin in-tegrity and become potential source of infection).	No infection or heals with no serious complications.
Delayed union/nonunion: failure of bone to heal within normal time re-lated to lack of use, inade-quate circulation, other complicating medical con-ditions such as diabetes or poor nutrition.	*Subjective data:* pain. *Objective data:* lack of callus formation on x-ray, poor alignment.	*Risk for injury* related to poor healing of bone frac-ture. *Impaired physical mobility* related to lower-limb frac-tures. *Dressing/grooming, bathing/ hygiene, self-care deficit* related to upper-limb fracture.	1. Maintain immobilization and alignment of affected limb. 2. Maintain adequate nutrition. 3. *Avoid* trauma to affected limb. 4. Monitor for circulatory or infec-tive complication. 5. Dietary instructions regarding foods containing *calcium* and *pro-tein* necessary for bone healing.	Bone heals. No complications noted. Pain decreases. Ambulation and self-care re-turn to preinjury status.

(continued)

	Assessment	Nursing Diagnosis/Analysis	Nursing Plan/Implementation	Evaluation
Skin breakdown (related to cast).	*Subjective data:* pain. *Objective data:* temperature and pulse elevated; erythema; edema—cast edges, exposed distal portion of limb, limb area within cast; drainage and foul odor from break in skin, may be under cast and stain through or exit at ends of cast; crepitus (crackling sound could indicate gas gangrene); hyperactive reflexes.	*Impaired skin integrity* related to cast trauma.	1. If open wound: verify tetanus administration; monitor site through cast window, change *dressing* daily and prn. 2. Apply lotion or cornstarch to exposed skin (no powder). 3. Petal tape edges of cast to reduce irritation. 4. Inspect skin for irritation, edema, odor, drainage—q2h initially, then q3h. 5. Instruct patient *not to* place any object under cast as skin abrasions may lead to decubitus ulcers. 6. Promote drying of cast by leaving it uncovered and exposed to air for 48 h, use *no plastic.* 7. Prevent indenting casts with fingertips or hard surface: place on pillows, use palms of hands when positioning affected limb. 8. *Avoid* excessive padding of Thomas splint in groin area—padding traps moisture, leading to skin breakdown.	No skin breakdown.
Duodenal distress (with spica cast): spica cast incorporates the trunk and affected limb and can cause respiratory or abdominal distress when edema is present under the cast or cast is too tight to allow for normal body functions.	*Subjective data:* anorexia, nausea, abdominal pain. *Objective data:* duodenal distress, vomiting, distention, cast too tight.	*Ineffective breathing pattern* related to pressure from cast. *Pain* related to abdominal distress from pressure. *Fear* related to cast constriction.	1. Place on firm mattress, use bed boards if necessary to reduce muscle spasm. 2. Maintain warmth by covering uncasted areas. 3. *Avoid* turning for first 8 h; *when turning:* use enough personnel to log-roll, *do not use* bar between legs while turning, support chest with pillows. 4. Monitor for signs of respiratory distress: increased respirations, apprehension. 5. Monitor for signs of duodenal distress: vomiting, distention; *if these signs occur:* place in *prone* position, have cast bivalved, may need NG tube, monitor for fluid imbalance. 6. Protect cast with nonabsorbent material during elimination.	Complications prevented or detected early enough to prevent serious damage.

Source: Lagerquist SL: *Little, Brown's NCLEX-RN Examination Review.* Boston: Little, Brown, 1996. P. 170–172.

b. Maintain skin integrity; check all bony prominences for evidence of pressure q4h and prn, depending on amount of pressure.

c. Monitor: *circulation* in, *sensation* of, and *motion* (CSM) of affected part q15min for first 4 h; q1h until 24 h; then q4h and prn, depending on amount of edema (Table 20.2).

d. Maintain mobility in unaffected limb and unaffected joints of affected limb by active and passive range of motion (ROM) exercises, prevent footdrop by using ankle-top sneakers.

☞ **2.** *Skin traction:*

  a. Maintain correct alignment:

    (1) If tape or moleskin is used, shave extremity and apply benzoin to improve adherence of strip and reduce itching.

    (2) Check apparatus for slippage, bunching; replace prn.

  b. Prevent tissue injury:

    (1) Check all bony prominences for evidence of pressure: q15min for first 4 h; q1h until 24 h; then q4h and prn, depending on amount of edema.

    (2) Nonadhesive traction may be removed q8h to check skin (e.g., *Bryant's*).

☞ **3.** *Skeletal traction:*

  a. Maintain affected part in optimal alignment:

    (1) Ropes on pulleys.

    (2) Weights hang free.

    (3) Position: *elevate* head of bed as prescribed.

    (4) Check knots routinely.

  b. Maintain skin integrity:

    (1) Frequent skin care.

TABLE 20.2 ✉ **ASSESSING NEURO-VASCULAR STATUS IN AN INJURED LIMB**

■ Assessing *circulation* to the limb:
  1. Warmth and color.
  2. Capillary refill.
  3. Peripheral pulse(s).

■ Assessing *nerve supply* to the limb
  1. Upper extremities:
    a. Sensory: pinprick over fingertips, dorsum of hand.
    b. Motor: dorsiflexion and palmar flexion of wrist.
  2. Lower extremities:
    a. Sensory: pinprick over heel and dorsum of foot.
    b. Motor: dorsiflexion and plantar flexion of foot.

Source: Caroline NL. *Emergency Care in the Street* (5th ed.)., Boston: Little, Brown, 1995.

---

    (2) Keep bed linens free of crumbs and wrinkles.

c. Prevent *infection:* special skin care to pin insertion site tid. Keep area around pins clean and dry. Utilize prescribed solution for cleansing.

d. Monitor: *circulation, sensation, motion* of affected part (see *Fracture care,* p. 223).

e. Maintain mobility in unaffected limb and unaffected joints; prevent footdrop of affected limb.

4. *Running traction:*

  a. Keep well centered in bed.

  b. *Position: elevate head of bed only* to point of countertraction.

  c. *No* turning from side to side—will cause rubbing of bony fragments.

  d. Check distal circulation frequently.

  e. Frequent back care to prevent skin breakdown.

  f. Fracture bedpan for toileting.

  g. *Avoid* excessive padding of splints in groin area to prevent tissue trauma.

☞ **5.** *Balanced suspension traction:*

  a. Maintain alignment and countertraction:

    (1) Ropes on pulleys.

    (2) Weights hang free.

    (3) *Position:* elevate head of bed as prescribed.

    (4) Check knots routinely.

  b. May move patient, but turn only slightly (*no more* than 30 degrees to *unaffected* side).

  c. Heel of affected leg *must* remain free of the bed.

  d. *20-degree angle* between thigh and bed.

  e. Check for pressure to popliteal area exerted by sling.

  f. Provide foot support to prevent footdrop.

  g. Maintain *abduction* of extremity.

  h. Check for signs of infection at pin insertion sites, cleanse tid as ordered.

  i. If tape or moleskin is used, shave extremity and apply benzoin to improve adherence of strip and reduce itching.

☞ **6.** *Cervical traction:*

  a. May be placed on specialized bed (e.g., *Stryker frame*).

  b. *Position:* maintain body alignment.

  c. Keep tongs free from bed, keep weights hanging freely to allow traction to function properly.

☞ **7.** *Halo traction:*

  a. Several times a day: check screws to the head and screws that hold the upper portion of the frame, to determine correct position.

  b. Pin sites cleansed tid with bacteriostatic solution to prevent infection.

  c. Monitor for signs of infection.

d. *Position* as any other patient in body cast, except *no pressure* on halo—pillows may be placed under abdomen and chest when patient is prone.

e. Institute ROM exercises to prevent contractures.

f. Turn frequently to prevent development of pressure areas.

g. Allow patient to verbalize about having screws placed in skull.

h. Postapplication nursing care same as that for pin insertion for other forms of traction.

☞ **8.** *External fixation devices:*

a. Pin care same as that for skeletal traction.

b. Teach clothing adjustment.

c. Teach to adjust for size of apparatus.

☞ **9.** *Internal fixation devices:*

a. Monitor for signs of infection/allergic reaction to materials used for maintenance of reduction (drainage, pain, increased temperature).

b. Position: as ordered to prevent dislocation.

☞ **10.** *Casts:*

a. Support drying cast on firm pillow, prevent finger imprints on cast.

b. *Position: elevate* limb to reduce edema.

c. Prevent complications of fractures, as listed.

d. Closely monitor: *circulation* (blanching, swelling, decreased temperature), *sensation* (absence of feeling, pain, burning), *motion* (inability to move digits of affected limb).

e. **Be prepared to notify MD or cut cast if circulatory impairment occurs.**

f. Protect skin integrity: *avoid* pressure from edges of cast, petal tape edges of cast as needed.

g. Monitor for signs of infection if skin integrity impaired.

☞ **C.** Goal: *provide care related to ambulation with crutches.*

1. See Table 20.3.

2. Measure crutches correctly (Table 20.4).

a. Subtract 16 in. from total height, top of crutch should be 2 in. below the axilla.

b. Complete extension of the elbows should be possible without axilla bar exerting pressure into the axilla.

c. Handgrip should be adjusted so that complete wrist extension is possible.

d. Instruct in correct body alignment:

(1) Head erect.

(2) Back straight.

(3) Chest forward.

(4) Feet 6–8 in. apart, wide base for support.

D. Goal: *provide safety measures related to possible complications following fracture* (see Table 20.1).

🏠 **E.** Goal: **health teaching.**

1. Explain and show apparatus before application, if possible.

TABLE 20.3   TEACHING CRUTCH WALKING

A. When only *one* leg can bear weight:
1. *Swing-to gait:* crutches forward; swing body to crutches:
   a. Move both crutches forward.
   b. Move both legs to meet the crutches.
   c. Continue pattern.
2. *Swing-through gait:* crutches forward; swing body through crutches:
   a. Move both crutches forward.
   b. Move both legs farther ahead than crutches.
   c. Continue pattern.
3. *Three-point gait:* crutches and *affected* extremity forward; swing forward, placing *nonaffected* foot ahead or between crutches:
   a. Both crutches and affected limb move at same time.
   b. Move both crutches and *affected* leg (e.g., left) ahead 6 in.
   c. Move *unaffected* leg (e.g., right) to same places as left and crutches.
   d. Continue pattern.
B. When *both* legs can move separately and bear some weight:
1. *Four-point gait:* right crutch forward, left foot forward; swing weight to right side while bringing left crutch forward, then right foot forward; gait simulates normal walking:
   a. Move right crutch forward 4–6 in.
   b. Move left foot forward same distances as right crutch.
   c. Move left crutch forward ahead of left foot.
   d. Move right foot forward to meet right crutch.
   e. Continue pattern.
2. *Two-point gait:* same as four-point gait but faster; one crutch and opposite leg moving forward at same time:
   a. Opposite crutch and limb move together.
   b. Move right crutch and left leg ahead 6 in.
   c. Move left crutch and right leg ahead.
   d. Continue pattern.
C. When patient is *unable* to walk: *tripod* gait: crutches forward at a wide distance; drag legs to point just behind crutches, balance, and repeat.

Source: Lagerquist SL: *Little, Brown's NCLEX-RN Examination Review.* Boston: Little, Brown, 1996. P. 173.

2. Pin care at least once daily to prevent granulation and cellulitis.

3. Correct position for rest/sleep and prevention of injury with halo traction—*no* pressure on halo.

4. Purpose of cast: to immobilize, to support body tissues, to prevent or correct deformities.

5. Teach signs and symptoms of complications to report related to cast care (i.e., numbness;

TABLE 20.4   MEASURING CRUTCHES CORRECTLY

1. Have patient lie on a flat surface. Measure from anterior fold of axilla to 4 in. lateral to heel.
2. Have patient stand. Measure from 1–2 in. below axilla to 2 in. in front of and 6 in. to the side of the foot.
3. Hand placement on bar of crutch: have patient stand upright, support body weight with hand on bar (not putting weight on axilla). Elbow flexion should be 30 degrees.
4. Slightly pad the shoulder rests of the crutches for general comfort.
5. Make sure there are nonskid rubber tips on the crutches.

Source: Lagerquist SL: *Little, Brown's NCLEX-RN Examination Review.* Boston, Little, Brown, 1996. P. 173.

odor; crack/break in cast; extremity cold, bluish).
6. Isometric exercises for use with affected joint.
7. *Safety measures with crutches:*
   a. Weight bearing on hands, *not* axilla.
   b. Position crutches 4 in. to side and 4 in. to front.
   c. Use short strides, looking ahead, *not* at feet.
   d. Prevent injury: if patient begins to fall, throw crutches to side to prevent falling on them; body should be relaxed.
   e. Check for environmental hazards: rugs, water spills.

⋈ VI. Evaluation/outcome criteria
   A. No injury or complications related to apparatus or immobilization (e.g., infection, tissue injury, altered circulation/sensation, dislocation).
   B. Bone remains in correct alignment and begins to heal.
   C. Demonstrates elevated limb position to relieve edema with casted extremity.
   D. Lists complications related to circulation and/or neurologic impairment and infection.
   E. Begins to use affected part.
   F. Demonstrates correct technique for ambulation with crutches—no pressure on axilla, utilizes strength of arms and wrists.
   G. No falls while using crutches.

Compartment Syndrome

An accumulation of fluid in the muscle compartment, resulting in an increase in pressure that reduces blood flow to the tissues; can lead to neuromuscular deficit, amputation, death.

   I. Risk factors:
   A. Fractures.
   B. Burns.

   C. Crushing injuries.
   D. Restrictive bandages.
   E. Cast.
   F. Prolonged lithotomy positioning.

   II. Pathophysiology: inability of the fascia surrounding the muscle group to expand to accommodate the increased volume of fluid → increased compartment pressure → impaired venous flow → continued arterial flow, increasing capillary pressure → pushing of fluid into the extravascular space → further increased intracompartment pressure → prolonged or severe ischemia → destruction of muscle and nerve cells; contracture; loss of function; necrotic tissue; infection; release of potassium, hydrogen, and myoglobin into bloodstream.

⋈ III. Assessment
   A. *Subjective data:*
      1. Severe, unrelenting *pain,* unrelieved by narcotics and associated with passive stretching of muscle.
      2. *Paresthesias.*
   B. *Objective data:*
      1. Edema, tense skin over limb.
      2. *Paralysis.*
      3. Decreased or absent peripheral *pulses.*
      4. Poor capillary refill.
      5. Limb temperature change (colder).
      6. Ankle-arm pressure index decreased: 0.4 indicates ischemia (see Chap. 3, Doppler ultrasonography, p. 27).
      7. Urine: decreased output (developing acute tubular necrosis), reddish brown.

⋈ IV. Analysis/nursing diagnosis
   A. *Pain* related to tissue swelling and ischemia.
   B. *Risk for injury* related to neuromuscular deficits.
   C. *Impaired physical mobility* related to contracture and loss of function.
   D. *Risk for infection* related to tissue necrosis.
   E. *Altered urinary elimination* related to acute tubular necrosis resulting from myoglobin accumulation.
   F. *Body image disturbance* related to limb disfigurement.

⋈ V. Nursing care plan/implementation
   A. Goal: *recognize early indications of ischemia.*
      1. Assess neurovascular status frequently (q1h): skin temperature, capillary refill, peripheral pulses, mobility, and sensation.
      2. Listen to patient complaints, report suspected complications.
      3. Report nonrelief of pain with narcotics.
      4. Recognize unrelenting pain with passive muscle stretching.
   B. Goal: *prevent complications.*
      1. Position. *elevate* injured extremity initially; if ischemia suspected, keep extremity at heart level to prevent compensatory increase in blood flow.
      2. *Avoid tight* bandages, splints, or casts.
      3. Monitor intravenous infusion for signs of infiltration.
      4. Prepare patient for *fasciotomy* (incision of skin and fascia to release tight compartment).

VI. Evaluation/outcome criteria
  A. Relief from pain, normal perfusion restored.
  B. Neurovascular status within normal limits.
  C. Retains function of limb, no contractures or infection.
  D. Compartment pressure returns to normal (<20 mm Hg).
  E. No systemic complications (e.g., normal cardiac and renal function, acid-base balance within normal limits).

Immobility

Impaired physical mobility or limitation of physical movement resulting from various causes that may be accompanied by many complications that can involve any or all of the major systems of the body. The complications are summarized in Table 20.5.

  I. Types of immobility:
  A. *Physical*—caused by limitation in physical movement or physiologic processes (e.g., breathing).
  B. *Intellectual*—caused by lack of knowledge (e.g., mental retardation, brain damage).
  C. *Emotional*—caused by highly stressed situations (e.g., after loss of loved person, diagnosis of terminal illness).
  D. *Social*—occurring when social interaction decreased due to separation from family when hospitalized or alone, as in old age.
  II. Risk factors:
  A. Pain, trauma, injury.
  B. Loss of body function or body part.
  C. Chronic disease.
  D. Emotional, mental illness; neglect.
  E. Malnutrition.
  F. Bed rest, traction, surgery, medications.
  III. Assessment
  A. *Subjective data: psychological/social effects* of immobility:
    1. Decreased motivation to learn, retention.
    2. Decreased problem-solving abilities.
    3. Diminished drives, hunger.
    4. Changes in body image, self-concept.
    5. Exaggerated emotional reactions, inappropriate to situation or person; aggression, apathy, withdrawal.
    6. Deterioration of time perception.
    7. Fear, anxiety, worthlessness related to change in role activities (e.g., when no longer employed).
  B. *Objective data: physical effects* of immobility:
    1. *Cardiovascular:*
      a. Orthostatic hypotension.
      b. Increased cardiac load.
      c. Thrombus formation.
    2. *Gastrointestinal:*
      a. Anorexia.
      b. Diarrhea.
      c. Constipation.

  3. *Metabolic:*
    a. Tissue atrophy and protein catabolism.
    b. Basal metabolic rate reduced.
    c. Fluid/electrolyte imbalances.
  4. *Musculoskeletal:*
    a. Demineralization (osteoporosis).
    b. Contractures and atrophy.
    c. Skin breakdown.
  5. *Respiratory:*
    a. Decreased respiratory movement.
    b. Accumulation of secretions in respiratory tract.
    c. Oxygen/carbon dioxide level imbalance.
  6. *Urinary:*
    a. Calculi.
    b. Bladder distention, stasis.
    c. Infection.
    d. Frequency.
  IV. Analysis/nursing diagnosis
  A. *Impaired physical mobility* related to specific patient condition.
  B. *Impaired skin integrity* related to physical immobilization.
  C. *Urinary retention* related to incomplete emptying of bladder.
  D. *Constipation* related to inactivity.
  E. *Risk for disuse syndrome* related to lack of ROM.
  F. *Bathing/hygiene self-care deficit* related to musculoskeletal impairment.
  G. *Sensory/perceptual alteration* related to complications of immobility.
  H. *Body image disturbance* related to physical limitations.
  V. Nursing care plan/implementation
  A. Goal: *prevent physical, psychological hazards.*
    1. Apply nursing measures to promote venous flow, muscle strength, endurance, joint mobility, skin integrity.
    2. Assess and counteract *psychological* effect of immobility (e.g., feelings of helplessness, hopelessness, powerlessness).
    3. Help maintain accurate sensory processing to prevent or lessen *sensory disturbances.*
    4. Help adapt to *altered body image* due to increased dependency, sensory deprivation, changes in status and power that accompany immobility.
    5. Offer counseling when sexual expression is impaired.
  B. Goal: **health teaching:** ways to prevent physical problems related to immobility (e.g., anticonstipation diet, ROM exercises, skin care); teach activities that encourage independence and provide sensory stimulation while immobile.
  VI. Evaluation/outcome criteria
  A. Minimal contractures, skin breakdown, muscle atrophy or loss of strength.
  B. Interest in self and environment, positive self-image.
  C. Returns to optimal level of physical activity.

TABLE 20.5 COMPLICATIONS OF IMMOBILIZATION

Disorder	Pathophysiology	▨ Assessment	▨ Analysis/Nursing Diagnosis	▨ Nursing Care Plan/ Implementation	▨ Evaluation/ Outcome Criteria
ORTHOSTATIC HYPOTENSION	A decrease in BP >30/15 mm Hg caused by failure of vasomotor responses to compensate for change from a recumbent to an upright position.	*Subjective data:* weakness, dizziness. *Objective data:* decreased BP >30/15 mm Hg measured 2 min after moving from a supine to a sitting or standing position; loss of muscle tone and strength; patient may faint.	*Decreased cardiac output* related to orthostatic hypotension. *Risk for injury* related to vertigo. *Activity intolerance,* related to dizziness.	*Prevent trauma due to sudden decrease in BP:* 1. Change position gradually. 2. Elastic stockings. 3. Leg exercises. 4. Dangle before getting up. 5. Tilt table. 6. Sitting and lying BP. 7. Monitor side effects of drugs. **Health teaching:** 1. Explain signs and symptoms to patient. 2. Encourage patient to dangle before standing. 3. Encourage slow movement from sitting to standing. 4. Exercises to maintain muscle tone.	Patient tolerates increased activity. No trauma occurs. BP remains within normal limits.
CARDIAC OVERLOAD	When the body is recumbent, some of the total blood volume that would be in the legs due to gravity is redistributed to other parts of the body, thereby increasing the circulating volume and increasing the workload of the heart; heart rate, which is decreased because blood is prevented from entering the thoracic vessels by pressure from the *Valsalva maneuver,* increases when normal breathing resumes.	*Subjective data:* fear, apprehension. *Objective data: Valsalva maneuver* (pressure against the closed glottis when breath is held) 10–20 times/h, when trying to move in bed; tachycardia; decreased exercise tolerance.	*Risk for injury* related to increased workload of heart. *Activity intolerance* related to increased workload of heart. *Fear* related to tachycardia.	*Prevent injury and further ischemic damage to cardiac tissue by decreasing workload of heart:* 1. Out of bed in chair when possible. 2. *Semirecumbent position* when in bed; pillows between legs when side-lying. 3. Exercises: passive and active ROM, isometric. 4. Encourage participation in self-care. 5. Turn every 2 h, dangle. 6. *Avoid* Valsalva maneuver, fatigue. 7. Minimize constipation. 8. Encourage slow, deep breathing when moving in bed. **Health teaching:** 1. Exhale while turning, don't hold breath. 2. Measures to conserve energy.	No complications noted. Patient tolerates increased activity. Heart rate within normal limits.

(continued)

	Assessment	Nursing diagnosis	Nursing interventions	Evaluation
THROMBUS FORMATION—Mass of blood constituents formed in the heart or blood vessels due to pooling of blood from lack of activity; increased viscosity related to dehydration or possible external pressure.	*Subjective data:* discomfort over involved vessel. *Objective data:* increased [RBC, venous stasis, hypercoagulability.]	*Altered peripheral tissue perfusion* related to obstructed vessel. *Risk for injury* related to emboli.	*Prevent injury by reducing risk factors and venous stasis:* 1. *Position:* change q1–2h. 2. Do *not* gatch bed (causes pressure against leg vessels). 3. *Increase fluid* intake. 4. Monitor coagulation lab values. 5. *Medications: anticoagulation* therapy, as prescribed for patients at risk (immobilized, trauma, low pelvic surgery). 6. Ambulate as soon as possible. **Health teaching:** 1. How to recognize signs of thrombophlebitis/thromboemboli. 2. Leg exercise program to strengthen muscles for improved tone, to prevent pooling of blood in vessels. 3. Precautions necessary when on anticoagulation therapy. 4. Side effects of anticoagulation therapy (bleeding from gums, body fluids, obvious bleeding).	No respiratory complications or excess secretions noted.
RESPIRATORY CONGESTION—decreased respiratory movements. Decreased thoracic movement due to restriction against bed or chair, lack of position change, restrictive clothing or binders/bandages, or abdominal distention.	*Subjective data:* dyspnea, pain. *Objective data:* immobilization of thorax or abdomen, due to position in bed; inability to cough or deep breathe; abdominal distention.	*Ineffective breathing pattern* related to splinting to reduce pain. *Ineffective airway clearance* related to retained secretions. *Impaired physical mobility* related to trauma.	*Prevent complications related to respiratory status:* 1. Maintain a clear airway, assist with *ventilation* prn. 2. Remove or minimize causes of dyspnea. 3. Conserve patient's energy (periods of rest and activity—patient able to cough more effectively when rested). 4. Incentive spirometry. *Promote comfort:* 1. Maintain hydration and nutrition. 2. *Position:* change q2h, out of bed in chair when possible (chest expansion greater when sitting in chair).	

(continued)

TABLE 20.5   COMPLICATIONS OF IMMOBILIZATION (Continued)

Disorder	Pathophysiology	⋈ Assessment	⋈ Analysis/Nursing Diagnosis	⋈ Nursing Care Plan/ Implementation	⋈ Evaluation/ Outcome Criteria
RESPIRATORY CONGESTION (continued)				**Health teaching:** 1. Methods to allay anxieties precipitated by dyspnea. 2. Effective breathing and coughing exercises.	
RESPIRATORY CONGESTION— pooled secretions.	Inability of cilia to move normal secretions out of bronchial tree due to ineffective coughing, lack of thoracic expansion, or effects of medications.	Subjective data: dyspnea, pain. Objective data: dehydration; drugs—anticholinergic, CNS depressants; anesthesia; inadequate coughing; stationary position.	Ineffective airway clearance related to pooled secretions. Impaired gas exchange related to ineffective coughing.	Prevent atelectasis, infection, stasis of air and secretions in lungs: 1. Maintain patent airway, cough, suction, change position. 2. See nursing care plan for Respiratory congestion related to decreased respiratory movements, p. 233. **Health teaching:** 1. Effective coughing techniques. 2. Importance of adequate hydration.	No respiratory complications. Patient coughs and removes secretions.
OXYGEN–CARBON DIOXIDE IMBALANCE	Imbalance in oxygen and carbon dioxide levels related to pulmonary congestion, ineffective breathing patterns, trauma, or effects of medications.	Subjective data: confusion, irritable, restless, dyspnea. Objective data: hypoxia, hypercapnia, cyanosis.	Impaired gas exchange related to immobilization.	Promote improved respirations: 1. Change position frequently. 2. Increase humidification. 3. Monitor side effects of administered medication, especially narcotics, barbiturates. 4. See nursing care plan for: Respiratory congestion related to decreased respiratory movements, p. 233.	No respiratory complications. Respiratory rate and depth are adequate for maintaining balance of oxygen and carbon dioxide.

(continued)

MALNUTRITION of immobilized adult.				No complications. Patient obtains/maintains normal weight. No tissue breakdown.

Lack of adequate dietary intake to maintain healthy tissue related to lack of food; lack of knowledge about food; problems with ingestion, digestion, or absorption; psychosocial factors that influence patient's motivation to eat.

Subjective data: anorexia, nausea; diet history validating lack of adequate nutritional intake; mental irritability.

Objective data:

1. Recent weight loss of >10%.
2. *Decreased:* healing ability, GI motility, absorption, secretion of digestive enzymes.
3. *Appearance:* listlessness, muscle weakness; posture—sagging shoulders, sunken chest.
4. Anthropometric data (measurement of size, weight, and body proportions) <85% of standard.
5. *Cardiovascular:* tachycardia (>100 beats/min) on minimal exertion; bradycardia at rest.
6. *Hair:* brittle, dry, thin.
7. *Skin:* dry, scaly.
8. Lack of financial resources: sociocultural influences.

9. *Decreased* blood values: serum albumin, ironbinding capacity, lymphocyte levels, hematocrit, and hemoglobin.

Altered nutrition, less than body requirements, related to decreased appetite.
Knowledge deficit related to nutrition requirements.

Improved nutritional intake to maintain basal metabolism requirements and replace losses from catabolism:

1. Provide balanced or prescribed diet, soft or ground food if cannot chew or is edentulous.
2. *Increase fluid* intake.
3. Attain/maintain normal weight.
4. Feed, assist with feeding, or place foods within patient's reach.

Promote comfort:

1. Mouth care: to facilitate mastication of food → improved digestion and absorption.
2. Relieve constipation (see nursing care plan for: Constipation, p. 236).
3. Observe for stomatitis; bleeding; changes in skin texture, color.
4. Medications: monitor nausea and vomiting side effects of prescribed medications; administer *antiemetics* as ordered to control nausea and vomiting.
5. Ambulate to alleviate flatulence and distention.
6. Alleviate pain and discomfort by providing distractions, increased social interactions, pleasant environment, backrubs; administering pain medications prn, as ordered.

Health teaching:

1. Diet and elimination.
2. See Appendix B for foods high in *protein* and *carbohydrate.*

(continued)

TABLE 20.5   COMPLICATIONS OF IMMOBILIZATION (Continued)

Disorder	Pathophysiology	⊠ Assessment	⊠ Analysis/Nursing Diagnosis	⊠ Nursing Care Plan/Implementation	⊠ Evaluation/Outcome Criteria
CONSTIPATION	Waste material in the bowel is too hard to pass easily, or bowel movements are so infrequent that patient has discomfort.	*Subjective data:* discomfort, pain, distress, pressure in the rectum; reported decrease in normal elimination pattern. *Objective data:* immobilization; hard-formed stool, possible palpable impaction; decreased bowel sounds; bowel elimination less frequent than usual.	*Constipation* related to decreased water and fiber intake. *Knowledge deficit* related to dietary and exercise requirements to prevent constipation.	*Promote normal pattern of bowel elimination:* 1. Administer: *stool softeners* or bulk *cathartics* as ordered; oil retention, soap suds *enemas* as ordered. 2. Encourage change of position and activity as tolerated. 3. Provide *high-bulk* diet. 4. *Increase fluid* intake. 5. Provide for privacy. 6. Encourage regular time for evacuation. **Health teaching:** 1. Dietary instructions regarding increased fiber. 2. Exercise program as tolerated. 3. Increase fluids.	Patient has normal bowel elimination pattern. No impactions. Increases fluid and fiber in diet.
OSTEOPOROSIS	Metabolic bone disorder in which there is a generalized loss of bone density due to an imbalance between bone formation and bone resorption; immobilization can cause calcium losses of 200–300 mg/d.	*Subjective data:* backache. *Objective data:* demineralization of bone seen on ⎍ x-ray; kyphosis; spontaneous fracture of bone.	*Pain* related to bone fractures or body structural changes.	*Prevent injury related to decreased bone strength:* 1. *Position:* correct body alignment, firm mattress. 2. Encourage self-care activities: plan maximal activity allowed by physical condition, muscle exercises against resistance as tolerated. 3. Rest/activity pattern: encourage ROM exercise, *avoid* fatigue. 4. Weight-bearing positions, tilt table. 5. *Diet:* high protein, vitamin C, calcium. 6. *Increase fluids* to prevent renal calculi (calcium from bones could cause kidney stones). **Health teaching:** 1. Dietary instructions, foods to include for high-protein, high-vitamin C, high-calcium diet. 2. Exercise program. 3. Signs and symptoms of renal calculi.	No fractures. No renal calculi. Incorporates dietary improvements in daily menu selection. Participates in exercise program on a regular basis.

(continued)

		Subjective/Objective data	Nursing diagnosis	Interventions	Outcomes
CONTRACTURES	Abnormal shortening of muscle tissue, rendering the muscle highly resistant to stretching; related to lack of active or passive ROM, or improper support and positioning of joints affected by arthritis or injury.	*Subjective data:* pain. *Objective data:* muscles—fixed, shortened, decreased tone; resistance of muscles to stretch; decreased ROM in affected limb.	*Impaired physical mobility* related to muscle weakness and contractures. *Pain* related to injury. *Self-care deficit* related to immobility.	*Prevent deformities:* 1. Active and/or passive ROM exercises. 2. *Position:* functional, correct alignment. 3. Footboard to prevent foot-drop. 4. *Avoid* knee gatch. **Health teaching:** 1. Importance of ROM exercises. 2. Correct anatomic positions.	ROM maintained. No deformities noted.
SKIN BREAKDOWN	Presence of risk factors that could lead to skin breakdown, (e.g., immobility, inadequate nutrition, lack of position changes).	*Subjective data:* fatigue, pain, inability to turn on own. *Objective data:* interruption of skin integrity, especially over ears, occiput, heels, sacrum, scrotum, elbows, trochanter, ischium, scapula; immobilization; malnutrition.	*Impaired skin integrity* related to lack of frequent position change.	*Prevent skin breakdown:* 1. Change position q1–2h and prn, out of bed when possible. 2. Protect from infection. 3. Increase dietary intake: *protein, carbohydrates.* 4. *Increase fluids.* *Assess for/reduce contributing factors known to cause decubitus ulcers:* incontinence, stationary position, malnutrition, obesity, sensory deficits, emotional disturbances, paralysis. *Promote healing:* 1. Wash gently, pat dry—to prevent skin abrasion. 2. Clean, dry, wrinkle-free bed linens and pads. 3. Massage skin with lotion that does *not* contain alcohol (alcohol dries skin). 4. Protect with "wafer barrier," alternating mattress, sheepskin pads, protectors, flotation devices. 5. *No* "doughnuts" or rubber rings (interfere with circulation of tissue within center of ring).	No skin breakdown.

(continued)

TABLE 20.5   COMPLICATIONS OF IMMOBILIZATION (Continued)

Disorder	Pathophysiology	⋈ Assessment	⋈ Analysis/Nursing Diagnosis	⋈ Nursing Care Plan/ Implementation	⋈ Evaluation/ Outcome Criteria
URINARY STASIS	Immobility leads to inability to completely empty the bladder, which increases risk for urinary tract infection and renal calculi.	*Subjective data:* pain, due to infection or renal calculi. *Objective data:* difficulty in urinating due to position or lack of privacy; infection related to catheter insertion or stasis of urine; hematuria.	*Altered urinary elimination* related to inability to empty bladder.	*Prevent urinary infections, stasis, or renal calculi:* 1. Increase activity as allowed. ☞ 2. Check for distended bladder. 3. *Increase fluids,* I&O. ● 4. *Diet: acid ash* to increase acidity, thereby preventing infection. ☞ 5. *Avoid* catheterization; use intermittent catheterization instead of Foley whenever possible or *Credé maneuver to empty bladder* (manual exertion of pressure on the bladder to force urine out). ☞ 6. Bladder training.	No urinary tract infections or evidence of renal calculi. Bladder emptied, no urinary stasis.

BP = blood pressure; ROM = range of motion; RBC = red blood cell count; CNS = central nervous system; GI = gastrointestinal; I&O = intake and output.

Source: Lagerquist SL: *Little, Brown's NCLEX-RN Examination Review.* Boston: Little, Brown, 1996. P. 162–166.

Osteoarthritis

Joint disorder characterized by degeneration of articular cartilage and formation of bony outgrowths at edges of weight-bearing joints.

I. **Pathophysiology:** excessive friction combined with risk factors → thinning of articular cartilage, narrowing of joint space, and loss of joint stability; erosion of cartilage → formation of shallow pits on articular surface, exposure of bone in joint space. Bone responds by becoming denser and harder.

II. **Risk factors:**
   A. Aging (>50 yr).
   B. Rheumatoid arthritis.
   C. Arteriosclerosis.
   D. Obesity.
   E. Trauma.
   F. Family history.

III. **Assessment**
   A. *Subjective data:*
      1. Pain, tender joints.
      2. Fatigability, malaise.
      3. Anorexia.
      4. Cold intolerance.
      5. Extremities: numb, tingling.
   B. *Objective data:*
      1. *Joints:*
         a. Enlarged.
         b. Stiff, limited movement.
         c. Swelling, redness, heat around affected joint.
         d. Shiny stretched skin over and around joint.
         e. Subcutaneous nodules.
      2. Weight loss.
      3. Fever.
      4. Crepitation (creaking or grating of joints).
      5. Deformities, contractures.
      6. Cold, clammy extremities.
      7. Lab data: *decreased* hemoglobin, *elevated* white blood cell count (WBC).
      8. Diagnostic tests: X-ray studies, thermography, arthroscopy (see Diagnostic Studies Box).

IV. **Analysis/nursing diagnosis**
   A. *Pain* related to friction of bones in joints.
   B. *Bathing/hygiene self-care deficit* related to decreased mobility of involved joints.
   C. *Risk for injury* related to fatigue.
   D. *Impaired physical mobility* related to stiff, limited movement.
   E. *Impaired home maintenance management* related to contractures.

V. **Nursing care plan/implementation**
   A. Goal: *promote comfort: reduce pain, spasms, inflammation, swelling.*
      1. Medications as prescribed:
         a. *Anti-inflammatory* agents: aspirin (Ecotrin), ibuprofen (Motrin), indomethacin (Indocin), corticosteroids.
         b. *Antimalarials:* chloroquine (Aralen), HCl/ hydroxychloroquine (Plaquenil), to relieve symptoms.

   2. Heat to reduce muscle spasm.
   3. Cold to reduce swelling and pain.
   4. Prevent contractures:
      a. Exercise.
      b. Bed rest on firm mattress during attacks.
      c. Splints to maintain proper alignment.
   5. *Position: elevate* extremity to reduce swelling.
   6. Rest.
   7. Assistive devices to decrease weight bearing on affected joints (canes, walkers.)
   B. Goal: **health teaching** *to promote independence.*
      1. Encourage self-care with assistive devices for activities of daily living.
      2. Activity, as tolerated, with ambulation-assistive devices.
      3. Scheduled rest periods.
      4. Correct body posture and body mechanics.
   C. Goal: *provide for emotional needs.*
      1. Accept feelings of frustration regarding long-term debilitating disorder.
      2. Provide diversional activities appropriate for age and physical condition to promote comfort and satisfaction.

VI. **Evaluation/outcome criteria**
   A. Remains independent as long as possible.
   B. No contractures.
   C. States comfort has improved.
   D. Uses methods that are successfully control pain.

Total Hip Replacement

Femoral head and acetabulum are replaced by a prosthesis, which is cemented into the bone with plastic cement. Performed to replace a joint with limited and painful function due to bony alkalosis and deformity, caused by degenerative joint disease. Goal of the surgery: restore or improve mobilization of hip joint, prevent complications of extended immobilization.

I. **Risk factors:**
   A. Rheumatoid arthritis.
   B. Osteoarthritis.
   C. Complications of femoral neck fractures (Table 20.6).
   D. Congenital hip disease.

II. **Analysis/nursing diagnosis**
   A. *Risk for injury* related to implant surgery.
   B. *Knowledge deficit* regarding joint replacement surgery.
   C. *Impaired physical mobility* related to major hip surgery.
   D. *Pain* related to surgical incision.
   E. *Risk for impaired skin integrity* related to immobility.

III. **Nursing care plan/implementation**
   A. **Preoperative care:**
      1. Goal: *prevent thrombophlebitis and pulmonary emboli.*
         a. Antiembolic stockings.
         b. *Increase fluid intake.*

TABLE 20.6   TYPES OF HIP FRACTURES

Type	✉ *Assessment*	*Treatment*	*Complications*
Femoral neck (intracapsular)	History of slight trauma Pain in groin and hip Pain with hip movement Usually occurs in women >60 yr Lateral rotation and shortening of leg with minimal deformity	Femoral head replacement with prosthesis, threaded pins Occasionally, primary total hip replacement	Avascular necrosis of femoral head Nonunion Pin complications Dislocation of prosthesis
Intertrochanteric (extracapsular)	History of direct trauma over trochanter Severe pain Tenderness over trochanter Usually women 60–85 yr or younger women with osteoporosis External rotation and shortening of leg with obvious deformity Loss of hip motion	Open reduction: internal fixation with nail, pin, compression plate with screw	Shortening of the leg Traumatic arthritis Pin migration, bending or breaking of pin Fracture impaction Loss of reduction Delayed union or nonunion of bone
Subtrochanteric (extracapsular)	History of direct trauma of great force Proximal leg pain Usually women >60 yr External rotation and shortening of leg with some deformity Large hematoma	Open reduction: internal fixation with intramedullary nail, sliding nail plates, and other fixed plates Closed reduction with nail insertion Closed intramedullary device (nail)	Shortening of the leg, metal fatigue Lateral displacement of proximal fragment Metal fatigue

Source: Dunajcik L. The hip: Nursing fracture patients to full recovery. *RN* 1989; 52(4):56–71.

2. Goal: *prevent infection.*
   ▬ a. *Antiinfectives* as ordered, given prophylactically.
   ☞ b. Assist patient with skin scrubs using antibacterial soap.
⌂ 3. Goal: **health teaching.**
   a. *Isometric exercises*—gluteal, abdominal, and quadriceps-setting; dorsiflexion and plantar flexion of the feet.
   b. Use of trapeze.
   c. Explain position of operative leg and hip postoperatively to prevent *adduction* and flexion.
   d. Transfer techniques—bed to chair and chair to crutches; dangle at bedside first time out of bed.
B. **Postoperative care:**
  1. Goal: *prevent respiratory complications.*
   a. Turn, cough, deep breathe.
   ☞ b. Incentive spirometry.

2. Goal: *prevent complications of shock or infection.*
   ☞ a. Check dressings for drainage q1h for first 4 h, then q4h and prn; may have Hemovac or other drainage tubes inserted in wound to keep dressing dry.
   b. Monitor intake and output, vital signs hourly for 4 h, then q4h and prn.
☞ 3. Goal: *prevent contractures, muscle atrophy:* initiate exercises as soon as allowed: isometric quadriceps, dorsiflexion and plantar flexion of foot, flexion and extension of the ankle.
  4. Goal: *promote early ambulation and movement.*
   a. Use trapeze.
   ☞ b. Transfer technique (pivot on unaffected leg), crutches/walker.
   c. Initiate progressive ambulation as ordered, ensure maximum extension of leg when walking.

d. Administer *anticoagulants* as ordered to prevent thromboemboli.

e. Recognize early side effects of medications and report appropriately.

5. Goal: *prevent constipation.*

a. *Increase fluid* intake.

b. Use fracture bedpan.

6. Goal: *prevent dislocation of prosthesis.*

a. Maintain *abduction* of the affected joint (prevent external rotation); *elevate head of bed,* turn according to physician's order. When turning to unaffected side, turn with abduction pillow between legs to maintain abduction.

b. *Buck's* extension or *Russell's* traction may be applied (temporary skin traction).

c. *Plaster booties* with an abduction bar may be used.

d. Use wedge-shaped *Charnley pillow* to *maintain abduction* between knees and lower legs.

e. Provide periods throughout day when patient lies flat in bed to *prevent hip flexion* and strengthen hip muscles.

f. Report signs of dislocation: *anteriorly*— knee flexes, leg turns outward, leg looks longer than other, femur head may be felt in groin area; *posteriorly*—leg turns inward, appears shorter than other, greater trochanter elevated.

7. Goal: *promote comfort.*

a. Initiate skin care, monitor pressure points for redness; back care q2h.

b. Alternating pressure mattress, sheepskin when sitting in chair.

8. Goal: **health teaching.**

a. Exercise program with written list of activity restrictions.

b. Methods to prevent hip adduction.

c. *Avoid* sitting for more than 1 h; stand, stretch, and walk frequently to prevent hip flexion contractures.

d. Advise *not to exceed 90 degrees of hip flexion* (dislocation can occur, particularly with posterior incisions), *avoid* sitting in low chairs.

e. Teach alternative methods of usual self-care activities to prevent hip dislocation—e.g., *avoid* bending from waist to tie shoes, sitting up straight in a low chair, using a low toilet seat.

f. *Avoid:* crossing legs, driving a car for 6 wk.

g. Wear support hose for 6 wk to enhance venous return and prevent thrombus formation.

IV. Evaluation/outcome criteria

A. Participates in postoperative nursing care plan to prevent complications.

B. Reports pain has decreased.

C. Ambulates with assistive devices.

D. Complications of immobility prevented.

E. Able to resume self-care activities.

Total Knee Replacement

Both sides of the joint are replaced by metal or plastic implants.

I. Analysis: see Total Hip Replacement, p. 239.

II. Nursing plan/implementation

A. See Total Hip Replacement, p. 239.

B. Goal: *to achieve active flexion beyond 70 degrees.*

1. *Immediately postoperatively:* may have continuous passive motion (CPM) device for flexion/ extension of affected knee. Maximum flexion: 110 degrees.

2. Monitor drainage in *Hemovac:* q15min for first 4 h, q1h until 24 h, then q4h and prn.

3. *Analgesics,* as ordered.

4. While dressings are still on: *quadriceps-setting exercises* for approximately 5 d (consult with physical therapist for specific instructions).

5. After dressings removed: *active flexion exercises.*

6. *Avoid* pressure on heel.

III. Evaluation/outcome criteria

A. No complications of infection, hemorrhage noted.

B. ROM of knee increases with exercises.

Amputation

Surgical removal of a limb due to trauma or circulatory impairment (gangrene). The amount of tissue amputated is determined by the severity of disease or trauma and the ability of the remaining tissue to heal.

I. Risk factors:

A. Atherosclerosis obliterans.

B. Uncontrolled diabetes mellitus.

C. Malignancy.

D. Extensive and intractable infection.

E. Severe trauma.

II. Assessment—*preoperative:*

A. *Subjective data:* pain in affected part.

B. *Objective data:*

1. Soft-tissue damage.

2. Partial or complete severance of a body part.

3. Lack of peripheral pulses.

4. Skin color changes, pallor → cyanosis → gangrene.

5. Infection, hemorrhage, or shock.

III. Analysis/nursing diagnosis

A. *Impaired physical mobility* related to lower-limb amputation.

B. *Body image disturbance* related to loss of body part.

C. *Pain* related to interruption of nerve pathways.

D. *Anxiety* related to potential change in life-style.

E. *Knowledge deficit* related to rehabilitation goals.

IV. Nursing care plan/implementation

A. Goal: *prepare for surgery, physically and emotionally.*

1. Validate that patient and family are aware that amputation of body part is planned.
2. Validate that informed consent is signed.
3. Allow time for grieving.
4. If time allows, prepare patient for postoperative phase (e.g., teach arm-strengthening exercises if lower limb is to be amputated, teach altered methods of ambulation).
5. Provide time to discuss feelings.
☞ 6. Prepare surgical site to decrease possibility of infection (e.g., shave, scrub as ordered).
7. Discuss postoperative expectations.

B. Goal: *promote healing postoperatively.*

☞ 1. Monitor respiratory status q1–4h and prn: rate, depth of respiration; auscultate for signs of congestion; question patient about chest pain (pulmonary emboli common complication).
2. Monitor for hemorrhage, keep tourniquet at bedside, keep Ace wrap secure.
● 3. Medicate for pain as ordered—patient may have phantom pain.
4. Support stump on pillow for first 24 h to reduce edema, **remove pillow** after 24 h to prevent contracture.
5. *Position: turn patient onto stomach* to prevent hip contracture.
☞ 6. ROM exercises for joint above amputation to prevent joint immobilization; strengthening exercises for arms, unaffected limbs, abdominal muscles.
☞ 7. **Stump care:**
  a. Early postoperative dressings changed prn.
  b. As incision heals, bandage is applied in cone shape to prepare stump for prosthesis: prevent edema
  c. Inspect for blisters, redness, abrasions.
  d. Remove stump sock daily and prn.
8. Assist in rehabilitation program.
☞ 9. **Prosthesis care:**
  a. Clean socket with damp cloth to prevent infection
  b. Instruct to wear prosthesis when out of bed to prevent swelling
  c. Follow up appointment with prosthetist yearly.

⋈ **V. Evaluation/outcome criteria**
  A. Begins rehabilitation program.
  B. No hemorrhage, infection.
  C. Adjusts to altered body image.

Gout

Disorder of purine metabolism; genetic disease believed to be transmitted by a dominant gene, characterized by recurrent attacks of acute pain and swelling of one joint (usually the great toe).

I. Pathophysiology: urate crystals and infiltrating leukocytes appear to damage the intracellular phagolysosomes → leakage of lysomal enzymes into the synovial fluid → tissue damage, joint inflammation.

II. Risk factors:
  A. Men.
  B. Age (>50 yr).
  C. Genetic/familial tendency.
  D. Prolonged hyperuricemia (*elevated* serum uric acid level).

⋈ **III. Assessment**
  A. *Subjective data:*
    1. Pain: excruciating.
    2. Fatigue.
    3. Anorexia.
  B. *Objective data:*
    1. Joint: erythema (redness), hot, swollen, difficult to move; skin stretched and shiny over joint.
    2. Subcutaneous nodules, trophi (deposits of urate) on hands and feet.
    3. Weight loss.
    4. Fever.
    5. Sensory changes, with cold intolerance.
    6. Lab data:
      a. Serum uric acid; *increased significantly* (6.5/dL in females, 7.5/dL in males) in *chronic* gout; only *slightly increased* in *acute* gout.
      b. WBC: 12,000–15,000/mm^3.
      c. Erythrocyte sedimentation rate: >20 mm/h.
      d. 24-h urinary uric acid: *slightly elevated.*
      e. Proteinuria (*chronic* gout).
      f. Axotemia (presence of nitrogen-containing compounds in blood) in *chronic* gout.

⋈ **IV. Analysis/nursing diagnosis**
  A. *Pain* related to inflammation and swelling of affected joint.
  B. *Impaired physical mobility* related to pain.
  C. *Knowledge deficit* related to diet restrictions and increased fluid needs.
  D. *Altered urinary elimination* related to kidney damage.

⋈ **V. Nursing care plan/implementation**
  A. Goal: *decrease discomfort.*
  ● 1. Administer antigout medications as ordered:
    a. Treatment of *acute attacks:* colchicine, phenylbutazone (Butazolidin), indomethacin (Indocin), allopurinol (Zyloprim).
    b. *Preventive* therapy: probenecid (Benemid), sulfinpyrazone (Anturane).
  2. Absolute rest of affected joint, then gradual increase in activities, to prevent complications of immobilization; at the same time, rest for comfort.
  B. Goal: *prevent kidney damage.*
    1. *Increase fluid* intake to 2000–3000 mL/d.
    2. Monitor urinary output.
  ⌂ **C.** Goal: **health teaching.**
    ● 1. Need for *low-purine diet* during acute attack

🔑 Summary of Key Points

1. Impaired musculoskeletal function affects a patient's ability to perform basic activities of daily living.
2. A nursing priority in patients with many medical-surgical disorders includes maintaining the ROM of the affected joints.
3. The greatest risk associated with a fracture is not the break itself, but the potential for it to injure nerves, blood vessels, and muscles that surround it. *Bone infection* is another risk.
4. Traction is applied *continuously* unless the physician orders that it be intermittent. *Suspension traction* allows for more movement and activity than running (straight) traction.
5. Regardless of the type of traction, the nurse must regularly assess the *circulation* and *sensation* in and *motor* function of the limb (CSM).
6. The ability to bear weight after surgery for a hip fracture is determined by the fixation procedure used.
7. Dislocation is more common in patients with a prosthesis as compared to those with fixation using a pin, nail, or screw. Remember *abduction*, not adduction, should be employed because bringing the limb closer to the body or "adding" to the body causes dislocation.
8. There are *three types of arthritis*—rheumatoid, osteo, and gouty. The causes are all *different*. However, all *cause* pain and joint immobility, and all are improved with weight loss and treatment with anti-inflammatory agents.
9. Osteoarthritis does *not* entail the *systemic* involvement of rheumatoid arthritis.
10. The greatest concern after a total hip and knee replacement is *contractures*. Maintaining limb extension or continuous passive motion is done to prevent this.
11. The nursing priorities after an amputation are: preventing edema, observing for bleeding, and then preventing limb contractures.

(see Purine-restricted diet in Appendix B, p. 325).
  2. Importance of *increased fluid in diet.*
  3. Signs and symptoms of increased disease.
  4. Dosage and side effects of prescribed medications.
▶ **VI. Evaluation/outcome criteria**
  A. Swelling decreased.
  B. Discomfort alleviated.
  C. Mobility returned to status before attack.
  D. Lab values return to normal.

〰 Diagnostic Studies

● **Arthroscopy**—examination of a joint through a fiberoptic endoscope called an *arthroscope*. Usually done in the operating room (same-day surgery) under aseptic conditions using a local anesthetic, although a general anesthetic may be used. A tourniquet is applied to reduce blood flow to the area while the scope is introduced through a cannula. Saline is used as the viewing medium. Biopsy or removal of loose bodies from the joint may be done. A compression dressing (e.g., Ace bandage) is applied afterward. Restrictions vary according to surgeon preference and nature of procedure. Weight bearing may be immediate or restricted for 24 h. Teach patient to observe for signs of infection.

Magnetic Resonance Imaging (MRI)
Noninvasive, nonionic technique produces cross-sectional images by exposure to magnetic energy sources. Provides superior contrast of soft tissue, including healthy, benign, and malignant tissue, along with veins and arteries; utilizes no contrast medium; takes 30–90 min to complete; patient must *stay still* for periods of 5–20 min at a time. *Patient preparation:* patient can take food and medications, except when undergoing low abdominal and pelvic studies (food/fluids withheld 4–6 h to decrease peristalsis). *Restrictions:* patients who have metal implants, permanent pacemakers, or implanted medication pumps such as insulin, or who are pregnant or on life support systems. Obese patients may not be able to undergo full-body MRI because they may not fit in the scanner tunnel.

💡 Study and Memory Aids

Compartment Syndrome—Characteristics: "Five P's"

Pain
Pale color
Pulselessness
Paralysis
Paresthesias

(Modified from Rogers P: *The Medical Students' Guide to Top Board Scores.* Boston: Little, Brown, 1992.)

✂ Traction: Nursing Care Plan—
"TRACTION"

Trapeze bar overhead to raise and lower upper body
Requires free-hanging weights for body alignment
Analgesia for pain, prn
Circulation (check color and pulse)
Temperature (check extremity)
Infection prevention
Output (monitor)
Nutrition (alteration related to immobility)

Source: Modified from Zerwekh J D, et al. *Memory Notebook of Nursing.* Dallas: Nursing Education Consultants, 1994. p 100.

🍎 Diet

Fractures: Diet to Promote Healing

↑ Bulk
Fluid
Fruits
Iron
Protein
Vitamins

💊 Drug Review

Fractures

Analgesics
Acetaminophen/codeine (Tylenol #1, #2, #3): 1–2
tablets q3–4 h, as needed
Meperidine HCl (Demerol): IM or SC, 50–150 mg
Morphine sulfate: IM or SC, 5–20 mg
Oxycodone/acetaminophen (Tylox, Percocet): 5 mg
q3–6h, as needed
Anticoagulants
Aspirin: 1.3 g/daily in 2–4 divided doses
Heparin sodium: IV, 1000 U/h; SC, 8000–10,000 U
q8h, adjusted according to partial thromboplastin
time (PTT)
Warfarin (Coumadin): 10–15 mg/d adjusted
according to prothrombin time (PT)
Stool softeners: Docusate (Colace): 50–500 mg/d

Osteoarthritis

Anti-inflammatories
Aspirin (Ecotrin): 2.6–6.2 g/d in divided doses
Ibuprofen (Motrin): 300–800 mg 3–4 times daily,
not to exceed 3200 mg/d

Indomethacin (Indocin): 25–50 mg 2–4 times daily
Antimalarials
Chloroquine (Aralen): up to 2.4 mg/kg/d
Hydroxychloroquine (Plaquenil): maintenance dose
200–400 mg/day
Steroids (should *never* be abruptly discontinued;
gradually taper dosage to prevent complications)
Dexamethasone (Decadron): 0.5–9 mg/d in single
or divided doses
Methylprednisolone (Medrol): 4–48 mg/d
Prednisone: 5–60 mg/d

Total Joint Replacement

Analgesics
Acetaminophen/codeine (Tylenol #1, #2, #3): 1–2
tablets q3–4h, as needed
Meperidine HCl (Demerol): IM or SC, 50–150 mg
Morphine sulfate: IM or SC, 5–20 mg
Oxycodone/acetaminophen (Tylox, Percocet): 5 mg
q3–6h, as needed
Anticoagulants
Aspirin: 1.3 g/d in 2–4 divided doses
Heparin sodium: IV, 1000 U/h; SC, 8000–10,000 U
q8h, adjusted according to PTT
Warfarin (Coumadin): 10–15 mg/d, adjusted
according to PT

Amputation

Analgesics
Acetaminophen/codeine (Tylenol #1, #2, #3): 1–2
tablets q3–q4h, as needed
Meperidine HCl (Demerol): IM or SC, 50–150 mg
Morphine sulfate: IM or SC, 5–20 mg
Oxycodone/acetaminophen (Tylox, Percocet): 5 mg
q3–6h, as needed

Gout

Allopurinol (Zyloprim): 200–800 mg/d
Colchicine: acute—0.5 mg–2 mg injected IV over
several minutes, then 0.5–10 mg q 6h until relief
obtained; Total dose should not exceed 4 mg during
any 24-h period.
Prophylaxis, up to 1–1.8 mg/d
Probenecid (Benemid): 250 mg bid for one week;
increase to 500 mg bid. *Do not exceed* 3 g/d.
Sulfinpyrazone (Anturane): 100–200 mg bid; increase
to 800 mg/d in 2 divided doses

Questions

1. The nurse tells the patient that to minimize a patient's claustrophobia in an MRI scanner, the technician will:
   1. Leave him alone in the room.
   2. Keep the air flow in the scan room cool.
   3. Give him a "Walk-man" to listen to music.
   4. Ask the patient to keep his eyes open so that he can see the room.
2. The most important exercise for rebuilding hip muscles to teach a patient who has undergone total hip replacement is to:
   1. Press the knee firmly backward into the bed.
   2. Alternately adduct and abduct the hip.
   3. Ride a stationary bicycle 20 to 30 minutes a day.
   4. Do slow deep-knee bends while holding onto a rail.
3. In the immediate period after a total knee replacement, it would be a priority for the nurse to assess the patient's:
   1. Bowel sounds.
   2. Pedal pulses.
   3. Urine output.
   4. Gag reflex.
4. Which nursing diagnosis would it be most important to identify when preparing to discharge a patient who has undergone a total hip replacement?
   1. Risk for injury.
   2. Impaired adjustment.
   3. Sleep pattern disturbance.
   4. Impaired physical mobility.
5. A patient who has fractured the left foot will be using crutches until a walking cast is applied. When teaching the patient the correct technique for the three-point gait, the instructions would include:
   1. Advancing the left crutch, then the right foot, followed by the right crutch, then the left foot.
   2. Moving the left crutch and right foot forward together, then the right crutch and left foot.
   3. Advancing both crutches forward, then swinging both legs forward.
   4. Moving both crutches and the injured leg forward, then moving the other leg.
6. A patient fractured his femur 3 days ago. The nurse would recognize the signs and symptoms of a fat embolism if the patient experienced:
   1. Disorientation, dyspnea, and tachycardia.
   2. Petechiae over the chest and bradycardia.
   3. Pain, swelling, and redness in the extremity.
   4. Cyanosis and Cheyne-Stokes breathing.
7. A patient is temporarily placed in Buck's extension traction while awaiting surgery for a fractured hip. The nurse would recognize a complication of the treatment if the following was noted:
   1. Redness and drainage at the pin site.
   2. Dusky color of the toes of the affected leg.
   3. Flushed skin over the fracture site.
   4. Dorsiflexion of the affected foot.
8. The nurse can tell a patient with degenerative joint disease that the most frequent side effect of the ibuprofen often used in its treatment can be minimized by:
   1. Taking the drug with meals.
   2. Drinking cranberry juice.
   3. Taking the drug at regular intervals.
   4. Taking the drug before meals.
9. During an acute flare-up of osteoarthritis, the patient should be advised to:
   1. Immobilize the affected joints.
   2. Continue passive range-of-motion exercises.
   3. Decrease the doses of prescribed medications.
   4. Stay out of the sun.
10. After removal of the dressing on a below-the-knee amputation, the nurse would wash the well-healed stump with:
    1. Soap and water.
    2. Lotion and water.
    3. Dilute hydrogen peroxide.
    4. Betadine solution.
11. Correct instructions on the use of a cane would include the importance of:
    1. Holding the cane on the same side as the affected leg.
    2. Moving the cane and the unaffected leg in unison.
    3. Using the cane on the side opposite the affected leg.
    4. Keeping the elbow flexed while bearing weight on the hand grip.
12. The nurse can explain to the patient that the purpose of wrapping an above-the-knee amputation with an elastic bandage 10 days after surgery is to:
    1. Promote muscle relaxation and comfort.
    2. Shape the stump in preparation for the prosthesis.
    3. Reduce edema in the thigh.
    4. Prevent bleeding from the incision.
13. A patient with osteoarthritis asks the nurse why she is not receiving prednisone as her friend with arthritis is. The best response for the nurse to make is that:
    1. Orally administered prednisone is not indicated for the treatment of osteoarthritis.
    2. Addiction to the drug is likely to occur.
    3. Weight gain is a side effect, and this may worsen her condition.
    4. Her friend's treatment is irrelevant.
14. Which crutch-walking gait should the nurse teach a patient who cannot put any weight on the affected leg?
    1. Two-point.
    2. Three-point.
    3. Four-point.
    4. Swing-through.

Answers/Rationale

1. **(2)** A patient undergoing MRI scanning must be able to tolerate very close surroundings. Keeping the room

---

Key to Codes

Nursing process: AS, assessment; **AN,** analysis; **PL,** planning; **IMP,** implementation; **EV,** evaluation. (See Appendix M for explanation of nursing process steps.)

Category of human function: 1, protective; **2,** sensory-perceptual; **3,** comfort, rest, activity, and mobility; **4,** nutrition; **5,** growth and development; **6,** fluid-gas transport; **7,** psychosocial-cultural; **8,** elimination. (See Appendix O for explanation.)

Client need: SECE, safe, effective care environment; **PhI,** physiologic integrity; **PsI,** psychosocial integrity; **HPM,** health promotion/maintenance. (See Appendix P for explanation.)

cool often helps reduce the closed-in feeling. Leaving the patient alone (**1**) may increase the feeling of claustrophobia. Talking to the technologist may help distract the patient from the claustrophobia during the procedure. *No metal,* such as that in a radio headset (**3**), can be in the area, or it may be pulled into the powerful magnet. Closing the eyes, *not* keeping them open (**4**), may help to decrease the patient's sense of closeness. **IMP, 3, SECE**

2. (**1**)   Pressing the knee firmly backward into the bed strengthens the quadriceps. Any exercise that involves adduction (**2**) or acute flexion of the hip (**3 and 4**) may cause the prosthesis to dislocate. **IMP, 3, PhI**

3. (**2**)   Pedal pulses, as well as skin color, capillary refill, warmth, movement, sensation, and ability to dorsiplantar flex the foot, are all assessment priorities, because the circulatory, sensory, and motor status of the operated limb is of the greatest importance to the success of the procedure. Bowel sounds (**1**), urine output (**3**), and the gag reflex (**4**) are all affected by general anesthesia and need to be assessed, but they are *not* as much of a priority. **AS, 3, PhI**

4. (**1**)   The priority in such a patient is to prevent injury. The ability to ambulate, get into and out of bed, and sit and stand without dislocating the prosthesis or falling must be determined before discharge. Problems adjusting (**2**) or sleeping (**3**) are not expected problems in such a patient. If they are present at discharge, they would probably only become a serious concern if they were prolonged. Immobility (**4**) would also be a concern at discharge, but the risk for injury as a result of the immobility would be a *more specific choice.* **AN, 3, SECE**

5. (**4**)   Moving both crutches is the first point; moving the injured leg is the second point; and moving the good leg is the third point. The other three options are the three other common types of crutch gaits: the four-point gait (**1**), the two-point gait (**2**), and the swing-through gait (**3**). **IMP, 3, SECE**

6. (**1**)   Fat emboli form when fat droplets are forced into the systemic circulation as pressure changes occur in the interior of the fracture; this causes pulmonary effusion and defective gas exchange, resulting in the signs and symptoms of hypoxia and tissue death. Petechiae (**2**) would be present, but *not* bradycardia. The fractured limb (**3**) would *not* be *directly* affected by the emboli. Cyanosis (**4**) would be present, but *not* Cheyne-Stokes breathing, which is an irregular breathing pattern often seen in elderly or head-injured patients. **AS, 3, PhI**

7. (**2**)   Buck's traction involves skin traction, and if it is too tight, there would be indications of circulatory impairment. There are *no pins* (**1**) with skin traction. Skin traction is usually applied distal to the fracture site, so there would be *no visible changes* at the site (**3**). If there were a problem with the foot position, it might be plantar flexion (foot drop), but *not dorsiflexion* (**4**). **AN, 3, PhI**

8. (**1**)   Taking the drug with food will minimize the gastrointestinal (GI) tract irritation that is a side effect of ibuprofen because the food protects the GI mucosa.

Another less common side effect is renal toxicity. Drinking cranberry juice (**2**) would be part of the treatment for *urinary* tract infection to make the urine more acidic. It is important to take most medication at a regular interval (**3**), but this does *not prevent* side effects. Taking it before meals (**4**) would *not minimize* the GI distress. **IMP, 3, PhI**

9. (**2**)   To preserve joint function even during a flare-up, the joint must be exercised. Pain medication should be taken before passive exercise, however. Osteoarthritis is the most common form of arthritis. Joint rest is important, but complete immobilization (**1**) would *contribute* to joint immobility. The doses of medications would more likely be *increased* than decreased (**3**). Avoiding sunlight (**4**) is called for in a patient with *systemic lupus erythematosus* who has joint pain. **IMP, 3, PhI**

10. (**1**)   No special cleansing agents are used, just soap and water. Lotion and water (**2**) may be used if there is dry skin. Hydrogen peroxide (**3**) is used as a wound antiseptic. Betadine (**4**) is used to clean the skin before invasive procedures. **IMP, 3, PhI**

11. (**3**)   The cane is used on the side *opposite* the affected leg providing better balance and support. It should *not* be used on the *same* side as the affected leg (**1**). The affected leg, *not* the unaffected leg (**2**), moves with the cane, and the weight is placed on the unaffected leg. The cane needs to be long enough to allow for elbow extension, *not* flexion (**4**). **IMP, 3, SECE**

12. (**2**)   The purpose of wrapping the stump changes during the postoperative period. The shape of the stump is now important to ensure the proper fit of the prosthesis. A change in the patient's position in bed and sitting in a chair would prevent contractures and increase comfort (**1**); a *bandage would not.* Elevation and wrapping would have been done to relieve edema (**3**) and minimize bleeding (**4**) in the *early* postoperative period. **PL, 3, PhI**

13. (**1**)   Orally administered steroids are not indicated for the treatment of osteoarthritis, which is *not a systemic* condition. The drug of choice for the relief of arthralgia and joint inflammation is *aspirin,* although a steroid may be injected locally. (The friend may have rheumatoid arthritis, which is a *systemic, autoimmune condition.*) Addiction (**2**) is *not* a concern with steroids. Weight gain (**3**) is a side effect of steroids and would aggravate the osteoarthritis, but that is *not the particular reason* it is not used. The response in option **4** does *not answer* the patient's question of why the treatment is different. **IMP, 3, PhI**

14. (**4**)   In the swing-through crutch gait, the weight is either on the unaffected limb or on both crutches, never on the affected limb. In the two-point gait (**1**), there is some weight placed bilaterally as the patient moves a crutch and the opposite limb together; however, most of the weight is on the crutch. In the three-point gait (**2**) there is partial weight bearing on both legs, but if necessary, there could be no weight on the affected leg. The four-point gait (**3**) involves weight bearing on both limbs, because the crutches and the limbs move independently. **IMP, 3, SECE**

Neurologic Disorders

Chapter Outline

Aphasia

Impaired ability to understand or use commonly accepted words or symbols; interferes with ability to speak, write, and/or read; usually occurs with right-sided hemiplegia in a cerebrovascular accident.

I. Types and pathophysiology:
A. *Receptive (sensory)*—lesion usually in Wernicke's area of temporal lobe; difficulty understanding spoken word (*auditory* aphasia) or written word (*visual* aphasia).
B. *Expressive (motor)*—lesion usually in Broca's area of frontal lobe; difficulty expressing thoughts in speech or writing (*motor* aphasia).

II. Risk factors:
A. Vascular disease of the brain (cerebrovascular accident).
B. Alzheimer's disease.
C. Sickle cell anemia.

✉ III. Analysis/nursing diagnosis
A. *Impaired verbal communication* related to cerebral cortex disorder.
B. *Powerlessness* related to inability to express needs/concerns.
C. *Impaired social interaction* related to difficulty communicating.

✉ IV. Nursing care plan/implementation: Goal: *assist with communication.*
A. Assess comprehension: use simple requests, write questions or use picture cards.
B. Stand on patient's unaffected side (stay within patient's visual field).
C. Talk slowly, clearly; do *not* shout or "talk down" (there is *no* intellectual impairment).
D. Use short, simple phrases; repeat words; ask questions needing one-word answers.
E. Use alternative ways to communicate: hand gestures, picture cards.
F. *Avoid* frustration for patient: do *not* force patient to repeat words, allow ample time to respond, anticipate needs.
G. Respond to patient's speech; if do not understand, tell patient; encourage patient to use other words.
H. Reinforce techniques taught by speech therapist.
I. Maintain one-way communication: receptive aphasia does *not* always accompany expressive aphasia.

✉ V. Evaluation/outcome criteria
A. Communication reestablished.
B. Minimal frustration exhibited.
C. Participates in speech therapy.

Traumatic Injuries to the Brain

I. Types:
  A. *Concussion*—transient disorder due to injury in which there is brief loss of consciousness due to paralysis of neuronal function; recovery is usually total.
  B. *Contusion*—structural alteration of brain tissue characterized by extravasation of blood cells (bruising); injury may occur on side of impact or on opposite side (when cranial contents shift forcibly within the skull with impact).
  C. *Laceration*—tearing of brain tissue or blood vessels caused by a sharp bone fragment or object or a tearing force.
  D. *Hematomas:*
    1. *Subdural*—blood from ruptured or torn vein collects between arachnoid and dura mater; may be acute, subacute, or chronic.
    2. *Extradural* (epidural)—blood clot located between dura mater and inner surface of skull; most often results from tearing of middle meningeal artery; **emergency condition.**

II. Pathophysiology of impaired central nervous system (CNS) functioning:
  A. Depressed neuronal activity in reticular activating system → depressed *consciousness* (Table 21.1).
  B. Depressed neuronal functioning in lower brain stem and spinal cord → depression of reflex activity → decreased eye movements, unequal pupils → decreased response to light stimuli → widely dilated and fixed *pupils.*
  C. Depression of respiratory center → altered respiratory pattern → decreased rate → *respiratory arrest.*

III. Risk factors: accidents—automobile, industrial and home, motorcycle, military.

◄ IV. Assessment
  A. *Subjective data:*
    1. Headache.
    2. Dizziness, loss of balance.
    3. Double vision.
    4. Nausea.
  B. *Objective data:*
    1. Laceration or abrasion around face or head; scalp vascular, *bloody* appearance with minor injuries.
    2. Drainage from ears or nose.
    3. Projectile vomiting, hematemesis.
    4. Vital signs indicating increased intracranial pressure (ICP) (see Increased Intracranial Pressure, p. 249).
    5. Neurologic:
      a. *Altered level of consciousness;* a numerical assessment, such as the *Glasgow Coma Scale* (Table 21.2), may be used. Generally, the lower the score, the poorer the prognosis.

TABLE 21.1	LEVELS OF CONSCIOUSNESS
Stage	*Characteristics*
Alertness	Aware of time and place
Automatism	Aware of time and place but demonstrates abnormal mood (euphoria to irritability)
Confusion	Inability to think and speak in coherent manner; responds to verbal requests but is unaware of time and place
Delirium	Restlessness and violent activity; may not comply with verbal instructions
Stupor	Quiet and uncommunicative; may appear conscious—sits or lies with glazed look; unable to respond to verbal instructions; bladder and rectal incontinence may occur
Semicoma	Unresponsive to verbal instructions but responds to vigorous or painful stimuli
Coma	Unresponsive to vigorous or painful stimuli

TABLE 21.2	GLASGOW COMA SCALE	
Best eye-opening responsive	Purposeful and spontaneous	4
	To voice	3
	To pain	2
	No response	1
	Untestable	U
Best verbal response	Oriented	5
	Disoriented	4
	Inappropriate words	3
	Incomprehensible sounds	2
	No response	1
	Untestable	U
Best motor response	Obeys commands	6
	Localizes pain	5
	Withdraws to pain	4
	Flexion to pain	3
	Extension to pain	2
	No response	1
	Untestable	U

b. *Pupils*—equal, round, react to light, *or* unequal, dilated, unresponsive to light.
c. *Extremities*—paresis or paralysis.
d. *Reflexes*—hypo- or hypertonia; *Babinski* present (flaring of great toe when sole is stroked).
e. See Diagnostic Studies Box, p. 254.

V. Analysis/nursing diagnosis
A. *Altered thought processes* related to brain trauma.
B. *Sensory/perceptual alteration* related to depressed neuronal activity.
C. *Risk for injury* related to impaired CNS functioning.
D. *Risk for aspiration* related to respiratory depression.
E. *Self-care deficit* related to altered level of consciousness.
F. *Risk for disuse syndrome* related to paresis or paralysis.

VI. Nursing care plan/implementation
A. Goal: *sustain vital functions and minimize or prevent complications.*
1. Patent airway: *endotracheal* tube or tracheostomy may be ordered.
2. *Oxygen:* as ordered (because hypoxia increases cerebral edema).
3. *Position:* semiprone or prone (*coma* position) with head level to prevent aspiration (*keep off back*); turn side to side to prevent stasis in lungs (see Positioning Box).
4. Vital signs as ordered.
5. *Neurologic check:* pupils, level of consciousness, muscle strength; report changes.
6. *Seizure precautions:* padded siderails.
7. Medications, as ordered:
  a. *Steroids* (dexamethasone [Decadron]).
  b. *Anticonvulsants* (phenytoin [Dilantin], phenobarbital).
  c. *Analgesics* (**morphine contraindicated**).
8. Cooling measures or hypothermia to reduce elevated temperature.
9. Assist with diagnostic tests:

a. *Lumbar puncture* (*contraindicated* with increased ICP).
b. *Electroencephalogram* (EEG).
10. *Diet:* NPO for 24 h, progressing to clear liquids if awake.
11. Fluids: IVs, *nasogastric tube* feedings, intake and output (I&O).
12. Monitor blood chemistries: sodium imbalance common with head injuries.
B. Goal: *provide emotional support and use comfort measures.*
1. Comfort: skin care, oral hygiene; sheepskins; wrinkle-free linen.
2. Eyes: lubricate q4h with artificial tears if periocular edema present.
3. Range of motion (ROM) exercises—passive, active; physical therapy as tolerated.
4. *Avoid* restraints.
5. Encourage verbalization of concerns about changes in body image, limitations.
6. Encourage family communication.

VII. Evaluation/outcome criteria
A. Alert, oriented—no residual effects (e.g., cognitive processes intact).
B. No signs of increased ICP (e.g., decreased respirations, increased systolic pressure with widening pulse pressure, bradycardia).
C. No paralysis—regains motor/sensory function.
D. Resumes self-care activities.

Increased Intracranial Pressure

Intracranial hypertension associated with altered states of consciousness.

I. Pathophysiology: increases in intracranial blood volume, cerebrospinal fluid (CSF), and/or brain tissue mass → cerebral distortion → increased ICP → impaired neural impulse transmission → cellular anoxia, atrophy.

II. Risk factors:
A. Congenital anomalies (hydrocephalus).
B. Space-occupying lesions (abscesses or tumors).
C. Trauma (hematomas or skull fractures).
D. Circulatory problems (aneurysms, emboli).
E. Inflammation (meningitis, encephalitis).

III. Assessment
A. *Subjective data:*
1. Headache.
2. Nausea.
B. *Objective data:*
1. Changes in level of consciousness.
2. Pupillary changes—unequal, dilated (side opposite to injury), unresponsive to light (*late sign*).
3. Vital signs—changes are variable (opposite of shock).
  a. Blood pressure—gradual or rapid elevation, widened pulse pressure.

POSITIONING THE UNCONSCIOUS PATIENT

Condition	Key Point	Rationale
Coma	Turn on side with head slightly *lowered*—"coma" position.	1. Important to let secretions drain out by gravity. 2. Must prevent aspiration.

Source: Jane Vincent Corbett, RN, MS, EdD, Professor, School of Nursing, University of San Francisco.

b. Pulse—bradycardia, tachycardia; significant sign is *slowing of pulse as blood pressure rises.*

c. Respiration—pattern changes (*Cheyne-Stokes*, apneusis, *Biot's*), deep and sonorous.

d. Temperature—moderate elevation.

4. Projectile vomiting.

5. See Diagnostic Studies section at the end of the chapter.

IV. Analysis/nursing diagnosis

A. *Altered cerebral tissue perfusion* related to increased ICP.

B. *Altered thought processes* related to cerebral anoxia.

C. *Ineffective breathing pattern* related to compression of respiratory center.

D. *Risk for aspiration* related to unconsciousness.

E. *Self-care deficit* related to altered level of consciousness.

F. *Impaired physical mobility* related to abnormal motor responses.

V. Nursing care plan/implementation: *promote adequate oxygenation and limit further impairment.*

A. Vital signs: report changes **at once.**

B. Patent *airway;* keep alkalotic, to prevent increased ICP resulting from elevated CO_2; hyperventilate if necessary.

C. Give medications as ordered:

1. *Hyperosmolar diuretics* (*mannitol*, urea) to reduce brain swelling.

2. *Steroids* (dexamethasone [Decadron]) for anti-inflammatory action.

3. *Antacids* or H_2 antagonist to prevent stress ulcer.

D. *Position:* elevate head of bed 30 degrees.

E. Fluids: *restrict*, strict I&O.

F. Cooling measures to reduce temperature, as fever increases ICP.

G. Prepare for surgical intervention (see Craniotomy, below).

VI. Evaluation/outcome criteria

A. No irreversible brain damage—regains consciousness.

B. Resumes self-care activities.

Craniotomy

Excision of a part of the skull (burr hole to several centimeters) for exploratory purpose and biopsy; to remove neoplasms, evacuate hematomas or excess fluid, control hemorrhage, repair skull fractures, remove scar tissue, repair or excise aneurysms, drain abscesses; produces minimal neurologic deficit.

I. Analysis/nursing diagnosis

A. *Altered cerebral tissue perfusion* related to edema.

B. *Altered thought processes* related to disorientation.

C. *Self-care deficit* related to continued neurologic impairment.

D. Also see analysis/nursing diagnosis for Traumatic Injuries to the Brain (pp. 248–249), Increased Intracranial Pressure (pp. 249–250), and Perioperative Nursing, p. 111.

II. Nursing care plan/implementation

A. **Preoperative care:**

1. Goal: *obtain baseline measurements.*

a. Vital signs.

b. Level of consciousness.

c. Mental, emotional status.

d. Pupillary reactions.

e. Motor strength, functioning.

2. Goal: *provide psychological support:* listen; give accurate, brief explanations.

3. Goal: *prepare for surgery.*

a. Cut hair, shave scalp (may be done in operating room).

b. Cover scalp with clean towel.

c. Administer *enema* and/or cathartics, as ordered.

d. Insert indwelling *Foley catheter,* as ordered.

B. **Postoperative care:**

1. Goal: *prevent complications and limit further impairment.*

a. *Vital signs* (**indications of complications**):

(1) Decreased blood pressure—*shock.*

(2) Widened pulse pressure—*increased ICP.*

(3) Respiratory failure—*compression* of medullary *respiratory* centers.

(4) Hyperthermia—disturbance of heat-regulating mechanism, *infection.*

b. *Neurologic:*

(1) Pupils—ipsilateral dilatation (increased ICP), visual disturbances.

(2) Altered level of consciousness.

(3) Altered cognitive or emotional status—disorientation common.

(4) Motor function and strength—hypertonia, hypotonia, seizures.

c. Blood gases, to monitor adequacy of ventilation.

d. Dressings: check frequently, aseptic technique, reinforce as necessary.

e. Observe for:

(1) CSF leakage (glucose-positive drainage from nose, mouth, ears)—*report immediately.*

(2) Periorbital edema—apply light ice compresses as necessary—remove crusts from eyelids.

f. Check integrity of seventh cranial nerve (facial)—incomplete closure of eyelids.

g. *Position:*

(1) *Supratentorial surgery* (cerebrum)—semi-Fowler's (*30-degree elevation*); may *not* lie on operative side.

(2) *Infratentorial* (brain stem, cerebellum)—*flat* in bed (prone), may turn to either side but *not* onto back.

h. Fluids: NPO for 24–48 h.

i. Medications as ordered:
   (1) *Osmotic diuretics* (mannitol).
   (2) *Corticosteroids* (dexamethasone [Decadron]).
   (3) *Mild analgesics* (do *not* mask neurologic or respiratory depression).
j. Orient frequently to person, time, place—to reduce restlessness, confusion.
k. Siderails up for safety.
l. *Avoid* restraints (may increase agitation and ICP).
m. Ice bags to head to reduce headache.
n. Activity: assist with ambulation.

2. Goal: *provide optimal supportive care.*
   a. Cover scalp once dressings are removed (scarves, wigs).
   b. Deal realistically with neurologic deficits—facilitate acceptance, adjustment, independence.

3. Goal: **health teaching.**
   a. Prepare for physical, occupational, and/or speech therapy, as needed.
   b. Activities of daily living.

III. Evaluation/outcome criteria
   A. Regains consciousness—is alert, oriented.
   B. Resumes self-care activities within limits of neurologic deficits.

Epilepsy

Seizure disorder characterized by sudden, transient aberration of brain function; associated with motor, sensory, autonomic, or psychic disturbances.

I. Seizure: involuntary muscular contraction and disturbances of consciousness resulting from abnormal electrical activity.

II. Risk factors:
   A. Brain injury.
   B. Infection (meningitis, encephalitis).
   C. Water and electrolyte disturbances.
   D. Hypoglycemia.
   E. Tumors.
   F. Vascular disorders (hypoxia or hypocapnia).

III. Generalized seizures:
   A. *Tonic-clonic* (grand mal) seizures:
      1. Pathophysiology: increased excitability of a neuron → possible activation of adjacent neurons → synchronous discharge of impulses → vigorous involuntary sustained muscle spasms (*tonic* contractions). Onset of neuronal fatigue → intermittent muscle spasms (*clonic* contractions) → cessation of muscle spasms → fatigue.
      2. Assessment
         a. *Subjective data*—aura: flash of light; peculiar smell, sound; feelings of fear; euphoria.
         b. *Objective data:*
            (1) *Convulsive stage*—tonic and clonic muscle spasms, loss of consciousness, breathholding, frothing at mouth, bit-

ing of tongue, urinary or fecal incontinence; lasts 2–5 min.
            (2) *Postconvulsion*—headache, fatigue (postictal sleep), malaise, vomiting, sore muscles, choking on secretions, aspiration.
            (3) See Diagnostic Studies Box, p. 254.
   B. *Absence* (petit mal) seizures:
      1. Pathophysiology: unknown etiology, momentary loss of consciousness (10–20 sec); usually no recollection of seizure; resumes previously performed action.
      2. Assessment—*objective data:*
         a. Fixation of gaze, blank facial expression.
         b. Flickering of eyelids.
         c. Jerking of facial muscle or arm.
   C. *Minor motor* seizures:
      1. *Myoclonic*—involuntary jerking contraction of major muscles, may throw person to the floor.
      2. *Akinetic*—momentary loss of muscle movement.
      3. *Atonic*—total loss of muscle tone, person falls to the floor.

IV. Partial (focal) seizures:
   A. *Partial motor*—arises from region in motor cortex (posterior frontal lobe); most commonly begins in upper extremities, spreading to face and lower extremities (*jacksonian march*); noting progression is important in identifying area of cortex involved.
   B. *Partial sensory*—sensory symptoms occur with partial seizure activity, vary with region in brain—transient.
   C. *Partial complex* (psychomotor)—arises out of anterior temporal lobe; frequently begins with an aura; characteristic feature is automatism (lip smacking, chewing, patting body, picking at clothes); lasts from 2–3 to 15 min; do *not* restrain.

V. Analysis/nursing diagnosis
   A. *Risk for injury* related to convulsive disorder.
   B. *Anxiety* related to sudden loss of consciousness.
   C. *Self-esteem disturbance* related to chronic illness.
   D. *Impaired social interaction* related to self-consciousness.

VI. Nursing care plan/implementation (generalized seizures):
   A. Goal: *prevent injury during seizure.*
      1. Do *not* force jaws open during convulsion.
      2. Do *not* restrict limbs—protect from injury, place something soft under head (towel, jacket, hands).
      3. Loosen constrictive clothing.
      4. Note time, level of consciousness, type and duration of seizure.
   B. Goal: *postseizure care:*
      1. *Turn on side* to drain saliva and facilitate breathing.
      2. *Suction* as necessary.
      3. Orient to time and place.
      4. Administer oral hygiene if tongue or cheek injured.

5. Check vital signs, pupils, level of consciousness.

C. Goal: *prevent or reduce recurrences of seizure activity.*

   1. Encourage patient to identify precipitating factors.

   2. Moderation in diet and exercise.

   3. Medications as ordered: phenytoin (Dilantin); phenobarbital; carbamazepine (Tegretol); primidone (Mysoline); trimethadione (Tridione)—petit mal only.

D. Goal: **health teaching.**

   1. Medications:

     a. Actions, side effects (apathy, ataxia, hyperplasia of gums).

     b. Complications with sudden withdrawal (*status epilepticus*).

   2. Attitude toward life and treatment, adhere to medication regimen.

   3. Clarify misconceptions, fears—especially about insanity, bad genes.

   4. Maintain activities, interests—*except* no driving until seizure free for period of time specified by state Department of Motor Vehicles.

   5. *Avoid:* stress, lack of sleep, emotional upset, alcohol.

   6. Relaxation techniques, stress-management techniques.

   7. Wear MedicAlert band or tag.

   8. Appropriate community resources.

VIII. Evaluation/outcome criteria

A. Avoids precipitating stimuli—achieves seizure control.

B. Complies with medication regimen.

C. Retains independence.

Transient Ischemic Attacks (TIAs)

Temporary, complete, or relatively complete cessation of cerebral blood flow to a localized area of brain, producing symptoms ranging from weakness and numbness to monocular blindness; an important precursor to cerebrovascular accident. Surgical intervention includes *carotid endarterectomy;* most common postoperative cranial nerve damage causes vocal cord paralysis or difficulty managing saliva and tongue deviation (cranial nerves VII, X, XI, XII); usually temporary; stroke may also occur.

Cerebrovascular Accident

Brain lesions resulting from damage to blood vessels supplying brain.

  I. Pathophysiology: reduced or interrupted blood flow → interruption of nerve impulses down corticospinal tract → decreased or absent voluntary movement on one side of the body (fine movements are more af-

fected than coarse movements); later, autonomous reflex activity → spasticity and rigidity of muscles.

  II. Risk factors:

A. Cerebral thrombosis (most common), embolism, hemorrhage.

B. Prior ischemic episodes (transient ischemic attacks [TIAs]).

C. Hypertension.

D. Oral contraceptives.

E. Emotional stress.

F. Family history.

G. Age.

H. Diabetes mellitus.

  III. Assessment

A. *Subjective data:*

   1. Weakness, sudden or gradual loss of movement of extremities on one side.

   2. Difficulty forming words.

   3. Difficulty swallowing (dysphagia).

   4. Nausea, vomiting.

   5. History of TIAs.

B. *Objective data:*

   1. Vital signs:

     a. Blood pressure—elevated, widened pulse pressure.

     b. Temperature—elevated.

     c. Pulse—normal, slow.

     d. Respiration—tachypnea, altered pattern, deep, sonorous.

   2. Neurologic:

     a. Altered level of consciousness.

     b. Pupils—unequal; vision—*homonymous hemianopia.*

     c. Ptosis of eyelid, drooping mouth.

     d. Paresis or paralysis (hemiplegia).

     e. Loss of sensation and reflexes.

     f. Incontinence of urine or feces.

     g. Aphasia (see p. 247).

   3. See Diagnostic Studies Box, p. 254.

  IV. Analysis/nursing diagnosis

A. *Impaired physical mobility* related to hemiplegia.

B. *Impaired swallowing* related to paralysis.

C. *Impaired verbal communication* related to aphasia.

D. *Risk for aspiration* related to unconsciousness.

E. *Sensory/perceptual alterations* related to altered cerebral blood flow, visual field blindness.

F. *Altered thought processes* related to cerebral edema.

G. *Self-care deficit* related to paresis or paralysis.

H. *Body image disturbance* related to hemiplegia.

I. *Total incontinence* related to interruption of normal nerve transmission.

J. *Impaired social interaction* related to aphasia or neurologic deficit.

K. *Risk for impaired skin integrity* related to immobility.

L. *Unilateral neglect* related to cerebral damage.

  V. Nursing care plan/implementation

A. Goal: *reduce cerebral anoxia.*

   1. Patent *airway:*

a. *Oxygen* therapy, as ordered, suctioning to prevent aspiration.
b. Turn, cough, deep breathe q2h to prevent aspiration pneumonia (high incidence).
2. Activity: bed rest, progressing to out of bed as tolerated.
3. *Position:*
  a. Maximize ventilation.
  b. Support with pillows when on side, use hand rolls and arm slings as ordered.

B. Goal: *prevent complications and maintain functioning.*
  1. Vital signs, neurologic checks.
  2. Medications, as ordered:
    a. *Antihypertensives* to prevent rupture.
    b. *Anticoagulants* to prevent thrombus.
  3. *Fluids:* IVs to prevent hemoconcentration, I&O, weigh daily.
  4. ROM exercises to prevent contractures, muscle atrophy, phlebitis.
  5. Skin care, position changes to prevent decubitus ulcers

C. Goal: *provide for emotional relaxation.*
  1. Identify grief reaction to changes in body image.
  2. Encourage expression of feelings, concerns.

D. Goal: *patient safety.*
  1. Identify existence of *homonymous hemianopia* (visual field blindness) and *agnosia* (disturbance in sensory information).
  2. Use siderails and assist as needed.
  3. Remind to walk slowly, take adequate rest periods, ensure good lighting, look where patient is going.

E. Goal: **health teaching.**
  1. Exercise routines.
  2. Diet: self-feeding, but assist as needed.
  3. Resumption of self-care activities.
  4. Use of supportive devices, transfer techniques.

VI. Evaluation/outcome criteria
  A. No complications (e.g., pneumonia).
  B. Regains functional independence—resumes self-care activities.
  C. Return of control over body functions (e.g., bowel, bladder, speech).

Bacterial Meningitis*

I. Pathophysiology
  A. Bacterial organism, commonly *H. influenza, S. pneumoniae, Neisseria meningitis,* or *S. aureus,* crosses blood–brain barrier into CNS. Organism migrates via subarachnoid space, producing an inflammatory response to the foreign substance in the pia mater, the arachnoid, the CSF, and the cerebral ventricles.

*Modified from Colombraro GC. Nursing Care of Children and Families. In *Little, Brown's NCLEX-RN Examination Review,* SL Lagerquist (ed). Philadelphia: Lippincott Raven, 1996. p 532–533.

II. Risk factors
  A. High population density (e.g., crowded living conditions).
  B. Basilar skull fracture.
  C. Brain or spinal surgery.
  D. Sinus or upper respiratory infection.
  E. Use of nasal sprays after sinus infection.
  F. Compromised immune system.

III. Assessment
  A. *Subjective data:*
    1. Abrupt onset: initial sign may be a seizure following an episode of upper respiratory tract infection/acute otitis media.
    2. Chills and fever.
    3. Vomiting.
  B. *Objective data:*
    1. Headache.
    2. Neck pain.
    3. Photophobia.
    4. Alterations in level of consciousness: delirium, stupor, increased ICP.
    5. Nuchal rigidity.
    6. Opisthotonos: head is drawn backward into overextension.
    7. Hyperactive reflexes related to CNS irritability.

IV. Analysis/nursing diagnosis
  A. *Risk for infection* related to communicability of meningitis.
  B. *Risk for injury* related to CNS irritability and seizures.
  C. *Pain* related to nuchal rigidity, opisthotonos, increased muscle tension.
  D. *Sensory/perceptual alterations* related to seizures and changes in level of consciousness.
  E. *Altered nutrition, less than body requirements,* related to fever and poor oral intake.
  F. *Knowledge deficit* regarding diagnostic procedures, condition, treatment, prognosis.

V. Nursing care plan/implementation
  A. Goal: *prevent spread of infection.*
    1. Institute universal precautions.
    2. Enforce strict handwashing.
    3. Institute and maintain *respiratory isolation* for minimum of 24 h after starting IV antibiotics, at which time patient is no longer considered to be communicable and patient can come off isolation.
    4. Instruct family when using isolation techniques.
    5. Identify family members and others at high risk: do cultures (e.g., *Haemophilus influenzae, Escherichia coli*); possibly begin prophylactic antibiotics (e.g., rifampin).
    6. Treat with IV antiinfectives, as ordered, as soon as possible after admission (after culture specimens are obtained); continue 10–14 d (until CSF culture is negative and there is clinical improvement). (See diagnostic studies for lumbar punctures.)

7. Anticipate large IV doses of medications only—administer slowly in dilute form to prevent phlebitis.
☞ 8. Maintain IV.
B. Goal: *promote safety and prevent injury/seizures.*
☞ 1. Maintain seizure precautions.
2. Place patient near nurses' station for maximum observation, provide private room for isolation.
3. Minimize stimuli: quiet, calm environment.
4. Restrict visitors to immediate family.
5. *Position:* head of bed slightly elevated to decrease ICP. (For opisthotonos: side-lying, for comfort and safety.)
C. Goal: *maintain adequate nutrition.*
1. NPO or clear liquids initially; supplement with IVs
2. Diet as tolerated—patient may experience anorexia (due to disease) or vomiting (due to increased ICP).
3. Monitor I&O, daily weights.
VI. Evaluation/outcome criteria
A. No spread of infection noted.
B. Safety maintained.
C. Adequate nutrition and fluid intake maintained.
D. Patient recovers without permanent neurologic damage (e.g., seizure disorders).

Encephalitis

Inflammation of the brain and its coverings, which usually results in prolonged coma.

I. Pathophysiology: brain tissue injury → release of enzymes that increase vascular dilatation, capillary permeability → edema → increased ICP → depression of CNS function.
II. Risk factors:
A. Syphilis.
B. Lead or arsenic poisoning.
C. Carbon monoxide.
D. Typhoid fever.
E. Measles, chickenpox.
F. Viruses.
III. Assessment
A. *Subjective data:*
1. Headache—severe.
2. Fever—sudden.
3. Nausea, vomiting.
4. Photophobia
5. Difficulty concentrating.
B. *Objective data:*
1. Altered level of consciousness.
2. Nuchal rigidity.
3. Tremors, facial weakness.
4. Nystagmus.
5. Elevated temperature.
6. *Lumbar puncture*—fluid cloudy; increased neutrophils, protein. See Diagnostic Studies.
7. Lab data: blood—slight to moderate leukocytosis (about 14,000/mm³).

IV. Analysis/nursing diagnosis
A. *Self-care deficit* related to altered level of consciousness.
B. *Risk for injury* related to coma.
C. *Sensory/perceptual alteration* related to brain tissue injury.
D. *Altered thought processes* related to increased ICP.
V. Nursing care plan/implementation
A. Goal: *support physical and emotional relaxation.*
1. Vital signs, neurologic signs, as ordered.
☞ 2. Seizure precautions.
☞ 3. *Position:* to maintain patent airway, prevent contractures, ROM exercises.
4. Medications as ordered:
a. *Analgesics* for pain.
b. *Antipyretics* for fever.
c. *Sedatives* for agitation.
d. *Anticonvulsants* for seizures.
e. *Antiinfectives* for infection.
f. *Osmotic diuretics* (mannitol) to reduce cerebral edema.
5. *No* isolation.
B. Goal: *health teaching:* self-care activities with residual motor and speech deficits, physical therapy.
VI. Evaluation/outcome criteria
A. Regains consciousness; is alert, oriented.
B. Performs self-care activities with minimal assistance.

Diagnostic Studies

Cerebral angiography—fluoroscopic visualization of the brain vasculature after injection of a contrast medium into the carotid or vertebral arteries; *used to* localize lesions (tumors, abscesses, intracranial hemorrhages, occlusions) that are large enough to distort cerebrovascular blood flow.
Brain scan—intravenous injection of a radioactive substance, followed by scanning that detects radioactivity.
1. *Increased* radioactivity at site of abnormality.
2. *Used to* detect: brain tumors, abscesses, hematomas, and arteriovenous malformations.
Electroencephalography—graphic record of the electrical potentials generated by the physiologic activity of the brain; *used to* detect surface lesions or tumors of the brain and epilepsy.
Echoencephalography—beam of pulsed ultrasound is passed through the head, and returning echoes are recorded graphically; *used to* detect: shifts in cerebral midline structures caused by subdural hematomas, intracerebral hemorrhage, or tumors.
Skull x-ray studies—outline configuration and density of brain tissues and vascular markings; *used to* determine the size and location of: intracranial calcifications, tumors, abscesses, or vascular lesions.
Computerized axial tomography (CAT or CT scan)—an x-ray beam sweeps around the body, allowing measurement of various tissue densities; provides clear radiographic definition of structures that are not visible by other techniques, permitting earlier diagnosis

☞ Summary of Key Points

1. Aphasic patients *can hear.* Speaking louder does not improve their comprehension.
2. With an aphasic patient, use nonverbal techniques, face the patient directly, speak slowly, repeat words, be patient and kind, and anticipate patient's needs to reduce his or her frustration.
3. Learn a mnemonic to help remember the cranial nerves.
4. Scalp wounds are very bloody but may actually be minor injuries.
5. With suspected head trauma, assess for signs of *hypoxia* and increasing *ICP.* The vital sign changes in increased ICP are the *opposite* of those seen in hypovolemic shock.
6. Pupil dilatation is a *late sign* of increased ICP. *A change of level of consciousness is the first indication* of a worsening of the patient's condition. Even a comatose patient will show a change in responsiveness. Use the *Glasgow Coma scale* to assess objectively.
7. The greatest concern with increased ICP is the amount of distortion and *anoxia* caused by the pressure.
8. *Pupil dilatation* occurs first in the pupil *opposite* the *side* of injury or hematoma.
9. Check any drainage from nose or ears for the presence of glucose, indicating a *CSF leak.*
10. Positioning and head elevation is determined by the type of surgery—*above or below the tentorium.*
11. The nursing priority during a seizure is to *protect the patient* from *injury.* Maintaining a patent airway is usually not possible. Clearing the airway after the seizure ends is important.
12. *Aspiration pneumonia* is a concern during the period immediately after a cerebrovascular accident. Positioning and careful observation of swallowing are important.
13. The amount of permanent disability is often not known for weeks after a cerebrovascular accident. Nursing care focuses on prevention of complications and maintenance of optimal functioning.
14. *Homonymous hemianopia* (visual field blindness) may be present, leading to accidents and behavior changes.
15. A *spinal headache* resulting from a lumbar puncture can be easily prevented by keeping the patient flat and well hydrated.

and treatment and more effective and efficient follow-up. Initial scan may be followed by "contrast enhancement," involving the IV injection of a contrast agent (iodine), followed by a repeat scan. *Patient preparation:* instructions for eating before test vary. *Clear liquids* up to 2 h before are usually permitted.

Lumbar puncture—puncture of the lumbar subarachnoid space of the spinal cord with a needle to withdraw samples of cerebral spinal fluid (CSF); *used to* evaluate CSF for infections and determine presence of hemorrhage. *Not done if ↑ ICP suspected.*

💡 Study and Memory Aids

Transient Ischemic Attacks: Assessment—"3 T's"

Temporary unilateral visual loss
Transient paralysis (one side)
Tinnitus → vertigo

Source: Modified from Zerwekh J D, et al. *Memory Notebook of Nursing.* Dallas: Nursing Education Consultants, 1994. p. 94.

● **Drug Review**

Traumatic Brain (Head) Injury

Analgesics (NO MORPHINE)
Acetaminophen/codeine (Tylenol #1, #2, #3): 1–2 tablets q3–4h, as needed
Meperidine HCl (Demerol): IM or SC, 50–75 mg
Oxycodone/acetaminophen (Tylox, Percocet): 5 mg q3–6h, as needed

Anticonvulsants
Phenobarbital: 60–250 mg/d in single or divided doses
Phenytoin (Dilantin): loading dose, 1 g or 20 mg/kg; maintenance dose, 300–400 mg

Steroids (should *never* be abruptly discontinued; gradually taper dose to prevent complications)
Dexamethasone (Decadron): 0.5–9 mg/d in single or divided doses
Methylprednisolone (Medrol): 4–48 mg/d
Prednisone (Deltasone): 5–60 mg/d

Increased Intracranial Pressure

Antiulceratives
Aluminum hydroxide gel (Amphojel): 5–10 mL q2–4h or 1 h pc
Calcium carbonate (Titralac): 1–2 g with water pc and hs
Magnesium and aluminum hydroxides (Maalox suspension): 5–30 mL pc and hs
Sucralfate (Carafate): 1 g qid
Histamine antagonists
Cimetidine (Tagamet): 300–600 mg q6h
Ranitidine (Zantac): 150 mg bid
Osmotic diuretics: Mannitol (Osmitrol): IV, 0.25–2 g/kg as 15%–25% solution over 30–60 min
Steroids (should *never* be abruptly discontinued; gradually taper dosage to prevent complications)
Dexamethasone (Decadron): 0.5–9 mg/d in single or divided doses

Craniotomy

Analgesics (NO MORPHINE)
Acetaminophen/codeine (Tylenol #1, #2, #3): 1–2 tablets q3–4h, as needed
Meperidine HCl (Demerol): IM or SC, 50–75 mg
Oxycodone/acetaminophen (Tylox, Percocet): 5 mg q3–6h, as needed
Osmotic diuretics: Mannitol (Osmitrol): IV, 0.25–2 g/kg as 15%–25% solution over 30–60 min
Steroids (should *never* be abruptly discontinued; gradually taper dose to prevent complications)
Dexamethasone (Decadron): 0.5–9 mg/d in single or divided doses

Epilepsy

Carbamazepine (Tegretol): 800–1200 mg/d in divided doses q6–8h
Phenobarbital: 60–250 mg/d in single or divided doses
Phenytoin (Dilantin): loading dose, 1 g or 20 mg/kg; maintenance dose, 300–400 mg
Primidone (Mysoline): 250 mg 3–4 times daily, *not to exceed* 2 g/d
Trimethadione (Tridione)—for petit mal seizures only: 900 mg in 3–4 divided doses with increases weekly of 300 mg to a total of 2400 mg per day.

Transient Ischemic Attacks

Agents administered to treat any existing medical condition.

Cerebrovascular Accident

Anticoagulants
Heparin sodium: IV, 1000 U/h; SC, 8000–10,000 U q8h, adjusted according to partial thromboplastin time
Warfarin (Coumadin): 10 mg/d, adjusted according to prothrombin time
Antihypertensive: Angiotensin-converting enzyme inhibitor (ACE)—Catopril (Capoten): 12.5–25 mg tid
Antiplatelet: Aspirin: 1–3 g/d in 2–4 divided doses

Encephalitis

Analgesics
Acetaminophen/codeine (Tylenol #1, #2, #3): 1–2 tablets q3–4h, as needed
Meperidine HCl (Demerol): IM or SC, 50–75 mg
Oxycodone/acetaminophen (Tylox, Percocet): 5 mg q3–6h, as needed
Anticonvulsants
Phenobarbital: 60–250 mg/d in single or divided doses
Phenytoin (Dilantin, diphenylhydantoin): loading dose, 1 g or 20 mg/kg; maintenance dose, 300–400 mg
Antiinfectives
Cephalexin (Keflex): 250–500 mg q6h
Cephalothin (Keflin): IV, 0.5–2 g q4–6h
Erythromycin: 250–500 mg q6–12h
Gentamicin (Garamycin): 3–5 mg/kg/d in divided doses
Penicillin G: 1.2 million U in single IM dose
Antipyretics: Aspirin: 325–1000 mg q4–6h, *not to exceed* 4 g/d
Osmotic diuretics: Mannitol (Osmitrol): IV, 0.25–2 g/kg as 15%–25% solution over 30–60 min
Sedatives
Phenobarbital: 30–120 mg/d in divided doses
Tranquilizers
Chlordiazepoxide HCl (Librium): 5–25 mg 3–4 times daily
Diazepam (Valium): 2–10 mg 2–4 times daily

Questions

1. Which of the following respiratory changes would the nurse see in a patient with increasing intracranial pressure (ICP)?
   1. Nasal flaring and sternal retractions.
   2. Slow, irregular respirations.
   3. Rapid, shallow respirations.
   4. Paradoxical chest movements.

2. Which nursing measure would prevent a further increase in ICP in a head-injured patient?
1. Positioning the patient flat in bed.
2. Turning the patient and having him cough and deep breathe every 3 hours.
3. Asking the patient to exhale while turning in bed.
4. Preventing the complications of immobility.

3. If a patient who has suffered a cerebrovascular accident (CVA) is found to have homonymous hemianopia, the nurse would know that the patient has:
1. Paralysis of limbs on one side of the body.
2. Visual field blindness.
3. Perceptual neglect of one side of body.
4. Deafness in one ear.

4. The nurse tells the daughter of a stroke victim that the most important aspect of rehabilitation after a CVA is:
1. Return of bowel and bladder continence.
2. Family or support persons' involvement.
3. Setting realistic goals for the patient.
4. Return of the long-term memory needed for learning.

5. The best way for the nurse to approach a patient with left homonymous hemianopia following a CVA would be to:
1. Speak to the patient while approaching from the left.
2. Stand at the foot of the patient's bed when talking.
3. Speak to the patient while approaching from the right.
4. Stand directly in front of the patient when talking.

6. A patient who has suffered a CVA pays little attention to her roommate and seems withdrawn. When the nurse enters the room, the patient is awake but does not respond until spoken to. The best explanation for her behavior is:
1. She does not remember the nurse's name.
2. She is angry she had the stroke.
3. CVAs frequently cause hearing impairment.
4. She may have visual field blindness.

7. While caring for a patient in the postanesthesia recovery room after a craniotomy, the nurse observes signs of increasing ICP. The first nursing action would be to:
1. Give the patient dexamethasone (Decadron) IV, as ordered.
2. Elevate the head of the patient's bed 30 degrees.
3. Contact the neurosurgeon for orders.
4. Assess the patient's bilateral pupillary reaction.

8. In providing health care teaching to a patient who is being discharged on dexamethasone (Decadron) therapy, the nurse should inform the patient that during long-term therapy he should observe a diet that is:
1. High in carbohydrates, sodium, and protein.
2. Low in carbohydrates and sodium and high in protein.
3. High in protein, calcium, and carbohydrates.
4. Low in potassium, protein, and carbohydrates.

9. The nurse knows that gentamycin, an aminoglycoside, may cause eighth cranial nerve damage. Which assessment finding would alert the nurse to this adverse effect?
1. Drooping eyelid.
2. Diplopia.
3. Tinnitus.
4. Dysphagia.

Answers/Rationale

1. (2) The respiratory change that occurs in the presence of increased ICP is often called ataxic or *Biot's breathing,* and it is a very irregular pattern that occurs with brainstem involvement. The other respiratory changes are characteristic of *other* potentially life-threatening conditions. Left ventricular *failure* would likely produce nasal flaring and sternal retractions **(1).** Rapid, shallow breathing **(3)** would be seen with *acute respiratory distress.* Paradoxical movements **(4)** occur in *flail chest.* **AS, 6, PhI**

2. (3) When such patients turn, they instinctively hold their breath (Valsalva maneuver); this increases the intrathoracic pressure and the ICP. Exhaling or breathing through the mouth prevents the *maneuver.* The head of the bed should be elevated 30 degrees, *not flat* **(1).** Preventing respiratory complications is important, but *coughing* **(2)** would only *increase* the ICP. Preventing the complications of immobility **(4)** is *too vague;* many such complications would not have any bearing on ICP. **IMP, 2, PhI**

3. (2) *Homonymous hemianopia* means defective vision or visual loss in the same half of the visual field of both eyes. Frequently the optic nerve is affected in CVA patients, and this causes visual field blindness. The nasal field of one eye and the temporal field of the other eye would be blind, as if a curtain had been drawn across half of each eye. Paralysis on one side **(1)** is *hemiplegia,* not hemianopia. CVA patients may also fail to perceive one side of the body **(3),** and this is *unilateral neglect.* Deafness or loss of hearing in one ear **(4)** is *hemianacusia,* and this may occur with damage to the eighth cranial nerve (the auditory/acoustic nerve). **AN, 2, PhI**

4. (2) Rehabilitation requires the help of family or support persons, because they can help provide the encouragement and assistance the patient needs during the process. The question does not provide any data about bowel and bladder control **(1),** so the rehabilitation needs in this regard are *not known.* However, the family would be critical to regaining control. Goals are set *with* the patient, not for the patient **(3).** There is also *no information* in the question about the patient's memory **(4),** but if there were a problem, the family would be the key to successful rehabilitation. **IMP, 2, HPM**

5. (3) The patient has left visual field blindness and can only see in the right visual fields of both eyes. Once the

---

Key to Codes

Nursing process: AS, assessment; **AN,** analysis; **PL,** planning; **IMP,** implementation; **EV,** evaluation. (See Appendix M for explanation of nursing process steps.)

Category of human function: 1, protective; **2,** sensory-perceptual; **3,** comfort, rest, activity, and mobility; **4,** nutrition; **5,** growth and development; **6,** fluid-gas transport; **7,** psychosocial-cultural; **8,** elimination. (See Appendix O for explanation.)

Client need: SECE, safe, effective care environment; **PhI,** physiologic integrity; **PsI,** psychosocial integrity; **HPM,** health promotion/maintenance. (See Appendix P for explanation.)

nurse is seen or heard approaching from the right, the patient can more easily turn his head to the right to see her than if she approaches from the left. The patient would *not see* anyone approaching *from the left* (**1**) or any item placed to the left side of the bedside table or on the left side of the bed. Options **2** and **4** do not explain how to approach the patient to avoid startling. **PL, 2, PhI**

6. (**4**)   There is decreased sensory stimulation as a result of visual field blindness, and the patient may appear withdrawn. Positioning the patient's bed so that the door and/or roommate are visible will enable the patient to be more responsive. The other explanations (**1, 2,** and **3**) are possible, but visual field blindness should be ruled out before they are considered. **AN, 2, PhI**

7. (**2**)   Head elevation of 30 degrees is considered the optimal position after supratentorial surgery, such as a craniotomy. ICP is not affected by atmospheric pressure in this position. The other measures may be taken if the signs and symptoms of increased ICP continue. Decadron (**1**) would reduce the cerebral *edema*. Contacting the MD (**3**) turns the decision-making process over to the MD and is usually *not* the *first nursing action*. Changes in pupillary reaction (**4**) would be a *late* sign of increased ICP. **IMP, 2, PhI**

8. (**2**)   The diet should be low in carbohydrates and sodium and high in protein, calcium, and potassium to counter the adverse effects of the drug. Option **1** is incorrect because CHO and sodium should be *low.* Option **3** is incorrect because CHO should be *low.* Option **4** is incorrect because potassium and protein should be *increased* in the diet. **IMP, 4, SECE**

9. (**3**)   Tinnitus, or ringing in the ears, occurs if there is damage to the acoustic (auditory) nerve, or cranial nerve VIII. Drooping eyelid (**1**) is due to damage to cranial nerve III (the oculomotor nerve), which also affects the pupillary response. Diplopia (**2**), or double vision, occurs as a result of weakness of the eye muscles; extraocular movements are controlled by cranial nerves III (oculomotor), IV (trochlear), and VI (abducens). Dysphagia, or difficulty swallowing (**4**), occurs with damage to cranial nerve X (the vagus nerve). **AS, 2, PhI**

Disorders of the Spinal Cord

Chapter Outline

Herniated/Ruptured Disk (Ruptured Nucleus Pulposus)

Strain or injury to a weakened cartilage between vertebrae can result in herniation of the nucleus, causing pressure on nerve roots in spinal canal, pain, and disability.

I. Pathophysiology: pulpy substance of disk interior (nucleus pulposus) bulges or ruptures through the outer annulus fibrosus → irritation and pressure on nerve endings in the spinal ligaments → muscle spasm and distortion of the joints of vertebral arches.

II. Risk factors:
   A. Strain as result of poor body mechanics.
   B. Trauma.
   C. History of back injuries.

III. Assessment:
   A. *Lumbar injuries* (90% of herniations):
      1. *Subjective data:*
         a. *Pain:* low back, radiating to buttocks, posterior thigh, calf; *relieved* by recumbency; *aggravated by* sneezing, coughing, flexion; sciatic pain continues even when back pain subsides.
         b. Numbness, tingling.
      2. *Objective data:*
         a. Muscle weakness: leg and foot.
         b. Inability to flex leg.
         c. Sensory loss: leg and foot.
         d. Alterations in posture: leans to side, unable to stand up straight.
         e. Edema: leg and foot.
         f. Positive *Lasègue's sign:* straight leg raising with hip flexed and knee extended produces sciatic pain.
         g. Diagnostic tests for cervical injuries (see Diagnostic Studies Box).
            (1) Spinal x-rays.
            (2) Computerized axial tomographic (CAT) scan.
            (3) Magnetic resonance imaging (MRI).
            (4) Myelography (less preferred than CAT scan or MRI).
            (5) Electromyography.
            (6) *Neurologic exam:* special attention to *sensory* status, including pain, touch, and temperature identification; and to *motor* status, including strength, gait, and reflexes.
   B. *Cervical injuries* (10% of herniations):
      1. *Subjective data:*
         a. *Pain:* upper extremities, radiating to hands and fingers; aggravated by coughing, sneezing, straining.
         b. Tingling, burning sensation in upper extremities and back of neck.
      2. *Objective data:*
         a. Upper extremities: weakness, atrophy.
         b. Neck: restricted movement.
         c. Same diagnostic tests as for lumbar injury (see above).

IV. Analysis/nursing diagnosis
   A. *Pain* related to pressure on nerve roots.
   B. *Fear* related to disease progression and/or potential surgery.
   C. *Knowledge deficit* related to correct body mechanics.

**CROSS-SECTION OF LUMBAR
VERTEBRA FROM ABOVE.**

D. *Impaired physical mobility* related to continued
pain.
E. *Sleep pattern disturbance* related to difficulty find-
ing comfortable position.
V. Nursing care plan/implementation
  A. Goal: *relieve pain and promote comfort.*
    1. *Bed rest* with bedboard.
    2. *Position—avoid* twisting.
      a. *Lumbar disk: William's* (head elevated 30
      degrees, knee gatch elevated to flatten the
      lumbosacral curve).
      b. *Cervical:* low Fowler's.
    3. Medications as ordered:
      a. *Analgesics.*
      b. *Muscle relaxants.*
      c. *Anti-inflammatories.*
      d. *Stool softeners.*
    3. Moist heat.
    4. Fracture bedpan.
    5. Gradual increase in activity.
    6. Apply brace for support.
    7. Apply traction prn for comfort.
    8. Prepare for surgery if medical regimen unsuc-
    cessful.
  B. Goal: **health teaching.**
    1. Correct body mechanics, keep back straight.
    2. Exercise program as symptoms decrease.
VI. Evaluation/outcome criteria
  A. Reports pain decreased.
  B. Mobility increased, normal body posture attained.

Laminectomy

Excision of dorsal arch of vertebrae with or without spinal
fusion of two or more vertebrae with a bone graft from iliac
crest, to stabilize spine.

I. Analysis/nursing diagnosis
  A. *Pain* related to edema resulting from surgery.
  B. *Impaired physical mobility* related to pain and dis-
  comfort resulting from surgery.
II. Nursing care plan/implementation
  A. Goal: *relieve anxiety.*

  1. Answer questions, explain routines.
  2. See General Postoperative Nursing Care,
  Chap. 9.
B. Goal: *prevent injury postoperatively.*
  1. Monitor vital signs:
    a. Neurologic signs (e.g., check sensation, mo-
    tor strength of limbs).
    b. Respiratory status (risk for *respiratory de-
    pression* with cervical laminectomy).
  2. Monitor intake and output (I&O) (*urinary retention* common, especially with cervical laminectomy); may need catheterization.
  Encourage fluids.
  3. Monitor bowel sounds (*paralytic ileus* common
  with lumbar laminectomy).
  4. Monitor dressing for possible bleeding.
  5. Bed *position* as ordered:
    a. *For lumbar laminectomy: head of bed flat;*
    supine with slight flexion of legs, with pil-
    low between knees for turning and side-
    lying position.
    b. *For cervical laminectomy: head of bed ele-
    vated,* neck immobilized with collar or sand
    bags.
  6. Encourage deep breathing to prevent respiratory complications.
  7. Prevent strain or flexion at surgical site: log-
  rolling with spinal fusion.
C. Goal: *promote comfort.*
  1. Administer *analgesics* because sciatic-type pain
  continues after lumbar surgery (arm pain after
  cervical surgery), due to edema resulting from
  trauma of surgery.
D. Goal: *prepare for early discharge:* Patients having
microsurgery for repair of herniated disk are usually discharged from the hospital 1 d postoperative;
teaching regarding allowed and restricted activities
must be done early.
E. Goal: **health teaching.**
  1. How to *turn and move* from side to side in
  one motion, *sit up,* and *get out of bed without
  twisting spine;* to get out of bed: raise head of
  bed while in side-lying position, then put feet
  over edge of bed, and stand.
  2. Proper positioning and *ambulation* techniques.
  3. Correct posture, *body mechanics,* activities to
  prevent further injury; increase activities according to tolerance.
  4. Physiotherapy; encourage compliance for full
  rehabilitation.
III. Evaluation/outcome criteria
  A. No respiratory, bowel, bladder complications
  noted.
    1. Lung sounds clear.
    2. Bowel sounds present, able to pass gas and
    feces.
    3. Urinary output adequate.
  B. Regains mobility.
  C. Comfort level increases: reports leg and back pain
  decreased.
  D. Demonstrates protective positioning and ambulation techniques.

Spinal Cord Injuries

Trauma from hyperextension, hyperflexion, axial compression, lateral flexion, or shearing of the spine.

I. Types:
  A. *C-1 and C-2 injury level*—resulting deficit:
    1. Phrenic nerve involvement.
    2. Diaphragmatic paralysis.
    3. Respiratory difficulties (require permanent ventilatory support).
    4. Possible quadriplegia.
    5. Possible death.
  B. *C-4 through T-1 injury level*—resulting deficit: possible quadriplegia.
  C. *Thoracic-lumbar injury level*—resulting deficit: possible paraplegia.

II. Pathophysiology: trauma → vertebral dislocation or fractures → cord trauma, compression or severance of the cord.

III. Risk factors
  A. Motor vehicle accidents.
  B. Athletic accidents (e.g., diving, surfing, contact sports).
  C. Falls.
  D. Gunshot wounds.

⋈ IV. Assessment
  A. *Subjective data:*
    1. Pain at the level of injury.
    2. Numbness/weakness, loss of sensation below level of injury.
    3. Psychological distress related to severity of injury and its effects.
  B. *Objective data:*
    1. Findings depend on extent of injury to spinal cord/spinal nerves.
    2. Paralysis: motor, sphincter.
      a. Initially a period of *flaccid paralysis* and loss of reflexes, called *spinal* or *neural shock.*
      b. *Incomplete injuries* may lead to loss of voluntary movement and sensory deficits below injury level (symptoms vary depending on injury).
      c. *Complete injury* leads to loss of function and all voluntary movement below level of injury.
    3. Respiratory distress.
    4. Alterations in temperature control.
    5. Alterations in bowel and bladder function.
    6. Involved muscles become spastic and hyperreflexic within days or weeks.
    7. Documentation via xrays of the spine, CAT scan and neurological examination.

⋈ V. Analysis/nursing diagnosis:
  A. *Ineffective breathing pattern* related to high-level injury.
  B. *Impaired physical mobility* related to injuries affecting lower limbs.
  C. *Fear* related to uncertain future health status.

  D. *Anxiety* related to loss of control over own activities of daily living.
  E. *Bathing/hygiene self-care deficit* related to injuries above T-1.
  F. *Impaired home maintenance management* related to quadriplegia or paraplegia.
  G. *Risk for altered body temperature* related to absence of sweating below level of injury.
  H. *Risk for injury* related to equipment necessary to accomplish daily activities.
  I. *Tactile sensory/perceptual alterations* related to injury level.
  J. *Body image disturbance* related to permanent change in physical status.

⋈ VI. Nursing care plan/implementation
  A. Goal: *maintain patent airway.*
    1. *Suction, cough, tracheostomy care, prn.*
    2. *Oxygen, ventilator care.*
    3. Monitor blood gas levels.
  B. Goal: *prevent further damage.*
    1. Immobilize spine.
    2. Firm mattress, *Stryker frame, Foster frame, CircO-electric* bed, traction, casts, braces, (see Fractures, p. 221).
    3. Skeletal traction via tongs: Crutchfield, Gardner-Wells (see Fractures, p. 221).
    4. Halo traction (see Fractures, p. 221).
  C. Goal: *relieve edema: anti-inflammatories, corticosteroids.*
  D. Goal: *relieve discomfort: analgesics, sedatives, muscle relaxants.*
  E. Goal: *promote comfort:*
    1. Maintain fluid intake: PO/IV, I&O.
    2. Increase nutritional intake.
    3. Prevent contractures and decubitus ulcers.
    4. Help patient deal with psychosocial issues (e.g., role changes).
    5. Begin rehabilitation plan.
  F. Goal: *prevent complications.*
    1. Monitor for spinal shock during initial phase of injury (see Spinal Shock, p. 262).
    2. Monitor for hyperreflexia with severed spinal cord injuries (see Autonomic Hyperreflexia, p. 262).
  G. Goal: health teaching.
    1. Self-care techniques for highest level of independence; include significant others in teaching.
    2. How to use ambulation-assistive devices (battery-operated wheelchair controlled by mouthpiece or hand controls, depending on level of paralysis).
    3. Identify community resources for follow-up care and career counseling.
    4. Signs and symptoms of autonomic hyperreflexia (see p. 262).
    5. Methods to prevent skin breakdown, infections of respiratory, urinary tract.
    6. Bowel, bladder program.

⋈VII. Evaluation/outcome criteria
  A. Complications avoided.

B. Accomplishes self-care to greatest ability for level for injury.
C. Participates in rehabilitation plan.
D. Grieves over loss and begins to integrate self into society.

Spinal Shock

Temporary flaccid paralysis and areflexia following a severe injury to the spinal cord.

I. Pathophysiology: squeezing or shearing of the spinal cord due to fractures or dislocation of vertebrae, interruption of sensory tracts, loss of conscious sensation, interruption of motor tracts, loss of voluntary movement, loss of facilitation, loss of reflex activity, loss of *muscle* tone, loss of stretch reflexes → bowel and bladder retention. Injury between T-1 and L-2, → loss of sympathetic tone and decrease in blood pressure. *Afferent* impulses are unable to *ascend* from below the injured site to the brain, and *efferent* impulses are unable to *descend* to points below the site.

II. Risk factors:
 A. Automobile/motorcycle accidents.
 B. Athletic accidents (e.g., diving in shallow water).
 C. Gunshot wounds.

III. Assessment
 A. *Subjective data:*
  1. Loss of sensation below level of injury.
  2. Inability to move extremities.
  3. Pain at level of injury.
 B. *Objective data:*
  1. *Neurologic:*
   a. *Absent:* pinprick, pressure, vibratory sensations below level of injury; reflexes below level of injury.
   b. Muscles: flaccid.
  2. *Vital signs:*
   a. Blood pressure (BP) decreased (loss of vasomotor tone below level of injury).
   b. Bradycardia.
   c. Elevated temperature.
   d. Respirations: may be depressed, possible respiratory failure if diaphragm involved.
  3. Absence of sweating below level of injury.
  4. Urinary retention.
  5. Abdominal distention: retention of feces, paralytic ileus.
  6. *Skin:* cold, clammy.

IV. Analysis/nursing diagnosis
 A. *Decreased cardiac output* related to loss of vasomotor tone below level of injury.
 B. *Ineffective breathing pattern* related to injuries involving diaphragm.
 C. *Impaired physical mobility* related to loss of voluntary movement of limbs.
 D. *Urinary retention* related to loss of stretch reflexes.
 E. *Fear* related to serious physical condition.
 F. *Risk for injury* related to potential organ damage if shock continues.

V. Nursing care plan/implementation
 A. Goal: *prevent injury related to shock.*

 1. Maintain patent airway: *intubation* and *mechanical ventilation* may be necessary with cervical spinal injuries because of involvement of diaphragm.
 2. Monitor vital signs; **profound hypotension** and **bradycardia** are **most dangerous aspects of spinal shock.**
 3. Administer blood/IV fluids, as ordered.
 4. Nutrition and hydration:
  a. NPO in acute stage: maintain nutrition by IV infusions as ordered.
  b. When allowed to eat: *high-protein, high-calorie, high-vitamin diet.*
 5. Maintain proper *position* to prevent further injury.
  a. Backboard is necessary to transport from place of injury.
  b. Support head in neutral alignment and prevent flexion.
  c. Skeletal traction is applied once diagnosis is made.
 6. Monitor urinary output q1h; may have *Foley catheter* while in shock; later, *intermittent* catheterization used as needed.
 7. Relieve bowel distention; use lubricant containing *anesthetic,* as necessary, when checking for or removing impaction.

VI. Evaluation/outcome criteria
 A. Complications are prevented.
 B. Body functions are maintained.

Autonomic Hyperreflexia (Autonomic Dysreflexia)

A group of spinal cord autonomic responses (symptoms) activated simultaneously; may occur when cord lesions are *above the sixth thoracic* vertebra; it is *most commonly* seen with cervical and high thoracic cord injuries; may occur up to 6 yr after injury. It is a pathologic reflex condition, which is an acute **medical emergency,** characterized by extreme hypertension and exaggerated autonomic responses to stimuli.

I. Pathophysiology: Stimulation of sensory receptors below the level of the cord lesion. The intact autonomic nervous system reflexively responds with an arteriolar spasm → increases blood pressure. When the hypertension is evident, the parasympathetic system is activated → heart rate decreases, but *visceral* and *peripheral* vessels do *not* dilate because efferent impulses cannot pass through the cord. The source of the stimulation, e.g., most commonly, distended bladder or rectum, must be corrected for autonomic hyperreflexia to be reversed.

II. Risk factors:
 A. Distention of bladder or rectum.
 B. Stimulation of skin (e.g., decubitus ulcers, wrinkled clothing).
 C. Stimulation of pain receptors.

III. Assessment
 A. *Subjective data:*
  1. Severe headache.

⊙━ Summary of Key Points

1. Slight *back elevation* (10–30 degrees) and slight *knee flexion* are often most comfortable for a patient with severe lumbar disk pain.
2. Surgery is done when the pain of a herniated disk is unrelieved and neurologic deficits increase. Microsurgery is now available, causing less trauma than the traditional laminectomy and spinal fusion.
3. *Log-rolling* is safest for turning the patient who has undergone back surgery, unless otherwise advised by the surgeon. It prevents twisting of the spine and pulling on the incision.
4. Assessment of *breathing effectiveness* is the *first priority* with a suspected spinal cord injury.

5. The patient must be observed initially for *spinal shock* after complete cord transection because *hypotension* can occur. Spinal shock may last days or months.
6. Autonomic hyperreflexia is a *life-threatening syndrome* for any patient with cord injuries from T-7 up. Reportedly this exaggerated sympathetic response can arise during at least the first 5 years after injury.
7. Although bladder and bowel distention are the most common causes of autonomic hyperreflexia, any noxious stimuli can cause a response.

---

    2. Blurred vision.
    3. Nausea.
    4. Restlessness.
    5. Flushed feeling.
  B. *Objective data:*
    1. Severe hypertension (systolic BP may reach 300 mm Hg).
    2. Bradycardia (30–40 beats/min).
    3. Profuse diaphoresis.
    4. *Flushing* of skin *above* level of injury.
    5. *Pale* skin *below* level of injury.
    6. Pilomotor spasm (goose flesh).
    7. Nasal congestion.
    8. Distended bladder, bowel.
    9. Skin breakdown.

⋈ **IV. Analysis/nursing diagnosis**
  A. *Hyperreflexia* related to high spinal cord injury.
  B. *Risk for injury* related to complications of hypertension, cerebrovascular accident.
  C. *Visual sensory/perceptual alteration* related to blurred vision.
  D. *Urinary retention* related to inability to empty bladder due to spinal injury.
  E. *Constipation* related to inability to establish successful bowel-training program.
  F. *Impaired skin integrity* related to immobility.

⋈ **V. Nursing plan/implementation**
  A. Goal: *decrease symptoms to prevent serious side effects.*
    1. *Elevate head of bed:* lowers BP in persons with high spinal cord injuries.
    2. Identify and correct source of stimulation if possible, notify physician.
    3. Monitor BP q15min and prn; uncontrolled hypertension can lead to cerebrovascular accident, blindness, death.
    4. Give medications as ordered: nitrates, nifedipine (Procardia), or hydralazine (Apresoline).
  B. Goal: *maintain patency of catheter.*

    1. Monitor output, palpate for distended bladder.
    2. Check for tubing kinks, irrigate catheter prn.
    3. Insert new catheter *immediately* if blocked.
    4. Culture if infection suspected.
  C. Goal: *promote regular bowel elimination.*
    1. Bowel training program.
      a. Establish a time schedule
      b. Increase *bulk* in diet
    2. Administer suppository, enemas, *laxatives* as ordered and prn.
    3. When checking for and/or *removing impaction,* first use *anesthetic* ointment (e.g., dibucaine [Nupercainal] ointment) to decrease irritation.
  D. Goal: *prevent decubitus ulcers.*
    1. Meticulous skin care.
    2. *Position:* change q1–2h.
    3. Flotation pads; alternating-pressure mattress on bed, wheelchair.
  E. Goal: **health teaching.**
    1. Risk factors that could trigger this condition.
    2. Methods to prevent situations that increase risk (e.g., bowel program, bladder program, skin care, position change schedule).

⋈ **VI. Evaluation/outcome criteria**
  A. BP remains within normal limits.
  B. No complications occur.

Diagnostic Studies

Electromyography (EMG) provides information necessary in diagnosing neuromuscular diseases. It measures and documents electrical currents produced by skeletal muscles. Needle electrodes are inserted into muscles, which then document electrical potential of each muscle on a screen and paper. The patient should *avoid* all stimulants for 24 h before the test. There may be some discomfort when the needles are inserted.

Myelogram—a contrast medium is injected through a lumbar-puncture needle into the subarachnoid space of the spinal column to visualize the spinal cord; *used to* detect herniated or ruptured intervertebral disks, tumors, or cysts that compress or distort spinal cord. ☞ *Nursing responsibilities:* with *water-soluble* contrast, *elevate* head of bed; with *oil* contrast, head of bed should be flat; check for bladder distention with metrizamide (water-soluble contrast agent); check vital signs every 4 h for 24 h.

Study and Memory Aids

• Diet

Spinal Shock

NPO/IV → ↑ Calories
Protein
Vitamins

• Drug Review

Herniated Intervertebral Disk

Analgesics
  Acetaminophen/codeine (Tylenol #1, #2, #3): 1–2 tablets q3–4h, as needed
  Meperidine HCl (Demerol): IM or SC, 50–75 mg
  Oxycodone/acetaminophen (Tylox, Percocet): 5 mg q3–6h, as needed
Anti-inflammatories
  Aspirin/ecotrin: 2.6–6.2 g/d in divided doses
  Ibuprofen (Motrin): 300–800 mg 3–4 times daily, not to exceed 3200 mg/d
  Indomethacin (Indocin): 25–50 mg 2–4 times daily
Muscle relaxants
  Baclofen (Lioresal): 5 mg 3 times daily, up to maximum of 80 mg/d
  Carisoprodol (Soma): 350 mg 3–4 times daily
  Cyclobenzaprine (Flexeril): 10 mg tid (20–40 mg/d, not to exceed 60 mg/d)
  Diazepam (Valium): 2–10 mg 2–4 times daily
Stool softeners: Docusate (Colace): 50–500 mg/d

Laminectomy

Analgesics
  Acetaminophen/codeine (Tylenol #1, #2, #3): 1–2 tablets q3–4h, as needed
  Meperidine HCl (Demerol): IM or SC, 50–75 mg
  Oxycodone/acetaminophen (Tylox, Percocet): 5 mg q3–6h, as needed

Spinal Cord Injury

Analgesics
  Acetaminophen/codeine (Tylenol #1, #2, #3): 1–2 tablets q3–4h, as needed
  Meperidine HCl (Demerol): IM or SC, 50–75 mg
  Oxycodone/acetaminophen (Tylox, Percocet): 5 mg q3–6h, as needed
Anti-inflammatories
  Aspirin/ecotrin: 2.6–6.2 g/d in divided doses
  Ibuprofen (Motrin): 300–800 mg 3–4 times daily, *not to exceed* 3200 mg/d
  Indomethacin (Indocin): 25–50 mg 2–4 times daily
Muscle relaxants
  Baclofen (Lioresal): 5 mg 3 times daily, up to maximum of 80 mg/d
  Carisoprodol (Soma): 350 mg 3–4 times daily
  Cyclobenzaprine (Flexeril): 10 mg tid (20–40 mg/d, not to exceed 60 mg/d)
Sedatives
  Chlordiazepoxide HCl (Librium): 5–10 mg 3–4 times daily
  Diazepam (Valium): 2–10 mg 2–4 times daily
Steroids (should *never* be abruptly discontinued; gradually taper dose to prevent complications):
  Dexamethasone (Decadron): 0.5–9 mg/d in single or divided doses

Autonomic Hyperreflexia

Hydralazine HCl (Apresoline): 10–50 mg qid
Nitroglycerin: 0.25–0.6 mg repeated q5min for 15 min for severe hypertension
Nifedipine (Procardia): 10–30 mg tid

Questions

1. A 72-year-old woman has undergone a lumbar laminectomy with spinal fusion 3 days earlier. The nurse teaches her that the correct way to get onto the bedpan is to:
   1. Lift herself up with an overhead trapeze and swing onto the bedpan.
   2. Turn to her side, then log-roll onto the bedpan.
   3. Have two nurses lift her onto the bedpan.
   4. Push down on the bed to raise herself onto the bedpan.
2. During a lumbar puncture the nurse's role is to:
   1. Hold the patient in the desired position.
   2. Check the patient's vital signs every 15 minutes.
   3. Remind the patient to breathe deeply to relax.
   4. Assess for indications of nerve damage.
3. Sciatic nerve involvement is suspected in a patient with a herniated disc. Which test would confirm the nerve problem?
   1. Straight-leg raising.
   2. Gluteal contraction.
   3. Pinprick over the gluteal area.
   4. Plantar flexion of the foot.

4. Which observations made by a patient preoperatively would provide the most useful information for the planning of care after a spinal fusion?
   1. Fears about surgery.
   2. Memories of previous hospitalizations.
   3. Preferred pain therapy.
   4. Currently experienced pain, muscle spasms, and numbness.

5. Which nursing action would be most helpful the first time a patient sits in a chair after surgery for a herniated disc?
   1. Teaching the patient relaxation techniques to use when getting out of bed.
   2. Using two people to transfer the patient to the chair.
   3. Bracing the patient's back with a rib support before the patient gets out of bed.
   4. Giving the patient the prescribed pain medication 30 minutes before getting out of bed.

6. An indication of adequate respiratory function in a patient with a cervical spinal cord injury would be:
   1. Use of accessory muscles.
   2. Nasal flaring.
   3. Diaphragmatic breathing.
   4. Swallowing air.

Answers/Rationale

1. **(2)** Log-rolling would not be required for a lumbar laminectomy alone, but the spinal fusion would require that a shearing motion be avoided during turning. The patient would therefore be taught to log-roll, and the nurse, or nurses, would assist her as needed. The key is having the patient roll as a single unit, avoiding the placement of stress on any particular area of the body. An *older* woman may *not* have the *arm strength* to lift

---

herself up **(1)** and may end up twisting. Lifting, even by the nurses **(3)**, would *not* ensure proper body mechanics. Pushing down on the bed **(4)** would again rely on arm strength and *may not be possible* for an *older* patient. **IMP, 3, PhI**

2. **(1)** The patient is placed on the side with the back arched, neck flexed, and knees drawn up; holding the patient still will ensure a safe procedure. Vital signs **(2)** would be assessed *before* and *after* the procedure, but it is not necessary to assess them every 15 minutes. Relaxation **(3)** would *not* reduce any discomfort, which is minimal, and deep breathing might cause too much movement. The site of a lumbar puncture is low enough that there is no danger of spinal cord injury, so assessment for nerve damage **(4)** is *unnecessary.* **IMP, 3, SECE**

3. **(1)** The sciatic nerve is the longest nerve in the body and is subjected to more trauma than any other nerve; any movement of the lower extremities stretches the nerve and would cause pain. Although the pain usually starts at the buttocks, contraction of the gluteal muscle **(2)** would *not* induce pain. Pinprick **(3)** is *too superficial* a stimulus. *Dorsiflexion,* rather than plantar flexion **(4)**, might elicit pain. **AS, 2, SECE**

4. **(4)** Postoperative care in this patient would include assessing the effectiveness of the surgery by comparing the degree of any postoperative discomfort with the patient's preoperative status. The observations in options 1 and 2 would be a source of increased preoperative anxiety, and this might influence the amount of anesthetic needed during surgery but would have less effect on the nature of postoperative care. If the surgery is successful, the degree of pain after surgery will be less, thus the patient would require a different approach to pain management **(3). AN, 2, PhI**

5. **(4)** Once the anesthetic wears off, there will be pain resulting from swelling; administering pain medication before the patient gets out of bed is recommended for any surgical patient. Relaxation techniques **(1)** do reduce pain, but the patient may be *too anxious* the *first time* out of bed to focus on such a technique. One nurse can assist the patient in transferring to a chair **(2)** but should be careful that this not involve twisting. A metal brace, corset, or cast may be used temporarily to support the patient's spine **(3)**, but it would *not* be *used* for the *first time* the patient gets out of bed. **IMP, 3, PhI**

6. **(3)** The diaphragm is a strong muscle and important to effective ventilation. The use of accessory muscles **(1)**, nasal flaring **(2)**, and swallowing air **(4)** would indicate *ineffective* breathing and respiratory difficulty. **EV, 2, PhI**

Degenerative Neurologic Disorders

Chapter Outline

Multiple Sclerosis

Progressive neurologic disease, common in northern climates, characterized by demyelination of brain and spinal cord, leading to degenerative neurologic function; chronic remitting and relapsing disease; cause unknown.

I. Pathophysiology: multiple foci (patches) of nerve degeneration throughout brain, spinal cord, optic nerve, and cerebrum → interruption (blockade) or distortion (slowing) of nerve impulses. Exacerbations aggravated by fatigue, chilling, and emotional distress.

II. Risk factors
   A. Northern climate.
   B. Onset age: 20–40 yr.
   C. Affects men and women equally.

III. Assessment
   A. *Subjective data:*
      1. Extremities: weak, numb, decreased sensation.
      2. Emotional instability, apathy, irritability, mood swings, fatigue.
      3. Eyes: diplopia (double vision), spots before eyes (*scotomas*), potential blindness.
      4. Difficulty swallowing.
   B. *Objective data:*
      1. Nystagmus (involuntary rhythmic movements of eyeball), decreased visual acuity.
      2. Inappropriate outbursts of laughing or crying (sometimes related to ingestion of *hot food*).
      3. Disorders of speech.
      4. Susceptibility to infections.
      5. Tremors to severe muscle spasms and contractures.
      6. Changes in muscular coordination; *gait:* ataxic, spastic.
      7. Changes in bowel habits (e.g., constipation).
      8. Urinary frequency, urgency.
      9. Incontinence: urine and feces.
      10. Lab tests: cerebrospinal fluid contains gamma globulin, IgG.

IV. Analysis/nursing diagnosis
   A. *Impaired physical mobility* related to changes in muscular coordination.
   B. *Self-esteem disturbance* related to chronic, debilitating disease.
   C. *Altered health maintenance* related to spasms and contractures.
   D. *Risk for impaired skin integrity* related to contractures.
   E. *Constipation* related to immobility.
   F. *Impaired swallowing* related to tremors.
   G. *Visual-sensory/perceptual alteration* related to nystagmus and decreased visual acuity.

V. Nursing care plan/implementation
   A. Goal: *maintain normal routine as long as possible.*
      1. Maintain mobility—encourage walking as tolerated, active and passive range of motion (*ROM*), exercises, splints to decrease spasticity.
      2. *Avoid* fatigue, infections.
      3. Frequent position changes to prevent skin breakdown, contractures; *position at night:* prone to minimize flexor spasms of knees and hips.
      4. Bowel/bladder training program to minimize incontinence.
      5. *Avoid* stressful situations.
   B. Goal: *decrease symptoms*—medications as ordered:
      1. Baclofen (Lioresal) for alleviating spasticity; *avoid* sudden withdrawal (which may cause hallucinations, rebound spasticity).
      2. *Steroids* during exacerbations.
      3. *Skeletal muscle relaxants:* Diazepam (Valium), dantrolene (Dantrium) to relieve muscle spasm.

4. *Anticonvulsants* and *antidepressants* for dyesthesias or neuralgias: carbamazepine (Tegretol), phenytoin (Dilantin), amitriptyline HCl, (Elavil).

C. Goal: **health teaching to** *prevent complications.*
   1. Signs and symptoms of disease, measures to prevent exacerbations.
   2. The way to monitor respiratory status to prevent infections.
   3. Importance of physical therapy to prevent contractures.
   4. Possible counseling or community support group for assistance in accepting long-term condition.
   5. Teach special skin care to prevent decubitus ulcers.
   6. Teach use of assistive devices to maintain independence.

VI. Evaluation/outcome criteria
   A. Establishes daily routine, adjusts to altered lifestyle.
   B. Injuries prevented, no falls.
   C. Urinary and bowel routines established, incontinence decreased.
   D. Infections prevented.
   E. Symptoms minimized by medications.

Myasthenia Gravis

Neuromuscular disease characterized by weakness and easy fatigability of facial, oculomotor, pharyngeal, and respiratory muscles.

   I. Pathophysiology: inadequate acetylcholine or excessive or altered cholinesterase → impaired transmission of nerve impulses to muscles at myoneural junction.
   II. Risk factors:
   A. Possible autoimmune reaction.
   B. Thymus tumor.
   C. Ages: 20–40 yr: affects more women than men.
   D. Older age groups: affects men and women equally.
   III. Assessment
   A. *Subjective data:*
      1. Diplopia (double vision).
      2. Severe generalized fatigue.
   B. *Objective data:*
      1. Muscle weakness: hands, arms affected first.
      2. Ptosis (drooping of eyelids), expressionless facies.
      3. Hypersensitivity to narcotics, barbiturates, tranquilizers.
      4. Abnormal speech pattern, with high-pitched nasal voice.
      5. Difficulty chewing/swallowing food.
      6. Decreased ability to cough and deep breathe, vital capacity.
      7. Positive *Tensilon* test (administration of edrophonium chloride, 10 mg IV, produces relief of symptoms within 30 sec).
      8. Positive *Prostigmin test* (neostigmine methylsulfate, 1.5 mg SC, produces relief of symp-

toms within 15 min, increased muscle strength within 30 min).
   IV. Analysis/nursing diagnosis
   A. *Ineffective breathing pattern* related to weakness.
   B. *Risk for injury* related to muscle weakness.
   C. *Activity intolerance* related to severe fatigue.
   D. *Bathing/dressing self-care deficit* related to progressive disease.
   E. *Impaired physical mobility* related to decrease in strength.
   F. *Anxiety* related to physical symptoms and disease progression.
   G. *Knowledge deficit* related to medication administration and expected effectiveness.
   V. Nursing care plan/implementation
   A. Goal: *promote comfort.*
      1. Passive and active ROM exercises, as tolerated, to increase strength.
      2. *Mouth* care: before and after meals.
      3. *Diet:* as tolerated; soft, pureed, or tube feedings.
      4. *Skin* care to prevent decubitus ulcers.
      5. *Eye care:* remove crusts, patch on affected eye prn.
      6. Monitor *respiratory* status: *suction* airway prn.
   B. Goal: *decrease symptoms.*
      1. Administer medications, as ordered:
         a. *Anticholinesterase* (neostigmine [Prostigmin], pyridostigmine) to elevate concentration of acetylcholine at myoneural junction.
         b. Give *before* meals to aid in chewing, *with* milk or food to decrease gastrointestinal (GI) symptoms; may be given parenterally.
   C. Goal: *prevent complications.*
      1. Respiratory assistance if breathing pattern not adequate.
      2. Monitor for choking/increased oral secretion.
      3. *Avoid:* narcotics, barbiturates, tranquilizers.
   D. Goal: *promote increased self-concept.*
      1. Encourage independence when appropriate.
      2. Encourage communication, provide alternative methods when speech pattern impaired.
   E. Goal: **health teaching.**
      1. Medication information:
         a. Adjust dosage to maintain muscle strength.
         b. Medication must be taken at prescribed time to *avoid:*
            (1) *Myasthenic crisis* (too little medication).
            (2) *Cholinergic crisis* (too much medication).
      2. *Signs and symptoms of crisis:* dyspnea, severe muscle weakness, respiratory distress, difficulty swallowing.
      3. Importance of preventing upper respiratory tract infections.
      4. Determine methods to conserve energy, maintain independence as long as possible, while *avoiding* overexertion.
      5. Refer to Myasthenia Gravis Foundation and other community agencies for assistance in reintegration into the community and plans for follow-up care.

VI. Evaluation/outcome criteria
   A. Independence maintained as long as possible.
   B. Respiratory arrest avoided.
   C. Infection avoided.
   D. Medication regimen followed and crisis avoided.

Parkinson's Disease

Progressive disease of the brain occurring in later life; characterized by stiffness of muscles, tremors.

   I. Pathophysiology: depigmentation of the substantia nigra of basal ganglia → decreased dopamine (neurotransmitter necessary for proper muscle movement) → decreased, slowed voluntary movement; wooden facies; difficulty initiating ambulation. Decreased inhibitions of alpha-motoneurons → increased muscle tone → rigidity of flexor and extensor muscles, tremors at rest.

   II. Risk factors:
   A. Age of onset: 50–60 yr.
   B. Affects men and women equally.
   C. Cause unknown, possibly connected to arteriosclerosis or viral infection.
   D. Drug-induced parkinsonian syndromes have been linked to:
      1. Phenothiazines.
      2. Reserpine (Serpasil).
      3. Butyrophenones (Haloperidol).

   III. Assessment
   A. *Subjective data:*
      1. Insomnia.
      2. Depression.
      3. Defects in judgment, emotional instability; intelligence *not* impaired.
   B. *Objective data:*
      1. Limbs, shoulders: stiff, resistant to passive ROM.
      2. Loss of coordination, muscular weakness with rigidity.
      3. Shuffling gait: difficulty initiating, then propulsive walking; trunk bent forward.
      4. Tremors: pill-rolling of fingers, to-and-fro head movements.
      5. Loss of postural reflexes.
      6. Weight loss, constipation.
      7. Difficulty maintaining social interactions because of impaired speech, lack of facial affect, drooling.
      8. Facies: wide-eyed, eye blinking, decreased facial expression.
      9. Akinesia (abnormal absence of movement).
      10. Excessive salivation, drooling.
      11. Speech: slowed, slurred.
      12. Judgment defective, intelligence intact.
      13. Heat intolerance.

   IV. Analysis/nursing diagnosis
   A. *Impaired physical mobility* related to loss of coordination.
   B. *Altered health maintenance* related to defective judgment.
   C. *Risk for injury* related to altered gait.

   D. *Dressing/grooming self-care deficit* related to muscular rigidity.
   E. *Sleep pattern disturbance* related to insomnia.
   F. *Body image disturbance* related to tremors and drooling.
   G. *Social isolation* related to altered physical appearance.
   H. *Altered nutrition, less than body requirements,* related to lack of appetite.
   I. *Impaired swallowing* related to excessive drooling.
   J. *Constipation* related to dietary changes.

   V. Nursing care plan/implementation
   A. Goal: *promote maintenance of daily activities.*
      1. ROM exercises, skin care, physical therapy.
      2. Encourage ambulation, discourage sitting for long periods.
      3. Assist with meals—*high protein, high calorie; soft diet;* small, frequent feedings; encourage increased fluids.
      4. Encourage compliance with medication regimen:
         a. *Dopamine agonists:*
            (1) Levodopa: given in increasing doses until symptoms are relieved; given *with food* to decrease GI symptoms. *Side effects:* nausea, vomiting, anorexia, postural hypotension, mental changes, cardiac arrhythmias. Levodopa helps restore dopamine in striated muscle.
            (2) Sinemet (carbidopa and levodopa): limits the metabolism of levodopa peripherally and provides more levodopa for the brain.
         b. *Anticholinergics:* effective in lessening muscle rigidity.
         c. *Antihistamines:* have mild central anticholinergic properties.
   B. Goal: *protect from injury.*
      1. Monitor blood pressure, side effects of medications (e.g., orthostatic hypotension).
      2. Monitor for GI disturbances.
      3. *Avoid* pyridoxine (vitamin B_6): cancels effect of levodopa.
      4. Levodopa *contraindicated* with:
         a. Glaucoma (causes increased intraocular pressure).
         b. Monoamine oxidase inhibitors (causes possible hypertensive crisis).
   C. Goal: **health teaching.**
      1. Teach patient, family about medications: dosage range, side effects, not discontinuing medications abruptly.
      2. Exercise program to maintain ROM and normal body posture; also get adequate rest to prevent fatigue.
      3. *Dietary adjustment and precautions* regarding cutting food in small pieces to prevent choking, taking fluid with food to facilitate swallowing.
      4. Importance of adding *roughage* to diet to prevent constipation.

5. Help patient, family adjust to this chronic debilitating illness.

VI. Evaluation/outcome criteria
  A. Activity level maintained.
  B. Symptoms relieved by medications, no drug interactions.
  C. Complications prevented.

Amyotrophic Lateral Sclerosis (ALS; Lou Gehrig's Disease)

Progressive degeneration of motoneurons within the brain and/or spinal cord, leading to death within 2–5 yr, usually from pneumonia resulting from respiratory or bulbar paralysis.

  I. Pathophysiology: myelin sheaths destroyed, replaced by scar tissue; involves lateral tracts of spinal cord, eventually medulla and ventral tracts.

 II. Risk factors:
  A. Affects more men than women.
  B. Onset usually in middle age.
  C. Viral infection possible causal agent.
  D. Possible familial or genetic component.

III. Assessment
  A. *Subjective data:*
    1. Early symptoms: fatigue, awkwardness.
    2. Dysphagia, dysarthria.
    3. Alert, no sensory loss.
  B. *Objective data:*
    1. Symptoms depend on which motoneurons affected.
    2. Decreased fine finger movement.
    3. Progressive muscular weakness, atrophy.
    4. Spasticity of flexor muscles, one side of body becomes more involved than other.
    5. Progressive respiratory difficulties → diaphragmatic paralysis.
    6. Progressive disability of upper and lower extremities.
    7. Tongue fasciculations.

IV. Analysis/nursing diagnosis
  A. *Ineffective airway clearance* related to difficulty coughing.
  B. *Ineffective breathing pattern* related to progressive respiratory difficulties and eventually respiratory paralysis.
  C. *Altered health maintenance* related to inability to perform self-care activities.
  D. *Impaired physical mobility* related to progressive muscular weakness.
  E. *Bathing/hygiene and dressing/grooming self-care deficit* related to neuromuscular impairment.
  F. *Powerlessness* related to progressive physical helplessness.
  G. *Impaired swallowing* related to disease progression.

 V. Nursing care plan/implementation
  A. Goal: *maintain independence as long as possible.*

  1. Assistance with activities of daily living (ADL); *splints, prosthetic devices* to support weak limbs and maintain mobility.
  2. Skin care to prevent decubitus.
  3. *Soft/liquid diet* to aid in swallowing, prevent choking; *suction* prn; *head of bed elevated* when eating.
  4. *Respiratory* assistance as needed, ventilators as disease progresses and diaphragm becomes involved.
  5. Arrange long-term care if home maintenance no longer feasible.
  6. Emotional support, when patient is alert; continue involving patient in decisions regarding care.

  B. Goal: **health teaching.**
    1. Skin care to prevent decubitus.
    2. Ramifications of disease, so patient and family can make decisions regarding future care, whether patient will remain at home as disease progresses or enter a long-term care facility.
    3. The way to use suction apparatus to clear airway.
    4. Care of nasogastric or gastrostomy feeding tube.

VI. Evaluation/outcome criteria
  A. Obtains physical and emotional support.
  B. Complications prevented in early stage of disease.
  C. Remains in control of ADL as long as possible.
  D. Skin breakdown prevented.
  E. Peaceful death.

Study and Memory Aids

● Diet

Myasthenia Gravis
Pureed
Soft
or
Tube feed

Parkinson's Disease	
Calories	
Fluids	
Frequent feeding	soft and bland
Protein	
Roughage	
Size of feedings	

☞ Summary of Key Points

1. Several degenerative disorders occur in young adults as early as 20–30 yr of age. Parkinson's disease is more common in adults over 60 yr.
2. *Visual* problems are often the *first indication* of multiple sclerosis.
3. Treatment for multiple sclerosis is *symptomatic* and designed to prevent complications, which may be fatal. Disease progression is *unpredictable.*
4. Muscle weakness resulting from myasthenia gravis increases with exercise and diminishes after rest.
5. Myasthenia gravis, like multiple sclerosis, often presents with *ocular* symptoms. The clinical course can vary greatly and may progress slowly or rapidly.
6. The nurse must be able to distinguish between a *myasthenic* and *cholinergic crisis.*
7. Parkinson's disease causes disability as a result of *tremors* and *rigidity.* Intellectual ability is usually *not* affected.
8. The *bowel- and bladder-related side* effects of anticholinergic drugs used to treat Parkinson's disease may be distressing to older adults.
9. ALS ends in death 2–5 yr after diagnosis. The cause of death is usually *pneumonia* secondary to ineffective respiratory function.
10. Nursing actions for a patient with ALS are *supportive.* Even after total debilitation the patient's *mental status* is *intact.*

● Drug Review

Multiple Sclerosis

Anticonvulsant
Carbamazepine (Tegretol): 200 mg bid; maintenance dose 800–1200 mg daily.
Phenytoin (Dilantin): 100 mg tid; maximum dose 600 mg daily.
Antidepressant
Amitryptyline HCL (Elavil): 75–100 mg in 1–4 divided doses; maintenance dose 40–100 mg daily.
Skeletal muscle relaxants
Baclofen (Lioresal): 5 mg 3 times daily, up to maximum of 80 mg/d (20 mg 4 times daily); optimal effect between 40–80 mg
Dantrolene (Dantrium): 25 mg/d; increase to 25 mg 2–4 times daily up to 100 mg 2–4 times daily (not to exceed 40 mg/d)
Diazepam (Valium): 2–10 mg 2–4 times daily
Steroids (should *never* be abruptly discontinued; gradually taper dose to prevent complications)
Dexamethasone (Decadron): 0.5–9 mg/d in single or divided doses
Methylprednisolone (Medrol): 4–48 mg/d
Prednisone: 5–60 mg/d.

Parkinson's Disease

Anticholinergics
Benzotropine (Cogentin): 0.5–6 mg/d in 1–2 divided doses
Biperiden (Akineton): 2 mg 3–4 times daily, *not* to exceed 16 mg/d
Trihexyphenidyl (Artane): 1–2 mg/d; increase by 2 mg q3–5 days; usual maintenance dose, 5–15 mg/d in 3–4 divided doses
Antihistamines
Chlorpheniramine maleate (Chlor-Trimeton): 2–4 mg tid
Diphenhydramine (Benadryl): 25–50 mg bid
Dopamine Agonists
Carbidopa/levodopa (Sinemet): 25–250 mg/d in 3–4 divided doses; can increase to 200/8000 mg/d
Levodopa (L-dopa): 500–1000 mg/d in divided doses q6–12h; increase by 100–750 mg/d q3–7 d until response reached; usual maintenance dose, should *not* exceed 18 g/d.
NO PYRIDOXINE (B$_6$)

Myasthenia Gravis

Anticholinesterase agent
Neostigmine (Prostigmin): 15 mg q3–4h; increase daily until optimal response achieved; usual maintenance dose, 150 mg/d (up to 375 mg may be needed)
Pyridostigmine (Mestinon): 60 mg 3 times/d, maintenance dose 60–1500 mg/d.

Questions

1. A 30-year-old woman with suspected myasthenia gravis is admitted to undergo testing to confirm or rule out the diagnosis. Which physical change would the nurse likely observe in the woman?
   1. Intention tremor.
   2. Muscle rigidity.
   3. Drooping eyelids.
   4. Hemiplegia.

2. Although the Tensilon (edrophonium) test is frequently used to establish the diagnosis of myasthenia gravis, the nurse should know that a more conclusive diagnosis is possible using neostigmine (Prostigmin) because:
   1. The desired effect occurs more rapidly.
   2. The desired effect lasts hours rather than minutes.
   3. The improvement is generalized, not just localized.
   4. The improvement is permanent, not temporary.

3. Which nursing diagnosis would be the greatest concern during the hospitalization of a patient with myasthenia gravis?
   1. Risk for activity intolerance.
   2. Pain.
   3. Impaired adjustment.
   4. Impaired memory.

4. Which drug would be contraindicated in a patient with myasthenia gravis?
   1. Nifedipine (Procardia).
   2. Furosemide (Lasix).
   3. Atropine.
   4. Potassium penicillin.

Answers/Rationale

1. **(3)** Myasthenia gravis is an autoimmune disease that presents with muscular weakness and fatigue resulting from a loss of acetylcholine receptors in the postsynaptic neurons of the neuromuscular junction. As a result, affected patients are often unable to keep their eyes open, chew, or swallow. Intention tremor **(1)** and muscle rigidity **(2)** would be seen in a patient with *Parkinson's* disease. Hemiplegia **(4)** would be seen in a patient who has had a *CVA*. **AS, 3, PhI**

2. **(2)** Neostigmine's effects last 2 to 4 hours, and edrophonium's effects only last 30 minutes. Testing with neostigmine would therefore permit more time to observe for an alleviation or worsening of symptoms. The onset of neostigmine's effects is slower, *not* more rapid **(1)**. *Both* drugs produce generalized effects **(3)**, and improvement is *temporary, not* permanent **(4)**. **AN, 3, SECE**

3. **(1)** The muscle weakness and fatigue, if not controlled with drug therapy, will interfere with basic activities, such as eating. The condition is *painless* **(2)**. There may be problems with adjustment **(3)** to the chronic illness, but the *priority* would be the activity intolerance. There is *no* memory impairment **(4)** in myasthenia. **AN, 3, SECE**

4. **(2)** The loss of potassium ions resulting from diuretic therapy may cause the muscle weakness to worsen. Nifedipine **(1)** may cause muscle cramping, but *not* weakness. Atropine **(3)** affects cardiac function, *not* skeletal muscle strength. Potassium penicillin **(4)** does *not* affect the potassium ion concentration. **IMP, 6, PhI**

Key to Codes

Nursing process: AS, assessment; **AN,** analysis; **PL,** planning; **IMP,** implementation; **EV,** evaluation. (See Appendix M for explanation of nursing process steps.)

Category of human function: 1, protective; **2,** sensory-perceptual; **3,** comfort, rest, activity, and mobility; **4,** nutrition; **5,** growth and development; **6,** fluid-gas transport; **7,** psychosocial-cultural; **8,** elimination. (See Appendix O for explanation.)

Client need: SECE, safe, effective care environment; **PhI,** physiologic integrity; **PsI,** psychosocial integrity; **HPM,** health promotion/maintenance. (See Appendix P for explanation.)

Neoplastic Disorders

Chapter Outline

The Cancer Patient

Cancer is a multisystem stressor. Regardless of the specific type of cancer, certain aspects of the disease and of nursing care are the same. The following principles apply universally and should be referred to when studying individual kinds of cancer.

I. Pathophysiology: result of altered cellular mechanisms. Several theories about causation, but current thinking is multiple causation. Alterations result in a progressive, uncontrolled multiplication of cells, with selective ability to invade and metastasize.

II. Risk factors
  A. Heredity (e.g., retinoblastoma).
  B. Familial susceptibility (e.g., breast cancer).
  C. Acquired diseases (e.g., ulcerative colitis).
  D. Virus (e.g., Burkitt's tumor).
  E. Environmental factors:
    1. Tobacco.
    2. Alcohol.
    3. Radiation.
    4. Occupational hazards.

  5. Drugs (e.g., immunosuppressive, cytotoxic).
  F. Age.
  G. Air pollution.
  H. Diet (e.g., *high animal protein*).
  I. Chronic irritation.
  J. Precancerous lesions (e.g., gastric ulcers).
  K. Stress.

III. Assessment
  A. Specific symptoms depend on the anatomic and functional characteristics of the organ or structure involved.
  B. Mechanical effects:
    1. *Pressure*—tumors growing in confined areas such as bone produce pain early, whereas tumors growing in expandable areas such as the abdomen may be undetected for some time.
    2. *Obstruction*—tumors that compress tubular structures such as the esophagus, bronchi, or lymph channels may cause symptoms such as swallowing difficulties, shortness of breath, edema. Symptoms depend on location of tumor and on the particular organ or structure being compressed.

3. *Interruptions of blood supply*—compression of blood vessels or diversion of blood supply may cause necrosis or ulceration or may precipitate hemorrhage.

C. Systemic effects:
   1. Anorexia, weakness, weight loss.
   2. *Metabolic* disturbances—malabsorption syndrome.
   3. *Fluid and electrolyte* imbalances.
   4. *Hormonal* imbalances—increased antidiuretic hormone (ADH), adrenocorticotropic hormone (ACTH), thyrotropin, or parathyroid hormone.
   5. Diagnostic tests:
      a. *Biopsy*—excision of part of tumor.
      b. *Needle biopsy*—aspiration of cells from subcutaneous masses or organs such as liver.
      c. *Exfoliative cytology*—scraping of any endothelium (cervix, mucous membranes) applied to slide.
      d. *X-rays*—detect tumor growth in gastrointestinal (GI), respiratory, renal systems.
      e. *Endoscopy*—visualization of body cavity through endoscope.
      f. *Computerized axial tomography* (CAT)—visualization of a body part whereby layers of tissue can be seen utilizing the very narrow beams of this type of x-ray equipment.
      g. *Magnetic resonance imaging (MRI)*—a scanning device using a magnetic field for visualization.
   6. Lab data:
      a. *Blood and urine tests*—refer to Appendix G for normal values.
      b. *Alkaline phosphates*—greatly *increased* in osteogenic carcinoma (>92 U/L).
      c. *Calcium—elevated* in multiple myeloma bone metastases (>10.5 mg/dL).
      d. *Sodium—decreased* in bronchogenic carcinoma (<135 mEq/L).
      e. *Potassium—decreased* in extensive liver carcinoma (<3.5 mEq/L).
      f. *Serum gastrin*—gauges gastric secretions. *Decreased* in gastric carcinoma. Normal value: 40–150 pg/mL.
      g. *Neutrophilic leukocytosis*—tumors.
      h. *Eosinophilic leukocytosis*—brain tumors, Hodgkin's disease.
      i. *Lymphocytosis*—chronic lymphocytic anemia.

IV. Analysis/nursing diagnosis
   A. *Pain* related to diagnostic procedures, pressure, obstruction, interruption of blood supply, or side effects of drugs.
   B. *Anxiety* related to fear regarding diagnosis or disease progression, treatment, and its known or expected side effects.
   C. *Altered nutrition, less than body requirements,* related to anorexia.
   D. *Risk for injury* related to radioactive contamination of excreta.

E. *Body image disturbance* related to loss of body parts, change in appearance as a result of therapy.
F. *Powerlessness* related to diagnosis and own perception of its meaning.
G. *Self-esteem disturbance* related to impact of cancer diagnosis.
H. *Risk for infection* related to immunosuppression resulting from radiation and chemotherapy.
I. *Altered urinary elimination* related to dehydration.
J. *Risk for injury* related to damage of normal tissue resulting from radiation source.
K. *Fluid volume deficit* related to nausea and vomiting.
L. *Diarrhea* related to irradiation of bowel.
M. *Constipation* related to dehydration.

V. Nursing care plan/implementation—general care of the cancer patient:
   A. Goal: *promote psychosocial comfort.*
      1. Assist with diagnostic workup by providing psychological support and information about diagnostic tests, diagnosis, treatment options.
      2. Reduce anxiety by listening, making referrals for special problems (peer support groups, self-help groups such as Reach to Recovery), supplying information, or correcting misinformation, as appropriate.
      3. Stress-management techniques.
      4. Nursing management related to depressed patient.
   B. Goal: *minimize effects of complications.*
      1. *Anorexia/anemia:*
         a. *Decrease anemia* by:
            (1) Providing well-balanced, *iron-rich,* small, frequent meals.
            (2) Administering supplemental vitamins and iron, as ordered.
            (3) Administering *packed red blood cells,* as ordered.
            (4) Maintaining *hyperalimentation,* as ordered.
         b. *Enhance nutrition* by providing nutritional supplements and a diet *high in protein,* necessary because of increased metabolism related to metastatic process. *Consult* with dietitian for suggestions about best food for individual patient.
      2. *Hemorrhage:* monitor *platelet* count and maintain platelet infusions, as ordered. Teach patient to monitor for any signs of bleeding.
      3. *Infection:* observe for signs of sepsis (changes in vital signs, temperature of skin, mentation, urinary output, or pain), monitor laboratory values, administer *antiinfectives* as ordered.
      4. *Pain and discomfort:* alleviate by frequent position changes, diversions, conversations guided imagery, relaxation, back rubs, *narcotics,* as ordered.
      5. Assist in adjusting to altered body image by encouraging expression of fears and concerns. *Don't* ignore patient's questions; give honest answers; be available.

C. Goal: general health teaching.
1. Self-care skills to maintain independence, e.g., patient who has a colostomy should know how to manage the colostomy before going home.
2. Importance of follow-up care and routine physical examinations to monitor for general health and possible signs of further disease.
3. Dietary instructions, adjustments necessary to maintain nutrition during and after treatment.
4. Health maintenance programs: teach hazards of tobacco and alcohol use; *avoid* high-fat, low-roughage diet.
5. Risk factors: family history, stress, age, diet, occupation, environment.

VI. General surgical intervention: surgery may be *curative* (when the lesion is localized or metastases to the lymph nodes are minimal) or *palliative* (to decrease symptomatology). (Also see The Perioperative Experience, p. 111, and specific types of cancer, following.)

A. Nursing care plan/implementation
1. **Preoperative care:**
   a. Goal: *prevent respiratory complications.*
      (1) Coughing and deep-breathing techniques.
      (2) *No* smoking for 1 wk before surgery.
   b. Goal: *counteract nutritional deficiencies.*
      (1) *Diet:*
         (a) High *protein,* high *carbohydrate* for tissue repair.
         (b) *Vitamin* and *mineral* supplements.
         (c) Hyperalimentation, as ordered.
      (2) Blood transfusions may be needed if counts are low.
   c. Goal: *reduce apprehension.*
      (1) Clarify postoperative expectations.
      (2) Explain care of ostomies or tubes.
      (3) Answer patient's questions honestly.
2. **Postoperative care:**
   a. Goal: *prevent complications.*
      (1) Monitor respiratory and hemodynamic status.
      (2) *Wound* care; active and passive *exercises* as allowed; *respiratory* hygiene; coughing, deep breathing, turning; fluids (see Postoperative Experience, p. 114).
   b. Goal: *alleviate pain and discomfort.*
      (1) Encourage early ambulation, depending on surgical procedure.
      (2) Administer prescribed medications, as needed.
      (3) Administer *stool softeners* and *enemas,* as ordered.
   c. Goal: **health teaching.**
      (1) Involve patient, significant others, family members in rehabilitation program.
      (2) Prepare for further therapies, such as radiation or chemotherapy.
      (3) Support groups, as appropriate: Reach to Recovery, Ostomy Associates, Laryngectomy Association.

(4) Develop skills to deal with disease progression if cure not realistic or metastasis evident (see X. Palliative care, p. 279).

VII. Chemotherapy: used as single treatment or in combination with surgery and irradiation, for early or advanced diseases. Antineoplastic agents' primary mode of action involves interfering with the supply and utilization of building blocks of nucleic acids as well as interfering with intact molecules of DNA or RNA, which are needed for replication and growth. *Bone marrow, hair follicles,* and the *GI tract* are three areas of the body in which cells are actively dividing; this is why *most side effects* are related to these areas of the body.

A. *Types:* alkylating agents, antimetabolites, antitumor antiinfectives, plant-derived alkaloids, enzymes, hormones. See Appendix D, Table D.4.
B. *Major problem:* lacks specificity, thus affecting normal as well as malignant cells.
C. *Major side effects:* bone marrow depression, stomatitis, nausea and vomiting, GI ulcerations, diarrhea, alopecia (Table 24.1).
D. *Routes of administration:* oral, intramuscular, intravenous (*Hickman or Groshong catheter*), subclavian lines, porta caths, peripheral, intraarterial (may have infusion pump for continuous or intermittent flow rate), intracavity (e.g., bladder through cystoscopy, Omaya reservoir). (See p. 97 for information about administration of IV chemotherapeutic agents.)
E. Nursing care plan/implementation
1. Goal: *assist with treatment of specific side effects.*
   a. *Nausea and vomiting—antiemetic* drugs and antacid therapy as ordered and scheduled; small, frequent, *high-calorie, high-potassium, high-protein* meals; include milk and milk products when tolerated for *increased calcium;* carbonated drinks; frequent mouth care; rest after meals; *avoid* food odors during preparation of meals; pleasant environment during meals; appropriate distractions; *IV* therapy; *nasogastric* tube for control of severe nausea or as route for *tube feeding* if unable to take food by mouth; *hyperalimentation.*
   b. *Diarrhea—low-residue diet; increased potassium; increased fluids;* atropine sulfate–diphenoxylate HCl (Lomotil) or kaolin-pectin (Kaopectate), as ordered; *avoid* hot or cold foods/liquids.
   c. *Stomatitis* (painful mouth)—soft toothbrushes or sponges (toothettes); mouth care q2–4h; *viscous lidocaine* HCl (Xylocaine), as ordered, before meals. Oral salt and soda mouth rinses; *avoid* commercial mouthwashes that contain high level of alcohol, which could be very irritating to mucous membranes. *Avoid* hot foods/liquids, include bland foods at cool temperatures; remove dentures if sores are under dentures; moisten lips with petroleum jelly.

TABLE 24.1 ⬤ **COMMON TOXICITIES OF ANTINEOPLASTIC AGENTS**

	Nausea and Vomiting	Mucositis	Diarrhea	Skin Reactions	Lung	Neurologic
Antimetabolites						
Cytosine arabinoside (low dose)	0	0	+	0	+	0
(moderate dose)	+ +	+	+ +	Alopecia	0	0
(high dose)	+ + +	+	+ +	Alopecia	0	Cerebellar
Fludarabine	+	0	0	0	0	0
5-Fluorouracil (low dose)	0	+	+	Phlebitis	0	Cerebellar
(moderate dose)	0	+ +	+ + +	Phlebitis	0	Cerebellar
(high dose)	0	+	+	Hand-foot syndrome	0	0
(with leucovorin)	0	+	+ + +	Hand-foot syndrome	0	0
Methotrexate	+	+ +	+ +	Dermatitis	+	0
with leucovorin	+ + +	+ + +	+ + +	Dermatitis	+	0
2-Deoxycoformycin	+	0	0	Erythema	0	Lethargy, coma
6-Mercaptopurine	+	0	0	Rash	0	0
Thioguanine	+	+	0	0	0	0
2-Chlorodeoxyadenosine	+	0	0	0	0	0
Alkylating agents						
Busulfan	0	+	0	Hyperpigmentation	0	0
Chlorambucil	0	0	0	0	+	0
Cyclophosphamide (low dose)	+	0	0	0	+	0
(moderate dose)	+ +	+	0	Alopecia	+	0
(high dose)	+ + +	+ +	+ + +	Alopecia	+	0
DTIC	+ + +	0	0	0	0	0
Ifosfamide	+ + +	0	0	Alopecia	0	Encephalopathy
Mechlorethamine	+ + +	+	+	Alopecia, rash	0	0
Melphalan	0	0	0	0	0	0
Nitrosoureas						
Carmustine (BCNU)	+ + +	0	0	0	+	0
Lomustine (CCNU)	+	0	0	0	0	0
Streptozocin	+ + +	0	0	0	0	0
Thiotepa	+ +	+ + +	+ + +	Alopecia, rash	0	0
Tumor antimicrobials						
Bleomycin	0	0	0	Erythema	+	0
Dactinomycin	+ +	+ +	0	Alopecia, rash	0	0
Daunorubicin	+ +	+	+	Alopecia, vesicant	0	0
Doxorubicin	+ +	+	+	Alopecia, vesicant	0	0
Idarubicin	+ +	+	+	Alopecia, vesicant	0	0
Mitomycin C	+	+	0	Vesicant	+	0
Mitoxantrone	+	+	+	Alopecia, vesicant	0	0
Plant alkaloids						
Etoposide	0	0	0	0	0	0
Vinblastine	+	+	0	Alopecia, vesicant	0	+
Vincristine	0	0	0	Vesicant	0	+ + Neuropathy
Taxol	+	0	0	Alopecia	0	Neuropathy
Other agents						
Carboplatin	+ +	0	0	0	0	0
Cisplatin	+ + +	0	0	0	0	+
Hydroxyurea	0	0	0	Skin atrophy	0	0
L-Asparaginase	0	0	0	0	0	Encephalopathy
Procarbazine	+	0	0	Rash	0	Encephalopathy

0 = none; + = mild; + + = moderate; + + + = severe.

Source: Adapted from Ewald G, McKenzie C (eds). *Manual of Medical Therapeutics.* Boston: Little, Brown, 1995.

d. *Skin care*—monitor: wounds that do not heal, infections (patient receives frequent sticks for blood tests and therapy); *avoid* sunlight; use sunblock, especially if receiving doxorubicin (Adriamycin).

☞ **e.** *Alopecia*—ice caps during therapy or tourniquet around forehead for 20 min before, during, and after infusion of a few drugs (as ordered by physician); be gentle when combing or lightly brushing hair; use wigs, night caps, scarves; provide frequent linen changes. Advise patient to have hair cut short before treatment with drugs known to cause alopecia (bleomycin, cyclosphosphamide, dactinomycin, daunorubicin HCl, doxorubicin HCl, 5-fluorouracil, ICRF-159, hydroxyurea, methotrexate, mitomycin, VP 16-213, vincristine).

🏠 **2.** Goal: **health teaching.**
   a. Educate patient and family to purpose of proposed drug regimen and anticipated side effects.
   b. Advise that frequent checks of hematologic status will be necessary (patient will undergo frequent IV sticks, lab tests).
   c. Advise patient and family of increased risk for infection (*avoid* uncontrolled crowds and individuals with upper respiratory tract infections or childhood diseases).
   d. Monitor injection site for signs of extravasation (infiltration) (site must be changed if leakage suspected, and guidelines to neutralize must be followed according to drug protocol).

☞ **F. Nursing precautions with chemotherapy**
   💊 **1.** Nurse should wear *gloves* and *mask* when preparing chemotherapeutic agents for administration.
   2. Drugs are toxic substance, nurses must take every precaution to handle them with care.
   3. When expelling air bubbles from syringes, care must be taken that the drugs are *not* sprayed into the atmosphere.
   4. Contaminated needles and syringes should be disposed of intact (to prevent aerosol generation) in plastic-lined box and incinerated. Disposable equipment should be used whenever possible.
   5. If skin becomes contaminated with a drug, wash under running water.
   6. Nurses should know the half-life and excretion route of the drugs being administered and take the special precautions necessary. For example, while the drug is actively being excreted, use *gloves* when touching *patient, stool, urine, dressings, vomitus,* etc.
   7. Nurses who are in the early phase of pregnancy should exercise caution when caring for patients receiving chemotherapeutic agents.

VIII. Radiation therapy: used in high doses to kill cancer cells or palliatively for pain relief. Side effects depend on site of therapy (vary in each person): nausea, vomiting, stomatitis, esophagitis, dry mouth, diarrhea, depression of bone marrow, suppression of immune response, decreased life span, sterility.

A. External radiation: cobalt or linear accelerator machine.
   1. *Procedure:* daily treatments, Monday through Friday, for prescribed number of times according to size and location of tumor (duration of treatment is usually 4–6 wk). Patient remains alone in room during treatment. (Nurse, therapist, family members cannot stay in room with patient during treatment due to radiation exposure). Patient instructed to lie still, so exactly same area irradiated each treatment. Marks (tattoos or permanent-ink marks) are made on skin to delineate area of treatment; marks must *not* be removed during entire treatment course.

✉ **2. Nursing care plan/implementation**
   a. Goal: *prevent tissue breakdown.*
      (1) Do *not* wash off site-identification marks (tattoos cannot be removed); dosage area is carefully calculated and must be exact for each treatment.
      (2) Assess skin daily and teach patient to do same (most radiation therapy is done on outpatient basis, so patient needs skills to manage independently).
      (3) Keep skin dry; cornstarch is usually the only topical application allowed:
      (4) *Contraindicated measures:*
         (a) Talcum powders, due to potential to alter radiation dose.
         (b) Lotions, due to increased moistening of skin.
         (c) Aloe preparations with alcohol, due to drying of skin. Check ingredients.
      (5) Reduce skin friction by *avoiding* constricting bedclothes or clothing and by using electric shaver.
☞   **(6)** Dress areas of skin breakdown with nonadherent dressing and paper tape.
   b. Goal: *decrease side effects of therapy.*
      (1) Provide meticulous oral hygiene.
   💊 **(2)** If diarrhea occurs, may need IV infusions, *antidiarrheal* medications; monitor bowel movements, possible adhesions resulting from surgery and radiation treatments.
      (3) Monitor vital signs, particularly respiratory function and blood pressure (sloughing of tissues puts patient at *risk for hemorrhage*).
   〰 **(4)** Monitor hematologic status—bone marrow depression can cause fatal toxicosis and sepsis.
☞   **(5)** Institute *reverse isolation* as necessary to prevent infections (reverse isolation usually instituted if <50% neutrophils).
   c. Goal: **health teaching.**
      (1) Instruct patient to *avoid:*

(a) *Strong sunlight;* must wear sunblock lotion, protective clothing over radiation site.

(b) *Extremes in temperature* to the area (hot-water bottles, ice caps).

(c) Synthetic, *nonporous* clothes *or tight* constrictive clothing over area.

(d) Eating 2–3 h *before* treatment and 2 h *after,* to decrease nausea; *do* give small, frequent meals *high* in *protein* and *carbohydrates* and *low* in *residue.*

(e) Strong *alcohol-base mouthwash;* use daily salt and soda mouthwash.

(f) *Fatigue,* an overwhelming problem. Need to pace themselves, nap; may need someone to drive them to therapy; can continue with usual activities as tolerated.

(g) *Crowds* and persons with upper respiratory tract infections or any other infections.

(2) Provide appropriate birth control information for patients of childbearing age.

B. **Internal radiation: sealed** (radium, iridium, cesium).

1. Used for localized masses (e.g., mouth, cervix, breast, testes). Due to exposure from radiation source, precautions must be taken while it is in place. Health care personnel and family must adhere to *principles of time, distance, and shielding to decrease exposure* (shortest amount of time possible, stay as *far away* as possible from the source of radiation, and wear *protective* lead apron, gloves). If source of radiation accidentally falls out, it should be picked up only with *forceps.* Radiation officer should be notified immediately. Patient should be in *private* room, and bed should be in the center of the room, if possible, to protect others. Unless the walls are lead lined, radiation will penetrate them; placing the bed in *center of room* will decrease exposure. Once the source of radiation has been removed, there is no radiation exposure from patient, excretions, or linens.

2. **Nursing care plan/implementation**

a. Goal: *assist with cervical radium implantation* (cervical radium is used here as the most common example of an internal radiation source).

(1) *Prior to insertion*—give douche, enema; perform perineal preparation; insert Foley catheter, as ordered.

(2) *After implantation*—check position of applicator q24h.

(a) Keep patient on bed rest in *flat position* to prevent displacing applicator (may turn to side for eating).

(b) Notify physician if temperature increases, nausea and/or vomiting occurs (indicate *radiation reaction* or *infection*).

(c) *After removal* of implant (48–144 h)—bathe, and douche patient; remove catheter, as ordered.

b. Goal: **health teaching.**

(1) Explain that nursing care will be limited to essential activities during postinsertion period.

(2) Signs and symptoms of complications, so patient can notify staff if something unusual happens (e.g., bleeding, radiation source falls out, fever).

3. **Nursing precautions for sealed internal radiation:**

a. **Never handle radium directly**—if applicators should accidentally be removed, pick up applicator by strings with long-handled forceps and **notify radiation officer.**

b. Linen must remain in patient's room and *not* be sent to laundry until source of radiation has been accounted for and returned to its container.

c. **Time, distance, and shielding** are factors that increase or decrease potential effects on personnel. Need to minimize exposure of nursing staff, patient's family, other health professionals. Nurses who may be *pregnant* should *not* care for patients with a radiation implant because of possible damage to the fetus from the radiation.

C. **Internal radiation: unsealed** (radioisotope/radionuclide).

1. Source of radiation is given orally or intravenously or instilled into a cavity as a liquid.

2. **Nursing care plan/implementation:** Goal: *reduce radiation exposure of others.*

a. *Isolate* patient, tag room with radioactivity symbol.

b. *Rotate* personnel to *avoid* overexposure (principles of *time, distance,* and *shielding*). Staff should use good handwashing technique. Patient should be in a room with running water. (Nurse who may be pregnant should *not* care for patient while radiation source still active.)

c. Encourage family to maintain telephone contact or use intercom, to decrease exposure to others.

d. Plan independent diversional activities.

3. **Specific nursing precautions** (post in chart, on patient's door).

a. *Radioactive iodine* (^{131}I): half-life—8.1 d; excreted in urine, saliva, perspiration, vomitus, feces.

(1) Wear *gloves* and isolation *gowns* when handling patient, excreta, or dressings directly.

(2) Collect *paper* plates, eating utensils, dressings, linen in impermeable bags; label and dispose of according to agency protocol.

(3) Collect excreta in *shielded* container and send to lab daily to monitor excretion rate and disposal.

b. *Radioactive phosphorus* (^{32}P): half-life—14 d; injected into cavity or given IV or orally.

(1) If injected into cavity, turn patient q10–15min for 2 h to ensure distribution.

(2) *No* radiation hazard unless leakage from instillation site or from patient's excreta, which are collected in *lead-lined containers* and brought to the radioisotope laboratory for disposal. Linen is collected in container, marked *radioactive*, and brought to the radioisotope lab for special handling.

(3) Seepage will stain linens *blue;* wear *gloves* when handling contaminated linens, dressings. Excreta disposed of as in (3) above.

c. *Radioactive gold* (^{198}Au): half-life—2.7 d; usually injected into pleural or abdominal cavity.

(1) May seep from instillation site or drainage tubes in cavity; stains *purple.*

☞ (2) Turn patient q15min for 2 h to ensure distribution.

(3) Same precautions regarding handling excreta as in a.(1) and b.(2).

☞ **D. Precautions for nurses:**

1. Use principles of *time, distance,* and *shielding* when caring for patients who are undergoing active radiation therapy.

2. Nurses who may be pregnant should *not accept* an assignment caring for patients who have an active radiation source in place.

3. Always use *gloves, gowns* to protect skin and clothing.

4. Wear detection *badge* to determine exposure to energy source.

IX. Immunotherapy: it has been hypothesized that clinical malignancy may occur as a result of failure of the immunologic surveillance system of the body to fight off cancer cells as they develop. The goal of immunotherapy is to immunize patients against their own tumors.

A. *Nonspecific* immunotherapy—encourages a host-immune response by use of an unrelated agent. BCG (bacillus Calmette-Guérin) vaccine and *Corynebacterium parvum* are the two agents used for this type of immunotherapy.

B. *Specific* immunotherapy—uses substances that are antigenically related to the tumor that stimulate a specific host-immune response.

C. *Side effects*—malaise, chills, nausea, vomiting, diarrhea; local reaction at site of injection, such as pruritus, scabbing.

D. Nursing care plan/implementation

1. Goal: *decrease discomfort associated with side effects of therapy.*

a. Identify measures to lessen side effects (see V. Nursing care plan/implementation—general care of the cancer patient, p. 274).

b. Know type of immunotherapy being used, adverse and desirable effects of therapy.

c. Administer fluids, encourage rest.

d. Administer acetaminophen, as ordered, to decrease flulike symptoms.

e. Administer *antiemetics,* as ordered, to control nausea.

f. Monitor for respiratory distress.

g. Administer *analgesics,* as ordered, to relieve pain.

2. Goal: **health teaching.**

a. Comfort measures to decrease side effects of therapy.

b. Expected and side effects of therapy.

c. Investigational nature of therapy.

d. Care of administration site.

e. Answer questions honestly.

X. Palliative care: When treatment has been ineffective in controlling the disease, the nurse must plan palliative, terminal care. Cure is not possible for such patients in an advanced phase of malignancy. Symptoms increase in severity; patients and family have many special problems.

A. General problems of terminal cancer patient:

1. *Cachexia:* progressive weakness, wasting, weight loss.

2. *Anemia:* leukopenia, thrombocytopenia, hemorrhage.

3. *GI tract disturbances:* anorexia, constipation.

4. *Tissue breakdown* leading to decubitus, seeping wounds.

5. *Urine:* retention, incontinence, renal calculi, tumor obstruction of ureters.

6. *Hypercalcemia* occurs in 10%–30% of patients.

7. *Pain* due to tumor growth, obstruction, vertebral compression, or secondarily to complications (e.g., decubitus, stiffened joints, stomatitis). Also neuropathy, due to prolonged use of neurotoxic chemotherapeutic agents such as vincristine.

8. *Fatigue:* major and debilitating problem.

B. Nursing care plan/implementation

1. Goal: *make patient as comfortable as possible;* involve nursing staff, family, support personnel, clergy, volunteers, support groups, hospice, etc.

a. *Nutrition:* obtain nutritional consultation; *high-calorie, high-protein diet;* small, frequent meals; blenderized or strained;

commercial nutritional supplements (Ensure, Vivonex, Sustacal).

☞ **b.** Prevent tissue breakdown and vascular complications: frequent turning, massage, air mattress, active and passive range of motion (ROM) exercises.

c. GI tract disturbances: observe for toxic reactions to therapy, particularly vomiting and diarrhea; administer medications: *antiemetics, antidiarrheal* agents, as ordered.

d. Relieve pain.

☞ **(1)** Use supportive measures such as massage, relaxation techniques, guided imagery, drugs for *pain* relief: administer codeine, fentanyl, aspirin–oxycodone HCl (Percodan), pentazocine (Talwin), morphine, methadone, as ordered.

(2) Monitor for side effects of narcotics: depressed respiratory status, constipation, anorexia.

2. Goal: *assist patient to maintain self-esteem and identity.*

a. Encourage self-care.

b. Spend time with patient; isolation is a great fear for the dying patient.

3. Goal: *assist patient with psychological adjustment.*

⋈ XI. Evaluation/outcome criteria

A. Tolerates treatment—complications of surgery are prevented, tolerates chemotherapy, completes radiation therapy.

B. Side effects of treatment are managed by effective nursing care and health teaching.

C. Maintains good nutritional status.

D. Uses effective coping mechanisms or seeks appropriate assistance to deal with psychosocial concerns.

E. Makes choices for follow-up care based on accurate information.

F. Finds methods to control pain and minimize discomfort.

G. Dignity maintained until death and/or during dying.

Lung Cancer

I. Pathophysiology: *squamous cell carcinoma:* undifferentiated, pleomorphic; accounts for 45%–60% of all cases of lung cancer; *small-cell (oat-cell) carcinoma:* small, dark cells located between cells of mucosal surfaces; characterized by early metastasis and poor prognosis; *large-cell (giant-cell) carcinoma:* located in the peripheral areas of the lung, has poor prognosis; *adenocarcinoma:* found in men and women; not necessarily related to smoking.

II. Risk factors:

A. Heavy cigarette smoking, 20-yr smoking history.

B. Exposure to certain industrial substances, such as *asbestos.*

C. Increased incidence in women during the last decade of life.

⋈ III. Assessment

A. *Subjective data:*

1. Dyspnea.

2. Pain: on swallowing; dull and poorly localized chest pain, referred to shoulders.

3. Anorexia.

4. History of cigarette smoking over a period of years; recurrent respiratory tract infections with chills and fever, especially pneumonia or bronchitis.

B. *Objective data:*

1. Wheezing, dry to productive persistent cough, hemoptysis.

2. Weight loss.

3. Positive diagnosis: cytology report of cells in tissue specimen obtained during bronchoscopy.

4. Signs of metastasis.

IV. Annual incidence: 178,100 new cases; 160,400 estimated deaths.

⋈ V. Analysis/nursing diagnosis

A. *Ineffective breathing pattern* related to pain.

B. *Impaired gas exchange* related to tumor growth.

C. *Pain* related to disease progression.

D. *Fear* related to uncertain future.

E. *Powerlessness* related to inability to control symptoms.

F. *Knowledge deficit* related to disease and treatment.

⋈ VI. Nursing care plan/implementation

A. Goal: *make patient aware of diagnosis and treatment options.*

1. Allow time to talk and to discuss diagnosis.

2. Patient makes informed decision regarding treatment.

B. Goal: *prevent complications related to surgery* for patient whose cancer is diagnosed early and for whom surgery is an option: wedge or segmental resection, lobectomy, or pneumonectomy are usual procedures.

☞ **1.** See Nursing care plan/implementation for the patient undergoing thoracic surgery, p. 68.

2. Monitor vital signs, including accurate respiratory assessment for respiratory congestion, blood loss, infection.

3. Assist patient to deep breathe, cough, change position.

C. Goal: *assist patient to cope with alternative therapies* when surgery is deemed not possible.

1. *Radiation therapy:* megavoltage x-ray, cobalt—usual form of radiation. (See Nursing care plan/implementation for the patient undergoing radiation therapy, p. 277.)

2. *Chemotherapy:*

a. Cyclophosphamide (Cytoxan), doxorubicin (Adriamycin), CCNU, methotrexate, vincristine sulfate (Oncovin) are the usual drugs given for lung cancer.

b. See Nursing care plan/implementation for the patient undergoing chemotherapy p. 275.

🏠 **D.** Goal: **health teaching.**
  1. Encourage patient to stop smoking to ensure best possible air exchange.
  ● 2. Encourage *high-protein, high-calorie diet* to counteract weight loss.
  3. *Force fluids* to liquefy secretions so they can be expectorated.
  4. Encourage adequate rest and activity to prevent problems of immobility.
  5. Desired effects and side effects of medications prescribed for therapy and pain relief.
  6. Coping mechanisms for maximal comfort and advanced disease (see X. Palliative care, p. 279).

🔖 **VII. Evaluation/outcome criteria**
  A. Copes with disease and treatment.
  B. Side effects of treatment are minimized by proper nursing management.
  C. Acid-base balance is maintained by careful management of respiratory problems.
  D. Patient is aware of the seriousness of the disease.

Colon and Rectal Cancer

I. Risk factors:
  A. Males.
  B. Middle age.
  C. Personal or family history of colon and rectal cancer.
  D. Personal or family history of polyps in the rectum or colon.
  E. Ulcerative colitis.
  F. Diet *high* in *beef* and *low* in *fiber.*
  G. *Gardner's syndrome* (multiple colonic adenomatous polyps, osteomas of the mandible or skull, multiple epidermoid cysts, or soft-tissue tumors of the skin).

II. Annual incidence: 131,200 new cases, 54,900 estimated deaths.

🔖 **III. Assessment**
  A. *Subjective data:*
    1. Change in bowel habits.
    2. Anorexia.
    3. Weakness.
    4. Abdominal cramping or vague discomfort with or without pain.
    5. Chills.
  B. *Objective data:*
    1. Diarrhea (pencil-like or ribbon-shaped feces) or constipation.
    2. Weight loss.
    3. Rectal bleeding, anemia.
    4. Fever.
    5. Signs of intestinal obstruction: obstipation, distention, pain, vomiting, fecal oozing.
    6. Diagnostic tests:

a. Digital examination reveals palpable mass if lesion is in ascending or descending colon.
b. Slides of stool specimen, for occult blood.
c. Proctoscopy.
d. Sigmoidoscopy.
e. Barium enema.
7. Lab data: occult blood, blood serotonin level *increased,* carcinoembryonic antigen; (CEA); *positive* radioimmunoassay of serum or plasma indicates presence of carcinoma or adenocarcinoma of colon; *positive* results after resection indicate return of tumor.

🔖 **IV. Analysis/nursing diagnosis**
  A. *Constipation or diarrhea* related to presence of mass.
  B. *Altered health maintenance* related to care of stoma.
  C. *Sexual dysfunction* related to possible nerve damage during radical surgery.
  D. *Body image disturbance* related to colostomy.

🔖 **V. Nursing care plan/implementation** (see also V. Nursing care plan/implementation—general care of the cancer patient, p. 274).
  A. *Radiation therapy:* to reduce tumor or for palliation.
  ● **B.** *Chemotherapy:* to reduce tumor mass and metastatic lesions.
    1. *Antitumor antiinfectives*—mitomycin C, doxorubicin HCl (Adriamycin).
    2. *Alkylating agents*—methyl-CCNU.
    3. *Antimetabolites*—5-fluorouracil.
    4. *Steroids* and *analgesics* for symptomatic relief.
  C. Prepare patient for surgery (colostomy), if necessary.

🔖 **VI. Evaluation/outcome criteria**
  A. Return of peristalsis and formed stool following resection and anastomosis.
  B. Adjusts to alteration in bowel elimination route following abdominoperineal resection (e.g., no depression, resumes life-style).
  C. Demonstrates self-care skills with colostomy.
  D. Makes dietary adjustments that affect elimination, as indicated.
  E. Identifies alternative methods of expressing sexuality, if needed.

Breast Cancer

I. Risk factors:
  A. Women >age 50 yr.
  B. Family history of breast cancer.
  C. Never bore children, or bore first child after age 30 yr.
  D. Had breast cancer in other breast.
  E. Menarche before age 11 yr.
  F. Menopause after age 50 yr.
  G. Excessive animal fat in diet.
  H. Exposure to endogenous estrogens.

II. Annual incidence: 181,600 new cases, 44,190 estimated deaths.

▶ **III. Assessment**
   A. *Subjective data:*
      1. Burning, itching of nipple.
      2. Reported painless lump.
   B. *Objective data:*
      1. Firm, nontender lump or mass.
      2. Asymmetry of breast.
      3. Nipple—retraction, discharge.
      4. Alteration in breast skin—redness, dimpling, ulceration.
      5. Palpation reveals lump.
      6. Diagnostic tests: mammography, needle biopsy, excisional biopsy—level of estrogen-receptor protein predicts response to hormonal manipulation of metastatic disease and may represent a prognostic indicator for primary cancer; measurement of carcinoembryonic antigen useful for patient with metastatic disease of the breast (see Diagnostic Studies Box, p. 287).

▶ **IV. Analysis/nursing diagnosis**
   A. *Risk for injury* related to surgical intervention.
   B. *Body image disturbance* related to effects of surgery, radiation therapy, or chemotherapy.
   C. *Altered sexuality patterns* related to loss of breast.

▶ **V. Nursing care plan/implementation** (see also V. Nursing care plan/implementation—general care of the cancer patient, p. 274).
   A. Goal: *assist through treatment protocol.*
      1. *Radiation therapy*—primary treatment; adjunctive, external, or implantation to primary lesion site or nodes.
      2. *Chemotherapy:*
         a. *Cytotoxic* agents to destroy tumor and control metastasis.
         b. *Alkylating* agents: cyclophosphamide (Cytoxan).
         c. *Antitumor antiinfectives:* doxorubicin (Adriamycin).
         d. *Antimetabolites:* fluorouracil, methotrexate (Amethopterin).
         e. *Plant alkaloids:* vincristine sulfate (Oncovin).
         f. *Hormones* to control metastasis, provide palliation: androgens, fluoxymesterone (Halotestin), testolactone (Teslac).
         g. *Antiestrogens:* tamoxifen citrate (Nolvadex).
         h. *Cortisols:* cortisone, prednisolone (Delta-Cortef), prednisolone acetate (Meticortelone), prednisone (Deltasone, Deltra).
         i. *Estrogens:* diethylstilbestrol.
      3. *Surgery:*
         a. Preoperative care:
            (1) Goal: *prepare for surgery—types:*
               (a) *Lumpectomy* (with or without radiation therapy)—used when lesion is small; section of breast is removed (often accompanied by ra-

diation therapy and then radium interstitial implant).
               (b) *Simple mastectomy*—breast removed, no alteration in nodes.
               (c) *Modified radical mastectomy*—breast, some axillary nodes, subcutaneous tissue removed; pectoralis minor muscle removed.
               (d) *Radical mastectomy*—breast, axillary nodes, and pectoralis major and minor muscles removed.
               (e) *Reconstructive surgery*—done at time of initial mastectomy or (most often) later, when other adjuvant therapy has been completed.
            (2) Goal: *promote comfort.*
               (a) Allow patient and family to express fears, feelings.
               (b) Provide correct information about diagnostic tests, surgical procedure, postoperative expectations.
         b. Postoperative care:
            (1) Goal: *facilitate healing.*
               (a) Observe pressure dressings for bleeding; will appear under axilla and toward the back.
               (b) Report if dressing becomes saturated, reinforce dressing as needed, monitor drainage from *Hemovac* or *suction pump.*
               (c) *Position:* semi-Fowler's to facilitate venous and lymphatic drainage; use pillows to *elevate affected arm* above right atrium, to prevent edema if nodes removed.
            (2) Goal: *prevent complications.*
               (a) Monitor vital signs for shock.
               (b) Use gloves when emptying drainage.
               (c) Maintain joint mobility—flexion and extension of fingers, elbow, shoulder.
               (d) ROM exercises, as ordered, to prevent ankylosis.
               (e) If skin graft done, check donor site and limit exercises.
            (3) Goal: *facilitate rehabilitation.*
               (a) Encourage patient, significant others, family to look at incision.
               (b) Involve patient in incisional care, as tolerated.
               (c) Refer to Reach to Recovery program of the American Cancer Society
               (d) Exercise program, hydrotherapy for postmastectomy patients, to reduce lymphedema.
            (4) Goal: **health teaching.**
               (a) Ways to avoid injury to affected area, ways to prevent lymphedema.
               (b) Exercises to gain full ROM.

(c) Availability of prosthesis, reconstructive surgery.

(d) Correct breast self-examination (BSE) technique (is at risk for breast cancer in remaining breast) (Figure 24.1). Best time for exam: premenopausal women, seventh day of cycle; postmenopausal women, same day each month.

▷◁ VI. Evaluation/outcome criteria

A. Identifies feelings regarding loss.

B. Demonstrates postmastectomy exercises.

C. Gives rationale for avoiding fatigue and avoiding constricting garments on affected arm; necessity for avoiding injury (cuts, bruises, burns) while carrying out activities of daily living.

D. Describes signs and symptoms of infection.

E. Demonstrates correct BSE technique.

FIGURE 24.1   BREAST SELF-EXAMINATION. (A) Examine breasts during bath or shower since flat fingers glide easily over wet skin. Use right hand to examine left breast and vice versa. (B) Sit or stand before a mirror. Inspect breasts with hands at sides, then raised overhead. Look for changes in contour or dimpling of skin. (C) Place hands on hips and press down firmly to flex chest muscles. (D) Lie down with one hand under head and pillow or folded towel under that scapula. (E) Palpate that breast with the other hand using concentric circle method. It usually takes three circles to cover all breast tissue. Include the tail of the breast and the axilla. Repeat with other breast. (F) End in a sitting position. Palpate the areola areas of both breasts, and inspect and squeeze nipples to check for discharge. *Source:* Lagerquist SL: *Little, Brown's NCLEX-RN Examination Review.* Boston: Little, Brown, 1996. P. 203.

Uterine (Endometrial) Cancer

Originates from epithelial tissues of the endometrium; second only to cervical cancer as cause of pelvic cancer. Slow growing, metastasizes late, responsive to therapy with early diagnosis, Pap test *not* as effective—more effective to have endometrial tissue sample (Tables 24.2 and 24.3). Table 24.4 summarizes the staging and other aspects of cervical cancer.

I. Risk factors:
   A. History of infertility (nulliparity).
   B. Failure of ovulation.
   C. Prolonged estrogen therapy.
   D. Obesity.
   E. Menopause after age 52 yr.
   F. Diabetes.

II. Annual incidence: 34,900 new cases; 6000 estimated deaths.

III. Assessment
   A. *Subjective data:*
      1. History of risk factor(s).
      2. Pain (late symptom).
   B. *Objective data:*
      1. Obese.
      2. Abnormal cells obtained by aspiration of endocervix or endometrial washings.
      3. Postmenopausal uterine bleeding.
      4. Abnormal menses, intermenstrual or unusual discharge.
      5. See Diagnostic Studies Box.

IV. Analysis/nursing diagnosis
   A. *Pain* related to surgery.
   B. *Risk for injury* related to surgery.
   C. *Body image disturbance* related to loss of uterus.

V. Nursing care plan/implementation (see also nursing care plan/implementation—general care of the cancer patient, p. 274):
   A. Goal: *assist patient through treatment protocol.*
      1. *Radiation therapy*—external and/or internal with poor surgical risk patient.
      2. *Chemotherapy*—to reduce tumors and produce remission of metastasis. *Antineoplastic* drugs: dacarbazine (DTIC), doxorubicin (Adriamycin), medroxyprogesterone acetate (Provera), megestrol acetate (Megace).
   B. Goal: *prepare patient for surgery—types:*
      1. *Subtotal hysterectomy:* removal of the uterus, cervical stump remains.
      2. *Total hysterectomy:* removal of entire uterus, including cervix (abdominally—approximately 70% of patients—or vaginally).
      3. *Total hysterectomy with bilateral salpingo-oophorectomy:* removal of entire uterus, fallopian tubes, ovaries.
   C. Goal: *reduce anxiety and depression:* allow for expression of feelings, concerns about femininity, role, relationships.
   D. Goal: *prevent postoperative complications.*
      1. *Catheter* care—temporary bladder atony may be present as a result of edema or nerve trauma, especially when vaginal approach is used.
      2. Observe for abdominal distention and hemorrhage:
         a. Auscultate for bowel sounds.
         b. Measure abdominal girth.
         c. Utilize *rectal tube* to decrease flatus.
      3. *Decrease pelvic congestion and prevent venous stasis.*

TABLE 24.2   PAPANICOLAOU SMEAR CLASSES

Class	Recommended Actions
I Normal	None
II Atypical cells, nonmalignant	Treat vaginal infections, repeat Pap smears
III Suspicious cells	Biopsy, dilatation & curettage
IV Abnormal cells; suspicious of malignancy	Biopsy, dilatation & curettage, conization
V Malignant cells present	See Table 24.3 for recommended treatment according to stage of invasion.

Source: Lagerquist SL: *Little, Brown's NCLEX-RN Examination Review.* Boston: Little, Brown, 1996. P. 203.

TABLE 24.3   UTERINE CANCER: RECOMMENDED TREATMENT, BY STAGE OF INVASION

Stage of Invasion	Recommended Treatment
0 (In situ) Atypical hyperplasia	Cryosurgery, conization
I Uterus is of normal size	Hysterectomy
II Uterus slightly enlarged, but tumor is undifferentiated	Radiation implant, x-ray; hysterectomy 4–6 wk after radiation therapy
III Uterus enlarged, tumor extends outside uterus	Radiation implant, total hysterectomy 4–6 wk after radiation therapy
IV Advanced metastatic disease	Radiation therapy, chemotherapy; progestin therapy to reduce pulmonary lesions

Source: Lagerquist SL: *Little, Brown's NCLEX-RN Examination Review.* Boston: Little, Brown, 1996. P. 204.

TABLE 24.4   INTERNATIONAL SYSTEM OF STAGING FOR CERVICAL CARCINOMA

Stage	Location	Prognosis	Treatment
0	In situ	Highly curable	Conization
I	Cervix	Cure rate decreases as stage progresses	Radiation therapy
II	Cervix to upper vagina		Radiation therapy
III	Cervix to pelvic wall or lower third of vagina		Surgical procedures: 1. Panhysterectomy, wide vaginal excision with removal of lymph nodes; ileal conduit
IV	Cervix to true pelvis, bladder, or rectum		2. Pelvic exenteration: a. Anterior: removal of vagina and bladder; ileal conduit b. Posterior: removal of rectum and vagina; colostomy c. Total: both anterior and posterior 3. Chemotherapy

Source: Lagerquist SL: *Little, Brown's NCLEX-RN Examination Review.* Boston: Little, Brown, 1996. P. 205.

     a. *Avoid* high Fowler's position.
     b. *Antiembolic* stockings, as ordered.
     c. Institute *passive leg* exercises.
     d. Apply *abdominal support*, as ordered.
     e. Encourage early ambulation.
  E. Goal: *support coping mechanisms* to prevent psychosocial response of depression: allow for verbalization of feelings.
  F. Goal: **health teaching** to prevent complication of hemorrhage, infection, thromboemboli.
    1. *Avoid:*
     a. Douching or coitus until advised by physician.
     b. Strenuous activity and work, for 2 mo.
     c. Sitting for long time and wearing constrictive clothing, which tend to increase pelvic congestion.
    2. Explain hormonal replacement therapy, if applicable; correct dosage, desired and side effects of prescribed medications.
    3. Explain:
     a. Menstruation will no longer occur.
     b. Importance of reporting symptoms (e.g., fever, increased or bloody vaginal discharge, hot flashes).
VI. Evaluation/outcome criteria
  A. Adjusts to altered body image.
  B. No complications—hemorrhage, shock, infection, thrombophlebitis.

Prostate Cancer

I. Risk factors:
  A. Men.
  B. Age >50 yr.
  C. Familial history.

  D. Geographic distribution, environmental (e.g., industrial exposure to cadmium).
  E. Diet high in fat.
II. Annual incidence: 334,500 new cases; 44,800 estimated deaths.
III. Assessment
  A. *Subjective data:*
    1. Difficulty in starting urinary stream, frequency, urgency.
    2. Pain due to metastasis in lower back, hip.
    3. Symptoms of cystitis.
  B. *Objective data:*
    1. Urinary: smaller, less forceful stream; terminal dribbling; nocturia; *retention* (inability to void after ingestion of alcohol or exposure to cold).
    2. Ultrasound, needle biopsy; tissue specimen shows cancer cells.
    3. Lab data: *elevated:* prostate-specific antigen (PSA); prostatic acid phosphatase.
IV. Analysis/nursing diagnosis
  A. *Altered urinary elimination* related to incontinence.
  B. *Altered sexuality pattern* related to surgery (nerve damage).
  C. *Body image disturbance* related to surgery.
V. Nursing care plan/implementation (see also nursing care plan/implementation—general care of the cancer patient, p. 274).
  A. Goal: *assist patient in advanced stage through treatment protocol.*
    1. *Radiation therapy*—alone or in conjunction with surgery.
    2. *Chemotherapy*—analgesics, antispasmodics, antiinfectives, adrenocortical hormones, and *cytotoxic* drugs in conjunction with orchiectomy, to limit production of androgens.
    3. *Surgery*—see Prostatectomy, p. 193.

A

B

Lump

FIGURE 24.2   TESTICULAR SELF-EXAMINATION. (A) Grasp testis with both hands; palpate gently between thumb and fingers. (B) Abnormal lumps or irregularities are reported to physician. *Source:* Lagerquist SL: *Little, Brown's NCLEX-RN Examination Review.* Boston: Little, Brown, 1996. P. 211.

VI. **Evaluation/outcome criteria:** see Prostatectomy, p. 193.

Bladder Cancer

The bladder is most common site of urinary tract cancer.

I. **Risk factors:**
   A. Contact with certain dyes.
   B. Cigarette smoking.

   C. Excessive coffee intake.
   D. Prolonged use of analgesics with *phenacetin.*
   E. Three times more common in males.
II. Annual incidence: 54,500 new cases; 11,700 estimated deaths.
III. **Assessment**
   A. *Subjective data:*
      1. Frequency, urgency.
      2. Pain: flank, pelvic; dysuria.
   B. *Objective data:*
      1. Painless hematuria (initially).
      2. Diagnostic tests:
         a. Cytoscopy, intravenous pyelography—mass or obstruction.
         b. Bladder biopsy, urine cytology—malignant cells.
      3. Lab data: urinalysis—*increased* red blood cells (men, >4.8/µL; women, >4.3/µL), erythrocytes (>30 mg/dL).
IV. **Analysis/nursing diagnosis**
   A. *Risk for injury* related to surgical intervention.
   B. *Altered urinary elimination* related to surgery.
V. **Nursing care plan/implementation** (see also care of the cancer patient, p. 274).
   A. Goal: *assist patient through treatment protocol.*
      1. *Radiation therapy*—cobalt, radioisotopes, radon seeds; often before surgery to slow tumor growth.
      2. *Chemotherapy:*
         a. *Antitumor antiinfectives:* doxorubicin HCl (Adriamycin).
         b. *Antimetabolites:* 5-fluorouracil.
         c. *Alkylating* agents: thiotepa.
         d. *Sedatives, antispasmodics.*
   B. Goal: *prepare patient for surgery*—types:
      1. *Transurethral fulguration or excision:* used for small tumors with minimal tissue involvement.
      2. *Segmental resection:* up to half the bladder may be resected.
      3. *Cystectomy with urinary diversion:* complete removal of the bladder, performed when disease appears curable.
   C. Goal: *assist with acceptance of diagnosis and treatment.*
   D. Goal: *prevent complications during postoperative period.*
      1. *Transurethral fulguration or excision:*
         a. Monitor for clots, bleeding, spasms.
         b. Maintain patency of *Foley catheter.*
      2. *Urinary diversion with stoma:*
         a. Protect skin, ensure proper fit of appliance—because constantly wet with urine (see also Ileal conduit, p. 192, and ostomies and stoma care, p. 174).
         b. Prevent infection by *increasing acidity* of urine and *increasing fluid* intake.
         c. **Health teaching.**
            (1) Self-care of stoma and appliance.
            (2) Expected and side effects of medications.
            (3) Importance of follow-up visits for early detection of metastasis.

VI. Evaluation/outcome criteria
   A. Accepts treatment.
   B. Utilizes prescribed measures to decrease side effects of surgery, radiation therapy, chemotherapy.
   C. Plans follow-up visits for further evaluation.
   D. Maintains dignity.

Laryngeal Cancer

I. Risk factors:
   A. Eight times more common in men.
   B. Occurs most often after age 60 yr.
   C. Cigarette smoking.
   D. Alcohol.
   E. Chronic laryngitis, vocal abuse.
   F. Family predisposition to cancer.
II. Annual incidence: 10,900 new cases; 4230 estimated deaths.
III. Assessment
   A. *Subjective data:*
      1. Dysphagia—pain in area of Adam's apple that radiates to ear.
      2. Dyspnea.
   B. *Objective data:*
      1. Persistent hoarseness.
      2. Cough and hemoptysis.
      3. Enlarged cervical nodes.
      4. General debility and weight loss.
      5. Foul breath.
      6. Diagnosis made by history, laryngoscopy with biopsy and microscopic study of cells.
IV. Analysis/nursing diagnosis
   A. *Impaired verbal communication* related to removal of larynx.
   B. *Body image disturbance* related to radical surgery.
   C. *Ineffective airway clearance* related to increased secretions through tracheostomy.
V. Nursing care plan/implementation (see also nursing care plan/implementation—general care of cancer patient, p. 274): treatment primarily surgical (see Laryngectomy, pp. 70–71); radiation therapy may also be indicated.
VI. Evaluation/outcome criteria: see Laryngectomy, pp. 70–71.

Additional Types of Cancer

See Table 24.5.

Diagnostic Studies

Mammography—examination of the breast with or without the injection of radiopaque substance into the ducts of the mammary gland; *used to* determine the presence of tumors or cysts. *Patient preparation:* no deodorant, perfume, powders, or ointment in under-arm area on day of x-ray. May be uncomfortable.

Thermography—a picture of the surface temperature of the skin using infrared photography (not ionizing radiation) detects the circulation pattern of areas in the breasts. Tumors produce more heat than normal breast tissue. Useful in patients with large tumors but may not detect small or deep lesions. Requires expensive equipment, and picture is difficult to interpret accurately.
Culdoscopy—surgical procedure in which a culdoscope is inserted into the posterior vaginal cul-de-sac; *used to* visualize: uterus, fallopian tubes, broad ligaments, and peritoneal contents.
Hysterosalpingography — X-ray examination of uterus and fallopian tubes after insertion of a radiopaque substance into the uterine cavity; *used to:* determine patency of fallopian tubes and detect abnormality in uterine cavity.
Breast biopsy—needle aspiration or incisional removal of breast tissue for microscopic examination; *used to* differentiate among: benign tumors, cysts, and malignant tumors in the breast.
Cervical biopsy and cauterization—removal of cervical tissue for microscopic examination and cautery; *used to* control bleeding or obtain additional tissue samples.
Uterotubal insufflation (Rubin's test)—injection of carbon dioxide into the cervical canal; *used to* determine fallopian tube patency.

Study and Memory Aids

Cancer: Focus of Patient Care—"CANCER"

Chemotherapy
Assess body image disturbance (related to alopecia)
Nutritional needs when nausea and vomiting are present
Comfort from pain
Effective response to treatment (Evaluate)
Rest (for patient and family)

Source: Modified from Zerweth, et al. *Memory Notebook of Nursing.* Dallas: Nursing Education Consultants, 1994. p. 31.

Diet

Cancer—Prior to Surgery

↓ Fat
    Carbohydrates
↑ Protein
    Roughage
    Iron

(*Study and Memory Aids continue on page 295*)

TABLE 24.5 SELECTED CANCER PROBLEMS

⊠ Assessment

	Subjective Data	Objective Data	Risk Factors	Annual Incidence	Specific Treatment
Gastrointestinal Tract					
Oral cancer	Difficulty chewing, swallowing, moving tongue or jaws; history of heavy smoking, drinking, or chewing tobacco.	Sore that bleeds and does not heal, persistent red or white patch, diagnosis by *biopsy*, early detection: dental checks.	Heavy smoking and drinking, user of chewing tobacco, men age >40 yr (affects twice as many men as women).	30,750 new cases; 8440 estimated deaths.	*Surgery*, with reconstructive surgery, useful for cure and palliatively (see nursing care plan/implementation for cancer patient having surgery, p. 275). *Radiation* using simulated computer localization to avoid destruction of normal tissue (see nursing care plan/implementation for patient having radiation therapy, p. 277).
Esophageal cancer	Dysphagia—difficulty swallowing, discomfort described as lump in throat, pressure in chest, pain; fatigue, lethargy, apathy, depression; anorexia.	Weight loss; regurgitation, vomiting; diagnostic tests—*barium swallow, esophagoscopy, biopsy*.	Age >50 yr, alcoholism, use of tobacco; increasing risk in nonwhite females, in people with achalasia (inability to relax lower esophagus with swallowing) or hiatal hernias.	12,500 new cases; 11,500 estimated deaths.	*Surgery*: resection with anastomosis or removal with gastrostomy. *Radiation*: best form of therapy. *Chemotherapy*: antineoplastic drugs *ineffective*; medications to reduce pain, discomfort, anxiety; see nursing care plan/ implementation for patient with cancer (p. 274); having radiation therapy (p. 277); having chemotherapy (p. 275); having surgery (p. 275).
Stomach cancer	Vague feeling of fullness, pressure, or epigastric pain following ingestion of food; anorexia, nausea, intolerance of meat; malaise.	Eructation, regurgitation, vomiting; melena, hematemesis, anemia; jaundice, diarrhea, ascites; big belly, upper gastric area; often palpable mass.	Men, lower socioeconomic classes, colder climates, early exposure to dietary carcinogens, *blood group A*, pernicious anemia, atrophic achlorhydric gastritis.	22,400 new cases; 14,000 estimated deaths.	*Surgery*: gastrectomy (see Gastric surgery, p. 163, for nursing care). *Radiation*: *not* as useful because dosage needed would cause side effects unlikely to be tolerated by patient. *Chemotherapy* alone or in conjunction with surgery: *antitumor antiinfectives, antimetabolites, nitrosoureas, hematinics* (see nursing care plan/implementation for patient having chemotherapy, p. 275).

Gastrointestinal Tract (continued)

	Symptoms	Detection	Risk factors	Incidence	Treatment
Pancreatic cancer	Anorexia, nausea; pain in upper abdomen, radiating to back; dyspnea.	Jaundice, vomiting, weight loss; determination of solid mass in area of pancreas by *computed tomographic scanning and ultrasound*; tissue identification by *thin-needle percutaneous biopsy.*	Excessive intake of alcohol; exposure to dry cleaning chemicals, gasoline, coffee and decaffeinated coffee; possibly diabetes and chronic pancreatitis.	27,600 new cases; 28,100 estimated deaths.	*Surgery:* removal (must then have supplemental *pancreatic enzymes*, some patients become insulin-dependent diabetics) or bypass to relieve obstruction (see nursing care plan/implementation for patient with diabetes, pp. 141–142). *Radiation:* intraoperative high dose to pancreatic tumors with external high beam; palliative radiation therapy for pain (see nursing care plan/implementation for patient having radiation therapy, p. 277); see nursing care plan/implementation for patient with cancer, (p. 273). *Chemotherapy: pain* relief, *antiemetics, insulin,* pancrelipase, 5-fluorouracil, cyclophosphamide, methotrexate, vincristine, mitomycin C (see nursing care plan/implementation for patient having chemotherapy, p. 275).

Skin

	Symptoms	Detection	Risk factors	Incidence	Treatment
Skin cancer: *basal cell*	Reported painless lesion.	Scaly plaques, papules that ulcerate; pale, waxy, pearly nodule or red, sharply outlined patch; unusual skin condition, change in size or color, or other darkly pigmented growth or mole.	Exposure to: sun, coal tar, pitch, arsenic compounds, creosote, radium; fair complexion.	900,000 new cases (40,300 of these are malignant melanoma; 7300 estimated deaths).	*Surgery:* electrodesiccation (dehydration of tissue by use of needle electrode); cryosurgery (destruction of tissue by application of extreme cold) (see nursing care plan/implementation—general care of the cancer patient, p. 273). *Radiation therapy* (see care of patient having radiation therapy, p. 277). *Prevention: avoid* sun from 10–3; use protective clothing, sunblock lotion.

(continued)

TABLE 24.5   SELECTED CANCER PROBLEMS (Continued)

	◢ Assessment				
	Subjective Data	Objective Data	Risk Factors	Annual Incidence	Specific Treatment
Nervous System					
Brain	*Headache:* steady, intermittent, severe (may be intensified by physical activity); nausea, lethargy, easy fatigability; forgetfulness, disorientation, impaired judgment; visual disturbances; blackouts.	Vomiting, may be projectile; sight loss, auditory changes; signs of increased intracranial pressure; seizures; paresthesia; behavior changes; *diagnostic studies*—computed tomography scan, arteriography, cytology of cerebrospinal fluid.	None known for primary tumors; brain is common site for metastasis.	17,600 new cases (brain and spinal cord); 13,200 estimated deaths.	*Surgery:* craniotomy with excision of lesion; ventricular shunt to allow for drainage of fluid (see nursing care plan/implementation for craniotomy, p. 250: see nursing care plan/implementation—general care of the cancer patient, p. 273). *Radiation:* cobalt (local or entire central nervous system), total brain irradiation causes alopecia, which may be permanent (see nursing care plan/implementation for patient having radiation therapy, p. 277); could be used alone, with surgery, or with chemotherapy. *Chemotherapy: antineoplastic alkylating agents; nitrosoureas* (cross blood-brain barrier to reduce tumor)—carmustine (BCNU), lomustine (CCNU), semustine (methyl-CCNU); *cerebral diuretics to reduce edema; anticonvulsants; analgesics; sedatives* (see nursing care plan/implementation for patient having chemotherapy, p. 275).
Endocrine					
Thyroid cancer	Painless nodule, dysphagia, dyspnea.	Enlarged thyroid, thyroid nodule; palpable thyroid, lymph nodes; hoarseness; hypofunctional nodule seen on isotopic imaging; *needle biopsy* for cytology studies.	Radiation exposure in childhood.	16,100 new cases; 1230 estimated deaths.	*Surgery:* total thyroidectomy, possible radical neck dissection (see Thyroidectomy, p. 203). *Radiation:* external or with radioactive iodine (131I) (see plan of care/implementation for patient having radiation therapy, p. 277). *Chemotherapy:* chlorambusil, doxorubicin, vincristine (Leukeran, Adriamycin, Oncovin, respectively) (see plan of care/implementation for patient having chemotherapy, p. 275).

Blood and Lymph Tissues

Hodgkin's disease

Fatigue, generalized pruritus, anorexia.

Painless enlargement of lymph nodes, especially in cervical area; fever; night sweats; hepatosplenomegaly; anemia; peak age of incidence, 15–35 yr; *diagnostic tests*—biopsy shows presence of *Reed-Sternberg cells; scans; x-rays; laparotomy.*

For young adults from 15–35 yr old; not clearly defined, some relationship to socioeconomic status; male-female ratio is 1.5 : 1; increased frequency among whites.

7500 new cases; 1480 estimated deaths.

Staging and treatment:

Stage I—involvement of a single node or a single node region; excision of lesion, and total nodal irradiation (see plan of care/implementation for patient having radiation therapy, p. 277).

Stage II—involvement of two or more lymph node regions on same side of diaphragm; excision of lesion and irradiation (see plan of care/implementation for patient having radiation therapy, p. 277).

Stage III—involvement of lymph node regions on both sides of the diaphragm, which may include the spleen; combination of radiation and chemotherapy.

Stage IV—involvement of one or more extralymphatic organs or tissues, with or without lymphatic involvement; treated with chemotherapy alone, radiation therapy alone, or both. Presence or absence of symptoms of night sweats, significant fever, and weight loss; treated with *chemotherapy,* MOPP protocol—*Mustargen* (mechlorethamine HCl, alkylating agent), Oncovin (vincristine, plant alkaloid), *procarbazine* (antineoplastic), prednisone (corticosteroid) (see plan of care/implementation for patient having chemotherapy, p. 275).

(*continued*)

TABLE 24.5   SELECTED CANCER PROBLEMS (Continued)

	◤ Assessment			
	Subjective Data	Objective Data	Risk Factors	Specific Treatment
Blood and Lymph Tissues (continued)				
Non-Hodgkin's lymphoma	Night sweats	Nontender lymphadenopathy, hepatomegaly, splenomegaly, fever of unknown origin, weight loss	Age, 50–60 yr	53,600 new cases; 23,800 estimated deaths.	Stage I—rarely observed, but remission possible with radiotherapy. Stage II—radiotherapy. Stage III and IV—combination chemotherapy with or without radiation therapy
Multiple myeloma	Weakness; history of frequent infections, especially pneumonias; severe bone pain on motion; neurologic symptoms, paralysis.	Fractures of long bones; deformity of sternum, ribs, vertebrae, pelvis; hepatosplenomegaly; renal calculi; renal insufficiency; anemia and bleeding tendencies; elevated uric acid.	Exposure to ionizing radiation; middle-aged or older females.	13,800 new cases; 10,900 estimated deaths.	Surgery: relieve spinal cord compression; orthopedic procedures to relieve or support bone problems (see nursing care plan/implementation for patients with internal fixation for fractures, Chap. 20; patient with spinal cord injuries when paralysis occurs, p. 261). Radiation: for some lesions (see nursing care plan/implementation for the patient having radiation therapy, p. 277). Chemotherapy: alkylating agents, antitumor antiinfectives, plant alkaloids, hormones—melphalan and prednisone (see nursing care plan/implementation for patient having chemotherapy, p. 275).

Urinary Organs
Kidney cancer

Anorexia, nausea, fatigue, abdominal or flank pain.

Painless, gross hematuria; firm, nontender, palpable kidney; vomiting and weight loss; *complications*—hypertension, nephrotic syndrome, lung metastasis; *lab and diagnostic tests*: intravenous pyelography, urinalysis—presence of red blood cells and albumin; complete blood count—*decrease* in red blood cells and leukocytes, *reduction* in serum albumin, *elevation* in alpha-globulin.

More common among men than women, whites than blacks; radiation exposure; possible familial influence; common site of metastatis from lung, breast. 28,800 new cases; 11,300 estimated deaths.

Surgery: nephrectomy (see pre/postoperative nursing care, pp. 111, 191).
Radiation: local as well as irradiation of metastatic sites when tumor is radiosensitive (see nursing care plan/implementation for patient having radiation therapy; p. 277).
Chemotherapy: plant alkaloids—vincristine (Oncovin); *antitumor antiinfectives*—dactinomycin (Actinomycin D), doxorubicin (Adriamycin); *alkylating agents*—cyclophosphamide (Cytoxan) (see nursing care plan/implementation for patient having chemotherapy, p. 275).

Genital Organs
Testicular cancer

Aching or dragging sensation in groin, usually painless.

Gynecomastia; enlargement, swelling, lump, hardening of testes; young adult male; early diagnosis—monthly testicular self-exam; See Figure 24.2.

Second most common malignancy among men between 25 and 40 yr; possibly exposure to chemical carcinogens; trauma, orchitis; gonadal dysgenesis; cryptorchidism (undescended testicles). 7200 new cases; 350 estimated deaths; 95%—100% 5-yr survival rate for early detected nonmetastatic lesions.

Surgery: orchiectomy (see nursing care plan/implementation for the pre- and postop patient, p. 111).
Radiation: see nursing care plan/implementation for patient having radiation therapy, p. 277.
Chemotherapy: chlorambucil (Leukeran), methotrexate, *steroids* (see nursing care plan/implementation for patient having chemotherapy, p. 275).

(continued)

TABLE 24.5   SELECTED CANCER PROBLEMS (Continued)

	▲ Assessment			
Subjective Data	Objective Data	Risk Factors	Annual Incidence	Specific Treatment

Genital Organs (continued)

Subjective Data	Objective Data	Risk Factors	Annual Incidence	Specific Treatment
Cervical cancer	Vague pelvic or low back discomfort, pressure, pain.	Intermenstrual postcoital, or postmenopausal bleeding; vaginal discharge—serosanguineous and malodorous hypermenorrhea; abdominal distention with urinary frequency; abnormal [MWv] *Pap smear* (see Table 24.2); recommended guidelines by American Cancer Society: Pap test annually; after 3 consecutive normal tests, MD may recommend less frequent testing; pelvic/uterine exam every 3 yr.	Early age at first intercourse; multiple sex partners; low socioeconomic status; exposure to herpes virus 2.	14,500 new cases; 4800 estimated deaths.	*Staging* (See Table 24.4): *Stage O*—carcinoma in situ; no distinct tumor observable; stage may last 8–10 yr; cure rate 100% following wedge or cone resection of cervix during childbearing years, or simple hysterectomy. *Stage I*—malignant cells infiltrate cervical mucosa; lesion bleeds easily; cure rate 80% with hysterectomy. *Stage II*—neoplasm spreads through cervical muscular layers, involves upper third of vaginal mucosa; cure rate 50% with radical hysterectomy. *Stage III*—neoplasm involves lower third of vagina; cure rate 25% with pelvic exenteration. *Stage IV*—involves metastasis to bladder, rectum, and surrounding tissues; considered incurable. *Radiation:* external and/or internal, in conjunction with surgery or alone, depending on stage of disease or condition of patient (see nursing care plan/implementation for patient having radiation therapy, p. 277). 💊 *Chemotherapy:* progestin, *antineoplastics,* megestrol (Megace), medroxyprogesterone (Curretab, Provera); *alkylating agents*—dacarbazine (DTIC).

☞ Summary of Key Points

1. The most important nursing function for a patient with cancer is teaching regarding prevention and detection, and, if treatment is necessary, symptom management.
2. Symptoms of cancer often do not appear until there is sufficient disease to produce *pressure, distortion, obstruction,* or *metabolic alterations.*
3. Side effects from radiation therapy are related to the size of the area being treated, the actual *part* of the body being irradiated, and the *total dose* of radiation.
4. Body excretions are *not radioactive* in patients undergoing treatment with a *sealed* source of radiation.
5. Skin redness is common with radiation therapy. Teach the patient how to care for the skin. *Avoid* products containing alcohol, even some aloe products.
6. Assure the patient fatigue is common during radiation and chemotherapy.
7. The carcinogenic risk to the nurse giving chemotherapy has not been proved conclusively, and suggested handling is controversial. However, antineoplastic agents are excreted in the patient's body fluids and feces, so *gloves* should definitely be worn.
8. Side effects from chemotherapy are numerous and vary depending on the antineoplastic agent. The most common is *decreased white blood* cell and *platelet count,* leading to *infection* and *bleeding.*
9. Nausea and vomiting are thought to be the side effects most dreaded by patients.
10. The negative impact cancer has on *body image* and *self-concept* is an area where the nurse can have a positive effect.

After Chemotherapy—To Combat Nausea

Calcium
Calories
Potassium
Protein

After Chemotherapy—To Combat Diarrhea

Fluids
Potassium
Residue
Hot foods
Foods with odors

Cancer—Palliative Care

Blenderized foods
Calories
Protein
Supplements

Radiation Therapy—To Decrease Nausea

Do not eat 2–3 hours *before* and 2 hours *after* treatment; then

Carbohydrates
Frequency
Protein
Residue
Size of feedings (small)

● Drug Review

Cancer

Antineoplastic medications listed in Appendix D.

Questions

1. Which position should the nurse place the arm of a patient in after a radical mastectomy of the right breast?
   1. Any position of comfort.
   2. Close to the chest.
   3. Elevated above the heart.
   4. Hyperextended to the side.
2. Postoperative exercises performed by the patient during the first 24 hours after a radical mastectomy of the left breast would include:
   1. Brushing her own hair with her left arm.
   2. Squeezing a rubber ball in her left hand.
   3. Pulling herself up in bed with a trapeze.
   4. Using her left hand to blow her nose.
3. The patient asks if she will be able to have visitors while receiving internal radiation therapy for cervical cancer. The best response is that:
   1. The threat to others is too great to allow visiting.
   2. Visiting is permitted on a limited basis, usually 30 minutes per day.
   3. There is no threat to the visitors, and therefore no restrictions.
   4. Only her husband may visit briefly every 24 hours.
4. What common systemic side effect of chemotherapy will the nurse observe in a patient receiving it?
   1. Ascites.
   2. Dysphagia.

3. Polycythemia.
4. Leukopenia.

5. A desired long-term goal of arm exercises after a mastectomy would include being able to:
   1. Squeeze a tennis ball with the affected hand.
   2. Brush the hair with the nonaffected arm.
   3. Cut meat on plate at meals.
   4. Raise both arms above head.

6. After a mastectomy the patient verbalizes concern about being unattractive to her husband. The best response to her concern would be:
   1. "Don't worry. After reconstruction you'll look like new."
   2. "Your feeling is normal after this kind of surgery."
   3. "I know he'll love you just the same as he did before the surgery."
   4. "Why do you feel so unattractive?"

7. The best nursing intervention for a patient who is having trouble accepting a mastectomy for removal of a malignant mass would be to:
   1. Ask the MD to talk to her about all the benefits of surgery.
   2. Tell her husband to tell her he still loves her as much as he did before the surgery.
   3. Have a member from a mastectomy support group visit her.
   4. Suggest that a psychiatric consultation be scheduled.

8. A patient receiving radiation therapy shows that he understands the nurse's teaching when he states:
   1. "I'll wash the area with soap and water."
   2. "I'll apply lotion to the affected area."
   3. "I'll massage the area vigorously."
   4. "I'll wear loose clothing over the area."

9. After chemotherapy, the patient's hematocrit is 25%, the hemoglobin level is 8.6 g/dL, the WBC is 600/mm³ and the platelet count is 10,000/mm³. The nurse would be alert to which manifestations of these laboratory findings?
   1. Mental confusion, headache, and blurred vision.
   2. Fatigue, alopecia, and stomatitis.
   3. Convulsions, tremors, and chills.
   4. Infection, respiratory arrest, and anorexia.

10. The patient returns from the post anesthesia recovery room (PAR) after a radical mastectomy of the right breast. An IV is running into the antecubital space of the left arm. Which technique is appropriate for drawing a blood sample needed for hemoglobin and hematocrit testing?
    1. Apply a tourniquet to the right arm and draw the sample.
    2. Do a fingerstick on the patient's left hand.
    3. Do a fingerstick on the patient's right hand.
    4. Call the MD to do an arterial stick.

Answers/Rationale

1. **(3)** To prevent lymphedema after a mastectomy and removal of the lymph nodes, the arm should be elevated to facilitate lymph drainage. In *none* of the other positions (**1**, **2**, and **4**) would the affected arm be placed *above the level of the heart*. **IMP, 3, PhI**

2. **(2)** During the early postoperative period, squeezing a ball in the hand of the affected arm would be done to begin strengthening the limb. Other exercises would be done *progressively*, from blowing her nose (**4**) to brushing her hair (**1**). The arm should *not* be raised *above* the shoulder until the drains are removed. Pulling herself up with a trapeze (**3**) would *not* be done during hospitalization because sufficient healing would not have occurred yet. *Mobility, not straining,* is the focus of exercises at this time. **IMP, 3, HPM**

3. **(2)** Radiation precautions include time, distance, and shielding; visitors to patients undergoing radiation therapy are protected in terms of the duration of exposure as well as distance from the patient, so limited visitation *is* permitted. Shielding is not routinely provided. No visitation (**1**) is an *extreme* restriction; no restrictions (**3**) is *unsafe;* and permitting only the husband to visit (**4**) is *too restrictive.* **IMP, 7, SECE**

4. **(4)** Chemotherapeutic agents suppress the body's normal immune response, resulting in a depressed white blood cell count (WBC), or leukopenia. This leaves the patient vulnerable to infection. Ascites (**1**) is associated with *liver* failure. Dysphagia (**2**), or difficulty swallowing, may occur in association with a *stroke* or *tumor.* Polycythemia (**3**), or an excessive number of immature *red* blood cells (RBCs), may be due to a primary problem in the *spleen* or a secondary problem stemming from *hypoxia.* **AS, 1, PhI**

5. **(4)** Exercises done after a mastectomy *progress* from squeezing a tennis ball, to brushing the hair, to being able to raise the arm, or arms, above the head, the latter signifying *maximum* mobility. Squeezing a tennis ball (**1**) is the *first* step, not the desired outcome. A *secondary* step would be brushing the hair with the *affected* arm, *not* the unaffected arm (**2**). Cutting meat (**3**) would *not* demonstrate the desired use of the affected arm. **EV, 3, PhI**

6. **(2)** The best response is to let the patient know that such feelings are normal and she may even feel depressed or angry. Allow patients time to verbalize their fears and anxieties; do not rush them if they show a desire to talk about their feelings regarding their surgery. Encourage them to ask questions. The nurse should *not* offer *uncertain assurances* (**1** and **3**). Even the most secure woman will experience a sense of loss and altered body image, so asking her why she feels this way (**4**) is *not therapeutic.* **IMP, 7, PsI**

7. **(3)** A group such as Reach for Recovery is designed to help women who have undergone a mastectomy

---

Key to Codes

Nursing process: AS, assessment; **AN,** analysis; **PL,** planning; **IMP,** implementation; **EV,** evaluation. (See Appendix M for explanation of nursing process steps.)

Category of human function: 1, protective; **2,** sensory-perceptual; **3,** comfort, rest, activity, and mobility; **4,** nutrition; **5,** growth and development; **6,** fluid-gas transport; **7,** psychosocial-cultural; **8,** elimination. (See Appendix O for explanation.)

Client need: SECE, safe, effective care environment; **PhI,** physiologic integrity; **PsI,** psychosocial integrity; **HPM,** health promotion/maintenance. (See Appendix P for explanation.)

meet common psychosocial, physical, and cosmetic needs. A hospital visit from the member of such a group may need to be authorized by the patient's physician, however. The difficulty accepting the mastectomy is normal. Knowing the benefits **(1)** does *not* compensate for the loss. Even with a supportive spouse **(2)**, the woman must grieve the loss over time. Because the grief is normal in the immediate postoperative period, a psychiatric consultation period, **(4)** would be *unnecessary* at *this* time. **IMP, 6, PsI**

8. **(4)** The patient should avoid wearing any clothing that will rub on the skin and cause it to break down. If washing of the skin is needed **(1)**, lukewarm water is used, as well as a hypoallergenic soap that is free of alcohol or perfume, to avoid possible irritation of reddened skin. Many lotions **(2)**, including some aloe products, contain alcohol, which is drying. Massaging or rubbing the radiated skin **(3)** may contribute to skin breakdown. **EV, 1, SECE**

9. **(1)** The patient has anemia (low RBC count), thrombocytopenia (low platelet count), and leukopenia (low WBC). The severe anemia and thrombocytopenia are the cause of the symptoms. Fatigue **(2)** would also be explained by the laboratory findings, *but* alopecia and stomatitis would be related to *drug toxicity*. Convulsions, tremors, and chills **(3)** would be seen if the patient had a fever resulting from a *severe infection*. Although the patient has an extremely low WBC and the risk of infection is great, the *low WBC alone would not* cause the symptoms. Anorexia **(4)** occurs as a result of chemotherapy, but *respiratory arrest* and, as already noted, *infection* are *not* related to the laboratory findings alone. **AS, 2, PhI**

10. **(2)** Capillary tubes of blood can be drawn from a fingerstick for these tests; in this case, the fingerstick should be done on the left hand. *No* blood pressure measurements, injections, IVs, or blood draws should be done or placed on the *right* arm (**1** and **3**), because these can cause circulatory impairment or infection in the limb. An arterial stick **(4)** is painful and *not* done for routine laboratory tests such as hemoglobin measurements and hematocrit determinations. **IMP, 1, SECE**

Emergency Nursing

Chapter Outline

Burns

Wounds caused by exposure to: excessive heat, chemicals, fire, steam, radiation, or electricity; most often related to carelessness or ignorance; 10,000–12,000 deaths annually; survival best at ages 15–45 yr and for burns covering less than 20% of total body surface.

I. Pathophysiology:

   A. *Emergent phase* (injury to 72 h): shock due to pain, fright, or terror → fatigue, failure of vasoconstrictor mechanisms → hypotension. Capillary dilatation, increased permeability → plasma loss to blisters, edema → hemoconcentration → hypovolemia → hypotension → decreased renal perfusion → renal shutdown.

   B. *Acute phase* (3–5 days): interstitial-to-plasma-fluid shift → hemodilution → hypervolemia → heart failure → pulmonary edema.

✉ **II. Assessment**

   A. *Subjective data:* how the burn occurred.

   B. *Objective data:*

   1. *Extent* of body surface involved: *"rule of nines"*—head and both upper extremities, 9% each; front and back of trunk, 18% each; lower extremities, 18% each; perineum, 1%. Requires adjustment for variation in size of head and lower extremities according to age. See text art at beginning of chapter.

   2. *Location*—facial, perineal, hand and foot burns associated with potentially more complications and fatalities because of poor vascularization.

   3. *Depth* of burn (Table 25.1).

   a. *First degree (superficial)*—epidermal tissue only, not serious unless large areas involved.

   b. *Second degree (shallow or deep partial thickness)*—epidermal and dermal tissue, hospitalization required if over 25% of body surface involved (major burn).

   c. *Third degree (full thickness)*—destruction of all skin layers, requires immediate hospitalization, involvement of 10% of body surface considered major burn.

   d. *Fourth degree (deep penetrating)*—skin and structures underneath.

   4. Indications of *airway burns* (e.g., singed nasal hair, brassy cough, sooty expectoration, increased mortality), edema may occur in 1 h.

   5. Poorer prognosis—*infants,* due to immature immune system and effects of fluid loss; *eld-*

TABLE 25.1	BURN CHARACTERISTICS ACCORDING TO DEPTH OF INJURY			
Classification	*Tissue Damage*	*Appearance*	*Pain*	*Clinical Course*
Superficial (*first* degree)	Epidermis	Mild to fiery red erythema; no blisters	Very painful	Ordinarily heals in 3–7 d.
Partial thickness: superficial or deep (*second* degree)	Epidermis and dermis	*Superficial:* mottled, moist, pink or red; may or may not blanch with pressure; usually blisters *Deep:* dry	*Superficial:* extreme pain and hypersensitivity to touch *Deep:* may or may not be painful	Healing takes 10–18 d; if infection develops in deep burn, it converts to full-thickness burn.
Full thickness (*third* degree)	All layers of skin and subcutaneous tissue	Charred and leathery or pale and dry	Usually absent.	Heals only with grafting or scarring.
°Fourth degree	All layers of skin and subcutaneous tissue, muscle, and bone	Black	Usually absent.	Heals only with grafting or scarring.

°Used in some classification systems. May require several days after a severe burn to determine fourth degree.

Source: Lagerquist SL: *Little, Brown's NCLEX-RN Examination Review.* Boston: Little, Brown, 1996. P. 96.

erly, due to degenerative diseases and poor healing.

6. Medical history—presence of hypertension, diabetes, alcohol abuse, or chronic obstructive pulmonary disease increases complication rate.

III. Analysis/nursing diagnosis

A. *Impaired skin integrity* related to thermal injury.

B. *Pain* (depending on type of burn) related to exposure of sensory receptors.

C. *Fluid volume excess or deficit* related to hemodynamic changes.

D. *Risk for infection* related to destruction of protective skin.

E. *Impaired gas exchange* related to airway injury.

F. *Body image disturbance* related to scarring, disfigurement.

G. *Ineffective individual or family coping* related to traumatic experience.

IV. Nursing care plan/implementation

A. Goal: *alleviate pain, relieve shock, and maintain fluid and electrolyte balance.*

1. Medications: give *narcotic* while physical exam is being completed and removing burned clothing.

2. Fluids: *IV* therapy (see Chap. 7, pp. 93, 96–97), colloids, crystalloids, or 5% dextrose according to burn formula.

3. Monitor hydration status:

a. Insert indwelling *catheter.*

b. Note color, odor, amount of urine; report fixed specific gravity—may indicate kidney problems.

c. *Strict* intake and output (I&O).

d. Check hematocrit (normal: men >40%; women >37%).

e. Weigh daily.

4. Soak: small burns may be soaked in cool saline.

B. Goal: *prevent physical complications.*

1. Vital signs: hourly; central venous pressure (CVP) for signs of shock or fluid overload.

2. Assess respiratory function (particularly with head, neck burns), patent airway, breath sounds.

3. Give medications, as ordered—*tetanus booster, antiinfectives* to prevent infection, *sedatives* and *analgesics, steroids, antipyretics—avoid* aspirin.

4. Isolation: protective, *strict* surgical asepsis (handwashing, protective clothing).

5. *Positioning:* turn q2h, prevent contractures—*Stryker frame* or circle bed if circumferential trunk burns present.

a. Head and neck burns—use pillows under shoulders only for *hyperextension* of neck.

b. Hand burns—use towel rolls or sandbags to align hands.

c. Upper-body burns—keep arms at 90-degree angle from body and slightly above shoulders.

d. Ankle and foot burns—allow feet to hang at 90-degree angle from ankles in *prone* position, use footboards to maintain angle in *supine* position, *elevate* to prevent edema.

e. *Traction* and *splints* to maintain positions.

f. Range of motion exercises according to

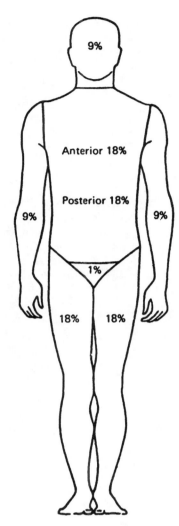

9%

Anterior 18%

Posterior 18%

9%   9%

1%

18%   18%

THE RULE OF NINES USED FOR ESTIMATING THE PERCENTAGE OF BODY BURNS IN THE ADULT.

therapy guidelines, usually several times per d; active exercises most beneficial.

6. *Diet:* initially NPO; begin oral fluids after bowel sounds return; do *not* give ice chips or free water, as these may contribute to electrolyte imbalance; food as tolerated—high *protein*, high *calorie* for energy and tissue repair (promote positive nitrogen balance).

7. Observe for:
   a. *Curling's (stress) ulcer*—sudden drop in hemoglobin, melena (give *antacids*, cimetidine, as ordered).
   b. Constriction due to *eschar* (circumferential or chest wall): prepare for *escharotomy* (lengthwise incisions)—painless procedure.

C. Goal: *promote emotional adjustment and provide supportive therapy.*
   1. Care by same personnel as much as possible, to develop rapport and trust.

2. Involve patient in care plans.
3. Answer questions clearly, accurately.
4. Encourage family involvement and participation.
5. Provide diversional activities and change furnishings or room adornments when possible, to prevent perceptual deprivation related to immobility.
6. Point out signs of progress (e.g., decreased edema, healing), as patient and family tend to become discouraged and cannot see progress.
7. Encourage self-care to highest level tolerated.
8. Anticipate psychological changes:
   a. *Acute period*—severe anxiety, mental confusion: orient to person, place, time; maintain eye contact; explain procedures.
   b. *Intermediate period*—reactions associated with pain, dependency, depression, anger: give medications to decrease pain; explain procedures; use other patients as models; have open, nonjudgmental attitude; use consistent approaches to care; contract with patient regarding division of responsibilities; encourage self-care.
   c. *Recuperative period*—grief process reactivated: anxiety, depression, anger, bargaining, as patient tries to cope with altered body image, leaving security of hospital, finances. Encourage verbalization; refer to self-help group to assist with adaptation.

D. Goal: *promote wound healing*—wound care:
   1. *Open method*—exposure of burns to drying effect of air; useful for burns of neck, face, trunk, perineum; eliminates painful dressing changes; *protective isolation* may be required.
   2. *Closed method*—pressure dressings applied to burned areas, particularly extremities; changed 1–3 times/d; if ordered, give *pain* medication 30 min before change; tubbing facilitates removal.
   3. *Topical antimicrobial therapies* (Table 25.2).
   4. *Tubbing and debridement:*
      a. Hydrotherapy—body temperature bath water; loosens dressings so they float off; soak 20–30 min; encourage limb exercises; do *not* leave unattended; loss of body heat may occur, with chilling and poor perfusion resulting.
      b. Removal of eschar (*debridement*)—done with forceps and curved scissors; medicate for pain before; use *sterile* technique; only loose eschar removed, to prevent bleeding; examine wound for infection, color change, decreased granulation—report changes immediately.
   5. Wound coverage, to decrease chances of infection:
      a. Temporary wound dressings (Table 25.3).
      b. *Autograft*—patient donates skin for wound coverage.
         (1) Types—free grafts (unattached to do-

TABLE 25.2   ◉ TOPICAL ANTIMICROBIALS USED IN BURN CARE

Agent	*Advantages*	*Disadvantages*	◉ *Nursing Implications*
Silver sulfadiazine 1% (Silvadene)	Broad spectrum Antifungal Nonstaining Relatively painless Usable without dressings No systemic metabolic abnormalities	Less eschar penetration than mafenide acetate Decreased granulocyte formation, transient leukopenia Macular rash	Check for allergy to sulfa
Mafenide acetate (Sulfamylon) cream or solution	Eschar penetration Effective with *Pseudomonas* Topical agent of choice for electrical burns Suitable for open method of treatment (cream) Used for gram-negative organisms	Severe pain and burning (lasts 30 min) Metabolic acidosis Carbonic anhydrase inhibitor Ineffective against fungi May cause hypersensitivity rash	Administer pretreatment *analgesic* Monitor for metabolic acidosis and hyperventilation Check for allergy to sulfa, observe for rash
Silver nitrate	Low cost Broad spectrum Effective with *Candida*	Continuous wet soaks Superficial penetration Black staining Stinging Electrolyte imbalances (low sodium, low chloride, low calcium, low potassium), alkalosis	Check serum electrolytes daily Rewet dressing q2h

Source: Lagerquist SL: *Little, Brown's NCLEX-RN Examination Review.* Boston: Little, Brown, 1996. P. 98.

nor site), pedicle grafts (attached to donor site).

(2) Procedure—general anesthesia; donor sites shaved and prepared; graft applied to granulation bed; face, hands, and arms grafted first.

☞ (3) *Post–skin-graft care:*

(a) Roll cotton-tipped applicator over graft to remove excess exudate; maintain dressings; use *aseptic* technique, apply heat lamps to dry donor sites.

(b) Third to fifth d—graft looks pink if it has taken.

(c) *Skeletal traction* may be applied, to prevent contractures.

(d) Elastic bandages may be applied for 6 mo to 1 yr, to prevent hypertrophic scarring.

🏠 **E.** Goal: **health teaching.**

1. Mobility needs: exercise, physical therapy, splints, braces.

2. Community resources: mental health practitioner or psychotherapist if needed for problems with self-image or sexual role; referrals as needed.

3. Techniques to camouflage appearance: slacks, turtlenecks, long sleeves, wigs, makeup.

◉ **V. Evaluation/outcome criteria**

A. Return of vital signs to preburn levels.

B. Minimal to no hypertrophic scarring.

C. Free of infection, demonstrates wound care.

D. Maintains functional mobility of limbs, no contractures.

E. Adjusts to changes in body image, no depression.

F. Regains independence; returns to work, social activities.

Emergency Nursing Procedures

I. Purpose—to initiate assessment and intervention procedures that will speed total care of the patient toward a successful outcome.

II. Emergency nursing procedures for adults are detailed in Table 25.4.

TABLE 25.3   TEMPORARY BURN DRESSINGS

Example	*Advantage*	*Disadvantage*	✉ *Nursing Implications*
Biologic			
Xenograft–pigskin	Promotes healing of clean wound, relieves pain, readily available, reduces water and heat loss	Easily digested by wound collagenase	Change q2–5d if over granulation tissue, overlap edges slightly, trim away when skin underneath has healed
Homograft–cadaver skin	Reduces water and heat loss, relieves pain, used with antimicrobial mesh, may be left in place for up to 8 d, debrides exudative wounds	May harbor disease	Observe for signs of infection
Amnion	Relieves pain, reduces water and heat loss, has bacteriostatic properties	Limited shelf life, requires special preparation for use	Change cover dressing q48h, leave on wound until it sloughs
Biosynthetic			
Biobrane	Protects from microbial penetration, decreases pain, promotes healing in partial-thickness burn	Not effective for preparing a granulation bed	Must be secured to skin ☞ with sutures, closure straps, tape, or staples; wrap with gauze; after 48 h, check for adherence; once adherence has occurred, may be left open to air; check for signs of infection

Source: Lagerquist SL: *Little, Brown's NCLEX-RN Examination Review.* Boston: Little, Brown, 1996. P. 98.

💡Study and Memory Aids

Trauma Care: Complications—"TRAUMA"

Thromboembolism/tissue perfusion, altered
Respiration, altered
Anxiety related to pain and prognosis
Urinary elimination, altered
Mobility impaired
Alterations in sensory-perceptual functions and skin integrity (infections)

Source: Lenaghan N. After the trauma. . . . Managing its effects down to the last letter. Nursing 92 March 1992, Pp 45–48.

Questions

1. A burn patient is admitted with a serum sodium level of 140 mEq/h. The nurse would attribute this normal laboratory finding on admission to the fact that:

   1. The anterior pituitary has released more antidiuretic hormone, thereby keeping the sodium level normal.
   2. Edema formation at the burn site has caused the serum sodium level to be normal.
   3. Sodium has been released from the damaged burned cells into the vascular compartment, keeping the level normal.
   4. An increase in the serum potassium level has caused aldosterone secretion to be depressed, thereby keeping the sodium level normal.

2. Because of the cellular damage resulting from a burn, the nurse can expect hyperkalemia to follow because there is:

   1. Edema formation at the burn site, causing the hemoconcentration of potassium.
   2. Release of the potassium from the cell into the vascular compartment.
   3. Decreased aldosterone secretion during physical stress.
   4. Excessive sodium loss, leaving a greater plasma concentration of potassium.

3. A male patient's bowel sounds are hypoactive after a blunt injury to the abdomen. The nurse would respond to this finding by:

TABLE 25.4   NURSING CARE OF THE ADULT IN MEDICAL AND SURGICAL EMERGENCIES

Condition	✉ *Assessment: Signs and Symptoms*	✉ *Prehospitalization Nursing Care*	✉ *In-Hospital Nursing Care*
Cardiovascular Emergencies			
Myocardial infarction—ischemia and necrosis of cardiac muscle secondary to insufficient or obstructed coronary blood flow.	*Prehospital:* *Chest pain:* viselike choking, unrelieved by rest or nitroglycerin. *Skin:* ashen, cold, clammy. *Vital signs:* pulse—rapid, weak, thready; increased rate and depth of respirations; dyspnea. *Behavior:* restless, anxious. *In hospital:* *C/V:* blood pressure and pulse pressure decreased. *Heart sounds:* soft; S_3 may be present. *Respirations:* fine basilar rales. 〰 *Lab:* ECG consistent with tissue necrosis (Q waves) and injury (ST segment elevation); serum enzymes *elevated*.	1. If coronary suspected, call physician, paramedic service, or emergency ambulance. 2. Calm and reassure patient that help is coming. 3. Place in *semi-Fowler's position.* 4. Keep patient warm but not hot.	1. Rapidly assess hemodynamic and respiratory status. 2. Start IV as ordered—usually 5% D/W per microdrip to establish lifeline for emergency drug treatment. ☞ 3. Draw blood for electrolytes, enzymes, as ordered. ☞ 4. Place on cardiac monitor. ⬭ 5. Relieve pain—morphine sulfate IV, as needed. 〰 6. Take 12-lead *ECG.* Once patient is stable, transfer to CCU.
Cardiac arrest—cardiac standstill or ventricular fibrillation secondary to rapid administration or overdose of anesthetics or narcotic drugs, obstruction of the respiratory tract (mucus, vomitus, foreign body), acute anxiety, cardiac disease, dehydration, shock, electrical shock, or emboli.	Cyanosis, gasping. *Respirations:* rapid, shallow, absent. *Pulse:* weak, thready, >120 beats/min, absent. *Muscle:* twitching. *Pupils:* dilated. *Skin:* cold, clammy. Loss of consciousness.	☞ **CPR:** 1. *Position:* flat on back. 2. Shake vigorously—establish unresponsiveness. 3. Call for help. 4. Tilt head back (chin lift). 5. Check for breathing—listen at mouth, look at chest, feel with cheek. **No breathing:** 1. Kneel close to head; place hand on forehead, bringing lower jaw forward and opening airway. 2. Pinch nostrils shut and blow two full breaths into patient's mouth. 3. Lips must form airtight seal. 4. Watch chest for adequate expansion, clear throat if indicated. 5. Check pulse—if present, breathe into mouth every 5 sec.	1. If monitored, note rhythm; call for help and note time. ☞ 2. Countershock if rhythm is ventricular fibrillation or ventricular tachycardia. ☞ 3. If countershock unsuccessful, begin CPR, as in prehospital care.

(continued)

TABLE 25.4   NURSING CARE IN MEDICAL AND SURGICAL EMERGENCIES (*Continued*)

Condition	◄ *Assessment: Signs and Symptoms*	◄ *Prehospitalization Nursing Care*	◄ *In-Hospital Nursing Care*
Cardiac arrest (continued)		**No heartbeat:** *Two-person CPR:* 80 chest compressions per minute, with one breath between every 5 compressions. *One-person CPR:* 80 chest compressions per minute, with two quick breaths between every 15 compressions. Check pulse at neck after 1 min and every few minutes thereafter. Check pupils to determine effectiveness of CPR—should begin to constrict. *If heartbeat returns:* Assist respiration and monitor pulse; continue CPR until help arrives.	*Two-person rescue:* *First person:* begins CPR as described in prehospital care. *Second person:* 1. Pages arrest team. ☞ 2. Brings defibrilaltor to bedside and *counter-shocks,* if indicated by rhythm. 3. Brings emergency cart to bedside. ☞ 4. *Suctions* airway, if indicated due to vomitus or secretions. ☞ 5. Bags patient with *100% O₂.* ☞ 6. Assist with *intubation* when arrest team arrives. ☞ 7. Establishes *IV* line if one is not available.
Shock—cellular hypoxia and impairment of cellular function secondary to trauma, hemorrhage, fright, dehydration, cardiac insufficiency, allergic reactions, septicemia, impairment of nervous system, poisons.	**Early shock:** *Sensorium:* conscious, apprehensive, restless; some slurring of speech. *Pupils:* dull but reactive to light. *Pulse:* <140 beats/min; amplitude full to mildly decreased. *Blood pressure:* normal to slightly decreased. *Neck veins:* normal to slightly flat in supine position; may be full in septic shock or grossly distended in cardiogenic shock. *Skin:* cool, clammy, pale. *Respirations:* rapid, shallow. *GI:* nausea, vomiting, thirst. *Renal:* urine output 20–40 mL/h.	☞ 1. Check breathing—clear airway if necessary; if no breathing, give *artificial respirations;* if breathing is irregular or labored, raise head and shoulders. ☞ 2. *Control bleeding* by placing pressure on the wound or at pressure points (proximal artery). 3. Make comfortable and reassure. 4. Cover lightly to prevent heat loss, but don't bundle up. 5. If neck of spine injury is suspected—do *not* move, unless victim in danger of more injury. If patient unconscious or has wounds of the lower face and jaw—place on *side* to promote drainage of fluids; position patient on *back* unless otherwise indicated.	1. Check vital signs rapidly—pulse, pupils, respirations. 2. Check airway; clear if necessary; PO₂ should be maintained above 60 mm Hg; *elevated* PCO₂ indicates need for intubation and ventilatory assistance. ☞ 3. Control gross bleeding. ☞ 4. Prepare for insertion of *intravenous line* and *central lines*—if abdominal injuries present. ☞ 5. *Peripheral line* should be placed in upper extremity if fluids being lost in abdomen. ☞ 1. Draw blood for specimens: Hgb, Hct, CBC, glucose, CO₂, sodium amylase, BUN, K⁺; type and cross-match, blood gases, enzymes, prothrombin times. ☞ 2. Prepare infusion of 5% D/NS *unless* hypernatremia suspected; dextran if blood loss.

(continued)

TABLE 25.4   **NURSING CARE IN MEDICAL AND SURGICAL EMERGENCIES (*Continued*)**

Condition	▶ Assessment: Signs and Symptoms	▶ Prehospitalization Nursing Care	▶ In-Hospital Nursing Care
Shock (continued)	**Severe or late shock:** *Sensorium:* confused, disoriented, apathetic, unresponsive; slow, slurred speech, often incoherent. *Pupils:* dilating, dilated, slow or nonreactive to light. *Pulse:* >150 beats/min, thready, weak. *Blood pressure:* 80 mm Hg or unobtainable. *Neck veins:* flat in a supine position—no filling; full to distended in septic or cardiogenic shock. *Skin:* cold, clammy, mottled; circumoral cyanosis, dusky, cyanotic. *Eyes:* sunken—vacant expression. *Renal:* urine output <20 mL/h.	1. *Raise* feet 6–8 in. unless patient has head or chest injuries; if victim becomes less comfortable, lower feet. 2. If patient complains of thirst, do *not* give fluids unless you are more than 6 h away from professional medical help; under *no* conditions give water to patients who are: unconscious, convulsing, or vomiting; appearing to need general anesthetic; or with a stomach, chest, or skull injury. 3. Be calm and confident, reassure patient help is on the way.	1. Assess and intervene as in early shock; then obtain information as to onset and past history. ☞ 2. *Catherize* and monitor patient urine output, as ordered. 〰 3. Take 12-lead ECG. ☞ 4. Insert *nasogastric tube* and assess aspirate for volume, color, and blood; save specimen if poison or drug overdose suspected. 5. *If CVP low*—infuse 200–300 mL over 5–10 min. *If CVP rises* sharply, fluid restriction necessary; if remains low, hypovolemia present. 〰 6. If patient febrile—*blood cultures* and *wound cultures* will be ordered. ⬭ 7. If urine output scanty or absent—give mannitol, as ordered.
Respiratory Emergencies *Choking*—obstruction of airway secondary to aspiration of a foreign object.	Gasping, wheezing; looks panicky, but can still breathe, talk, cough. *Cough:* weak, ineffective; breathing sounds like high-pitched crowing. *Color*—white, gray, blue. Difficulty speaking, clutches throat.	Do not interfere if coughing; do *not* slap on back; watch closely, call for assistance. **Victim standing, sitting and conscious:** ☞ Perform *obstructed airway maneuver* (formerly Heimlich): stand behind victim, wrap arms around waist, place fist against abdomen, and with your other hand, press it into the victim's abdomen with a quick upward thrust until the obstruction is relieved or the victim becomes unconscious. **Victim lying down:** ☞ Roll the victim onto his or her back, straddle the victim's thighs, place heel of hand in the middle of abdomen, place other hand on top of the first, stiffen arms and deliver 6–10 abdominal thrusts.	As in prehospital care. As in prehospital care.

(continued)

TABLE 25.4   NURSING CARE IN MEDICAL AND SURGICAL EMERGENCIES (*Continued*)

Condition	✖ Assessment: Signs and Symptoms	✖ Prehospitalization Nursing Care	✖ In-Hospital Nursing Care
Choking (continued)		**Unconscious victim:** ☞ Try to ventilate; if unsuccessful, deliver abdominal thrusts using technique described for conscious victim; probe mouth for foreign objects; keep repeating above procedure until ventilation occurs; as victim becomes more deprived of air, muscles will relax and maneuvers that were previously unsuccessful will begin to work; when successful in removing obstruction, give two breaths; check pulse; start CPR if indicated. ☞ On **obese or pregnant victims:** use chest thrusts instead of abdominal thrusts. **You are victim and alone:** Place your two fists for abdominal thrusts; bend over back of chair, sink, etc., and exert hard, repeated pressure on abdomen to force object up; push fingers down your throat to encourage regurgitation.	☞ As in prehospital care; when probing mouth for foreign object, *turn* head to side, unless patient has neck injury; in event of neck injury, *raise* the arm opposite you and *roll* the head and shoulders as a unit, so that head ends up supported on the arm.
Acute respiratory failure— sudden onset of an abnormally low Po$_2$ (<60 mm Hg) and/or high Pco$_2$ (>60 mm Hg) secondary to lung disease or trauma, peripheral or central nervous system depression, cardiac failure, severe obesity, airway obstruction, environmental abnormality.	*Hypoxia:* *Sensorium:* acute apprehension. *Respiration:* dyspnea; shallow, rapid respirations. *Skin:* circumoral cyanosis; pale, dusky skin and nailbeds. *C/V:* slight hypertension and tachycardia, or hypotension and bradycardia. *Hypercapnia.* *Sensorium:* decreasing mentation, headache. *Skin:* flushed, warm, moist. *C/V:* hypertension, tachycardia	☞ If you suspect respiratory distress, call physician; calm and reassure patient; place in a chair or *semisitting position;* keep warm but *not* hot; phone for ambulance; if respirations cease or patient becomes unconscious, clear airway and commence *respiratory resuscitation;* check pulse; initiate *CPR* if necessary; continue resuscitation until help arrives.	Check patient's ability to speak; maintain airway by placing in *high Fowler's position;* check vital signs: BP, pulse rate and rhythm, temperature, skin color, rate and depth of respirations. Prepare for intubation if: 1. Patient has flail chest. 2. Patient is comatose without gag reflex. 3. Has respiratory arrest; maintain mouth to mouth until intubation. 4. Pco$_2$ > 55 mm Hg. 5. Po$_2$ < 60 mm Hg. 6. FiO$_2$ > 50% using nasal cannula, catheter, or mask 7. Respiratory rate >36 breaths/min

(continued)

TABLE 25.4   NURSING CARE IN MEDICAL AND SURGICAL EMERGENCIES (*Continued*)

Condition	◁ Assessment: Signs and Symptoms	◁ Prehospitalization Nursing Care	◁ In-Hospital Nursing Care
Acute respiratory failure (continued)			☞ *After intubation:* 1. Check bilateral lung sounds. 2. Observe for symmetric lung expansion. ☞ 3. Maintain humidified oxygen at lowest FIO_2 possible to achieve PO_2 of 60 mm Hg. ☞ *Improve ventilation (decrease PCO_2) by:* 1. Liquefying secretions—oral and parenteral fluids; if intubated, frequent instillations of normal saline or sodium bicarbonate. 2. Frequent *suctioning*. 3. *IPPB* indicated if tidal volume ↓. 4. Chest *physiotherapy*. ⬭ Administer *drugs*, as ordered: *sympathomimetics, xanthines, antiinfectives*, and *steroids*. 〰 Monitor: arterial blood gases, electrolytes, Hct, Hgb, and WBC. *Do not:* 1. Administer sedatives. 2. Correct acid-base problems without monitoring electrolytes. 3. Overcorrect PCO_2. 4. Leave patient alone while oxygen therapy is initiated. Once patient is stable, transfer to ICU.
Near-drowning—asphyxiation or partial asphyxiation due to immersion or submersion in a fluid or liquid medium.	**Conscious victim:** Acute anxiety, panic. Increased rate of respirations. Pale, dusky skin. **Unconscious victim:** Shallow or no respirations. Weak or no pulse.	**Conscious victim:** 1. Try to talk victim out of panic so can find footing and way to shore. 2. Utilize devices such as poles, rings, clothing to extend to victim; do *not* let panicked victim grab you; do *not* attempt swimming rescue unless specially trained. 3. If you suspect head or neck injury—handle carefully, floating victim back to shore with body and head as straight as possible; do *not* turn head or bend back.	**Nonsymptomatic near-drowning victim:** 〰 1. Draw blood for arterial blood gases with patient breathing room air. 〰 2. PA and lateral chest *x-ray*. ☞ 3. Auscultate lungs. 4. Admit to hospital for further evaluation if: a. PO_2 < 80 mm Hg. b. pH < 7.35. c. Pulmonary infiltrates present, or auscultation reveals crackles. d. Victim inhaled fluids containing chlorine, hydrocarbons, sewage, or hypotonic or fresh water.

(continued)

TABLE 25.4	NURSING CARE IN MEDICAL AND SURGICAL EMERGENCIES (*Continued*)		
Condition	⋈ *Assessment: Signs and Symptoms*	⋈ *Prehospitalization Nursing Care*	⋈ *In-Hospital Nursing Care*
Near-drowning (continued)		**On shore:** 1. Check breathing. 2. Lay victim flat on back; cover and keep warm. 3. Calm and reassure victim. 4. Do *not* give food or water. 5. Get to medical assistance as soon as possible. ☞ 6. *If unconscious and not breathing,* begin sequence for CPR; compress water from abdomen *only* if interfering with ventilation attempts. ☞ 7. *If airway obstructed,* reposition head; attempt to ventilate; perform 6–10 abdominal thrusts; sweep mouth deeply; attempt to ventilate; repeat until successful. ☞ 8. Once ventilation established, check pulse; if absent, begin chest compressions as in CPR, one-person or two-person rescue. 9. Continue CPR until victim revives or help arrives. 10. If victim revives, cover and keep warm; reassure victim help is on the way. 11. Rescue personnel can further assist emergency room personnel by: a. Documenting prehospital resuscitation methods used. ☞ b. Immobilizing victims suspected of cervical spine injuries. c. Utilizing a sterile container to take a sample of immersion fluid. ☞ d. Taking on-scene arterial blood gas sample for later analysis.	**Symptomatic near-drowning victim:** ☞ 1. Provide basic or advanced cardiac life support. ☞ 2. Provide clear airway and adequate ventilation by: a. *Suctioning* airway. b. Inserting artificial *airway* and attaching it to *ventilator,* as indicated. c. Inserting *nasogastric tube* to suction to minimize aspiration of vomitus. 3. Monitor ECG continuously. ☞ 4. Start IV infusion of 5% D/W at keep-open rate for *fresh water near-drowning;* 5% D/NS in *salt water near-drowning.* ☞ 5. Assist with insertion of *CVP* and *Swan-Ganz* catheter to guide subsequent infusion rates. ◗ 6. Administer drugs, as ordered: *anticonvulsants, steroids, antiinfectives, stimulants, antiarrhythmics.* 7. Provide rewarming if hypothermia present. ☞ 8. Insert *Foley* to assess kidney output, as fresh water near-drowning causes renal tubular necrosis due to RBC hemolysis. Transfer to ICU when stabilized.

(continued)

TABLE 25.4   NURSING CARE IN MEDICAL AND SURGICAL EMERGENCIES (Continued)

Condition	✉ Assessment: Signs and Symptoms	✉ Prehospitalization Nursing Care	✉ In-Hospital Nursing Care
Systemic Injuries *Multiple traumas.*	*Sensorium:* alert, disoriented, stuporous, comatose.	1. *Don't* move patient unless you must, to prevent further injury; send for help.	1. Assess vital functions.
	Respirations: increased rate, depth; shallow; asymmetric; parodoxical breathing; mediastinal shift; gasping, blowing.	☞ 2. Check breathing—give *mouth-to-mouth* resuscitation if indicated.	☞ 2. Establish airway; *ventilate* with Ambu-bag, volume-cycled ventilator.
	C/V: signs of shock (see pp. 305–306).	3. Check for bleeding.	☞ 3. Draw arterial blood gases.
	Abdomen: contusions, pain, abrasions, open wounds, rigidity, increasing distention.	☞ 4. *Control bleeding* by applying pressure on wound or on pressure points (artery proximal to wound).	☞ 4. Control bleeding.
	Skeletal system: pain, swelling, deformity, inappropriate or no movement.	☞ 5. Use tourniquet *only* if above pressure techniques fail to stop severe bleeding.	☞ 5. Support circulation by *closed-chest massage.*
	Neurologic: pupils round, equal, reactive to light; ipsilateral dilatation and unresponsive; fixed and dilated bilaterally.	6. Check for shock (pulse, pupils, skin color) and other injuries.	☞ 6. Prepare *infusions* of dextran, blood, crystalloids.
	Bilateral movement and sensation in all extremities.	7. Fractures: keep open-fracture area clean.	7. Assess for other injuries: head injuries—suspect cervical neck injury with all head injuries.
	Progressive contralateral weakness.	8. Do *not* try to set bone.	
	Loss of voluntary motor function.	☞ 9. If patient must be moved—*splint* broken bones with splints that extend past the limb joints; tie splints on snugly but not so tight as to cut off circulation.	☞ 8. Place sandbags to immobilize head and neck.
	See *Sensorium* for level of consciousness.		☞ 9. Do *mini-neurologic exam:* level of consciousness, pupils, bilateral movement, and sensation.
		10. Check peripheral pulses.	10. Get history—time of injury, any loss of consciousness, any drug ingestion.
		☞ 11. If head or back injury suspected—keep body straight; move only with help.	☞ 11. Stop bleeding on or about head.
		12. Reassure patient that help is on the way.	☞ 12. Apply ice to contusions and hematomas.
			13. Check for bleeding from nose, pharynx, ears.
			14. Check for cerebrospinal fluid from ears or nose.
			☞ 15. Assist with spinal tap if ordered.
			16. Keep accurate I&O.
			17. Protect from injury if restless; seizures: orient to time, place, person.
			⬤ 18. Administer *steroids, diuretics,* as ordered.
			☞ 19. *Check for signs of increasing intracranial pressure:* slowing pulse and respiration, widened pulse pressure, decreasing mentation.

(continued)

TABLE 25.4   Nursing Care in Medical and Surgical Emergencies (*Continued*)

Condition	◄ Assessment: Signs and Symptoms	◄ Prehospitalization Nursing Care	◄ In-Hospital Nursing Care
Spinal injuries.			1. Assess and support vital functions as above.
			☞ 2. *Immobilize*—no flexion or extension allowed.
			☞ 3. **If in respiratory distress**—*nasotracheal intubation* or *tracheostomy* to *avoid* hyperextending neck.
			☞ 4. *Check for level of injury and function,* asking patient to:
			a. Lift elbow to shoulder height (C-5).
			b. Bend elbow (C-6).
			c. Straighten elbow (C-7).
			d. Grip your hand (C8–T1).
			e. Lift leg (L-3).
			f. Straighten knee (L-4, L-5).
			g. Wiggle toes (L-5).
			h. Push toes down (S-1).
			5. If patient **comatose**—sternum with knuckles:
			a. If all extremities move, severe injury unlikely.
			b. If one side moves and other does not, potential hemiplegia.
			c. If arms move and legs don't, lower spinal cord injury.
			● 6. Administer *steroids,* as ordered.
			7. Assist with application of skull tongs—*Vinke* or *Crutchfield.*
			☞ 8. Maintain *IV* infusions.
			☞ 9. Insert *Foley* as indicated.
			☞ 10. Assist with *dressing* of open wounds.

(continued)

1. Ignoring the finding, because all men have hypoactive bowel sounds.
2. Notifying the MD immediately, because hypoactive bowel sounds are a sign of impending complications.
3. Planning to reassess the abdomen again in 1 hour, because stress can cause hypoactive bowel sounds.
4. Giving the prescribed medications as ordered to stimulate gastrointestinal motility.

4. Before giving a patient a first dose of cefoxitin (Mefoxin), the most important nursing action is to:
   1. Explain the potential side effects.
   2. Record the patient's baseline vital signs.
   3. Determine whether the patient has any known allergies to the agent.
   4. Check the patient's hearing and kidney function.

TABLE 25.4   NURSING CARE IN MEDICAL AND SURGICAL EMERGENCIES (*Continued*)

Condition	▶ Assessment: Signs and Symptoms	▶ Prehospitalization Nursing Care	▶ In-Hospital Nursing Care
Chest injuries.			1. Note color and pattern of respirations, position of trachea.
			☞ 2. Auscultate lungs and palpate chest for: crepitus, pain, tenderness, position of trachea.
			☞ 3. Place gauze soaked in petroleum jelly over open pneumothorax (sucking chest wound) to seal hole and decrease respiratory distress.
			☞ 4. Assist with tracheostomy if indicated.
			5. Prepare for insertion of chest tubes if pneumothorax or hemothorax present.
Abdominal injuries.			1. Observe for rigidity.
			2. Check for hematuria.
			☞ 3. Auscultate for bowel sounds.
			4. Assist with *paracentesis* to confirm bleeding in abdominal cavity.
			5. Prepare for exploratory laparotomy.
			☞ 6. Insert *nasogastric tube*— to detect presence of UGI bleeding.
			7. Monitor vital signs.
			If organs protruding:
			1. *Flex* patient's *knees.*
			☞ 2. Cover intestines with sterile towel soaked in saline.
			3. Do *not* attempt to replace organs.
Fractures.			⬤ 1. Administer *tetanus toxoid*, as ordered.
			2. Observe for pain, peripheral pulses, pallor, loss of sensation and/or movement.
			☞ 3. Assist with wound cleansing, casting, x-rays, reduction.
			4. Prepare for surgery if indicated.
			5. Monitor vital signs.

(continued)

TABLE 25.4   NURSING CARE IN MEDICAL AND SURGICAL EMERGENCIES (*Continued*)

Condition	◄ Assessment: Signs and Symptoms	◄ Prehospitalization Nursing Care	◄ In-Hospital Nursing Care
Burns—tissue trauma secondary to scalding fluid or flame, chemicals, or electricity.	*Superficial (first degree):* Erythema and tenderness. Usually sunburn.	☞ Relieve pain by applying cold, wet towel or cold water (not iced).	☞ 1. Cleanse thoroughly with mild detergent and water. ☞ 2. Apply gauze or sterile towel. ⬬ 3. Administer *sedatives, narcotics,* as ordered. 4. Arrange for follow-up care, or prepare for admission if burn ambulatory care impractical.
	Partial thickness (second degree): Swelling, blisters; moisture due to escaping plasma.	1. Douse with cold water until pain relieved. 2. Blot skin dry and cover with clean towel. 3. Do *not* break blisters, remove pieces of skin, or apply antiseptic ointments. 4. If arm or leg burned, keep *elevated.* 5. Seek medical attention if *second-degree* burns: a. Cover 15% of body surface in adult. b. Cover 10% of body surface in children. c. Involve hands, feet, or face.	⬬ 1. Check tetanus immunization status. ⬬ 2. Administer *sedatives* or *narcotics,* as ordered. ☞ 3. Assess respiratory and hemodynamic status; *oxygen* or ventilatory assist as indicated, *intravenous* infusions as ordered to combat shock. 4. Remove all clothing from burn area. ☞ 5. Using *aseptic technique,* cleanse burns with antiseptic followed by soap and water, and irrigate with normal saline.
	Full thickness (third degree): White, charred areas.	1. *Don't* remove charred clothing. 2. Cover burned area with clean towel, sheet. 3. *Elevate* burned extremities. ☞ 4. Apply cold pack to hand, face, or feet. 5. *Sit up* patient with face or chest wound to assist respirations. ☞ 6. Maintain *airway.* 7. Observe for shock. 8. *Do not:* a. Put ice water on burns or immerse wounds in ice water— may increase shock. b. Apply ointments. 9. Calm and reassure victim. 10. Get medical help promptly. 11. *If* patient conscious, not vomiting, and medical assistance is more than 6 h away: may give sips of weak solution of *salt, soda,* and *water.*	1. Do *not* break blebs or attempt debridement. ☞ 2. Assist with application of *dressings,* as ordered. 3. Maintain frequent checks of vital signs, urine output. 4. Provide psychological support—explain procedures, orient, etc. ☞ 5. Assist with application of *splints* as ordered. 6. Administer *tetanus* immune globulin or toxoid as ordered. 7. Assist with transfer to hospital unit.

(continued)

TABLE 25.4   NURSING CARE IN MEDICAL AND SURGICAL EMERGENCIES (*Continued*)

Condition	◣ *Assessment: Signs and Symptoms*	◣ *Prehospitalization Nursing Care*	◣ *In-Hospital Nursing Care*
Burns (continued)	*Fourth degree:* Black.	Same as full thickness.	
	Chemical burns.	☞ 1. Flush with copious amounts of water. 2. Get rid of clothing over burned area.	☞ 1. Flush with copious amounts of water. 💊 2. Administer *sedation* or *narcotics,* as ordered.
	Burns of the eye: Acid.	☞ 1. Flush eye with water for at least 15 min. ☞ 2. Pour water from inside to outside of eye to *avoid* contaminating unaffected eye. 3. Cover—seek medical attention at once.	☞ 1. Irrigate with water; *never* use neutralizing solution. 💊 2. Instill 0.5% tetracaine, as ordered. ☞ 3. Apply patch.
	Alkali (laundry detergent or cleaning solvent).	1. *Don't* allow patient to rub eye. ☞ 2. Flush eye with water for at least 30 min. 3. Cover—seek medical attention at once.	As above for acid.
Abdominal Emergencies			
Aortic aneurysm—rupture or dissection.	Primarily males > age 60 yr. Sudden onset of excruciating pain: abdominal, lumbosacral, groin, or rectal. Orthopnea, dyspnea. Fainting, hypotension; if dissecting, marked hypertension may be present. Palpable, tender, pulsating mass in umbilical area. Femoral pulse present; dorsalis pedes—weak or absent.	1. Notify physician. 2. Lay patient *flat* or *raise head* if in respiratory distress. 3. Cover—keep warm but *not* hot. ☞ 4. Institute shock measures (see pp. 305–306). 5. Calm, reassure that help is on the way.	1. Assess respiratory and hemodynamic status. ☞ 2. Institute shock measures if indicated. 3. Evaluate and compare peripheral pulses. 〰 4. Assist with *x-rays.* 5. Assist with emergency preoperative treatment.
Blunt injuries—spleen	Left upper quadrant pain, tenderness and moderate rigidity; left shoulder pain (*Kehr's sign*). Hypotension; weak, thready pulse; increased respirations (shock).	☞ 1. Lay patient *flat.* ☞ 2. Institute shock measures.	1. Assess respiratory and hemodynamic status: ☞ a. Maintain *airway* and *ventilation* as indicated. ☞ b. Institute *infusions* of colloids and/or crystalloids, as ordered. ☞ c. Insert both *CVP* and *arterial monitoring lines.* ☞ d. Insert *Foley* catheter. 2. Prepare for splenectomy.

(continued)

TABLE 25.4 NURSING CARE IN MEDICAL AND SURGICAL EMERGENCIES (*Continued*)

Condition	◁ Assessment: Signs and Symptoms	◁ Prehospitalization Nursing Care	◁ In-Hospital Nursing Care
Eye and Ear Emergencies			
Chemical burns	*See Burns.*	*See Burns.*	*See Burns.*
Blunt injuries secondary to flying missiles (e.g., balls, striking face against car dashboard).	Decreased visual acuity, diplopia, blood in anterior chamber. Pain, conjunctiva reddened, edema of eyelids.	1. Prevent victim from rubbing eye. ☞ 2. Cover with patch to protect eye. 3. Seek medical help immediately.	📈 1. Test visual acuity of each eye using *Snellen* or *Jaeger* chart. 📈 2. Assist with *fluorescein* administration—to facilitate identifying breaks in cornea.
Sharp ocular trauma—secondary to small or larger foreign bodies.	Reports of feeling something hit eye. Pain, tearing, reddened conjunctiva. Blurring of vision. Foreign object may be visible.	1. Keep victim from rubbing eye. ☞ 2. Cover very lightly—do *not* apply pressure.	📈 1. Check visual acuity in both eyes. 2. Check pupils. ⬭ 3. Instill 1% tetracaine HCl, as ordered, to relieve *pain*. ⬭ 4. Administer *antiinfective* drops or ointment, as ordered. ☞ 5. Apply eye patch. 6. Provide instructions for subsequent care and follow-up.
Foreign bodies in ears— beans, peas, candy, foxtails, insects.	Decreased hearing; pulling, poking at ear and ear canal; buzzing, discomfort	1. Do *not* attempt to remove object. 2. Seek medical assistance.	1. Inspect ear canal. ☞ 2. Assist with sedating patient—*restraint* may be necessary. 3. Assist with procedures to remove object: a. Forceps or curved probe for *foxtails, irregularly shaped* objects b. 10F or 12F catheter with tip cut squarely off and attached to suction to remove *round* object. ☞ 4. Irrigate external auditory canal to flush out *insects*, materials that do not absorb water; do *not* irrigate if danger of perforation.

C/V cardiovascular; CPR = cardiopulmonary resuscitation; D/W; dextrose in water; ECG = electrocardiogram; CCU = cardiac care unit; Hgb = hemoglobin; Hct = hematocrit; CBC = complete blood count; BUN = blood urea nitrogen; D/NS = dextrose in normal saline; GI = gastrointestinal; CVP = central venous pressure; IPPB = intermittent positive-pressure breathing; WBC = white blood cell count; ICU = intensive care unit; PA = posteroanterior; RBC = red blood cell; I&O = intake and output; UGI = upper GI tract.

Source: Lagerquist SL: Little, Brown's NCLEX-RN Examination Review. Boston: Little, Brown, 1996. P. 212–222.

☞ Summary of Key Points

1. When faced with an emergency situation, the nurse must set priorities. Think "patient safety"—assess *airway, breathing, circulation, neurologic function,* and *pain.*
2. The age of a burn victim affects the severity and prognosis: The *very young* and the *elderly* are at greater risk for complications and death.
3. During the *first 48–72* h after a burn, the maintenance of adequate *perfusion* is the *priority.*
4. Even though body weight is the best indication of hydration status, *urine output* is more easily determined during early treatment. The expected output is *75–100 mL/h.*
5. The *cause* of the burn is important in determining related injuries, such as smoke inhalation.
6. The skin is the body's first line of defense against infection. A burn significantly compromises that protective mechanism.
7. Extensive burns (>20%–25%) increase the likelihood of multisystem complications such as *paralytic ileus, hypothermia, renal failure,* and *stress ulcers.*
8. IV drugs such as *morphine sulfate are* necessary for pain management when skin and muscle have been extensively destroyed and there is the potential for ileus.
9. The plan of care in a burn victim must also focus on preventing or minimizing potential *contractures* and *hypertrophic scarring.*
10. Even though physical healing may have occurred, further nursing interventions may be required to promote *emotional healing.*

Answers/Rationale

1. **(2)** The serum sodium level is influenced by the shift of water into the tissues that occurs in burns; the normal value in this patient is most likely due to the shift of water only to the site of the burn injury, rather than also to a loss of sodium. The serum value may actually rise as the serum sodium concentration increases. The posterior pituitary, *not* the anterior pituitary **(1)**, stimulates the release of antidiuretic hormone. Potassium, *not* sodium **(3)**, is released from destroyed cells. An increased potassium level **(4)** or a decreased sodium level *stimulates* aldosterone secretion. **AN, 6, PhI**

2. **(2)** Cell damage causes potassium, an intracellular ion, to be released, which increases the serum level. Edema formation **(1)** increases the *sodium, not* the potassium, level. During physical stress **(3)** there is an increase in *sodium* and water retention resulting from the *increase*

in the secretion of aldosterone. Sodium is an extracellular ion, and potassium is an intracellular ion; if sodium is lost **(4)**, the potassium level does *not* automatically increase. With burns there is a movement of water into the tissues, and the serum sodium level appears normal. **AN, 6, PhI**

3. **(3)** When such physical stress occurs, there is an increased sympathetic response, which decreases blood flow to the gut; as a result, peristalsis would be diminished or stop. Blunt trauma to the abdomen may result in shearing, crushing, or compressing forces, requiring continued assessment. There are *no* differences between the sexes in terms of bowel sounds **(1)**. The patient is still under observation, and additional data should be gathered *before* notifying the MD **(2)**. Drug therapy **(4)** is *not* indicated at this time, given the normal response of the body to stress. **AN, 8, PhI**

4. **(3)** Medication allergies, which are potentially life-threatening, must be identified during the admitting history. In addition to allergies to cephalosporins such as cefoxitin, there are cross-over allergies between penicillins and cephalosporins, so it is also important for the nurse to find out whether the patient is taking a penicillin. This is a *priority question;* although a knowledge of the side effects **(1)** is important, this is *not* the greatest concern. Side effects include nausea, vomiting, diarrhea, and rashes. Recording the patient's baseline vital signs **(2)** is *not specifically required* for patients receiving cephalosporin. Hearing and renal problems **(4)** are associated with the use of *aminoglycosides,* such as gentamycin. **IMP, 1, PhI**

Key to Codes

Nursing process: AS, assessment; **AN,** analysis; **PL,** planning; **IMP,** implementation; **EV,** evaluation. (See Appendix M for explanation of nursing process steps.)

Category of human function: 1, protective; **2,** sensory-perceptual; **3,** comfort, rest, activity, and mobility; **4,** nutrition; **5,** growth and development; **6,** fluid-gas transport; **7,** psychosocial-cultural; **8,** elimination. (See Appendix O for explanation.)

Client need: SECE, safe, effective care environment; **PhI,** physiologic integrity; **PsI,** psychosocial integrity; **HPM,** health promotion/maintenance. (See Appendix P for explanation.)

Common Acronyms and Abbreviations

Appendix A

This list provides a review of need-to-know acronyms and abbreviations used in charting, verbal directives, and study guides.

ā	Before (*ante*)
Ab	Antibody/Abortion
AAA	Abdominal aortic aneurysm
Abd	Abdomen/Abdominal
ABG	Arterial blood gas
ac	Before meals (*ante cibum*)
ADH	Antidiuretic hormone
ad lib	As much as desired (*ad libitum*)
ADLs	Activities of daily living
AFB	Acid-fast bacillus
Afib	Atrial fibrillation
Aflutter	Atrial flutter
AFP	Alpha-fetoprotein
AG	Antigen
AIDS	Acquired immunodeficiency syndrome
A-K (or AKA)	Above-the-knee (amputation)
ALL	Acute lymphocytic (lymphoblastic) leukemia
ALT	Alanine Aminotransferase (formerly SGPT)
AMA	Against medical advice
A&O × 3	Alert, oriented to person, place, time
AP	Anteroposterior/Alkaline phosphatase
aPPT	Activated partial thromboplastin time
ARC	AIDS-related complex
ARDS	Adult respiratory distress syndrome
ARF	Acute renal failure
ASA	Acetylsalicylic acid (aspirin)
ASAP	As soon as possible
ASD	Atrial septal defect
AST	Aspartate aminotransferase (formerly SGOT)
AV	Atrioventricular/Arteriovenous/Aortic valve
AVB	Atrioventricular block
AVM	Arteriovenous malformation
AVR	Atrial valve replacement
bid	Twice daily (*bis in die*)
BK (or BKA)	Below-the-knee (amputation)
BM	Bowel movement/Bone marrow

BMR	Basal metabolic rate
BP	Blood pressure
BPH	Benign prostatic hypertrophy (hyperplasia)
bpm	Beats per minute
BUN	Blood urea nitrogen
c̄	With (*cum*)
CA	Carcinoma/Cancer
CABG	Coronary artery bypass graft operation (× 1, 2, 3, 4 = number of grafts)
CAD	Coronary artery disease
CAPD	Continuous ambulatory peritoneal dialysis
CBC	Complete blood count
CC	Chief complaint
CCU	Cardiac (intensive) care unit
CF	Cystic fibrosis
CHD	Congenital heart disease
CHF	Congestive heart failure (now called HF—heart failure)
CK	Creatine kinase
CMV	Cytomegalovirus
CNS	Central nervous system/Coagulase-negative *Staphylococcus*
C/O	Complains of
CO_2	Carbon dioxide
COPD	Chronic obstructive pulmonary disease
CPAP	Continuous positive airway pressure
CPK	Creatine phosphokinase (now creatine kinase)
CPR	Cardiopulmonary resuscitation
CRF	Chronic renal failure/Cardiac risk factors
CRP	C-reactive protein
CSF	Cerebrospinal fluid
CSMs	Circulation sensation motion checks
CT	Computed tomography
CVA	Cerebrovascular accident/Costovertebral angle
CVP	Central venous pressure
Δ	Change (Greek letter delta)
DBM	Diabetes mellitus (also called DM)
D/C	Discharge/Discontinue
D&C	Dilatation and curettage
DI	Diabetes insipidus

Source: Fine P. *The Wards: An Introduction to Clinical Clerkships.* Boston: Little, Brown, 1994.

DIC	Disseminated intravascular coagulation		**HR**	Heart rate
Dig	Digitalis		**hs**	Bedtime (*hora somni*)
DM	Diabetes mellitus (also called DBM)		**HTN**	Hypertension
DNR	Do not resuscitate		**Hx**	History
DOA	Dead on arrival			
DOB	Date of birth		**ICP**	Intracranial pressure
DOE	Dyspnea on exertion		**ICU**	Intensive care unit
DPT	Diphtheria, pertussis, and tetanus		**I&D**	Incision and drainage
DRG	Diagnosis-related group		**IDDM**	Insulin-dependent diabetes mellitus
DTs	Delirium tremens		**Ig**	Immunoglobulin
DTR	Deep tendon reflex		**IM**	Intramuscular
DVT	Deep vein thrombosis		**INH**	Isoniazid
D₅W/D5W	5% dextrose in water		**I&O**	Intake and output
Dx	Diagnosis		**IPPB**	Intermittent positive-pressure breathing
			IUD	Intrauterine device
ECG	Electrocardiogram (purist's version)		**IV**	Intravenous
Echo	Echocardiogram		**IVC**	Inferior vena cava
ECT	Electroconvulsive therapy		**IVP**	Intravenous pyelogram/Intravenous push
EDB	Estimated date of birth			
EEG	Electroencephalogram		**IZ**	Immunization
EKG	Electrocardiogram (common version)		**JRA**	Juvenile rheumatoid arthritis
EMG	Electromyogram		**JVD**	Jugular venous distention
EMT	Emergency medical technician			
ENT	Ear, nose, and throat		**KUB**	Kidneys, ureters, and bladder (flat/upright abdominal x-ray)
EOM	Extraocular movement			
ER	Emergency room		**KVO**	Keep vein open
ESR	Erythrocyte sedimentation rate			
ETOH	Alcohol (ethanol)		**LLL**	Left lower (lung) lobe
			LLQ	Left lower quadrant
FB	Foreign body		**LMP**	Last menstrual period
FBS	Fasting blood sugar		**LOC**	Loss of consciousness/Level of consciousness
FEV₁	Forced expiratory volume in 1 second			
FRC	Functional residual capacity		**LPN**	Licensed practical nurse
FTT	Failure to thrive		**LUL**	Left upper (lung) lobe
FUO	Fever of unknown origin		**LUQ**	Left upper quadrant
FVC	Forced vital capacity		**LVN**	Licensed vocational nurse
Fx	Fracture			
			MAP	Mean arterial pressure
g	Gram		**MCL**	Midclavicular line
G	Gravida		**Med**	Medication
GB	Gallbladder		**MI**	Myocardial infarction
GC	Gonococcus/Gonorrhea		**MMR**	Measles, mumps, and rubella
GI	Gastrointestinal		**MODS**	Multiple organ dysfunction syndrome
GT	Gastric tube		**MOM**	Milk of magnesia
GTT	Glucose tolerance test		**Mono**	Mononucleosis
gtt(s)	Drop(s) (*guttae*)		**MR**	Mitral regurgitation/Mental retardation
GU	Genitourinary		**MRI**	Magnetic resonance imaging
GYN	Gynecologic		**MRSA**	Methicillin-resistant *Staphylococcus aureus*
			MS	Mental status/Mitral stenosis/Multiple sclerosis/Morphine sulfate
HAV	Hepatitis A virus			
HBV	Hepatitis B virus		**MVA**	Motor vehicle accident
HCG	Human chorionic gonadotropin		**MVR**	Mitral valve replacement
Hct	Hematocrit			
HDL	High-density lipoprotein		**NA**	Not applicable
HEENT	Head, eyes, ears, nose, and throat		**NG**	Nasogastric
Hgb	Hemoglobin		**NIDDM**	Non–insulin-dependent diabetes mellitus
HgbA₁C	Glycosylated hemoglobin			
HIV	Human immunodeficiency virus		**NL**	Normal
HMO	Health maintenance organization			
HOB	Head of bed			

noc	Night (nocturnal)
NPH	Neutral-protamine-Hagedorn (inter-mediate-acting insulin)
NPO	Nothing by mouth (*nil per os*)
NS	Normal saline
NSAID	Nonsteroidal anti-inflammatory drug
NSR	Normal sinus rhythm
NTG	Nitroglycerin
N/V	Nausea, vomiting
NVD	Nausea, vomiting, and diarrhea
O$_2$	Oxygen
OB	Obstetrics
OD	Right eye (*oculus dexter*)/Overdose
OOB	Out of bed/Out of breath
O&P	Ova and parasites
OR	Operating room
OS	Left eye (*oculus sinister*)
OT	Occupational therapy
OU	Both eyes (*oculo utro*)
P	Para/Pulse
p̄	Post (after)
PA	Posteroanterior/Physician's assistant/ Pulmonary artery
PaCO$_2$	Arterial partial pressure of carbon di-oxide
PAF	Paroxysmal atrial fibrillation
PAO$_2$	Alveolar oxygen pressure
PaO$_2$	Arterial partial pressure of oxygen
PAR	Post-anesthesia recovery
PAS	Para-aminosalicylic acid
PAT	Paroxysmal atrial tachycardia
pc	After meals (*post cibum*)
PCA	Patient-controlled analgesia (pump)/ Patient care assistant
PCP	*Pneumocystis carinii* pneumonia/Phen-cyclidine
PDA	Patent ductus arteriosus
PEEP	Positive end-expiratory pressure
PERRL(A)	Pupils equally round and reactive to light (and accommodation)
pH	Hydrogen ion concentration
PID	Pelvic inflammatory disease
PIN	Prostatic intraepithelial neoplasia
PKU	Phenylketonuria
PMI	Point of maximum impulse
PMS	Premenstrual syndrome
PND	Paroxysmal nocturnal dyspnea
PO	By mouth (*per os*)
PPD	Purified protein derivative (TB skin test)
PPO	Preferred provider organization
prn	When necessary (*pro re nata*)
PSA	Prostate-specific antigen
Pt	Patient
PT	Prothrombin time/Physical therapy
PTA	Prior to admission
PTCA	Percutaneous transluminal coronary angioplasty
PTT	Partial thromboplastin time
PUD	Peptic ulcer disease
PVC	Premature ventricular contraction

q	Each, every (*quaque*)
qd	Each day (*quaque die*)
qhs	Every night before sleep (*quaque hora somni*)
qid	Four times a day (*quarter in die*)
qod	Every other day
R	Respirations
RA	Rheumatoid arthritis/Right atrium
RBC	Red blood cell
RDS	Respiratory distress syndrome
RHD	Rheumatic heart disease
RLL	Right lower (lung) lobe
RLQ	Right lower quadrant
RML	Right middle (lung) lobe
R/O	Rule out
ROM	Range of motion
ROS	Review of systems
RUL	Right upper (lung) lobe
RUQ	Right upper quadrant
Rx	Prescription/Therapy/Treatment
s̄	Without (*sine*)
S$_1$	First heart sound
S$_2$	Second heart sound
S$_3$	Third heart sound
S$_4$	Fourth heart sound
SBE	Subacute bacterial endocarditis
SC	Subcutaneously
SGA	Small for gestational age
SIADH	Syndrome of inappropriate antidiuretic hormone
SICU	Surgical intensive care unit
SIRS	Systemic inflammatory response
SL	Sublingually
SLE	Systemic lupus erythematosus
SOB	Short(ness) of breath
SQ	Subcutaneously
SR	Sinus rhythm
S/S	Signs, symptoms
Stat	Immediately (*statim*)
STD	Sexually transmitted disease
SVG	Spontaneous vaginal delivery
SVT	Supraventricular tachycardia
Sx	Symptoms
T	Temperature
T&A	Tonsillectomy and adenoidectomy
TB	Tuberculosis
TIA	Transient ischemic attack
tid	Three times a day (*ter in die*)
TKO	To keep open
TLC	Total lung capacity/Tender loving care
TPN	Total parenteral nutrition
TPR	Temperature, pulse, and respirations
TSH	Thyroid-stimulating hormone
TURP	Transurethral resection of prostate
TV	Total volume/Tidal volume
Tx	Treatment

UA	Urinalysis	**VC**	Vital capacity
UGI	Upper gastrointestinal	**Vfib (VF)**	Ventricular fibrillation
UOQ	Upper outer quadrant	**VS**	Vital signs
UQ	Upper quadrant	**VSD**	Ventricular septal defect
URI	Upper respiratory (tract) infection		
UTI	Urinary tract infection	**WBC**	White blood count/White blood cells
UV	Ultraviolet	**WNL**	Within normal limits
		w/o	Without

Review of Nutrition

Nutritional Needs of the Elderly

I. *Calories*—1500–2000 kcal/d to maintain ideal weight; 15–20% of calories from protein sources (Table B.1).
II. *High fiber*—prevents or alleviates constipation and dependence on laxatives.
III. *Sodium*—3–4 g/d according to cardiac and renal status.
IV. *Fats*—limit to help retard the development of cancer, atherosclerosis, obesity, and other diseases.
V. *Fluids*—6–8 glasses/d.
VI. *Common deficiencies:* calories, calcium, folic acid, thiamine, vitamins A and D, zinc.
VII. Factors contributing to food preferences:
    A. Physical ability to prepare, shop for, and eat food.
    B. Income.
    C. Availability of food if dependent on others.
    D. Food intolerances.
VIII. Table B.2 provides interventions for *common eating problems in the elderly.*

Religious Considerations in Meal Planning

See Table B.3.

I. *Orthodox Jews:*
    A. Kosher meat and poultry.
    B. *No* shellfish or pork products.
    C. Milk and dairy products *cannot* be consumed with meat or poultry, require separate utensils.
II. *Conservative* and *Reform Jews:* dietary practices may vary from religious laws.
III. *Muslims: no* pork or alcohol.
IV. *Hindus:* vegetarians (cows are sacred).
V. *Seventh-day Adventists:*
    A. Vegetarianism is common (lacto-ovo).
    B. *No* shellfish or pork products.
    C. *Avoid* stimulants (coffee, tea, other caffeine sources).
    D. *No* alcohol.
VI. *Mormons:* no coffee, tea, or alcohol.

Special Diets

I. **Low-carbohydrate diet**—*ketogenic:* low carbohydrate, high fat; *dumping syndrome:* low carbohydrate, high fat, high protein.
II. **Gluten-free diet**—elimination of all foods made from oats, barley, wheat, rye; used for *celiac* disease.
III. **High-protein diet**—lean meat, cheese, green vegetables.
    A. *Nephrotic syndrome* (may also be on low-sodium diet).
    B. *Acute leukemia* (combined with high-calorie and soft-food diets).
    C. *Neoplastic* disease.
IV. **Low-protein diet:**
    A. Usually accompanied by high-carbohydrate diet and normal fats and calories.
    B. Renal failure, uremia, anuria, acute glomerulonephritis.
V. **Low-sodium diet:**
    A. Heart failure.
    B. Nephrotic syndrome.
    C. Acute glomerulonephritis (varies with degree of oliguria).

Common Therapeutic Diets

See Table B.4.

I. **Clear-liquid diet:**
    A. *Purpose:* relieve thirst and help maintain fluid balance.
    B. *Use:* postoperatively and after acute vomiting or diarrhea.
    C. *Foods allowed:* carbonated beverages; coffee (caffeinated and decaffeinated); tea; fruit-flavored drinks; strained fruit juices; clear, flavored gelatins; broth, consommé; sugar; popsicles, commercially prepared clear liquids, and hard candy.
    D. *Foods avoided:* milk and milk products, fruit juices with pulp, fruit.
II. **Full-liquid diet:**
    A. *Purpose:* provide an adequately nutritious diet for patients who cannot chew or who are too ill to do so.

TABLE B.1   MEDIAN HEIGHTS AND WEIGHTS AND RECOMMENDED ENERGY INTAKE

| Category | Age (y) or Condition | Weight | | Height | | REE (kcal/d) | Average Energy Allowance (kcal)[a] | | |
		kg	lb	cm	in.		Multiples of REE	Per kg	Per day[b]
Males	11–14	45	99	157	62	1440	1.70	55	2500
	15–18	66	145	176	69	1760	1.67	45	3000
	19–24	72	160	177	70	1780	1.67	40	2900
	25–50	79	174	176	70	1800	1.60	37	2900
	51+	77	170	173	68	1530	1.50	30	2300
Females	11–14	46	101	157	62	1310	1.67	47	2200
	15–18	55	120	163	64	1370	1.60	40	2200
	19–24	58	128	164	65	1350	1.60	38	2200
	25–50	63	138	163	64	1380	1.55	36	2200
	51+	65	143	160	63	1280	1.50	30	1900

[a] In the range of light to moderate activity, the coefficient of variation is ±20%.

[b] Figure is rounded.

The data in this table are based on the desirable weights for adults for the mean heights of men (70 in.) and women (64 in.) between the ages of 18 and 34 y as surveyed in the United States population (HEW/NCHS data). The energy allowances for the young adults are for men and women doing light work. The allowances for the two older age groups represent mean energy needs over these age spans, allowing for a 2% decrease in basal (resting) metabolic rate per decade and a reduction in activity of 200 kcal/d for men and women between 51 and 75 years of age, 500 kcal for men over 75, and 400 kcal for women over 75. The customary range of daily energy output for adults is based on a variation in energy needs of ±400 kcal at any one age, emphasizing the wide range of energy intakes appropriate for any group of people.

REE = resting energy expenditure.

Source: Food and Nutrition Board, National Research Council. *Recommended Dietary Allowances* (10th ed.) Washington, DC: National Academy of Sciences, 1989.

TABLE B.2   DIETARY INTERVENTIONS FOR EATING PROBLEMS OF THE ELDERLY

Problem	Rationale	◄ Dietary Interventions
Difficulty chewing	Missing or ill-fitting dentures	Provide liquid, semisolid, mashed, or chopped foods as tolerated
Difficulty swallowing	Paralysis related to stroke	Thickened and gelled liquids are usually better tolerated than thin liquids; baby food can be used as a nutritious thickener. *Avoid* overuse of puréed foods because of the negative connotations associated with it
Lack of appetite	Depression Acute or chronic disease Loss of sense of smell and taste Side effect of medication Loneliness Early satiety	Offer small, frequent meals Solicit food preferences Allow plenty of time to eat Because appetite is usually greatest in the morning, emphasize a nutritious breakfast Encourage group eating
Impaired ability to feed self	Poor vision Arthritis of the hands, stroke	Describe the meal and how it is arranged on the plate. Assist the patient by opening packages of bread and crackers, buttering bread and vegetables, cutting meat, and opening milk cartons Assess the patient's ability to grasp utensils and guide food to the mouth Refer the patient to an occupational therapist to evaluate the need for assistive devices or retraining

Source: Dudek S. *Nutrition Handbook for Nursing Practice.* 2nd edition Philadelphia: Lippincott, 1993 P. 340. Reprinted by permission of J.B. Lippincott Company.

TABLE B.3   ETHNIC FOOD PATTERNS — SELECTED EXAMPLES

Ethnic Group	Cultural Food Patterns	Dietary Excesses or Omissions
Mexican (native)	Basic sources of protein—dry beans, flan, cheese, many meats, fish, eggs Chili peppers and many deep-green and yellow vegetables Fruits include zapote, guava, papaya, mango, citrus Tortillas (corn, flour); sweet bread; fideo; tacos, burritos, enchiladas	Limited meats, milk, milk products Some use flour tortillas more than the more nutritious corn tortillas Excessive use of lard (manteca), sugar. Tendency to boil vegetables for long time
Filipino (Spanish-Chinese influence)	Most meats, eggs, nuts, legumes Many different kinds of vegetables Large amounts of rice and cereals	May limit meat, milk, and milk products (the latter may be due to lactose intolerance) Tend to prewash rice Tend to fry many foods
Chinese (mostly Cantonese)	Cheese, soybean curd (tofu), many meats, chicken and pigeon eggs, nuts, legumes Many different vegetables, leaves, bamboo, sprouts Rice and rice-flour products; wheat, corn, millet seed; green tea Mixtures of fish, pork, and chicken with vegetables—bamboo shoots, broccoli, cabbage, onions, mushrooms, pea pods	Tendency among some immigrants to use excess grease in cooking May be low in protein, milk, and milk products (the latter may be due to lactose intolerance) Often prewash rice Large amounts of soy and oyster sauces, both of which are high in salt
Puerto Rican	Milk with coffee Pork, poultry, eggs, dried fish; beans (habichuelas) Viandas (starchy vegetables, starchy ripe fruits). Avocados, okra, eggplant, sweet yams. Rice, cornmeal	Utilize large amounts of lard for cooking Limited use of milk and milk products Limited amounts of pork and poultry
African American	Milk with coffee Pork, poultry, eggs, fish Fruit: strawberries, watermelon Vegetables: turnip, mustard, collard greens, kale, sweet potatoes Cereals (including grits, hominy, corn bread, hot breads) Molasses (dark molasses is especially good source of calcium, iron, vitamins B_1 and B_2 and niacin)	Limited use of milk group (lactose intolerance) Extensive use of frying, "smothering," simmering for cooking Large amounts of fat: salt pork, bacon drippings, lard, gravies Possibly limited use of citrus and enriched breads
Middle Eastern (Greek, Syrian, Armenian)	Yogurt Predominantly lamb, nuts, dried peas, beans, lentils Deep-green leaves, vegetables, dried fruits Dark breads, cracked wheat	Tend to use excessive sweeteners, lamb fat, olive oil Tend to fry meats and vegetables Insufficient milk and milk products (almost no butter—use olive oil, which has no nutritive value except for calories) Deficiency of fresh fruits

(continued)

TABLE B.3   ETHNIC FOOD PATTERNS (*Continued*)

Ethnic Group	*Cultural Food Patterns*	*Dietary Excesses or Omissions*
Middle European (Polish)	Cream with coffee Many milk products Pork, chicken Root vegetables (potatoes), cabbage, fruits Wheat products, noodles, dumplings, bread Sausages, smoked and cured meats	Tend to use *excessive* sweets and to overcook vegetables *Limited* amounts of fruits (citrus), raw vegetables, meats
Native American (American Indian— much variation)	If "Americanized," eat milk and milk products Variety of meats: game, fowl, fish Nuts, seeds, legumes Variety of vegetables, some wild; roots Variety of fruits, some wild; rose hips; Variety of breads, including tortillas, cornmeal, rice	*Nutrition-related problems:* obesity, diabetes, dental problems, iron deficiency anemia; alcoholism *Limited* quantities of high-protein foods depending on availability (flocks) and economic situation *Excessive* use of sugar
Italian	Staples are pasta with sauces; bread; eggs; cheese; tomatoes and vegetables such as artichokes, eggplant, greens, zucchini Only small amount of meat is used	*Limited* use of whole grains *Insufficient* servings from milk group Tendency to *overcook* vegetables Enjoy sweets

Source: Lagerquist SL: *Little, Brown's NCLEX-RN Examination Review.* Boston: Little, Brown, 1996. P. 242.

B. *Use:* acute infection with fever, gastrointestinal upsets, after surgery as a progression from *clear liquids.*

C. *Foods allowed:* clear liquids, milk drinks, cooked cereals, custards, ice cream, sherbets, eggnog, all strained fruit juices, vegetable juices, creamed vegetable soups, puddings, mashed potatoes, instant breakfast drinks, yogurt, mild cheese sauce or pureed meat, seasonings.

D. *Foods avoided:* nuts, seeds, coconut, fruit, jam, marmalade.

III. Soft diet:

A. *Purpose:* provide adequate nutrition for those who have trouble chewing.

B. *Use:* patients with no teeth or ill-fitting dentures; transition from full-liquid to general diet; those who cannot tolerate highly seasoned, fried, or raw foods following acute infections or gastrointestinal disturbances, such as gastric ulcer or cholelithiasis.

C. *Foods allowed:* very tender minced, ground, baked, broiled, roasted, stewed, or creamed beef, lamb, veal, liver, poultry, or fish; crisp bacon or sweetbreads; cooked vegetables; pasta; all fruit juices; soft raw fruits; soft breads and cereals; all desserts that are soft; cheeses.

D. *Foods avoided:* coarse whole-grain cereals and breads; nuts; raisins; coconut; fruits with small seeds; fried foods; high-fat gravies or sauces; spicy salad dressings; pickled meat, fish, or poultry; strong cheeses; brown or wild rice; raw vegetables

as well as lima beans and corn; spices such as horseradish, mustard, catsup; popcorn.

IV. Sodium-restricted diet:

A. *Purpose:* reduce sodium content in the tissues and promote excretion of water.

B. *Use:* heart failure, hypertension, renal disease, cirrhosis, toxemia of pregnancy, cortisone therapy.

C. *Modifications:* mildly restrictive 2-g sodium diet to extremely restricted 200-mg sodium diet.

D. *Foods avoided:* table salt; *all commercial* soups, including bouillon; gravy, catsup, mustard, meat sauces; soy sauce; buttermilk, ice cream, sherbet; sodas; beet greens, carrots, celery, chard, sauerkraut, spinach; *all canned* vegetables; frozen peas; all baked products containing salt, baking powder, or baking soda; potato chips and popcorn; fresh or canned shellfish; *all cheeses;* smoked or commercially prepared meats; salted butter or margarine; bacon; olives; commercially prepared salad dressings.

V. Renal diet

A. *Purpose:* control protein, potassium, sodium, and fluid levels in body.

B. *Use:* acute and chronic renal failure, hemodialysis.

C. *Foods allowed:* high-biologic proteins such as meat, fowl, fish, cheese, dairy products—range, 20–60 mg/d. Potassium is usually limited to 1500 mg/d. Vegetables such as cabbage, cucumber, and peas are lowest in potassium. Sodium is restricted to 500 mg/d. See Sodium-restricted diet. Fluid intake is restricted to the daily urine volume plus 500 mL, which represents insensible water loss. Fluid intake measures water in fruit, vegetables, milk, meat.

   D. *Foods avoided:* cereals, bread, macaroni, noodles, spaghetti, avocados, kidney beans, potato chips, raw fruit, yams, soybeans, nuts, gingerbread, apricots, bananas, figs, grapefruit, oranges, percolated coffee, Coca-Cola, Orange Crush, sport drinks, and breakfast drinks such as Tang or Awake.

VI. High-protein, high-carbohydrate diet:

   A. *Purpose:* corrects large protein losses and raises the blood albumin level. May be modified to include low-fat, low-sodium, low-cholesterol diets.

   B. *Use:* burns, hepatitis, cirrhosis, pregnancy, hyperthyroidism, mononucleosis, protein deficiency due to poor eating habits, geriatric patients with poor food intake, nephritis, nephrosis, liver and gallbladder disorders.

   C. *Foods allowed:* general diet with added protein. In adults, high-protein diets usually contain 135–150 g of protein.

   D. *Foods avoided:* restrictions depend on modifications added to the diet. These modifications are determined by the patient's condition.

VII. Purine-restricted diet:

   A. *Purpose:* designed to reduce the amount of consumed uric acid–producing foods.

   B. *Use:* high uric acid retention, uric acid renal stones, gout.

   C. *Foods allowed:* general diet plus 2–3 quarts of liquid daily.

   D. *Foods avoided:* cheese containing spices or nuts, fried eggs, meat, liver, seafood, lentils, dried peas and beans, broth, bouillon, gravies, oatmeal and whole wheats, pasta, noodles, alcoholic beverages. *Limited* quantities of meat, fish, seafood allowed.

VIII. Bland diet:

   A. *Purpose:* provision of a diet low in fiber, roughage, mechanical irritants, chemical stimulants.

   B. *Use:* ulcers (gastric and duodenal), gastritis, hyperchlorhydria, functional GI disorders, gastric atony, diarrhea, spastic constipation, biliary indigestion, hiatal hernia.

   C. *Foods allowed:* varied to meet individual needs and food tolerances.

   D. *Foods avoided:* fried foods, including eggs, meat, fish, seafood; cheese with added nuts or spices; commercially prepared luncheon meats; cured meats such as ham; gravies and sauces; raw vegetables; potato skins; fruit juices with pulp; figs; raisins; fresh fruits; whole wheats; rye bread; bran cereals; rich pastries; pies; chocolate; jams with seeds; nuts; seasoned dressings; caffeinated coffee; strong tea; cocoa; alcoholic and carbonated beverages; pepper.

IX. Low-fat, cholesterol-restricted diet:

   A. *Purpose:* reduce hyperlipidemia, provide dietary treatment for malabsorption syndromes and patients having acute intolerance to fats.

   B. *Use:* hyperlipidemia, atherosclerosis, pancreatitis, cystic fibrosis, sprue, gastrectomy, massive resection of the small intestine, cholecystitis.

   C. *Foods allowed:* nonfat milk; low-carbohydrate, low-fat vegetables; most fruits; breads; pastas; cornmeal; lean meats; unsaturated fats such as corn oil; desserts made without whole milk; unsweetened carbonated beverages.

   D. *Foods avoided:* whole milk and whole milk or cream products, avocados, olives, commercially prepared baked goods such as donuts and muffins, poultry skin, highly marbled meats, shellfish, fish canned in oil, nuts, coconut, commercially prepared meats, butter, ordinary margarines, olive oil, lard, pudding made with whole milk, ice cream, candies with chocolate, cream, sauces, gravies, commercially fried foods.

X. Diabetic diet:

   A. *Purpose:* maintain blood glucose as near normal as possible, prevent or delay onset of diabetic complications.

   B. *Use:* diabetes mellitus.

   C. *Foods allowed:* composed of 50%–60% carbohydrates, 25%–30% fats, 12%–20% protein. Foods are divided into groups from which exchanges can be made. Coffee, tea, broth, bouillon, spices, and flavorings can be used as desired. Exchange groups include milk, vegetables, fruit, starch/bread (includes starchy vegetables), meat (divided into lean, medium fat, and high fat), and fat exchanges. The number of exchanges allowed from each group is dependent on the total number of calories allowed. Nonnutritive sweeteners (asparatame) if desired. Nutritive sweeteners (sorbitol) in moderation with controlled, normal-weight diabetics.

   D. *Foods avoided:* concentrated sweets or regular soft drinks.

XI. Acid and alkaline ash diet:

   A. *Purpose:* furnish a well-balanced diet in which the total acid ash is greater than the total alkaline ash each day.

   B. *Use:* retard the formation of renal calculi. The type of diet chosen depends on laboratory analysis of the stones.

   C. *Acid and alkaline ash food groups:*

      1. *Acid ash:* meat, whole grains, eggs, cheese, cranberries, prunes, plums.

      2. *Alkaline ash:* milk, vegetables, fruit (except cranberries, prunes, plums).

      3. *Neutral:* sugars, fats, beverages (coffee, tea).

   D. *Foods allowed:* all the patient wants of the following.

      1. Breads: any, preferably whole grain; crackers; rolls.

      2. Cereals: any, preferably whole grain.

      3. Desserts: angel food or sunshine cake; cookies made without baking powder or soda; cornstarch pudding; cranberry desserts; custards; gelatin desserts; ice cream; sherbet;

TABLE B.4   HOT-COLD THEORY OF DISEASE TREATMENT*

Hot Diseases or Conditions	Cold Diseases or Conditions	Hot Foods	Cold Foods	Hot Medicines and Herbs	Cold Medicines and Herbs
Infections	Cancer	Chocolate	Fresh vegetables	Penicillin	Bicarbonate of soda
Kidney diseases	Earache	Cheese	Tropical fruits	Aspirin	Milk of magnesia
Diarrhea	Rheumatism	Temperate-zone fruits	Dairy products	Castor oil	Sage
Rashes and other skin eruptions	Tuberculosis	Chili peppers	Low-prestige meats (goat, fish, chicken)	Cod liver oil	Linden
Sore throat	Common cold	Cereal grains		Iron preparations	Orange flower water
Warts	Headache	Goat milk	Honey	Vitamins	
Constipation	Paralysis	High-prestige meats (beef, water fowl, mutton)	Raisins	Anise	
Ulcers	Stomach cramps		Bottled milk	Cinnamon	
Liver complaints	Teething		Barley water	Garlic	
	Menstrual period	Oils	Cod	Mint	
	Joint pain	Hard liquor		Ginger root	
	Malaria	Aromatic beverages		Tobacco	
	Pneumonia	Coffee			
		Onions			
		Peas			
		Eggs			

*A Latin American, particularly Puerto Rican, approach to treating diseases. A "hot" disease is treated with "cold" treatments (foods, medicines) and vice versa.

Source: Reprinted with permission from Wilson HS, Kneisl CR. *Psychiatric Nursing (2nd ed). Mento Park, CA: Additon-Wesley, 1983. P. 774*

plum or prune desserts; rice or tapioca pudding.

4. Fats: any, such as butter, margarine, salad dressings, Crisco, Spry, lard, salad oils, olive oil.

5. Fruits: cranberries, plums, prunes.

6. Meat, eggs, cheese: any meat, fish, or fowl, two servings daily; at least one egg daily.

7. Potato substitutes: corn, hominy, lentils, macaroni, noodles, rice, spaghetti, vermicelli.

8. Soup: broth as desired, other soups from foods allowed.

9. Sweets: cranberry or plum jelly, sugar, plain sugar candy.

10. Miscellaneous: cream sauce, gravy, peanut butter, peanuts, popcorn, salt, spices, vinegar, walnuts.

E. *Restricted foods:* no more than the amount allowed each day.

1. Milk: 1 pint daily (may be used in other ways than as beverage).

2. Cream: ⅓ cup or less daily.

3. Fruits: one serving of fruit daily (in addition to the prunes, plums, cranberries); certain fruits listed under *Foods avoided* below are *not allowed at any time.*

4. Vegetables, including potatoes: two servings daily; certain vegetables listed under *Foods avoided* below are *not allowed at any time.*

F. *Foods avoided:*

1. Carbonated beverages, such as ginger ale, cola, root beer.

2. Cakes or cookies made with baking powder or soda.

3. Fruits: dried apricots, bananas, dates, figs, raisins, rhubarb.

4. Vegetables: dried beans, beet greens, dandelion greens, carrots, chard, lima beans.

5. Sweets: chocolate or candies other than those listed under *Foods allowed* above; syrups.

6. Miscellaneous: other nuts, olives, pickles.

XII. **High-fiber diet:**

A. *Purpose:* soften stool, exercise digestive tract muscles, speed passage of food through digestive tract to prevent exposure to cancer-causing agents in food, lower blood lipid levels, prevent sharp rise in blood glucose level after eating.

B. *Use:* diabetes, hyperlipidemia, constipation, diverticulosis, anticarcinogenic (colon).

C. *Foods allowed:* recommended intake about 6 g of crude fiber daily: all bran cereals; watermelon, prunes, dried peaches, apple with skin; parsnips, peas, brussels sprouts; sunflower seeds.

XIII. **Low-residue (low-fiber) diet:**

A. *Purpose:* reduce stool bulk and slow transit time.

B. *Use:* bowel inflammation during acute diverticulitis or ulcerative colitis, preparation for bowel surgery, esophageal and intestinal stenosis.

C. *Foods allowed:* eggs; ground or well-cooked tender meat, fish, poultry; milk; mild cheeses;

TABLE B.5   PHYSIOLOGIC FUNCTIONS AND DEFICIENCY SYNDROMES OF COMMON VITAMINS

Nutrient	Functions	Signs of Deficiency
Fat-Soluble Vitamins		
Vitamin A	Essential for formation and maintenance of epithelial cells; essential for normal function of the retina and the synthesis of rhodopsin (visual purple)	Night blindness; xerosis and softening of the cornea; dry, bumpy skin
Vitamin D	Necessary for absorption and metabolism of calcium and phosphorus; important for the formation of normal teeth and bones	Rickets in children; osteomalacia in adults
Vitamin E	Antioxidant that protects red blood cells from hemolysis; utilized in epithelial tissue maintenance and prostaglandin synthesis	Increased hemolysis of red blood cells, macrocytic anemia, increased capillary fragility
Vitamin K	Essential for the formation of prothrombin and other clotting factors by the liver	Hypoprothrombinemia; hemorrhagic disease in newborns
Water-Soluble Vitamins		
Vitamin C	Essential for the formation of collagen; promotes healing of wounds and fractures; reduces susceptibility to infections; promotes the absorption of iron; necessary for the conversion of folic acid and folinic acid, tryptophan to serotonin, and cholesterol to bile salts; may play a role in resistance to certain types of cancer	Scurvy—petechiae and ecchymoses, joint pain, delayed wound healing, gingivitis, bleeding gums, loss of teeth
Vitamin B_1 (thiamine)	Coenzyme in carbohydrate metabolism; essential for normal nerve function	Beriberi—peripheral neuropathy, muscle cramping, paresthesia, muscle degeneration, and heart failure
Vitamin B_2 (riboflavin)	Coenzyme in cellular metabolism and respiration; essential for healthy eyes	Red conjunctivae; fissures at corners of mouth, around nose and ears, on tongue; magenta tongue
Vitamin B_3 (niacin)	Coenzyme in the metabolism of carbohydrates and amino acids; essential for the synthesis of fatty acids and cholesterol and the conversion of phenylalanine to tyrosine	Pellagra—cracks in skin and lips; red lesions of hands, feet, face, and neck; dementia
Vitamin B_6 (pyrodoxine)	Coenzyme in protein metabolism and several other enzymatic reactions; necessary for the formation of norepinephrine, epinephrine, tyramine, dopamine, serotonin	Seborrheic dermatitis, cheilosis, peripheral neuritis, convulsions
Vitamin B_9 (folic acid)	Essential for DNA synthesis and normal maturation of red blood cells	Megaloblastic and macrocytic anemia; reduced platelet levels
Vitamin B_{12} (cyanocobalamin)	Coenzyme in protein metabolism; essential for red blood cell formation and maintenance of myelin sheaths of nerves	Pernicious anemia, progressive neuropathy owing to demyelination

Source: Shlafer M, Marieb E. *The Nurse, Pharmacology and Drug Therapy.* Menlo Park, CA: Addison-Wesley, 1993.

strained fruit juice (except prune); cooked or canned apples, apricots, peaches, pears; ripe bananas; strained vegetable juice; canned, cooked, or strained asparagus, beets, green beans, pumpkin, acorn squash, spinach; white bread; refined cereals (Cream of Wheat).

Food List for Ready Reference in Menu Planning

I. High-cholesterol foods—over 50 mg/100 g portion: beef, butter, cheese, egg yolks, fish, kidney, liver, pork, veal.

II. High-sodium foods—over 500 mg/100 g portion: *bacon*—cured, Canadian; baking powder; *beef*—corned, cooked, canned, dried, creamed; biscuits, baking powder; bouillon cubes; bran with added sugar and malt; bran flakes with thiamine; raisins; *breads*—wheat, French, rye, white, whole wheat; butter; *cheese*—cheddar, Parmesan, Swiss, pasteurized American; cocoa; cookies—gingersnaps; corn flakes; cornbread; *crackers*—graham, saltines; margarine; *milk*—dry, skim; mustard; oat products; olives—green, ripe; peanut butter; pickles—dill; popcorn with oil and salt; *salad dressing*—blue cheese, Roquefort, French, Thousand Island; *sausages*—bologna, frankfurters; soy sauce; catsup; tuna in oil.

III. High-potassium foods—more than 400 mg/100 g portion: almonds; bacon, Canadian; baking powder, low sodium; *beans*—white, lima; *beef*—hamburger; fruits, fruit juices; bran with sugar and malt; *cake*—fruitcake, gingerbread; cashew; chicken, light meat; cocoa; coffee, instant; cookies—gingersnaps; dates; garlic; *milk*—skim, powdered; peanuts, roasted; peanut butter; peas; pecans; potatoes, boiled in skin; scallops; tea, instant; tomato puree; turkey, light meat; veal; walnuts, black; yeast, brewers.

IV. Foods high in B vitamins (see Table B.5):
   A. *Thiamine:* pork, dried beans, dried peas, liver, lamb, veal, nuts, peas.
   B. *Riboflavin:* liver, poultry, milk, yogurt, whole-grain cereals, beef, oysters, tongue, fish, cottage cheese, veal.
   C. *Niacin:* liver, fish, poultry, peanut butter, whole grains and enriched breads, lamb, veal, beef, pork.

V. Foods high in vitamin C (see Table B.5): oranges, strawberries, dark-green leafy vegetables, potatoes, grapefruit, tomato, cabbage, broccoli, melons, liver.

VI. Foods high in iron, calcium, and residue:
   A. *Iron: breads*—brown, corn, ginger; fish, tuna; poultry; organ meats; whole-grain cereals; shellfish; egg yolk; *fruits*—apples, berries; *dried fruits*—dates, prunes, apricots, peaches, raisins; *vegetables*—dark-green leafy, potatoes, tomatoes, rhubarb, squash; molasses; dried beans and peas; peanut butter; brown sugar; noodles; rice.
   B. *Calcium: milk*—dry, skim, whole, evaporated, buttermilk; *cheese*—American, Swiss, hard; *vegetables*—kale; turnip greens; mustard greens; collards; tofu.
   C. *Residue:* whole-grain *cereals*—oatmeal, bran, shredded wheat; *breads*—whole wheat, cracked wheat, rye, bran muffins; *vegetables*—lettuce, spinach, Swiss chard, raw carrots, raw celery, corn, cauliflower, eggplant, sauerkraut, cabbage; *fruits*—bananas, figs, apricots, oranges.

VII. Foods to be used in low-protein and low-carbohydrate diets
   A. *Low protein°:* milk—buttermilk, reconstituted evaporated, low sodium, skim, dry; *meat*—chicken, lamb, turkey, beef (lean), veal; *fish*—sole, flounder, haddock, perch; *cheese*—cheddar, American, Swiss, cottage; eggs; *fruits*—apples, grapes, pears, pineapple; *vegetables*—cabbage, cucumbers, lettuce, tomatoes; *cereals*—cornflakes, puffed rice, puffed wheat, farina, rolled oats.
   B. *Low carbohydrate: all meats; cheese*—hard, soft, cottage; eggs; *shellfish*—oysters, shrimp; *fats*—bacon, butter, French dressing, salad oil, mayonnaise, margarine; *vegetables*—asparagus, green beans, beet greens, broccoli, brussels sprouts, cabbage, celery, cauliflower, cucumber, lettuce, green pepper, spinach, squash, tomatoes; *fruits*—avocados, strawberries, cantaloupe, lemons, rhubarb.

VIII. Food guide pyramid—guide to daily food selection (Figure B-1).
   A. *Fats, oils:* use sparingly.
   B. *Milk group:* two to three servings.
   C. *Meat group:* two to three servings.
   D. *Fruit group:* two to four servings.
   E. *Vegetable group:* three to five servings.
   F. *Bread/cereal group:* six to 11 servings.

° These proteins are allowed in various amounts in controlled-protein diets for renal decompensation.

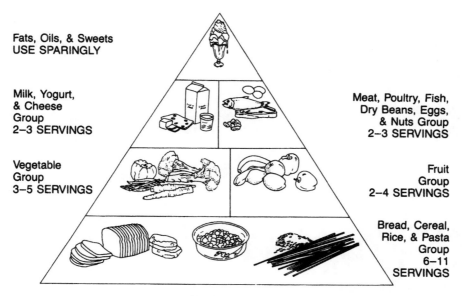

FIGURE B-1. FOOD GUIDE PYRAMID—GUIDE TO DAILY FOOD CHOICES. (From U.S. Department of Agriculture.)

● Index to Diets

For a quick review, use this appendix to locate special dietary considerations covered in this text as they pertain to specific medical conditions.

⟜ Review of Pharmacology

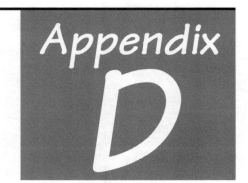
Appendix D

Absorption Rates

Table D.1.

Common Drugs

Table D.2.

Adrenergics
Adrenocortical steroids
Analgesics
Antianemics
Antianginals
Antiarrhythmics
Antiasthmatics
Anticholinergics
Anticoagulants
Anticoagulant antidotes
Anticonvulsants
Antidiarrheals
Antiemetics
Antifungals
Antigout
Antihistamines
Antihyperglycemics
Antihypertensives
Antiinfectives
Antilipemics
Antiplatelets
Antituberculosis
Antiulceratives
Antivirals
Bronchodilators
Calcium channel blockers
Cardiac glycosides
Cholinergic drugs
Cholinergic miotics
CNS stimulants
Decongestants
Diuretics
Emetics
Enzymes
Expectorants
Fibrinolytic agents
Fibrinolytic antidote
Hormones
Mucolytic agents

Muscle relaxants
Narcotic antagonists
Sedatives and hypnotics
Thyroid hormone inhibitor
Thyroid hormone replacement

Food and Drug Considerations

Table D.3.

Classification of Anticancer Drugs

Table D.4.

Properties of Selected Anti-inflammatory Agents

Table D.5.

TABLE D.1	**RATES OF ABSORPTION BY DIFFERENT ROUTES**
Route of Administration	*Time Until Drug Takes Effect**
Topical	Hours to days
Oral	30–90 min
Rectal	5–30 min (unpredictable)
Subcutaneous injection	15–30 min
Intramuscular injection	10–20 min
Sublingual tablet	3–5 min
Sublingual injection	3 min
Inhalation	3 min
Endotracheal	3 min
Intravenous	30–60 sec
Intracardiac	15 sec

*In a healthy person with normal perfusion.

Source: Caroline NL. *Emergency Care in the Streets* (5th ed). Boston: Little, Brown, 1995.

TABLE D.2   COMMON DRUGS

Drug and Dosage	Use	Action	▷◁ Assessment: Side Effects
ADRENERGICS **Alpha and beta agonists** Epinephrine (Adrenalin)—SC or IM 0.1–1 mg in 1:1000 solution; IV—intracardiac 1:10,000 solution; ophthalmic 1:1000–1:50,000 solution	Asystole, bronchospasm, anaphylaxis, glaucoma	Stimulates pacemaker cells; inhibits histamine and mediates bronchial relaxation; ↓ intraocular pressure	Ventricular arrhythmias, fear, anxiety, anginal pain, decreased renal blood flow, burning of eyes, headache

NURSING IMPLICATIONS: Use *TB syringe* for greater accuracy; *massaging* injection site hastens action; repeated injections may cause tissue necrosis; *avoid* injection in buttocks because bacteria in area may lead to gas gangrene; may make mucous plugs in lungs more difficult to dislodge.

Drug and Dosage	Use	Action	Assessment: Side Effects
Norepinephrine (Levophed)—IV 8–12 µg/min titrated to desired response	*Acute* hypertension, cardiogenic shock	Increases rate and strength of heart beat; increases vasoconstriction	Palpitations, pallor, headache, hypertension, anxiety, insomnia, dilated pupils, nausea, vomiting, glycosuria, tissue sloughing

NURSING IMPLICATIONS: Observe vital signs, mentation, skin temperature, and color (earlobes, lips, nailbeds); tissue necrosis occurs with infiltration; *antidote* is *phentolamine* 5–10 mg in 10–15 mL normal saline.

Drug and Dosage	Use	Action	Assessment: Side Effects
Beta agonists Dobutamine (Dobutrex)—IV 2.5–15 µg/kg/min	Acute heart failure	Stimulates cardiac contractile force (positive inotropy); fewer changes in heart rate than dopamine or isoproterenol	Tachycardia, arrhythmias

NURSING IMPLICATIONS: Mix with 5% dextrose; do *not* dilute until ready to use; *protect from light;* administer with *infusion pump;* check vital signs *constantly; extravasation* can produce tissue necrosis; see Norepinephrine.

Drug and Dosage	Use	Action	Assessment: Side Effects
Dopamine (Intropin)—IV 0.5–5 µg/kg/min titrated to desired response (10–30 min. intervals) maintenance at 20 µg/kg/min or less	Acute heart failure	↑ Cardiac contractility; ↑ renal blood flow	Ectopic beats, nausea, vomiting, tachycardia, anginal pain, dyspnea, hypotension

NURSING IMPLICATIONS: Monitor vital signs, urine output, and signs of peripheral ischemia; will cause *tissue sloughing* if infiltration occurs.

Drug and Dosage	Use	Action	Assessment: Side Effects
Isoproterenol (Isuprel)—10–15 mg sublingually; IV 0.5–5.0 µg/min in solution	Cardiogenic shock, heart block, bronchospasm—asthma, emphysema	↑ Cardiac contractility: facilitates AV conduction and pacemaker automaticity	Tachyarrhythmias, hypotension, headache, flushing of skin, nausea, tremor, dizziness

NURSING IMPLICATIONS: Monitor vital signs, ECG: oral inhalation solutions must *not* be injected.

Drug and Dosage	Use	Action	Assessment: Side Effects
ADRENOCORTICAL STEROIDS Cortisone acetate—PO or IM 20–100 mg qd in single or divided doses	ACTH insufficiency, rheumatoid arthritis, allergies, ulcerative colitis, nephrosis	Anti-inflammatory effect of unknown action	Moon facies, hirsutism, thinning of skin, striae, hypertension, menstrual irregularities, delayed healing, psychoses

NURSING IMPLICATIONS: Give oral form *pc,* with snack at bedtime; give deep IM (*never* deltoid); monitor vital signs; observe for behavior changes; skin care and activity to tolerance; 🍎 *diet*—salt restricted, high protein, KCl supplement; protect from injury.

(continued)

TABLE D.2   COMMON DRUGS (*Continued*)

Drug and Dosage	Use	Action	✉ Assessment: Side Effects
ADRENOCORTICAL STEROIDS (*continued*)			
Desoxycorticosterone acetate (hydrocortisone)—IM 1–5 mg	Addison's disease, burns, surgical shock, adrenal surgery	Promotes resorption of sodium; restores plasma volume, BP, and electrolyte balance	Edema, hypertension, pulmonary congestion, hypokalemia
NURSING IMPLICATIONS: *Salt restriction* according to BP readings; monitor vital signs; *weigh* daily.			
Dexamethasone (Decadron)—PO 0.75–9.0 mg qd; IM or IV 4–20 mg qd	Addison's disease, allergic reactions, leukemia, Hodgkin's disease, iritis, dermatitis, rheumatoid arthritis	Anti-inflammatory effect	See Cortisone acetate
NURSING IMPLICATIONS: *Contraindicated* in tuberculosis; see Cortisone acetate for nursing implications.			
Methylprednisolone sodium (Solu-Medrol)—IV, IM 10–40 mg, slowly	Glucocorticoid, corticosteroid	See Dexamethasone	See Dexamethasone
NURSING IMPLICATIONS: See Dexamethasone.			
Prednisone—PO 2.5–15.0 mg qd	Rheumatoid arthritis, cancer therapy	Anti-inflammatory effect of unknown action	Insomnia, gastric distress
NURSING IMPLICATIONS: See Cortisone acetate.			
ANALGESICS			
Acetaminophen (Tylenol, Datril, Panadol)—PO 325–650 mg q4h	Simple fever or pain	Analgesic and antipyretic actions; *no* anti-inflammatory or anticoagulant effects	No remarkable side effects when taken for a short period
NURSING IMPLICATIONS: Consult with physician if no relief after 4 d of therapy.			
Aspirin (acetylsalicylic acid)—PO or rectal 0.3–0.6 g	Minor aches and pains, fever of colds and influenza, rheumatoid arthritis, anticoagulant therapy	Selectively depresses subcortical levels of CNS	Erosive gastritis with bleeding, coryza, urticaria, nausea, vomiting, tinnitus, impaired hearing, respiratory alkalosis
NURSING IMPLICATIONS: Administer *with food or after meals;* observe for nasal, oral or subcutaneous *bleeding;* push *fluids;* check Hct, Hgb, prothrombin times frequently; *avoid* use in children with flu.			
Codeine—PO, IM, or SC 15–60 mg (gr ¼ to 1)	Control pain, may be used during the puerperium	Nonsynthetic narcotic analgesic	Of little use during labor, allergic response, constipation, GI upset
NURSING IMPLICATIONS: Note response to the medication; less respiratory depression; preferred for head injury patient.			
Ecotrin (enteric-coated aspirin)	See Aspirin	See Aspirin	See Aspirin
NURSING IMPLICATIONS: See Aspirin.			

(continued)

TABLE D.2   COMMON DRUGS (*Continued*)

Drug and Dosage	Use	Action	◄ Assessment: Side Effects
ANALGESICS (*continued*) Ibuprofen (Motrin)—300–800 mg oral 3–4/d, *not to exceed* 3200 mg/d	Nonsteroidal anti-inflammatory, *antirheumatic* used for chronic arthritis pain	Inhibition of prostaglandin *synthesis or release*	GI upset, leukopenia, sodium/*water retention*

NURSING IMPLICATIONS: Give on *empty stomach* for best result; may mix with food if GI upset severe; teach caution when using other medications.

Drug and Dosage	Use	Action	Assessment: Side Effects
Etodolac (Lodine)—PO 400–1200 mg/d, 300–400 mg q6–8h	Management of osteoarthritis, mild to moderate pain	Inhibits prostaglandin synthesis, suppression of inflammation and pain (NSAID)	Dyspepsia, asthma, drowsiness, dizziness, rash, tinnitus, anaphylaxis

NURSING IMPLICATIONS: Give 30 min *before or 2 h after* meals for rapid effect; may be taken *with* food to decrease GI irritation.

Drug and Dosage	Use	Action	Assessment: Side Effects
Fentanyl transdermal (Duragesic)—25–100 µg/h	Chronic pain; *not* recommended for postoperative pain	Binds to opiate receptors in the CNS to alter response and perception of pain	Drowsiness, confusion, weakness, constipation, dry mouth, nausea, vomiting, anorexia, sweating

NURSING IMPLICATIONS: Apply to *upper* torso, flat, nonirritated surface; when applying, hold firmly with palm of hand 10–20 sec.

Drug and Dosage	Use	Action	Assessment: Side Effects
Hydromorphone (Dilaudid)—PO 2–4 mg q3–6h; IM 1–2 mg q3–6h up to 2–4 mg q4–6h; IV 0.5–1.0 mg q3h	Moderate to severe pain, antitussive	Binds to opiate receptors in the CNS, alters perception and response to pain	Sedation, confusion, hypotension, constipation

NURSING IMPLICATIONS: Give PO with *food or milk;* give 2 mg IV over 3–5 min; *fluids, bulk,* and laxatives to minimize constipation.

Drug and Dosage	Use	Action	Assessment: Side Effects
Indomethacin (Indocin)—PO 25 mg 3–4/d; increase to max 200 mg daily in divided doses	Rheumatoid arthritis, bursitis, gouty arthritis	Antipyretic/anti-inflammatory action, inhibits prostaglandin biosynthesis	GI distress, GI bleeding, rash, headache, blood dyscrasias, corneal changes

NURSING IMPLICATIONS: Monitor GI side effects; administer *after* meals for best effect or *with* food, milk, or antacids if GI symptoms severe.

Drug and Dosage	Use	Action	Assessment: Side Effects
Ketorolac (Toradol)—PO 10 mg q4–6h; IM 30–60 mg initially, then 15–30 mg q6h; ophthalmic 1 gtt qid for 1 wk	Short-term management of pain, ocular itching due to allergies (NSAID)	Inhibits prostaglandin synthesis producing peripherally mediated analgesia, antipyretic/anti-inflammatory	Drowsiness, dizziness, dyspnea, prolonged bleeding time, dyspepsia

NURSING IMPLICATIONS: May be given routinely or prn; *advise* dentist or MD before any procedure.

Drug and Dosage	Use	Action	Assessment: Side Effects
Meperidine HCl (Demerol)—PO or IM 50–100 mg q3–4h	Pain due to trauma or surgery, allays apprehension prior to surgery	Acts on CNS to produce analgesia, sedation, euphoria, respiratory depression	Palpitations, bradycardia, hypotension, nausea, vomiting, syncope, sweating, tremors, convulsions

NURSING IMPLICATIONS: Check *respiratory rate* and depth before giving drug; give IM, as *subcutaneous* administration is *painful* and can cause local irritation.

(*continued*)

TABLE D.2   COMMON DRUGS (*Continued*)

Drug and Dosage	Use	Action	◁ Assessment: Side Effects
ANALGESICS (*continued*)			
Morphine SO$_4$—PO 10–30 mg (Roxanol, MS Contin); SC 8–15 mg; IV 4–10 mg; rectal 10–20 mg	Control pain and relieve fear, apprehension, restlessness, as in pulmonary edema	Depresses CNS reception of pain and ability to interpret stimuli, depresses respiratory center in medulla	Nausea, vomiting, flushing, confusion, urticaria, depressed rate and depth of respirations, decreased blood pressure

NURSING IMPLICATIONS: Check rate and depth of *respirations* before administering drug; observe for gas pains and *abdominal distention;* smaller doses for aged; monitor vital signs; observe for *postural hypotension.*

Naproxen (Naprosyn)—PO 250–500 mg bid	Mild to moderate pain, dysmenorrhea, rheumatoid arthritis, osteoarthritis (NSAID)	Inhibits prostaglandin synthesis, suppresses inflammation	Headache, drowsiness, dizziness, nausea, dyspepsia, constipation, bleeding

NURSING IMPLICATIONS: Take with a full glass of *water; avoid* exposure to sun.

Oxycodone HCl (Percodan, Tylox)—PO 3–20 mg; SC 5 mg	Controls pain; 5–6 times more potent than codeine	Less potent and addicting than morphine; for moderate pain—peak action 1 h	See Morphine SO$_4$

NURSING IMPLICATIONS: Administer per order and observe for effect.

Pentazocine (Talwin)—PO 50–100 mg; IM 30–60 mg q3–4h	Relief of moderate to severe pain	Narcotic antagonist, opioid antagonist properties, equivalent to codeine	Respiratory depression, nausea, vomiting, dizziness, light-headedness, seizures

NURSING IMPLICATIONS: Monitor *respirations,* BP; *caution* with patients with MI, head injuries, COPD.

ANTACIDS (see Antiulceratives)

ANTIANEMICS			
Ferrous SO$_4$ (Feosol, Fer-in-Sol)—adults, PO 300 mg–1.2 g qd	Iron deficiency anemia; prophylactically during infancy, childhood, pregnancy	Corrects nutritional iron deficiency anemia	Nausea, vomiting, anorexia, constipation, diarrhea, yellow-brown discoloration of eyes, teeth

NURSING IMPLICATIONS: To minimize GI distress, give *with* meals; do *not* give with antacids or tea, liquid form should be taken through straw to prevent *staining* of teeth; *causes dark-green/black stool.*

ANTIANGINALS			
Atenolol (Tenormin)—PO 50–150 mg daily; IV 5 mg initially, wait 10 min, then another 5 mg	Hypertension, angina, arrhythmias	Blocks beta$_1$ (cardiac) adrenergic receptors	Fatigue, weakness, bradycardia, heart failure, pulmonary edema

NURSING IMPLICATIONS: Give 1 mg/min IV; check vital signs; assess for signs of fluid *overload.*

Isosorbide dinitrate (Isordil, Isorbid)—sublingual 2.5–10.0 mg q5–10 min for 3 doses; PO 5–20 mg initially, 10–40 mg q6h	Acute angina, *long-term* prophylaxis for angina, heart failure	Produces vasodilation, decreases preload	Headache, dizziness, hypotension, tachycardia

NURSING IMPLICATIONS: *Avoid* eating, drinking, or smoking until sublingual tablets are dissolved; change positions *slowly;* aspirin or acetaminophen for headache.

(continued)

TABLE D.2   COMMON DRUGS *(Continued)*

Drug and Dosage	Use	Action	◀ Assessment: Side Effects
ANTIANGINALS *(continued)*			
Nitroglycerin—sublingual 0.25–0.6 prn; transdermal (patch) 2.5–15.0 mg/d; topical 2–3 in. q8h; IV 10–20 μg/min	Angina pectoris; adjunctive treatment in MI, heart failure, hypertension (IV form)	Directly relaxes smooth muscle, dilating blood vessels; lowers peripheral vascular resistance; increases blood flow	Faintness, throbbing headache, vomiting, flushing, hypotension, visual disturbances

NURSING IMPLICATIONS: Instruct patient to *sit* or *lie down* when taking drug, to reduce *hypotensive* effect; onset 1–3 min; may take 1–3 doses at 5-min intervals to relieve pain; up to *10/d* may be allowed; if headache occurs, tell patient to expel tab as soon as pain relief occurs; keep drug at bedside or on person; watch *expiration* dates—tabs lose potency with exposure to air and humidity; *alcohol* ingestion soon after taking may produce *shocklike syndrome* from drop in BP; *smoking* causes vasoconstricting effect; causes burning under tongue; may crush between teeth to ↑ absorption.

ANTIARRHYTHMICS			
Bretylium (Bretylol)—IV 0.5–10 mg/kg q6h; IM 5–10 mg/kg (max 250 mg in one site)	Ventricular fibrillation, ventricular tachycardia	Inhibits norepinephrine release from sympathetic nerve endings, increased fibrillation threshold	Worsening of arrhythmia; tachycardia and increased BP *initially*; nausea, vomiting, hypotension *later*

NURSING IMPLICATIONS: Monitor BP and cardiac status closely; *rotate* IM injection sites; no more than 5 mL/site.

Diphenylhydantoin (Dilantin)—PO 100–200 mg 3–4 times daily; IV loading dose 10–15 mg/kg (*not* to exceed 50 mg/min), 50–100 mg over 5–10 min	Digitalis toxicity, ventricular ectopy	Depresses pacemaker activity in SA node and Purkinje tissue without slowing conduction velocity	Severe pain if administered in small vein; ataxia, vertigo, nystagmus, seizures, confusion, skin eruptions, hypotension if administered too fast

NURSING IMPLICATIONS: With IV use monitor vital signs; observe for *CNS* side effects; have O₂ on hand; *seizure precautions* (padded siderails, nonmetal airway, suction, mouth gag); also see Anticonvulsants.

Lidocaine HCl—IV 50–100 mg, bolus; 1–4 mg/kg/min, IV drip	Ventricular tachycardia, PVCs	Depresses myocardial response to abnormally generated impulses	Drowsiness, dizziness, nervousness, confusion, paresthesias

NURSING IMPLICATIONS: Check *apical and radial pulses* for deficits; observe for signs of *CNS* toxicity; monitor ECG for *prolonged PR* interval.

Procainamide HCl (Pronestyl)—PO, IM 500–1000 mg 4–6 times qd; IV 1 g q 5 min until arrhythmia is suppressed	Atrial and ventricular arrhythmias, PVCs, *overdose* of digitalis, general anesthesia	Depresses myocardium, lengthens conduction time between atria and ventricles	Polyarthralgia, fever, chills, urticaria, nausea, vomiting, psychoses, rapid decrease in BP

NURSING IMPLICATIONS: Check pulse rate *before* giving; monitor heart action during IV administration.

Propranolol HCl (Inderal)—0.5–3.0 mg, IV push (up to 3 mg); 20–60 mg orally 3–4 times daily	Ventricular ectopy, angina *unresponsive* to nitrites, paroxysmal atrial tachycardia, hypertension	Beta-adrenergic blocker, ↓ cardiac contractility, ↓ heart rate, ↓ myocardial oxygen requirements	Bradycardia, hypotension, vertigo, paresthesia of hands

NURSING IMPLICATIONS: Instruct patient to take pulse *before* each dose; do *not* give to patients with history of asthma or chronic obstructive pulmonary disease (COPD); *no* smoking, as hypertension may occur.

(continued)

TABLE D.2   COMMON DRUGS (*Continued*)

Drug and Dosage	Use	Action	✉ Assessment: Side Effects
ANTIARRHYTHMICS (continued)			
Quinidine SO$_4$—PO 0.2–0.6 g q2h, loading dose; 400–1000 mg tid–qid, maintenance; IV 5–10 mg/kg over 30–60 min	Atrial fibrillation, PAT, ventricular tachycardia, PVCs	Lengthens conduction time in atria and ventricles, blocks vagal stimulation of heart	Nausea, vomiting, diarrhea, vertigo, tremor, headache, abdominal cramps, AV block, cardiac arrest

NURSING IMPLICATIONS: *Count pulse before* giving; report changes in rate, quality, or rhythm; give drug *with food;* monitor BP daily; *supine* during IV administration.

ANTIASTHMATICS			
Cromolyn sodium—inhale, 1 cap 4 times qd	Perennial bronchial asthma (*not* acute asthma or status asthmaticus)	Inhibits release of bronchoconstrictors—histamine and SRS-A; suppresses allergic response	Cough, hoarseness, wheezing, dry mouth, bitter aftertaste, urticaria, urinary frequency

NURSING IMPLICATIONS: Instruct on *use of inhaler*—exhale; tilt head back; inhale rapidly, deeply, steadily; remove inhaler; exhale—repeat until dose is taken; gargle or drink water after treatment.

ANTICHOLINERGICS			
Atropine SO$_4$—0.3–1.2 mg PO, SC, IM, or IV; ophthalmic 0.5%–1.0% up to 6 times qd	Peptic ulcer, spasms of GI tract, Stokes-Adams syndrome; control excessive secretions during surgery	Blocks parasympathomimetic effects of acetylcholine on effector organs	Dry mouth; tachycardia, blurred vision, drowsiness; skin flushing; urinary retention; *contraindications:* glaucoma, paralytic ileus

NURSING IMPLICATIONS: Observe for postural *hypotension* in ambulating patients; administer cautiously in aged; monitor vital signs for *pulse* and *respiratory* rate changes.

Propantheline bromide (Pro-Banthine)—PO 15 mg qid; IM or IV 30 mg	Decreases hypertonicity and hypersecretion of GI tract, ulcerative colitis, peptic ulcer	Blocks neural transmission at ganglia of autonomic nervous system and at parasympathetic effector organs	Nausea, gastric fullness, constipation, mydriasis

NURSING IMPLICATIONS: Give *before* meals; observe urinary output to *avoid retention*, particularly in elderly; mouth care pc will relieve dryness; *contraindicated* with glaucoma.

Tincture of belladonna—0.3–0.6 mL tid	Hypermotility of stomach; bowel, biliary, and renal colic; prostatitis	Blocks parasympathomimetic effects of acetylcholine	Dry mouth, thirst, dilated pupils, skin flushing, elevated temperature, delirium

NURSING IMPLICATIONS: Administer 30–60 min *before* meals; observe for side effects; *physostigmine salicylate* is antidote.

ANTICOAGULANTS			
Heparin—initial dose: IV 5,000 U followed by 20,000–40,000 U infusion over 24h	Acute thromboembolic *emergencies*	Prevents thrombin formation	Hematuria, bleeding gums, ecchymosis

NURSING IMPLICATIONS: Observe clotting times—should be 20–30 min; antagonist is *protamine sulfate.*

(continued)

TABLE D.2   COMMON DRUGS (*Continued*)

Drug and Dosage	Use	Action	◄ Assessment: Side Effects
ANTICOAGULANTS (*continued*)			
Warfarin sodium (Coumadin)—initial dose, PO 10–15 mg; maintenance dose, PO 2–10 mg qd	Venous thrombosis, atrial fibrillation with embolization, pulmonary emboli, myocardial infarction	Depresses liver synthesis of prothrombin and factors VII, IX, X	Minor or major hemorrhage, alopecia, fever, nausea, diarrhea, dermatitis
NURSING IMPLICATIONS: Drug effects last 3–4 d; antagonist is *vitamin K; avoid* foods high in vitamin K; *no* aspirin.			
ANTICOAGULANT ANTIDOTES			
Protamine SO$_4$ 1%—IV 10 mg/mL *slowly;* 1 mg/ 100 U heparin	*Overdose* of heparin	Positive electrostatic charge inactivates negatively charged heparin molecules	Excessive coagulation, hypotension, bradycardia, dyspnea
NURSING IMPLICATIONS: *Slow* IV; no more than 50 mg in 10-min period; monitor vital signs continuously; Check activated partial thromboplastin time for effectiveness.			
Vitamin K$_1$ (AquaMEPHY-TON, Konakion)—PO, IM, SC 2.5–25.0 mg; 0.5–1.0 mg in newborns	Warfarin hypoprothrombinemia, hemorrhagic disease in newborns	Counteracts the inhibitory effects of oral anticoagulants on hepatic synthesis of vitamin K–dependent clotting factors	Flushing, hypotension, allergic reactions, reappearance of clotting problems (high doses)
NURSING IMPLICATIONS: Give IV only *if absolutely necessary; dilute* with preservative-free 0.9% NaCl, D$_5$W, or D$_5$NaCl; protect solution *from light;* repeated injection may cause redness and pain; check PT for drug effect.			
ANTICONVULSANTS			
Clonazepam (Klonopin)—PO 1.5 mg in 3 doses initially, 0.5–1.0 mg q third d	Absence (petit mal) seizures, myoclonic seizures	Produces anticonvulsant and sedative effects in the CNS; mechanism unknown	Drowsiness, ataxia, behavioral changes
NURSING IMPLICATIONS: Give *with* food; evaluate *liver, CBC,* and *platelets; Avoid* abrupt withdrawal—may cause *status epilepticus.*			
Diazepam (Valium)—PO 2–10 mg bid–qid; IM or IV 5–10 mg	All types of seizures	Induces calming effect on limbic system, thalamus, hypothalamus	Drowsiness, ataxia, and paradoxical increase in excitability of CNS
NURSING IMPLICATIONS: IV may cause *phlebitis;* give IV injection *slowly,* as respiratory arrest can occur; inject IM *deeply* into tissue.			
Ethosuximide (Zarontin)—PO 500 mg/d, increase by 250 mg/d until effective	Absence seizures	Depresses motor cortex and reduces CNS sensitivity to convulsive nerve stimuli	GI distress: nausea, vomiting, cramps, diarrhea, anorexia; blood dyscrasias
NURSING IMPLICATIONS: Administer *with* meals; regular *CBC;* precautions to prevent injury from drowsiness.			
Magnesium SO$_4$—PO 1–5 g; IM or IV 1–4 g at rate of 1.5 mL/min	Control seizures in pregnancy, epilepsy; relief of acute constipation; reduces edema, inflammation, and itching of skin; may inhibit preterm contractions	Depresses CNS as well as smooth, cardiac, and skeletal muscle; promotes osmotic retention of fluid	Flushing, sweating, extreme thirst, complete heart block, dehydration, depressed or absent reflexes, ↓ respirations
NURSING IMPLICATIONS: If given IV, monitor vital signs *continuously;* I&O; do *not* give during the 2 h preceding delivery; observe mother and newborn for signs of toxicity if given near delivery.			

(continued)

TABLE D.2 Common Drugs (*Continued*)

Drug and Dosage	Use	Action	◀ Assessment: Side Effects
ANTICONVULSANTS (*continued*)			
Phenytoin or diphenylhydantoin (Dilantin) SO₄ —PO 30–100 mg 3–4 times qd; IM 100–200 mg 3–4 times qd; IV 150–250 mg	Psychomotor epilepsy, convulsive seizures, ventricular arrhythmias	Depresses motor cortex by preventing spread of abnormal electrical impulses	Nervousness, ataxia, gastric distress, nystagmus, slurred speech, hallucinations, gingival hyperplasia

NURSING IMPLICATIONS: Give *with* meals *or* pc; frequent and diligent mouth care; advise patient that urine may turn *pink to red-brown;* teach patient signs of adverse reactions; mix IV with normal saline (precipitates with 5% D/W).

Drug and Dosage	Use	Action	Assessment: Side Effects
Primidone (Mysoline)— PO 100–375 mg, increase over 10 d	Tonic-clonic, focal, or local seizures	Inhibits abnormal brain electrical activity, dose-dependent CNS depression	Excessive sedation or ataxia, vertigo

NURSING IMPLICATIONS: Careful neurologic, cardiovascular, and respiratory assessment; have resuscitation equipment available.

Drug and Dosage	Use	Action	Assessment: Side Effects
Valproic acid (Depakene) —PO 15 mg/kg/d, increase up to 60 mg/kg/d	Absence, tonic-clonic, myoclonic, focal, or local seizures	Inhibits spread of abnormal discharges through brain	Nausea, vomiting, diarrhea (disappear over time); drowsiness or sedation if taken in combination with other anticonvulsants

NURSING IMPLICATIONS: Assess responses; monitor *blood levels;* precautions against excessive sedation; *discourage alcohol* use.

Drug and Dosage	Use	Action	Assessment: Side Effects
ANTIDIARRHEALS			
Diphenoxylate HCl with atropine sulfate (Lomotil)—PO 5–10 mg tid–qid	Diarrhea	Increases intestinal tone and decreases propulsive peristalsis	Rash, drowsiness, dizziness, depression, abdominal distention, headache, blurred vision, nausea

NURSING IMPLICATIONS: May *potentiate* action of barbiturates, opiates, and other depressants; closely observe patients receiving these drugs, and administer *narcotic antagonists* such as levallorphan (Lorfan) tartrate, naloxone HCl (Narcan), and nalorphine HCl (Nalline) as ordered; administer cautiously to patients with hepatic dysfunction—may precipitate *hepatic coma.*

Drug and Dosage	Use	Action	Assessment: Side Effects
Kaolin with pectin (Kaopectate)—adults, PO 60–120 mL after each bowel movement	Diarrhea	Reported to absorb irritants and soothe	Granuloma of the stomach

NURSING IMPLICATIONS: Do *not* administer: for more than 2 *d;* in presence of *fever;* or to children *younger than 3 yr.*

Drug and Dosage	Use	Action	Assessment: Side Effects
Paregoric or camphorated opium tincture—5–10 mL q2h, *not* more than qid	Diarrhea	Acts directly on intestinal smooth muscle to increase tone and decrease propulsive peristalsis	Occasional nausea; prolonged use may produce dependence

NURSING IMPLICATIONS: Contains approximately 1.6 mg morphine or 16 mg opium and is subject to federal narcotic regulations; administer with partial glass of *water* to facilitate passage into stomach; observe number and consistency of stools—discontinue drug as soon as diarrhea is controlled; keep in tight *light-resistant* bottles.

(continued)

TABLE D.2   COMMON DRUGS (*Continued*)

Drug and Dosage	Use	Action	⋈ Assessment: Side Effects
ANTIEMETICS			
Chlorpromazine (Thorazine)—preop IM 12.5–25.0 g 1–2 h before; IV 25–50 mg; PO 10–25 mg q4–6h; IM 25–50 mg q3–4h; suppository 50–100 mg q6–8h	Nausea, vomiting, hiccups, preoperative sedation, psychoses	Alters the effects of dopamine in the CNS; anticholinergic, alpha-adrenergic blocker	Sedation, extrapyramidal reactions, dry eyes, blurred vision, hypotension, constipation, dry mouth, photosensitivity

NURSING IMPLICATIONS: Keep *flat* 30 min after IM injection; change positions slowly; frequent mouth care; may turn urine *pink* to *red-brown.*

Prochlorperazine dimaleate (Compazine)—5–30 mg qid PO, IM, rectal	Nausea, vomiting, retching	See Trimethobenzamide HCl	Drowsiness, orthostatic hypotension, palpitations, blurred vision, diplopia, headache

NURSING IMPLICATIONS: Use *cautiously* in: children, pregnant women, and patients with liver disease.

Trimethobenzamide HCl (Tigan)—250 mg qid, PO, IM, rectal	Nausea, vomiting	Suppresses chemoreceptors in the trigger zone located in the medulla oblongata	Drowsiness, vertigo, diarrhea, headache, hypotension, jaundice, blurred vision, rigid muscles

NURSING IMPLICATIONS: Give *deep IM* to prevent escape of solution; can cause edema, pain, and burning.

ANTIFUNGAL			
Amphotericin B (Fungizone)—IV 5 mg/ 250 mL dextrose over 4–6h (to 1 mg/kg body weight)	*Severe* fungal infections, histoplasmosis	Fungistatic or fungicidal; binds to sterols in cell membrane, altering cell permeability	Febrile reactions: chills, nausea and vomiting, muscle/ joint pain; renal damage; hypotension; tachycardia; arrhythmias, hypokalemia

NURSING IMPLICATIONS: Monitor for side effects; *thrombophlebitis* at IV site; BUN > 40 mg/dL; creatinine 3 mg/dL or >; stop drug because of *nephrotoxicity.*

Ketoconazole (Nizoral)—oral 200–400 mg daily	Histoplasmosis, *systemic* fungal infections	Antifungal	Headache, fatigue, dizziness; nausea and vomiting; decreased libido, impotence; gynecomastia, esp. in males

NURSING IMPLICATIONS: Administer *with* food; *avoid* concomitant use of antacids, H_2 blockers; advise to report side effects.

Nystatin (Nilstat, Mycostatin)—PO, rectal, vaginal 100,000– 1,000,000 U 3–4 times qd	Skin, mucous membrane infections (*Candida albicans*); oral thrush; vaginitis; intestinal candidiasis	Fungistatic and fungicidal; binds to sterols in fungal cell membrane	Nausea, vomiting, GI distress, diarrhea

NURSING IMPLICATIONS: *Oral* use—clear mouth of food; keep medication in mouth several minutes before swallowing; *vaginal*—usually requires 2-wk therapy; continue use during menses; consult physician before using anti-infective douches; determine predisposing factors to infection (diabetes, pregnancy, antiinfectives, tight-fitting nylon pantyhose).

(continued)

TABLE D.2   COMMON DRUGS (*Continued*)

Drug and Dosage	Use	Action	◀ Assessment: Side Effects
ANTIGOUT Allopurinol (Lopurin, Zyloprim)—PO 100 mg initially; 300 mg daily with meals or pc	Primary hyperuricemia, secondary hyperuricemia with cancer therapy	Lowers plasma and urinary uric acid levels; *no* analgesic, anti-inflammatory, or uricosuric actions	Rash, itching, nausea, vomiting, anemia, drowsiness

NURSING IMPLICATIONS: Report side effects, particularly *rash*, as drug must be stopped; *avoid* driving or other complex tasks until drug effects known; give at least *3000 mL* fluid daily; minimum urine output of *2000 mL/d;* keep urine neutral or *alkaline* with sodium bicarbonate or potassium citrate; use *cautiously* with: liver disease, impaired renal function, history of peptic ulcers, lower GI disease, or bone marrow depression.

Drug and Dosage	Use	Action	Assessment: Side Effects
Colchicine—PO 1.0–1.2 mg acute phase; 0.5–2.0 mg nightly with milk or food; IV 1–2 mg initially	Gouty arthritis, acute gout	Inhibits leukocyte migration and phagocytosis in gouty joints; nonanalgesic, nonuricosuric	Nausea, vomiting, diarrhea, abdominal pain, peripheral neuritis, bone marrow depression (sore throat, bleeding gums, sore mouth), tissue and nerve necrosis with IV use

NURSING IMPLICATIONS: Do *not* dilute IV form with normal saline or 5% dextrose—use *sterile water* to prevent precipitation; infuse over 3–5 min IV; potentiate drug action with ● *alkaline ash foods* (milk, most fruits and vegetables).

Drug and Dosage	Use	Action	Assessment: Side Effects
Probenecid (Benemid)—PO 0.25–0.50 g twice daily pc	*Chronic* gouty arthritis, *no* value in acute; adjuvant therapy with penicillin to increase plasma levels	Inhibits renal tubular resorption of uric acid; *no* analgesic or anti-inflammatory activity; competitively inhibits renal tubular secretion of penicillin and many weak organic acids	Headache, nausea, vomiting, anorexia, sore gums, urinary frequency, flushing

NURSING IMPLICATIONS: Give *with* food, milk, or prescribed antacid; *3000 mL/d fluids; avoid* alcohol, which increases serum urates; do *not* take with aspirin—inhibits action of drug; *renal* function and *hematology* should be evaluated frequently; during acute gout, give with colchicine.

Drug and Dosage	Use	Action	Assessment: Side Effects
ANTIHISTAMINES Astemizole (Hismanal)—PO 10 mg/d	Relief of allergic symptoms (rhinitis, urticaria), less sedating	Blocks the effects of histamine	Drowsiness, headache, fatigue, stimulation, dry mouth, rash, increased appetite (none of these are frequent)

NURSING IMPLICATIONS: Take *1 h before* or *2 h after* eating; good oral hygiene; may need to *reduce calories.*

Drug and Dosage	Use	Action	Assessment: Side Effects
Chlorpheniramine maleate (Chlor-Trimeton)—PO 2–4 mg tid–qid; SC, IM, or IV 10–20 mg	Asthma, hay fever, serum reactions, anaphylaxis	Inhibits action of histamine	Nausea, gastritis, diarrhea, headache, dryness of mouth and nose, nervousness, irritability

NURSING IMPLICATIONS: IV may *drop BP*; give *slowly; caution* patient about drowsiness.

(continued)

TABLE D.2   COMMON DRUGS (Continued)

Drug and Dosage	Use	Action	▶ Assessment: Side Effects
ANTIHISTAMINES (continued)			
Diphenhydramine HCl (Benadryl)—PO 25–50 mg tid–qid; IM or IV 10–20 mg	Allergic and pyrogenic reactions, motion sickness, radiation sickness, hay fever, Parkinson's disease	Inhibits action of histamine on receptor cells, decreases action of acetylcholine	Sedation, dizziness, inability to concentrate, headache, anorexia, dermatitis, nausea, diplopia, insomnia

NURSING IMPLICATIONS: *Avoid* use in newborn or premature infants and patients with glaucoma; supervise ambulation; *caution* against driving or operating mechanical devices; excitation or hallucinations may occur in children.

Drug and Dosage	Use	Action	Assessment: Side Effects
Terfenadine (Seldane)— PO 60 mg 2 times daily	Relief of allergic symptoms, nasal and dermatoses	Blocks the effects of histamine	Drowsiness, sedation, headache, nausea, abdominal pain, dry mouth

NURSING IMPLICATIONS: Risk of *arrhythmias* if taking certain antibiotics; *false-negative skin test* reactions; take *with* food or milk.

Drug and Dosage	Use	Action	Assessment: Side Effects
ANTIHYPERGLYCEMICS **Sulfonylureas**			
Acetohexamide (Dymelor) —PO 200–1500 mg qd; 1–2/d; duration 12–24 h	*Oral* hypoglycemic, antidiabetic	Lowers blood glucose by stimulating insulin release from beta cells; effective only if pancreas has ability to produce insulin	Hypoglycemia (profuse sweating, hunger, headache, nausea, confusion, ataxia, coma), skin rashes, bone marrow depression, liver toxicity

NURSING IMPLICATIONS: Drug therapy *must* be combined with *diet* therapy, *weight* control, and planned, graded *exercise; alcohol intolerance* may occur (*disulfiram reaction*—flushing, pounding headache, sweating, nausea, vomiting); should *not* be taken at bedtime unless specifically ordered (nocturnal hypoglycemia more likely); take at *same time* each day; *contraindicated* in: liver disease, renal disease, pregnancy.

Drug and Dosage	Use	Action	Assessment: Side Effects
Chlorpropamide (Diabinese)—PO 100–1,000 mg; 1/d; duration 30–60 h	See Acetohexamide	See Acetohexamide	See Acetohexamide

NURSING IMPLICATIONS: See Acetohexamide.

Drug and Dosage	Use	Action	Assessment: Side Effects
Tolazamide (Tolinase)— PO 100–500 mg; 1/d; duration 10–14 h	See Acetohexamide	See Acetohexamide	See Acetohexamide

NURSING IMPLICATIONS: See Acetohexamide.

Drug and Dosage	Use	Action	Assessment: Side Effects
Tolbutamide (Orinase)— PO 500–3000 mg; 2–3/d; duration 6–12 h	See Acetohexamide	See Acetohexamide	See Acetohexamide

NURSING IMPLICATIONS: See Acetohexamide.

Drug and Dosage	Use	Action	Assessment: Side Effects
Insulin—rapid acting			
Crystalline zinc (*Regular*) (Humulin R) (clear)— onset 0.5–1.0 h; peak 2–4 h; duration 6–8 h	*Poorly controlled* diabetes, trauma, surgery, coma	Enhances transmembrane passage of glucose into cells; promotes carbohydrate, fat, and protein metabolism	Hypoglycemia (profuse sweating, nausea, hunger, headache, confusion, ataxia, coma), allergic reaction at injection site

NURSING IMPLICATIONS: Monitor blood and urine for *glucose* and *acetone* levels; insulin currently being used can be kept at *room temperature for 1 mo;* refrigerate stock insulin only; *rotate* injection sites; cold insulin leads to: *lipodystrophy,* reduced absorption, and local reaction; *only* form of insulin that is given IV.

(continued)

TABLE D.2   COMMON DRUGS (*Continued*)

Drug and Dosage	Use	Action	⋈ Assessment: Side Effects
ANTIHYPERGLYCEMICS (*continued*)			
Prompt insulin zinc suspension (Semilente) purified pork (cloudy)—onset 1–2 h; peak 4–10 h; duration 12–16 h	Patients *allergic* to Regular; used in combination with longer-lasting insulin	See Crystalline zinc (Regular)	See Crystalline zinc (Regular)

NURSING IMPLICATIONS: See Crystalline zinc (Regular); compatible with all Lente preparations.

Insulin—intermediate acting NPH insulin (isophane insulin suspension) purified pork (Humulin N⁺) (cloudy)—onset 1–2 h; peak 5–12 h; duration 18–24 h	Patients who can be controlled by *one dose* per day	See Crystalline zinc (Regular)	See Crystalline zinc (Regular)

NURSING IMPLICATIONS: Gently rotate vial between palms, invert several times to mix; do *not* shake; see Crystalline zinc (Regular).

Insulin zinc suspension (Lente insulin) (cloudy)—onset 1–3 h; peak 6–12 h; duration 18–24 h	Patients *allergic* to NPH	See Crystalline zinc (Regular)	See Crystalline zinc (Regular)

NURSING IMPLICATIONS: See Crystalline zinc (Regular).

Insulin—slow acting PZI (Protamine zinc insulin suspension) (cloudy)—onset 4–8 h; peak 14–24 h; duration 24–36 h	*Rarely* used, only if uncontrolled by other types	See Crystalline zinc (Regular)	See Crystalline zinc (Regular)

NURSING IMPLICATIONS: Between-meal snacks may be necessary; *bedtime snacks* are essential; see Crystalline zinc (Regular).

Extended insulin zinc suspension (Ultralente) purified beef (cloudy)—onset 4–8 h; peak 12–24 h; duration 36 h	Often *mixed* with Semilente for 24-h curve	See Crystalline zinc (Regular)	See Crystalline zinc (Regular)

NURSING IMPLICATIONS: See Crystalline zinc (Regular).

ANTIHYPERTENSIVES			
Captopril (Capoten)—PO 50 mg tid	Hypertension, heart failure	Prevents production of angiotensin II, vasodilation	Hypotension, loss of taste perception, proteinuria, rashes

NURSING IMPLICATIONS: Monitor vital signs and weight; take 1 h *before* and 2 h *after* meals; change positions slowly; *avoid* salt and salt substitutes.

Guanfacine HCl (Tenex)—PO 1 mg daily to maximum dose of 3 mg/d	Hypertension, in combination with thiazidelike diuretics	Centrally acting alpha₂-adrenergic receptor agonist	Drowsiness, weakness, dizziness, dry mouth, constipation, impotence

NURSING IMPLICATIONS: Warn patient *not* to drive or perform activities requiring alertness; take at *bedtime* to minimize sedation; monitor BP and pulse.

(continued)

TABLE D.2   COMMON DRUGS (*Continued*)

Drug and Dosage	Use	Action	◁ Assessment: Side Effects
ANTIHYPERTENSIVES (*continued*)			
Guanethidine SO$_4$ (Ismelin)—PO 10–50 mg qd in divided doses	Severe to moderately severe hypertension	Blocks norepinephrine at postganglionic synapses	Orthostatic hypotension, diarrhea, inhibition of ejaculation

NURSING IMPLICATIONS: *Postural hypotension* is marked in the morning and *accentuated* by hot weather, alcohol, and exercise; teach to rise slowly, with assistance.

Hydralazine HCl (Apresoline)—PO 10–50 mg qid	Moderate hypertension	Dilates peripheral blood vessels, increases renal blood flow	Palpitations, tachycardia, angina pectoris, tremors, depression

NURSING IMPLICATIONS: Encourage moderation in exercise and identification of stressful stimuli.

Methyldopa (Aldomet)—PO 500 mg–2 g in divided doses	Severe to moderately severe hypertension	Inhibits formation of dopamine, a precursor of norepinephrine	Initial drowsiness, depression with feelings of unreality, edema, jaundice, dry mouth

NURSING IMPLICATIONS: *Contraindicated* in acute and chronic liver disease; encourage *not* to drive car if drowsy.

Phentolamine HCl (Regitine)—PO 50 mg 4–6 doses daily; IV, IM, or local 5–10 mg, diluted in minimum 10 mL normal saline	Prevents dermal necrosis; hypertensive crisis; diagnosis of pheochromocytoma	Blocks alpha-adrenergic receptors	Weakness, dizziness, orthostatic hypotension, nausea, vomiting, abdominal pain

NURSING IMPLICATIONS: When giving parenterally, patient should be *supine;* monitor for overdose (precipitous *drop* in BP); do *not* give with epinephrine.

Reserpine (Serpasil)—PO 0.25 mg qd	Mild and moderate hypertension	Depletes catecholamines and decreases peripheral vasoconstriction, heart rate, BP	Depression, nasal stuffiness, increased gastric secretions, rash, pruritus

NURSING IMPLICATIONS: Watch for signs of *mental depression;* closely monitor pulse rates of patients also receiving digitalis; *avoid* alcohol.

Timolol (Timoptic)—PO 20–40 mg/d; ophthalmic 1 gtt 1–2 times/d	Hypertension, migraine, glaucoma	Blocks stimulation of myocardial (beta$_1$) and pulmonary/vascular (beta$_2$) receptors	Fatigue, weakness, depression, insomnia, peripheral vasoconstriction, diarrhea, nausea, vomiting

NURSING IMPLICATIONS: Check vital signs and for evidence of heart failure; do *not* take if pulse <50 beats/min; *avoid:* over-the-counter cold remedies, coffee, tea, and cola.

ANTI-INFECTIVES			
Cefazolin (Ancef, Kefzol)—IM or IV 250 mg–1.5 g q6–12h	*Staphylococcus aureus, Escherichia coli, Klebsiella,* group A and B *Streptococcus; Pneumococcus*	Bactericidal	Allergic reaction, urticaria, rash, abnormal bleeding

NURSING IMPLICATIONS: See Penicillin; may cause *false-positive* lab tests (Coombs', urine glucose); oral probenecid may be taken *concurrently* to prolong effects of drug.

(continued)

TABLE D.2   COMMON DRUGS (*Continued*)

Drug and Dosage	Use	Action	◅ Assessment: Side Effects
ANTI-INFECTIVES (continued)			
Cephalexin (Keflex)—PO 1–4 g/d in 2–4 equally divided doses	Infections caused by gram-positive cocci; infections: respiratory, biliary, urinary, bone, septicemia, abdominal; surgical prophylaxis	Bactericidal effects on susceptible organisms, inhibition of bacterial cell wall synthesis	Nausea, vomiting; urticaria, toxic paranoid reactions, dizziness, increased alkaline phosphatase, nephrotoxicity, bone marrow suppression

NURSING IMPLICATIONS: Peak blood levels delayed when given with food; *report:* nausea, flushing, tachycardia, headache; monitor for *nephrotoxicity* and for bleeding.

Cephalothin (Keflin, Seffin)—IM, IV 2–12 g/d in 4–6 equally divided doses	Same as Cephalexin except *not* recommended for biliary tract infections	Same as Cephalexin	Same as Cephalexin

NURSING IMPLICATIONS: Same as Cephalexin; *pain* at site of IM; given in *large* muscle; *rotate* sites.

Ciprofloxacin (Cipro)—PO 250–750 mg q12h; IV 200–400 mg q12h; ophthalmic 1–2 gtt q15–30 min, then 4–6 times daily	Lower respiratory tract infections; skin, bone, joint infections; UTI	Inhibits bacterial DNA synthesis	Restlessness, nausea, diarrhea, vomiting, abdominal pain

NURSING IMPLICATIONS: Give PO on an *empty* stomach unless GI irritation occurs, then take with food; *do not* take with milk or yogurt; IV over 60 min.

Clarithromycin (Biaxin)—PO 250–500 mg q12h	Upper respiratory including streptococcal pharyngitis and sinusitis; lower respiratory tract bronchitis, pneumonia.	Bacteriostatic; gram-positive and gram-negative bacteria. *Not* effective against MRSA.	Headache, diarrhea, nausea, abnormal taste, abdominal pain.

NURSING IMPLICATIONS: Give around the clock without regard for meals. Food slows but does *not* decrease absorption.

Cloxacillin (Tegopen)—PO 250–500 mg q6h	Penicillinase-producing staphylococci infections: respiratory, sinus, skin	Binds to bacterial cell wall, leading to cell death	Nausea, vomiting, diarrhea, rashes, allergic reactions, seizures (high doses)

NURSING IMPLICATIONS: *Give around the clock* on an *empty* stomach; observe for signs of *superinfection* (black, furry tongue, vaginal itching, loose stools).

Co-trimoxazole (Bactrim, Septra)—PO 160 mg twice daily or 20 mg/kg/d for *Pneumocystis carinii* pneumonia	Acute otitis media, urinary tract infection, shigellosis, *P. carinii* pneumonia, prostatitis	Bacteriostatic, anti-infective; antagonizes folic acid production; combination of sulfamethoxazole and trimethoprim	Hypersensitivity; see Sulfisoxazole

NURSING IMPLICATIONS: IV administration can cause phlebitis and *tissue damage* with extravasation.

Erythromycin—adults, PO 250 mg q6h; children, PO 30–50 mg/kg qd	Pneumonia, pelvic inflammatory disease, intestinal amebiasis, ocular infections; used *if allergic* to penicillin	Inhibits protein synthesis of microorganism, more effective against gram-positive organisms	Abdominal cramping, distention, diarrhea

NURSING IMPLICATIONS: Be sure culture and sensitivity done *before* treatment; give on *empty* stomach 1 h before or 3 h after meals; do *not* crush or chew tabs; do *not* give with fruit juice.

(continued)

TABLE D.2   COMMON DRUGS (*Continued*)

Drug and Dosage	Use	Action	⊠ Assessment: Side Effects
ANTI-INFECTIVES (*continued*)			
Gentamicin (Garamycin)— IM, IV 3–5 mg/kg/d in 3–4 divided doses; topical: skin, eye	Serious gram-negative bacillary infections; possible *S. aureus,* uncomplicated urinary tract infections	Bactericidal effects on susceptible gram-positive and gram-negative organisms and mycobacteria	Serious toxic effects: kidneys, ear; causes muscle weakness/ paralysis

NURSING IMPLICATIONS: Monitor *plasma* levels (peak is 4–10 μg/mL); patients with burns, cystic fibrosis may need higher doses.

Drug and Dosage	Use	Action	Assessment: Side Effects
Penicillin—penicillin G, penicillin G potassium, penicillin G procaine, ampicillin	*Streptococcus; Staphylococcus; Neisseria gonnorhoeae, Treponema pallidum*	Primarily bactericidal	Dermatitis, delayed or immediate anaphylaxis

NURSING IMPLICATIONS: Outpatients should be observed for *20 min after injection;* hospitalized patients should be observed at frequent intervals for 20 min after injection.

Drug and Dosage	Use	Action	Assessment: Side Effects
Pentamidine (Pentam)— IV 4 mg/kg once daily; inhale 300 mg via nebulizer	Prevention or treatment of *P. carinii* pneumonia	Appears to disrupt DNA or RNA synthesis to protozoa	Anxiety, headache, bronchospasm, cough, hypotension, arrhythmias, nephrotoxicity, hypoglycemia, leukopenia, thrombocytopenia, anemia, chills

NURSING IMPLICATIONS: Assess for infection and respiratory status; unpleasant metallic taste may occur (not significant).

Drug and Dosage	Use	Action	Assessment: Side Effects
Sulfisoxazole (Gantrisin), sulfamethizole (Thiosulfil), sulfisomidine (Elkosin)	Acute, chronic, and recurrent urinary tract infections	Bacteriostatic, bactericidal	Nausea, vomiting, oliguria, anuria, anemia, leukopenia, dizziness, jaundice, skin rashes, photosensitivity

NURSING IMPLICATIONS: Maintenance of *blood levels* very important; encourage *fluids* to prevent crystal formation in kidney tubules—push up to *3000 mL/d.*

Drug and Dosage	Use	Action	Assessment: Side Effects
Tetracyclines—chlortetracycline (Aureomycin), doxycycline (Vibramycin hyclate), oxytetracycline (Terramycin), and tetracycline HCl (Sumycin)	Broad-spectrum antibiotic	Primarily bacteriostatic	GI upsets such as diarrhea, nausea, vomiting; sore throat; black, hairy tongue; glossitis; inflammatory lesions in anogenital region

NURSING IMPLICATIONS: *Phototoxic* reactions have been reported; patients should be advised to stay out of direct sunlight, and medication should *not* be given with milk or snacks, as food interferes with absorption of tetracyclines, do *not* give to pregnant women and children under 8 yr.

Drug and Dosage	Use	Action	Assessment: Side Effects
Trimethoprim (TMP)/ sulfamethoxazole (SMZ) (Bactrim)—PO 15–20 mg/kg/d in 3–4 divided doses q6–8h for >72 months; IV 8–10 mg/kg TMP/40–50 mg/kg SMZ q6–12h	Bronchitis, *Shigella* enteritis, otitis media, *P. carinii* pneumonia, urinary tract infection, traveler's diarrhea	Combination inhibits the metabolism of folic acid in bacteria, bactericidal	Nausea, vomiting, rashes, phlebitis at IV site, aplastic anemia, hepatic necrosis

NURSING IMPLICATIONS: Check IV site frequently; do *not* give IM; give PO on *empty* stomach; take *around the clock; avoid* exposure to sun.

(continued)

TABLE D.2   COMMON DRUGS *(Continued)*

Drug and Dosage	Use	Action	◀ Assessment: Side Effects
ANTILIPEMICS			
Cholestyramine (Questran) —PO 4 g 1–6 times/d	Hypercholesterolemia, pruritus from increased bile	Binds bile acids in GI tract, increased clearance of cholesterol	Nausea, constipation, abdominal discomfort

NURSING IMPLICATIONS: Take *before* meals; *do not* take with other medications; give others 1 h before or 4–6 h after.

Drug and Dosage	Use	Action	Assessment: Side Effects
Gemfibrozil (Lopid)—PO 1200 mg/d	Hypercholesterolemia	May inhibit peripheral lipolysis and reduce triglyceride synthesis in liver	GI upset: abdominal pain, epigastric pain, diarrhea, nausea, vomiting; rash; headache; dizziness; blurred vision

NURSING IMPLICATIONS: Use *caution* when driving or doing tasks requiring alertness; take *before* meals.

Drug and Dosage	Use	Action	Assessment: Side Effects
Lovastatin (Mevacor)—PO 20–80 mg/d with evening meal	Primary hypercholesterolemia	Inhibits enzyme that catalyzes synthesis of cholesterol; decreases synthesis of low-density lipoproteins (LDLs)	Headache, constipation, diarrhea, altered taste, blurred vision, muscle cramps

NURSING IMPLICATIONS: Give *with* food; *restrict* fat, cholesterol, carbohydrate, and alcohol in diet.

Drug and Dosage	Use	Action	Assessment: Side Effects
Niacin (vitamin B_3, nicotinic acid)—PO 1.5–6.0 g	Hypercholesterolemia	Decreases liver's production of LDLs and synthesis of triglycerides	GI upset, flushing, pruritus, hyperuricemia, hyperglycemia

NURSING IMPLICATIONS: Take the drug *with* meals; prevent flushing by taking an *aspirin 30 min before;* monitor closely during *first year* of therapy.

Drug and Dosage	Use	Action	Assessment: Side Effects
ANTIPLATELET			
Dipyridamole (Persantine) —PO 70–100 mg 4 times/d; IV 570 µg/kg	Prevent thromboembolism, surgical graft patency, *diagnostic* agent in myocardial perfusion studies	Decrease platelet aggregation, coronary vasodilator	Headache, dizziness, hypotension, nausea; MI, arrhythmias with IV

NURSING IMPLICATIONS: Take at *evenly* spaced intervals; *avoid* use of alcohol; if no GI irritation, take 1 h before or 2 h after meals.

Drug and Dosage	Use	Action	Assessment: Side Effects
ANTITUBERCULOUS *First-line drugs*			
Isoniazid—5–10 mg/kg up to 300 mg PO or IM	Tuberculosis	Suppresses or interferes with biosynthesis, bacteriostatic	Peripheral neuritis, hepatitis, hypersensitivity

NURSING IMPLICATIONS: Give pyridoxine (vitamin B_6) 10 mg as *prophylaxis* for neuritis; 50–100 mg as treatment.

Drug and Dosage	Use	Action	Assessment: Side Effects
Ethambutol—15–25 mg/kg PO			Optic neuritis (*reversible* with discontinuation of drug; very rare at 15 mg/kg), skin rash

NURSING IMPLICATIONS: Use with caution with *renal* disease or when *eye testing* is not feasible; used in combination *with* other drug.

Drug and Dosage	Use	Action	Assessment: Side Effects
Rifampin—10–20 mg/kg up to 600 mg PO			Hepatitis, febrile reaction, purpura (rare)

NURSING IMPLICATIONS: *Orange* urine color; *negates* effect of birth control pills.

(continued)

TABLE D.2 COMMON DRUGS (*Continued*)

Drug and Dosage	Use	Action	⋈ Assessment: Side Effects
ANTITUBERCULOUS (*continued*)			
Streptomycin—15–20 mg/kg up to 1 g IM			*Eighth cranial* nerve damage, *nephrotoxicity*
NURSING IMPLICATIONS: Use with caution in *older* patients or those with *renal* disease.			
Pyrazinamide—15–30 mg/kg up to 3 g PO			Hyperuricemia, hepatotoxicity
NURSING IMPLICATIONS: Combination with an aminoglycoside is bactericidal.			
ANTIULCERATIVES			
Aluminum hydroxide gel (Amphojel)—PO 5–10 mL q2–4h or 1 h pc	Gastric acidity, peptic ulcer, phosphatic urinary calculi, ↓ phosphorus level in chronic renal failure	Buffers HCl in gastric juices without interfering with electrolyte balance	Constipation and fecal impaction
NURSING IMPLICATIONS: *Shake well* before administering; encourage *fluids* to prevent impaction and milk-alkali syndrome.			
Calcium carbonate (Titralac)—PO 1–2 g taken with H_2O after meals and at bedtime	Peptic ulcer and chronic gastritis	Reduces hyperacidity	Constipation or laxative effect
NURSING IMPLICATIONS: See Aluminum hydroxide gel.			
Cimetidine (Tagamet)—PO 300–600 mg q6h (qid); IM, IV 300 mg q6h	Duodenal ulcers, gastroesophageal reflux disease (GERD), gastric hypersecretion, esophagitis	Inhibits action of histamine at H_2 receptor site, inhibits gastric secretion; neutralizes and absorbs excess acid	Confusion, dizziness, nausea, rash, diarrhea, constipation, hypermagnesemia
NURSING IMPLICATIONS: Give *with* meals or immediately *after; avoid* smoking. *Avoid* prolonged administration in patients with renal insufficiency.			
Magnesium and aluminum hydroxides (Maalox suspension)—PO 5–30 mL pc and hs	Gastric hyperacidity, peptic ulcer, heartburn	Neutralizes and binds acids	Constipation, fecal impaction
NURSING IMPLICATIONS: Encourage fluid intake; *contraindicated* for debilitated patients or those with renal insufficiency.			
Omeprazole (Prilosec)—PO 20 mg qd for 4–8 wk (maximum 40 mg/d)	Gastroesophageal reflux (GERD), duodenal ulcers, gastric hyperacidity.	Prevents transport of hydrogen ions into gastric lumen.	Adominal pain, acid regurgitation, headache, dizziness, drowsiness
NURSING IMPLICATIONS: Give *before* meals, preferably in morning. Do *not* crush, open, or chew capsules. May give with antacids.			
Ranitidine (Zantac)—PO 150 mg bid; IM 50 mg q6–8h; IV 50 mg q6–8h	Duodenal ulcer, gastric ulcer, GERD, gastric hypersecretion	Inhibits action of histamine at H_2 receptor site, inhibits gastric acid secretion	Headache, malaise, nausea, constipation, diarrhea
NURSING IMPLICATIONS: Food does *not* affect absorption; give 1 h *apart* from antacids; *smoking* interferes with action			

(*continued*)

TABLE D.2　Common Drugs (*Continued*)

Drug and Dosage	Use	Action	◨ Assessment: Side Effects
ANTIULCERATIVES (*continued*)			
Sucralfate (Carafate)—PO 1 g qid	Prevention and treatment of duodenal ulcer	Reacts with gastric acid to form a thick paste that adheres to the ulcer surface	Constipation

NURSING IMPLICATIONS: Give 1 h *before* meals and at *bedtime; do not* crush or chew tablets; take *antacids* 30 min before or 1 h after sucralfate; increase *fluids and dietary* bulk.

ANTIVIRALS			
Acyclovir (Zovirax)—PO 200 mg, 3–5 times/d; IV 5 mg/kg q8h over 1 h; topical 6 times daily for 1 wk	Herpes simplex (1) (2)	Converts to an active cytotoxic metabolite that inhibits viral DNA replication	Headache, nausea and vomiting, diarrhea, increased serum BUN and creatinine

NURSING IMPLICATIONS: Measure I&O q8h; ensure adequate *hydration;* assess for common side effects; apply topical with *finger cot* or rubber glove; refer for counseling.

Zidovudine (AZT Retrovir) —PO 200 mg q4h	AIDS and related disorders	Inhibits replication of HIV	Blood disorders, especially anemia and granulocytopenia; headache; nausea; insomnia; myalgia

NURSING IMPLICATIONS: Monitor for signs of *opportunistic infection* and adverse drug effects; drug must be taken *around* the clock; regular *blood tests* (q2wk).

BRONCHODILATORS			
Albuterol (Ventolin)—PO 2–6 mg 3–4 times/d; inhale q4–6h or 2 puffs 15 min before exercise	Bronchodilator	Results in accumulation of cyclic adenosine monophosphate at beta-adrenergic receptors	Nervousness, restlessness, tremor, hypertension, nausea

NURSING IMPLICATIONS: Give *with* meals; allow 1 min *between* inhalations; rinse mouth with water *after* inhalation.

Aminophylline—PO 250 mg bid–qid; rectal 250–500 mg; IV 250–500 mg over 10–20 min	*Rapid* relief of bronchospasm; asthma; pulmonary edema	Relaxes smooth muscles and increases cardiac contractility; interferes with resorption of Na^+ and Cl^- in proximal tubules	Nausea, vomiting, cardiac arrhythmias, intestinal bleeding, insomnia, restlessness, rectal irritation from suppository

NURSING IMPLICATIONS: Give orally *with or after meals;* monitor *vital signs* for changes in BP and pulse; *weigh* daily; IM injections are painful.

Ephedrine SO_4—PO, SC, or IM 25 mg tid–qid	Asthma, allergies, bradycardia, nasal decongestant	Relaxes hypertonic muscles in bronchioles and GI tract	Wakefulness, nervousness, dizziness, palpitations, hypertension

NURSING IMPLICATIONS: Monitor vital signs; *avoid* giving dose near bedtime; *check urine* output in older adults.

Isoproterenol HCl (Isuprel)—inhalation of 1:100 or 1:200 solution	Mild to moderately severe asthma attack, bronchitis, pulmonary emphysema	Relaxes hypertonic bronchioles	Nervousness, tachycardia, hypertension, insomnia

NURSING IMPLICATIONS: Monitor vital signs *before and after* treatment; teach patient how to use nebulizer.

(continued)

TABLE D.2   COMMON DRUGS (*Continued*)

Drug and Dosage	Use	Action	◄ Assessment: Side Effects
BRONCHODILATORS (*continued*)			
Theophylline—PO 400 mg/d in divided doses; max. adult dose: 900 mg divided dose	Treatment/prevention of emphysema, asthma (broncho-constriction); chronic bronchitis	Bronchodilation	Restlessness, increased respiration/heart rate, palpitations, arrhythmias, nausea and vomiting, increased urine output → dehydration

NURSING IMPLICATIONS: Monitor theophylline levels: *10–20/µg/mL;* monitor signs of toxicity; take with 8 oz water or *with* meals to decrease GI symptoms.

Terbutaline (Brethine)— PO 2.5–5.0 mg q6h (*not* to exceed 20 mg/24 h); SC 0.25 mg, repeat 15– 30 min (*not* to exceed 0.5 mg/h); inhalation—2 puffs (0.2-mg each) q4–6h	Bronchospasm	See Isoproterenol HCl	See Isoproterenol HCl

NURSING IMPLICATIONS: See Isoproterenol HCl.

CALCIUM CHANNEL BLOCKERS			
Diltiazem (Cardizem)— PO 30–120 mg 3–4 times/d; IV 5–15 mg/h	Angina, hypertension, atrial arrhythmias	Inhibits excitation-contraction; decreased SA, AV node conduction	Headache, fatigue, arrhythmias, edema, hypotension, constipation, rash

NURSING IMPLICATIONS: May take *with* meals; take pulse; do *not* give drug if pulse <50 beats/min; change positions *slowly;* may take nitroglycerin sublingually concurrently.

Nicardipine (Cardene)— PO 20–40 mg tid	Angina, hypertension	Inhibits excitation-contraction	Dizziness, light-headedness, headache, peripheral edema, flushing

NURSING IMPLICATIONS: Give on an *empty* stomach; chest pain may occur 30 min after dose (temporary, from *reflex tachycardia*).

Nifedipine (Procardia)— PO 10–30 mg tid (*not* to exceed 180 mg/d); sublingual 10 mg repeated in 15 min	Angina, hypertension	Vasodilation	Dizziness, light-headedness, giddiness, headache, nervousness, nasal congestion, sore throat, dyspnea, cough, wheezing, nausea, flushing, warmth

NURSING IMPLICATIONS: May take *with* meals; make position changes *slowly;* angina may occur 30 min after dose (temporary).

Verapamil HCl (Calan, Isopten)—PO 240–480 mg, 3–4 times/d; IV 75– 150 µg/kg over 2 min	Angina, supraventricular arrhythmias, essential hypertension	Inhibits calcium movement into smooth-muscle cells, lowers pressure by reducing cardiac contractility	Constipation, AV block, hepatotoxicity

NURSING IMPLICATIONS: Monitor vital signs and ECG for *bradycardia* and *arrhythmias;* observe for *jaundice, abdominal pain;* encourage *fluids* and *bulk-forming* foods.

(continued)

TABLE D.2   COMMON DRUGS (Continued)

Drug and Dosage	Use	Action	▶ Assessment: Side Effects
CARDIAC GLYCOSIDES			
Digitoxin—digitalizing dose: PO 200 μg twice/ d; IM or IV 200–400 μg; maintenance dose: PO 50–300 μg qd	Heart failure, atrial fibrillation and flutter, supraventricular tachycardia	Increases force of cardiac contractility, slows heart rate, decreases right atrial pressures, promotes diuresis	Arrhythmias, nausea, vomiting, anorexia, malaise, color vision (yellow or blue)

NURSING IMPLICATIONS: Hold medication if pulse rate less than *60* or over *120* beats/min; encourage ● foods high in *potassium* (e.g., bananas, orange juice); observe for signs of electrolyte depletion, apathy, disorientation, and anorexia.

Digoxin (Lanoxin)—digitalizing dose: PO 10–15 μg/kg; IM or IV 0.6–1 mg/kg; maintenance dose: PO 125–375 μg qd	See Digitoxin	See Digitoxin	See Digitoxin

NURSING IMPLICATIONS: See Digitoxin.

CHEMOTHERAPY (see Tables 24.1, p. 278; D.4, p. 363; D.5, p. 364)

CHOLINERGIC DRUGS			
Bethanechol Cl (Urecholine)—PO, 5–30 mg; SC, 2.5–5.0 mg; neostigmine bromide (Prostigmin) —PO, 10–30 mg; IM or SC 0.25–1.00 mg	Postoperative abdominal atony and distension; bladder atony with retention; postsurgical or postpartum urinary retention; myasthenia gravis	Increases GI and bladder tone; decreases sphincter tone	Belching, abdominal cramps, diarrhea, nausea, vomiting, incontinence, profuse sweating, salivation, and respiratory depression

NURSING IMPLICATIONS: Check *respirations;* have urinal or bedpan close at hand and answer calls quickly; atropine SO₄ is the *antidote* for cholinergic drugs

Edrophonium (Tensilon) —IV 2 mg; IM 10 mg	Diagnosis of myasthenia gravis; reversal of neuromuscular blockers	Inhibits breakdown of acetylcholine; anticholinesterase, cholinergic	Excess secretions, bronchospasm, bradycardia, abdominal cramps, vomiting, diarrhea, excess salivation, sweating

NURSING IMPLICATIONS: Effects last up to 30 min; give IV *undiluted* with *TB* syringe

Neostigmine (Prostigmin) —PO 15 mg q3–4h; SC, IM 0.5 mg	Myasthenia gravis, postoperative bladder distention, urinary retention, reversal of neuromuscular blockers	Inhibits breakdown of acetylcholine; cholinergic	Excess secretions, bronchospasm, bradycardia, abdominal cramps, nausea, vomiting, diarrhea, excess salivation, sweating

NURSING IMPLICATIONS: Take oral form *with* food or milk; with chewing difficulty, take 30 min before eating

CHOLINERGIC MIOTICS			
Pilocarpine HCl—1–2 gtts 1–2% solution up to 6 times/d. Physostigmine salicylate (Eserine)—0.1 mL of 0.25–10.00% solution; *not* more than qid	Chronic open-angle and acute angle-closure glaucoma	Contraction of the sphincter muscle of iris, resulting in miosis	Brow ache, headache, ocular pain, blurring and dimness of vision, allergic conjunctivitis, nausea, vomiting, and profuse sweating; bronchoconstriction in patients with bronchial asthma

NURSING IMPLICATIONS: Initially the medication may be irritating; teach proper *sterile* technique for instilling drops— *wipe excess* solution to prevent systemic symptoms; *discard cloudy* solutions

(continued)

TABLE D.2   COMMON DRUGS (*Continued*)

Drug and Dosage	Use	Action	▶◀ Assessment: Side Effects
CHOLINERGIC MIOTICS (*Continued*)			
Pyridostigmine (Mestinon) —PO 60 mg/d; IM, IV 2 mg q2–3h; maintenance: 60–150 mg/d	Myasthenia gravis, reversal of neuromuscular blockers	Inhibits breakdown of acetyl-choline and prolongs its effects	See Neostigmine
NURSING IMPLICATIONS: See Neostigmine			
CNS STIMULANTS			
Amphetamine SO$_4$—PO 5–60 mg qd in divided doses	Mild depressive states; narcolepsy; postencephalitic parkinsonism; obesity control; minimal brain dysfunction in children (attention deficit disorder)	Raises BP, decraeses sense of fatigue, elevates mood	Restlessness, dizziness, tremors, insomnia; increases libido; suicidal and homicidal tendencies; palpitations; angina pain
NURSING IMPLICATIONS: Give *before* 4 P.M. to avoid sleep disturbance; *dependence on* drug may develop; *contraindicated* with: MAO inhibitors, hyperthyroidism, and psychotic states			
Methylphenidate hydrochloride (Ritalin)—PO 0.3 mg/kg/d or adults 20–60 mg in divided doses	Childhood hyperactivity; narcolepsy; MBD (attention deficit disorder) in children	Mild CNS and respiratory stimulation	Anorexia, dizziness, drowsiness, insomnia, nervousness, BP and pulse changes
NURSING IMPLICATIONS: To avoid insomnia take last dose *4–5 h before* bedtime; monitor vital signs; check *weight* 2–3 times weekly and report losses			
DECONGESTANTS			
Phenylephrine (Neo-Synephrine, Sinex)—SC, IM 2–5 mg q10–15 min (*not* to exceed 5 mg); IV 40– 60 µg/min; nasal 2–3 gtts or 1–2 sprays q3– 4h; ophthalmic 3 gtt/d	Shock, hypotension, decongestant, adjunct to spinal anesthesia, mydriatic	Constricts blood vessels by stimulating alpha adrenergic receptors	Dizziness, restlessness, dyspnea, tachycardia, arrhythmias; ophthalmologic— burning, photophobia, tearing
NURSING IMPLICATIONS: Check for correct concentration; protect eyes from *light sensitivity;* blow nose *before* using; *rebound congestion* will occur with prolonged use			
Pseudoephedrine (Sudafed)—PO 60 mg q4–6h	Nasal congestion, allergies, chronic ear infections	Produces vasoconstriction in respiratory tract and possibly bronchodilation	Nervousness, anxiety, palpitations, anorexia
NURSING IMPLICATIONS: Give at least *2 h before* bedtime to minimize *insomnia*			
DIURETICS			
Acetazolamide (Diamox)— PO 250–1000 mg/d; IV 500 mg	Glaucoma; heart failure; convulsive disorders	Weak diuretic; produces acidosis; self-limiting effect; increases bicarbonate excretion	Electrolyte depletion symptomatology—lassitude, apathy, decreased urinary output, and mental confusion
NURSING IMPLICATIONS: Weigh *daily;* I&O; assess edema; give *early* in day to allow sleep at night; observe for side effects; replace electrolytes as ordered			

(continued)

TABLE D.2 COMMON DRUGS (*Continued*)

Drug and Dosage	Use	Action	✉ Assessment: Side Effects
DIURETICS (continued)			
Ethacrynic acid (Edecrin) —PO 50–200 mg qd in divided doses	Pulmonary edema; ascites; edema of heart failure	Inhibits the reabsorption of NA$^+$ in the ascending loop of Henle	Nausea, vomiting, diarrhea, hypokalemia, hypotension, gout, dehydration, deafness, and metabolic acidosis

NURSING IMPLICATIONS: Assess for *dehydration*—skin turgor, neck veins; hypotension; *KCl* supplement

Furosemide (Lasix)—PO 40–80 mg qd in divided doses	Edema and associated heart failure; cirrhosis; renal disease; nephrotic syndrome; hypertension	Inhibits Na$^+$ and Cl$^-$ reabsorption in the loop of Henle	Dermatitis, pruritus, paresthesia, blurring of vision, postural hypotension, nausea, vomiting, diarrhea, dehydration, electrolyte depletion, and hearing loss (usually reversible)

NURSING IMPLICATIONS: Assess for: weakness, lethargy, leg cramps, anorexia; *peak* action in 1–2 h; duration 6–8 h; do *not* give at bedtime; supplementary *KCl* indicated; may induce *digitalis toxicity*

Hydrochlorothiazide (Hydro-DIURIL and Esidrix 25–100 mg tid)—PO Diuril 0.5–1.0 g qd	Edema; heart failure; Na$^+$ retention in steroid therapy; hypertension	Inhibits sodium chloride and water reabsorption in the distal ascending loop and the distal convoluted tubule of the kidneys	Hypokalemia, nausea, vomiting, diarrhea, dizziness, and paresthesias; may accentuate diabetes

NURSING IMPLICATIONS: Watch for *muscle weakness;* give well-diluted *potassium chloride* supplement; *monitor* urine for changes in sugar and acetone

Osmotic diuretic 30% urea, 10% invert sugar, 20% mannitol	Cerebral edema	Hypertonic solution that kidney tubules cannot reabsorb, thereby causing obligatory water loss	↑ Extracellular fluid volume

NURSING IMPLICATIONS: Usually *Foley* catheter required; monitor *cardiac and respiratory* status

Spironolactone (Aldactone) —PO 25 mg bid–qid	Cirrhosis of liver; when other diuretics are ineffective	Inhibits effects of aldosterone in distal tubules of kidney	Headache, lethargy, diarrhea, ataxia, skin rash, gynecomastia

NURSING IMPLICATIONS: Potassium-sparing drug; do *not* give supplemental KCl; monitor for signs of electrolyte imbalance

EMETICS			
Ipecac syrup—PO 15–30 mL for emesis, followed by 1–2 glasses H$_2$O (adults and children >1 yr); 5–10 mL followed by ½–1 glass H$_2$O (children <1 yr)	*Emergency* emetic for poison ingestion	NH$_4$ ions cause gastric irritation	Violent emesis, tachycardia, decreased BP, and dyspnea

NURSING IMPLICATIONS: *Contraindicated* in liver and renal disease; if given for emesis, follow dose with as much *water* as patient will drink

(*continued*)

TABLE D.2   COMMON DRUGS (*Continued*)

Drug and Dosage	Use	Action	⋈ Assessment: Side Effects
ENZYMES			
Pancrelipase (Viokase)—adults, PO 325 mg–1 g qd, during meals; children, PO 300–600 mg tid	Chronic pancreatitis; cystic fibrosis; gastrectomy; pancreatectomy; sprue	Assists in digestion of starch, protein, and fats; decreases nitrogen and fat content of stool	Anorexia, nausea, vomiting, diarrhea, buccal/anal soreness (infants), sneezing, skin rashes, diabetes

NURSING IMPLICATIONS: May be taken *with* antacid or cimetidine; do *not* crush or chew tabs; *monitor* I&O, weight; be alert for signs of diabetes; children may use sprinkles

EXPECTORANTS			
Guaifenesin (Robitussin) 100–400 mg q4h	Respiratory congestion	Increases expectoration by causing irritation of gastric mucosa; reduces adhesiveness/surface tension of respiratory tract fluid	Low incidence of GI upset; drowsiness

NURSING IMPLICATIONS: Encourage to stop smoking; increase *fluid* intake; respiratory hygiene

Terpin hydrate—PO 5–10 mL q3–4h	Bronchitis; emphysema	Liquefies bronchial secretions	Nausea, vomiting, and gastric irritation

NURSING IMPLICATIONS: Give undiluted; *push* fluids

FIBRINOLYTIC AGENTS			
Alteplase, recombinant (Activase, tPA)—IV bolus, 15 mg over 1–2 min; then 50 mg over 30 min; then 35 mg over 60 min; 100 mg over 90 min	Acute MI; under investigation for pulmonary emboli, deep vein thrombosis, and peripheral artery thrombosis	Promotes conversion of plasminogen to plasmin, which is fibrinolytic	Internal or local bleeding; urticaria; dysrhythmias related to reperfusion; hypotension, nausea, and vomiting

NURSING IMPLICATIONS: Assess for signs of *reperfusion* (relief of chest pain, no ST segment elevation); observe for *bleeding; avoid* IM injection; *do not* mix other meds in line

Streptokinase IV—1.5 million IU diluted to 45 ml infused over 60 min	Lysis of pulmonary or systemic emboli or thrombi; acute MI	Reacts with plasminogen, dissolves fibrin clots	Prolonged coagulation; allergic reactions; mild fever

NURSING IMPLICATIONS: Monitor for signs of excessive *bleeding*, particularly at injection sites; *avoid* nonessential handling of patient

Urokinase—IV 4400 IU/kg over 10 min; 1.0–1.8 mL of 5000 IU/mL into catheter	Massive pulmonary emboli, coronary artery thrombi, occluded IV catheter	Directly activates plasminogen	Bleeding, anaphylaxis, rash

NURSING IMPLICATIONS: Vital signs; check *q15min* for bleeding during first h; *q15–30min for 8 h;* have *epinephrine* ready

FIBRINOLYTIC ANTIDOTE			
Aminocaproic acid (Amicar)—PO, IV 5 g loading dose; 1 g/h to 30 g in 24 h	Management of streptokinase or urokinase overdose	Inhibits plasminogen activator and antagonizes plasmin	Hypotension; bradycardia; cardiac arrhythmias

NURSING IMPLICATIONS: Give *slowly* IV to prevent side effects; *not* recommended for DIC

(continued)

TABLE D.2   COMMON DRUGS (*Continued*)

Drug and Dosage	Use	Action	◀ Assessment: Side Effects
MUCOLYTIC AGENTS			
Acetylcysteine (Mucomyst) —1–10 mL of 20% solution per nebulizer tid	Emphysema; pneumonia; tracheostomy care; atelectasis; cystic fibrosis	Lowers viscosity of respiratory secretions by opening disulfide linkages in mucus	Stomatitis, nausea, rhinorrhea, bronchospasm

NURSING IMPLICATIONS: Observe *respiratory rate;* maintain open airway with suctioning as necessary; observe asthmatics carefully for *increased bronchospasm;* discontinue treatment immediately if this occurs; odor disagreeable initially

Drug and Dosage	Use	Action	Assessment: Side Effects
MUSCLE RELAXANTS			
Baclofen (Lioresal)—5 mg tid up to 10–20 mg 4/d maintenance dose	Relief of spasticity of multiple sclerosis, spinal cord injury	Centrally acting skeletal-muscle relaxant; depresses polysynaptic afferent reflex activity at spinal cord level	Pruritis, tinnitus; N/V, diarrhea or constipation; drowsiness

NURSING IMPLICATIONS: Administer *with* food if GI symptoms; monitor for safety when ambulating; do *not* discontinue abruptly

Drug and Dosage	Use	Action	Assessment: Side Effects
Dantrolene sodium (Dantrium)—25 mg/day to 25 mg bid–qid to 100 mg qid max	See Baclofen	see Baclofen	See Baclofen

NURSING IMPLICATIONS: See Baclofen

Drug and Dosage	Use	Action	Assessment: Side Effects
NARCOTIC ANTAGONISTS			
Naloxone (Narcan) HCl— IV 0.1–0.2 mg repeated	Reverses respiratory depression due to narcotics	Reverses respiratory depression of morphine SO_4, meperidine HCl, and methadone HCl; does not itself cause respiratory depression, sedation, or analgesia	No known side effects

NURSING IMPLICATIONS: Note time, type of narcotic, dosage received; *not* useful with *CNS depression from other* drugs; respiratory depression *may return;* monitor closely

Drug and Dosage	Use	Action	Assessment: Side Effects
SEDATIVES AND HYPNOTICS			
Chlordiazepoxide (Librium) HCl—PO 5–10 mg; IM or IV 50–100 mg	Psychoneuroses; preoperative apprehension; chronic alcoholism; anxiety	CNS depressant resulting in mild sedation; appetite stimulant; and anticonvulsant	Ataxia, fatigue, blurred vision, diplopia, lethargy, nightmares, and confusion

NURSING IMPLICATIONS: Ensure anxiety relief by allowing patient to verbalize feelings; advise patient to *avoid* driving and alcoholic beverages

Drug and Dosage	Use	Action	Assessment: Side Effects
Chloral hydrate—PO 250 mg tid; hypnotic: PO 0.5–1.0 g; rectal supplement 0.3–0.9 g	Sedation for elderly; delirium tremens; pruritus; mania; barbiturate and alcohol withdrawal	Depresses sensorimotor areas of cerebral cortex	Nausea, vomiting, gastritis; pinpoint pupils; delirium; rash; decreased BP, pulse, respirations, and temperature; hepatic damage

NURSING IMPLICATIONS: *Caution*—should *not* be taken in combination with *alcohol;* dependency is possible

(continued)

TABLE D.2   COMMON DRUGS (Continued)

Drug and Dosage	Use	Action	◄ Assessment: Side Effects
SEDATIVES AND HYPNOTICS (continued)			
Diazepam (Valium)—PO 2–10 mg tid–qid; IM or IV 2–10 mg q3–4h	Anxiety disorders; alcohol withdrawal; adjunctive therapy in seizure disorders; status epilepticus; tetanus; preoperative or preprocedural sedation (also see Midazolam)	Induces calming effect on limbic system, thalamus, and hypothalamus	CNS depression—sedation or ataxia (dose related); dry mouth; blurred vision; mydriasis; constipation; urinary retention

NURSING IMPLICATIONS: *Do not* mix with other drugs; IM injection painful; observe for *phlebitis;* monitor response; measures to ensure patient safety (e.g., falls); high potential for *abuse; contraindicated* in acute angle-closure glaucoma and porphyria

Flurazepam (Dalmane)— PO >15 yr, 30 mg hs; elderly or debilitated, 15 mg hs	Hypnotic	Fastest acting; see Diazepam	See Diazepam

NURSING IMPLICATIONS: See Diazepam

Hydroxyzine pamoate (Vistaril)—PO 25–100 mg qid	See Chlordiazepoxide (Librium); antiemetic in postoperative conditions; adjunctive therapy	CNS relaxant with sedative effect on limbic system and thalamus	Drowsiness, headache, itching, dry mouth, and tremor

NURSING IMPLICATIONS: Give *deep IM only; potentiates* action of warfarin (Coumadin), narcotics, and barbiturates

Lorazepam (Ativan)—PO 1–2 mg bid–tid (up to 10 mg); 2–4 mg hs; IM 4 mg max; IV 2 mg max	Anxiety disorders; insomnia; alternative to diazepam for status epilepticus; preanesthesia	See Diazepam	See Diazepam

NURSING IMPLICATIONS: See Diazepam

Meprobamate (Equanil, Miltown)—PO 400 mg tid–qid	Anxiety; stress; absence seizures	See Hydroxyzine pamoate (Vistaril)	Voracious appetite, dryness of mouth, and ataxia

NURSING IMPLICATIONS: Older patients prone to drowsiness and hypotension; observe for *jaundice*

Midazolam (Versed)—IM 0.05–0.08 mg/kg; IV 0.1–0.15 mg kg	Preanesthesia; prediagnostic procedures; induction of general anesthesia	Penetrates blood-brain barrier to produce sedation and amnesia	Respiratory depression; apnea; disorientation and behavioral excitement

NURSING IMPLICATIONS: Monitor ventilatory status and oxygenation; prevent injuries from CNS depression; nonirritating to vein

Phenobarbital Na—sedative, PO 20–30 mg tid; hypnotic, PO 50–100 mg; IV or IM 100–300 mg. Butabarbital NA (Butisol), pentobarbital Na (Nembutal), secobarbital Na (Seconal)	Preoperative sedation; emergency control of convulsions; absence seizures	Depresses CNS, promoting drowsiness	Cough, hiccups, restlessness, pain, hangover, and CNS and circulatory depression

NURSING IMPLICATIONS: Observe for *hypotension* during IV administration; put up siderails on bed of older patients; observe for increased *tolerance*

(continued)

TABLE D.2 COMMON DRUGS (*Continued*)

Drug and Dosage	Use	Action	▶ Assessment: Side Effects
SEDATIVES AND HYPNOTICS (*continued*)			
Promethazine (Phenergan) 25–50 mg IV, IM, PO	Preoperative sedation; postoperative sedation	Antihistaminic; sedative, antiemetic, antimotion sickness	Drowsiness, coma, hypo/hypertension; leukopenia; photosensitivity; irregular respirations; blurred vision; urinary retention; dry mouth, nose, throat

NURSING IMPLICATIONS: Administer oral med *with* food, milk; IM *deep* into large muscles, rotate sites; verify compatibility with other drugs; *safety* concerns due to sedative effect

THYROID HORMONE INHIBITOR			
Lugol's solution—PO 2–6 drops tid 10 d prior to thyroidectomy	To reduce size, vascularity of thyroid before thyroid surgery; emergency treatment of thyroid storm; or control of hyperthyroid symptoms after radioiodine (^{131}I) therapy	Inhibits thyroid hormone secretion, synthesis	GI distress, stains teeth; increased respiratory secretions; rashes, acne

NURSING IMPLICATIONS: *Dilute in juice,* give through *straw;* bloody diarrhea/vomiting indicates acute poisoning

Propylthiouracil—PO 300–400 mg/d, divided initial dose; 100–150 mg/d maintenance dose; methimazole (Tapazole) 15–60 mg/d initial dose; 5–15 mg/d maintenance dose	Hyperthyroidism; return patient to euthyroid state; also used preoperatively	Inhibits functional thyroid hormone synthesis by blocking reactions; responsible for iodide conversion to iodine; inhibition of T_4 conversion to T_3	Blood dyscrasias; hepatotoxicity; hypothyroidism

NURSING IMPLICATIONS: Teach importance of compliance with med protocol; *avoid* 🍎 iodine-rich foods (seafood, iodized salt); caution when using other drugs

Saturated potassium iodide (SSKI)—300 mg tid–qid	Same as Lugol's solution	Same as Lugol's solution	Same as Lugol's solution

NURSING IMPLICATIONS: Same as Lugol's solution

THYROID HORMONE REPLACEMENT			
Levothyroxine (Levothroid, Synthroid)—PO 0.05–0.10 mg/d oral; 200–500 µg IV	Hypothyroidism	Replacement therapy to alleviate symptoms	Symptoms of hyperthyroidism
	Myxedema coma	Emergency replacement therapy	

NURSING IMPLICATIONS: Teach signs and symptoms of hyper/hypothyroidism; monitor bowel activity; teach diet to combat constipation; keep meds in tight *light-proof* containers; 🍎 *avoid foods* that inhibit thyroid secretion (turnips, cabbage, carrots, peaches, peas, strawberries, spinach, radishes)

Liothyronine (Cytomel)—PO 25 µg/d to maintenance dose 25–75 µg	Mild hypothyroidism in adults	Replacement therapy	See Levothyroxine

NURSING IMPLICATIONS: See Levothyroxine

TABLE D.3   GUIDE TO IMPORTANT FOOD AND DRUG CONSIDERATIONS

Key to Nursing Implications
(with codes for medication administration records):
1. Take with food or milk (F-M).
2. Take on empty stomach (1 hour ac or 2 to 3 hours pc).
3. Don't drink milk or eat other dairy products (M-D).
4. Take with full glass of water (+ H_2O).
5. Take before meals (½ hour ac).
6. May take without regard to meals (OK c̄ meals).

A
acebutolol 6
Achromycin V 2, 3
allopurinol 1
Amcill 2
aminophylline 1
amiodarone 1
amoxicillin 6
amoxicillin/clavulanate 6
Amoxil 6
ampicillin 2
aspirin 1
Augmentin 6
Azo Gantrisin 4, 6
Azolid 1

B
Bactrim 4, 6
Benemid 4
bisacodyl 3
Butazolidin 1

C
Capoten 2
captopril 2
Carafate 2
Carprofen 1
Ceclor 6
cefaclor 6
Ceftin 6
cefuroxime axetil 6
cephalexin 6
chlorothiazide 1
cimetidine 1
Cipro 6
ciprofloxacin 6
Cleocin 4, 6
clindamycin 4, 6
cloxacillin sodium 2
Cloxapen 2
ColBENEMID 1, 4
Cordarone 1

co-trimaxazole 4, 6
Cuprimine 2

D
Declomycin 2, 3
Deltasone 1
demeclocycline 2, 3
Depen 2
Desyrel 1
dicloxacillin sodium 2
diflunisal 1
Diuril 1
Dolobid 1
Donnatal 5
Dopar 1
doxycycline hyclate 3, 6
Dulcolax 3
Dynapen 2

E
Ecotrin 3
E.E.S. 2
E-Mycin 6
enalapril 6
ERYC 2
Ery-Tab 6
Erythrocin 2
erythromycin estolate 6
erythromycin ethylsuccinate 6
erythromycin stearate 2
etretinate 1

F
famotidine 6
Feldene 1
ferrous sulfate 3
Flagyl 1
flecainide 6
fluoxetine 6
Fulvicin 1
Furadantin 1

G
Gantrisin 4, 6
glycopyrrolate 5
Grifulvin V 1
Grisactin 1
griseofulvin 1

H
Hydropres 1
Hytrin 6

I
Ilosone 6
Indocin 1
indomethacin 1
INH 2
isoniazid 2

K
Kaon 1
Kay Ciel 1
Keflex 6
ketoconazole 1
ketoprofen 1
K-Lor 1
K-Lyte 1

L
Larodopa 1
Larotid 6
levodopa 1
Lincocin 2
lincomycin 2
lisinopril 6
Lorelco 1
lovastatin 1

M
Macrodantin 1
Marax 1
methysergide maleate 1
metronidazole 1
Mevacor 1
mexiletine 1
Mexitil 1
Minocin 3, 6
Minocyline 3, 6

N
nafcillin 2
nitrofurantoin 1
nitrofurantoin macrocrystals 1
Nizoral 1
norfloxacin 2, 4
Noroxin 2, 4

O
Omnipen 2
Orazinc 3
Orudis 1
oxacillin sodium 2
oxytetracycline 2, 3

P
penicillamine 2
penicillin G (oral) 2
penicillin V 6
Pen-Vee K 6
Pepcid 6
phenylbutazone 1
pindolol 6
piroxicam 1
Polycillin 2
potassium chloride 1
prednisone 1
Prinivil 6

Pro-Banthine 5
probenecid 4
probucol 1
procainamide 6
Pronestyl 6
propantheline bromide 5
Prostaphlin 2
Prozac 6

R
ranitidine 6
Raudixin 1
rauwolfia serpentina 1
Regroton 1
reserpine 1
Rifadin 2
rifampin 2
Rimactane 2
rimadyl 1
Robinul 5

S
Sansert 1
Sectral 6
Septra 4, 6
Ser-Ap-Es 1
Serpasil 1
Sinemet 1
Slow-K 1
Somophyllin 1
sucralfate 2
sulfisoxazole 4, 6
Sumycin 2, 3

T
Tagamet 1
Tambocor 6
Tedral 1
Tegison 1
terazosin 6
Terramycin 2, 3
tetracycline HCl 2, 3
Theobid 6
Theo-Dur 6

U
Unipen 2

V
Vasotec 6
V-Cillin K 6
Vibramycin 3, 6
Visken 6

Z
Zantac 6
Zestril 6
zinc sulfate 3
Zyloprim 1

Source: McGavin K. 10 Golden rules for administering drugs safely. *Nursing 88*, 18(8):40, 1988.

TABLE D.4   CLASSIFICATION OF THE ANTICANCER DRUGS

I. Alkylating agents
  A. Nitrogen mustards
    1. Mechlorethamine hydochloride (*Mustargen,* HN$_2$, nitrogen mustard)
    2. Cyclophosphamide (*Cytoxan*)
    3. Chlorambucil (*Leukeran*)
    4. Melphalan (*Alkeran, L-PAM,* L-phenylalanine mustard)
    5. Ifosfamide (*Ifex*)
  B. Alkyl sulfonates
    1. Busulfan (*Myleran*)
  C. Nitrosoureas
    1. Carmustine (BCNU, *BiCNU*)
    2. Lomustine (CCNU, *CeeNU*)
    3. Semustine (methyl-CCNU)
    4. Streptozocin (*Zanosar,* streptozotocin)
  D. Ethylenimines
    1. Thiotepa
  E. Triazenes
    1. Dacarbazine (*DTIC-Dome*)

II. Antimetabolites
  A. Folate antagonist
    1. Methotrexate (*Folex, Mexate*)
  B. Purine analogues
    1. Thioguanine (6-TG, 6-thioguanine)
    2. Mercaptopurine (6-MP, *Purinethol*)
    3. Fludarabine (*Fludara*)
    4. Pentostatin (deoxycoformycin, *Nipent*)
    5. Cladribine (2-chloro-deoxyadenosine, *Leustatin*)
  C. Pyrimidine analogues
    1. Cytarabine (cytosine arabinoside, *Cytosar-U,* ara-C)
    2. Fluorouracil (5-FU, 5-fluorouracil)

III. Antiinfectives
  A. Anthracyclines
    1. Doxorubicin hydrochloride (*Adriamycin*)
    2. Daunorubicin (daunomycin, *Cerubidine*)
    3. Idarubicin (*Idamycin*)
  B. Bleomycins
    1. Bleomycin sulfate (*Blenoxane*)
  C. Mitomycin (mitomycin C, *Mutamycin*)
  D. Dactinomycin (actinomycin D, *Cosmegen*)
  E. Plicamycin (*Mithracin*)

IV. Plant-derived products
  A. Vinca alkaloids
    1. Vincristine (*Oncovin*)
    2. Vinblastine (*Velban*)
  B. Epipodophyllotoxins
    1. Etoposide (VP-16, *Vepesid*)
    2. Teniposide (VM-26, *Vumon*)
  C. Taxanes: paclitaxel (*Taxol*)

V. Enzymes
  A. L-Asparaginase (*Elspar*)

VI. Hormonal agents
  A. Glucocorticoids
  B. Estrogens/antiestrogens
    1. Tamoxifen citrate (*Nolvadex*)
    2. Estramustine phosphate sodium (*Emcyt*)
  C. Androgens/antiandrogens
    1. Flutamide (*Eulexin*)
  D. Progestins
  E. Luteinizing hormone–releasing hormone (LH-RH) antagonists
    1. Buserelin (*Suprefact*)
    2. Leuprolide (*Lupron*)
  F. Octreotide acetate (*Sandostatin*)

VII. Miscellaneous agents
  A. Hydroxyurea (*Hydrea*)
  B. Procarbazine (*N*-methylhydrazine, *Matulane, Natulan*)
  C. Mitotane (o,p′-DDD, *Lysodren*)
  D. Hexamethylmelamine (HMM)
  E. Cisplatin (*cis*-platinum II, *Platinol*)
  F. Carboplatin (*Paraplatin*)
  G. Mitoxantrone (*Novantrone*)

VIII. Monoclonal antibodies

IX. Immunomodulating agents
  A. Levamisole (*Ergamisol*)
  B. Interferons
    1. Interferon alfa-2a (*Roferon-A*)
    2. Interferon alfa-2b (*Intron A*)
  C. Interleukins: aldesleukin (interleukin-2, IL-2, *Proleukin*)

X. Cellular growth factors
  A. Filgrastim (G-CSF, *Neupogen*)
  B. Sargramostim (GM-CSF, *Leukine, Prokine*)

Source: Craig C, Stitzel R. *Modern Pharmacology.* Boston: Little, Brown, 1994.

TABLE D.5 PROPERTIES OF SELECTED ANTI-INFLAMMATORY AGENTS

Specific Group	Analgesic	Antipyretic	Anti-inflammatory	Uricosuric
Salicylate derivatives				
Acetylsalicylic acid (aspirin)	°	°	°	°
Pyrazolone derivatives				
Phenylbutazone	°	°	°	°
Oxyphenbutazone	°	°	°	°
Sulfinpyrazone	0	0	0	°
Paraaminophenol derivatives				
Acetaminophen	°	°	0	0
Phenacetin	°	°	0	0
Propionic acid derivatives				
Ibuprofen	°	°	°	0
Naproxen	°	°	°	0
Fenoprofen	°	°	°	0
Flurbiprofen	°	°	°	0
Ketoprofen	°	°	°	0
Newer drugs				
Indomethacin	°	°	°	0
Sulindac	°	0	°	0
Mefenamic acid	°	0	°	0
Tolmetin	°	°	°	0
Diflunisal	°	0	°	0
Piroxicam	°	°	°	0
Diclofenac	°	°	°	0
Etodolac	°	0	°	0
Nabumetone	°	°	°	0

° = possesses the property assigned; 0 = lacks the property assigned.

Source: Ebadi M. *Pharmacology* (2nd ed). Boston: Little, Brown, 1993.

Quick Guide to Common Clinical Signs

Appendix E

Many clinical signs have been named for the physicians who first described them or the phenomena they resemble. Following is a list of 25 of the most common clinical signs for use as a quick reference as you review.

Babinski reflex   dorsiflexion of the big toe after stimulation of the lateral sole; associated with *corticospinal* tract lesions.

Blumberg's sign   transient pain in the abdomen after approximated fingers pressed gently into abdominal wall are suddenly withdrawn—rebound tenderness; associated with *peritoneal inflammation.*

Brudzinski's sign   flexion of the hip and knee induced by flexion of the neck; associated with *meningeal* irritation.

Chvostek's sign   facial muscle spasm induced by tapping on the facial nerve branches; associated with *hypocalcemia.*

Cheyne-Stokes respiration   rhythmic cycles of deep and shallow respiration, often with apneic periods; associated with *central nervous system respiratory center dysfunction.*

Coppernail's sign   ecchymoses on the perineum, scrotum, or labia; associated with *fracture* of the *pelvis.*

Cullen's sign   bluish discoloration of the umbilicus; associated with acute *pancreatitis* or *hemoperitoneum,* especially *rupture of fallopian tube* in ectopic pregnancy.

Doll's eye sign   dissociation between the movements of the head and eyes: as the head is raised, the eyes are lowered, and as the head is lowered, the eyes are raised; associated with global-diffuse disorders of the *cerebrum.*

Fluid wave sign   transmission across the abdomen of a wave induced by snapping the abdomen; associated with *ascites.*

Goldstein's sign   wide distance between the great toe and the adjoining toe; associated with *cretinism* and *trisomy 21.*

Homans' sign   pain behind the knee, induced by dorsiflexion of the foot; associated with peripheral vascular disease, especially *venous thrombosis* in the calf.

Kehr's sign   severe pain in the left upper quadrant, radiating to the top of the shoulder; associated with *splenic rupture.*

Kernig's sign   inability to extend leg when sitting or lying with the thigh flexed on the abdomen; associated with *meningeal* irritation.

Knie's sign   unequal dilatation of the pupils; associated with *Graves' disease.*

Kussmaul's respiration   paroxysmal air hunger; associated with acidosis, especially *diabetic ketoacidosis.*

Lasègue's sign   straight leg raising with hip flexed and knee extended will elicit sciatic pain; associated with *herniated lumbar disc.*

McBurney's sign   tenderness at McBurney's point (located two-thirds of the distance from the umbilicus to the anterior-superior iliac spine); associated with *appendicitis.*

Murphy's sign   pain on taking a deep breath when pressure is applied over the gallbladder; associated with *gallbladder disease.*

Osler's sign   small painful erythematous swellings in the skin of the hands and feet; associated with *bacterial endocarditis.*

Psoas sign   pain induced by hyperextension of the right thigh while lying on the left side; associated with *appendicitis.*

Setting-sun sign   downward deviation of the eyes so that each iris appears to "set" beneath the lower lid, with white sclera exposed between it and the upper lid; associated with *increased intracranial pressure* or irritation of the brain stem.

Simian crease   transverse palmar crease; associated with *Down syndrome*

Tinel's sign   tingling sensation felt from light percussion on the radial side of the palmaris longus tendon; associated with *carpal tunnel syndrome.*

Trousseau's sign   carpopedal spasm develops when BP cuff is inflated above systolic pressure for 3 minutes; associated with *hypocalcemia.*

Williamson's sign   markedly diminished blood pressure in the leg as compared with that in the arm on the same side; associated with *pneumothorax* and *pleural effusions.*

Source: Macklis RM, et al. *Introduction to Clinical Medicine* (3rd ed). Boston: Little, Brown, 1994.

Index to Common Diagnostic Tests and Procedures

Appendix F

For a quick review, use this index to locate 105 selected diagnostic tests and procedures covered in this book as they relate to specific conditions

Test/Procedure (*continued*)	Condition	Page(s)
Cholangiography	Biliary disorders (bile ducts)	146
Cholecystography	Gall bladder disorders	146
Computerized axial tomography (CAT or CT) scan	Brain tumor	292
	Cancer	256, 276
	Herniated disk; spinal cord injuries	261, 263
Culdoscopy	Gyn conditions	289
Cystography	Bladder conditions	195
Cystoscopy	Bladder, urethra conditions	195
Doppler flow meter	Varicose veins	14
Doppler ultrasonography	Arterial and venous blood flow measurement	27
Echocardiography	Heart studies	40
Echoencephalography	Brain lesions	256
8-hr IV ACTH test	Adrenal cortex disorders (Addison's, Cushing's)	205, 206, 207
Electrocardiography (ECG)	Air embolus	101
	Assessment (routine)	5
	Cardiac dysrhythmias	29
	Hyperkalemia	89
	Hypokalemia	89
	Myocardial infarct	37
	Pericarditis	26
	Post-cardiac catheterization	23, 25, 27
	Shock	108
Electroencephalography (EEG)	Brain injury, traumatic	251, 256
Electromyography	Herniated/Ruptured disk	261, 265
Endometrial washing	Uterine cancer	286
Endoscopy	Cancer of body cavity; ulcers	161, 276
Esophagoscopy	Gastric disorders	165
Excisional biopsy	Breast cancer	284
Exfoliative cytology	Cancer of cervix	276
Eye exam	Older adult	3–4
Fasting blood sugar (FBS)	Diabetes	141, 146
Fluoroscopy (also see upper, lower GI series)	Gastric disorders	164
Gastric analysis	Gastric disorders, e.g., ulcers	78, 161, 165
Gastric lavage	Pulmonary infections	78
Gastroscopy	Stomach disorders	165
Glasgow Coma Scale	Brain injury, traumatic	250
Glucose test of cerebrospinal fluid	Post-op craniotomy	252
Glucose tolerance test	Diabetes	146
Hepatoportography	Hepatic disorders	155
Hysterosalpingography	Uterine conditions	289
Intravenous pyelography (IVP)	Pyelonephritis	183, 195
	Renal calculi	191
Intravenous urography (IVU)	Kidney/ureter function	195
Joint Aspiration	Lyme disease	137
Kidney, ureter, bladder x-ray (KUB)	Renal system conditions	195
Laryngoscopy (with biopsy)	Laryngeal cancer	289
Liver biopsy	Liver conditions	155
Lower gastrointestinal series	Colon cancer	164
Lumbar puncture	Brain injury, traumatic	251
	Encephalitis	256
Lung scan	Pulmonary emboli or tumor	78
Magnetic resonance imaging (MRI)	Cancer; musculoskeletal disorders	243, 276
Mammography	Breast lesions	284, 289
Mantoux tuberculin test	TB	61
Multiple gaited acquisition scan (MUGA)	Cardiac conditions	26
Myelography	Herniated/Ruptured disk; spinal cord tumors	261, 266

Test/Procedure	Condition	Page(s)
Needle biopsy	Breast cancer	276, 284
Neurologic exam	Assessment, physical	3
	Craniotomy, post-operative	252
	CVA	254
	Herniated ruptured disk	261
	Traumatic injury to the brain	250
Neurovascular assessment	Injured limb	224
Pap test (Papanicolaou smear)	Cervical cancer	286, 296
Paracentesis	Ascites	154, 156
Pericardiocentesis	Cardiovascular system assessment	41
Peritoneoscopy	Liver and peritoneum conditions	155
Phlebography	Lower limb vascular assessment	14, 16
Phonocardiography	Heart studies	40
Postprandial blood sugar test (2 hr) (PPBS)	Diabetes; older adult assessment	4, 146
Proctoscopy	Colon and rectal cancer; hernia; hemorrhoids	175, 177, 283
Prostigmin test	Myasthenia Gravis	270
Pulmonary angiography	Emphesema, pulmonary embolism, tumors	78
Pulmonary function studies		
Forced expiratory volume (FEV)	ARDS	65, 77–78
Maximum breathing capacity (MBC)	Asthma	64
Residual volume	Bronchitis	64
Total lung capacity,	Cardiac surgery, preop	24
Vital capacity (VC)	Emphysema	62
Radioactive iodine (iodine 131) uptake test	Hyper/hypothyroidism	201, 204, 207
Renal angiography	Renal cysts, hypertension, tumors	195
Renal biopsy	Kidney disorders	195
Rinne test	Otosclerosis	2, 213
Romberg's test	Pernicious Anemia	50
Schilling test	Pernicious Anemia	51
Sigmoidoscopy	Colon and rectal cancer; diverticulosis, ulcerative colitis	171, 172, 283
Skin test	Histoplasmosis	60
Skull x-rays	Intracranial lesions, vascular tumors	256
Small-bowel biopsy	Celiac disease	169, 177
Snellen eye exam	Eye injury	317
Sputum culture	Histoplasmosis	60
	Pneumonia	58
	TB	61, 78
Sputum smear	Respiratory system cancer; TB	61, 78
Stool specimens	Celiac disease; gastric disorders	165, 169
Tensilon test	Myasthenia Gravis	270
Thermography	Breast cancer	289
Thoracentesis	Air in pleural space (Pneumothorax)	78
Tonometry	Glaucoma	215
Tourniquet test	Idiopathic thrombocytopenia purpura	53
Trendelenburg test	Varicose veins	14
Ultrasonography	Thyroid, kidney, liver, uterus, gallbladder conditions	146
Upper gastrointestinal series	Ulcer (gastric, duodenal)	161, 164
Uterotubal insufflation (Rubin's test)	Fallopian tube disorders	289
Weber's test	Ear assessment	2, 213

Laboratory Values

Appendix **G**

Use this chart as a quick overview of lab values: both normal and conditions that result in high or low values.

Test	Normal Values	Possible Significance	
		Increases	**Decreases**
HEMATOLOGY			
Aspartate amino-transferase (AST)—*formerly* called serum glutamic oxaloacetic transaminase (SGOT)	*Men:* 10–40 U/L *Women:* 9–25 U/L	Myocardial infarction, cardiac surgery, hepatitis, cirrhosis, trauma, Severe burns, progressive muscular dystrophy, infectious mononucleosis, acute renal failure.	Uremia, chronic dialysis, ketoacidosis
Bleeding time—indicator of hemostatic efficiency	1–9 min	Hemorrhagic purpura, acute leukemia, aplastic anemia, disseminated intravascular coagulation, oral anticoagulant therapy.	
Hematocrit—volume of packed red blood cells per dL of blood	*Men:* 45% (38%–54%) *Women:* 40% (36%–47%)	Dehydration, polycythemia, congenital heart disease.	Anemia, leukemia, hemorrhage, dietary deficiencies.
Hemoglobin—oxygen-combining protein	*Men:* 14–18 g/dL *Women:* 12–16 g/dL	Same as for Hematocrit.	Same as for Hematocrit.
Partial thromboplastin time (PTT)—tests coagulation mechanism, stage I deficiencies	*APTT:* 30–40 sec *PTT:* 60–70 sec	Deficiency of Factors VIII, IX, X, XI, XII; anticoagulant therapy.	Extensive cancer, disseminated intravascular coagulation
Platelets—thrombocytes	150,000–400,000/mm³	Polycythemia, postsplenectomy, anemia.	Leukemia, aplastic anemia, cirrhosis, multiple myeloma, chemotherapy.
Prothrombin time–tests extrinsic clotting, stages II and III	11–15 sec	Anticoagulant therapy, disseminated intravascular coagulation, hepatic disease, malabsorption.	Digitalis therapy, diuretic reaction, vitamin K therapy
Red blood cell count—number of circulating erythrocytes in 1 µL of whole blood	*Men:* 4.5–6.2 million/µL *Women:* 4.0–5.5 million/µL	Polycythemia vera, anoxia, dehydration.	Leukemia, hemorrhage, anemias, Hodgkin's disease

Test	Normal Values	Possible Significance	
		Increases	*Decreases*
Sedimentation rate—speed at which red blood cells settle in uncoagulated blood	*Men:* 0–15 mm/h *Women:* 0–20 mm/h	Acute bacterial infection, cancer, infectious disease, numerous inflammatory states	Polycythemia vera, sickle cell anemia
White blood cell count—number of leukocytes in 1 mm³	5000–10,000/mm³	Leukemia, bacterial infection, severe sepsis	Viral infection, overwhelming bacterial infection, lupus erythematosus, antineoplastic chemotherapy
White blood cell differential—enumeration of individual leukocyte distribution:			
Neutrophils	55%–70%	Bacterial infection, tumor, inflammation, stress, drug reaction, trauma, metabolic disorders	Acute viral infection, anorexia nervosa, radiation therapy, drug induced, alcohol ingestion
Eosinophils	1%–4%	Allergic disorder, parasitic infestation, eosinophilic leukemia	Acute or chronic stress; excess ACTH, cortisone, or epinephrine; endocrine disorder
Basophils	25–100 µL, or 0–1%	Myeloproliferative disease, leukemia	Anaphylactic reaction, hyperthyroidism, radiation therapy, infections, pregnancy, aging
Lymphocytes	20%–40%	Chronic lymphocytic leukemia, infectious mononucleosis, chronic bacterial infection, viral infection	Leukemia, systemic lupus erythematosus, immune deficiency disorders
BLOOD CHEMISTRY **Alkaline phosphatase (ALP)**	30–85 mIU/mL	Hyperparathyroidism, Paget's disease, cancer with bone metastasis, obstructive jaundice, cirrhosis, infectious hepatitis, rickets	Malnutrition, scurvy, celiac disease, chronic nephritis, hypothyroidism
Amylase	53–123 IU/L	Acute pancreatitis, mumps, duodenal ulcer, pancreatic cancer, perforated bowel, renal failure	Advanced chronic pancreatitis, chronic alcoholism
Bilirubin, serum	*Direct:* 0.1–0.3 mg/dL *Indirect:* 0.2–0.8 mg/dL *Total:* 0.1–1.0 mg/dL	Massive hemolysis, low-grade hemolytic disease, cirrhosis, obstructive liver disease, hepatitis, biliary obstruction, erythroblastosis fetalis	
Calcium, serum	9–10.5 mg/dL; 4.5–5.6 mg/dL, ionized	Hyperparathyroidism, multiple myeloma, bone metastasis, bone fracture, thiazide diuretic reaction, milk-alkali syndrome	Hypoparathyroidism, renal failure, pregnancy, massive transfusion
Carbon dioxide	24–30 mEq/L	Emphysema, salicylate toxicity, vomiting	Starvation, diarrhea
Chloride, serum	90–110 mEq/L	Hyperventilation, diabetes insipidus, uremia	Heart failure, pyloric obstruction, hypoventilation, vomiting, chronic respiratory acidosis

Test	Normal Values	Possible Significance	
		Increases	Decreases
Cholesterol (total serum)	<200 mg/dL	Hypercholesterolemia, hyperlipidemia, myocardial infarction, uncontrolled diabetes mellitus, high-cholesterol diet, atherosclerosis, stress, glomerulonephritis (nephrotic stage), familial	Malnutrition, cholesterol-lowering medication, anemia, liver disease, hyperthyroidism
Creatinine, serum	*Men:* 0.6–1.2 mg/dL *Women:* 0.5–1.1 mg/dL	Chronic glomerulonephritis, nephritis, heart failure, muscle disease	Debilitation
Creatine kinase (CK) (creatine phosphokinase [CPK])	*Men:* 12–70 U/mL (55–170 U/L) *Women:* 10–55 U/mL (30–135 U/L)	Acute myocardial infarction, acute cerebrovascular accidents, convulsions, surgery, muscular dystrophy, hypokalemia	
Isoenzymes:			
CPK-MM/CK-MM	100%	Muscular dystrophy, delirium tremens, surgery, hypokalemia, crush injuries, hypothyroidism	
CPK-MB/CK-MB	0%	Acute myocardial infarction, cardiac defibrillation, myocarditis, cardiac ischemia	
CPK-BB/CK-BB	0%	Pulmonary infarction, brain surgery, cerebrovascular accident, pulmonary embolism, seizures, intestinal ischemia	
Fibrinogen, serum	0.2–0.4 g/dL or 200–400 mg/dL	Pneumonia, acute infection, nephrosis, rheumatoid arthritis	Cirrhosis, toxic liver necrosis, anemia, disseminated intravascular coagulation, advanced carcinoma
Glucose (fasting)	80–120 mg/dL	Acute stress, Cushing's syndrome, hyperthyroidism, acute or chronic pancreatitis, diabetes mellitus, hyperglycemia	Addison's disease, liver disease, reactive hypoglycemia, pituitary hypofunction
Glycosylated hemoglobin (HbA$_{1c}$)	4.0%–7.0%	Newly diagnosed or poorly controlled diabetes mellitus	
Iron-binding capacity (total)	25–420 µg/L	Lead poisoning, hepatic necrosis	Iron deficiency anemia, chronic blood loss
Lactate dehydrogenase (LDH)	40–90 U/L, 115–225 IU/L LDH-1: 17%–27% LDH-2: 27%–37% LDH-3: 18%–25% LDH-4: 3%–8% LDH-5: 0%–5%	Myocardial infarction, pernicious anemia, chronic viral hepatitis, pneumonia, pulmonary emboli, CVA, renal tissue destruction, leukemia, non-Hodgkin's lymphoma, shock, trauma	

Test	Normal Values	Possible Significance	
		Increases	Decreases
Phosphorus (inorganic), serum	3.0–4.5 mg/dL	Chronic glomerular disease, hypoparathyroidism, milk-alkali syndrome, sarcoidosis	Hypoparathyroidism, rickets, osteomalacia, renal tubular necrosis, malabsorption syndrome, vitamin D deficiency
Potassium, serum	3.5–5.0 mEq/L	Diabetic ketosis, renal failure, Addison's disease, excessive intake	Thiazide diuretics, Cushing's syndrome, cirrhosis with ascites, hyperaldosteronism, steroid therapy, malignant hypertension, poor dietary habits, chronic diarrhea, diaphoresis, renal tubular necrosis, malabsorption syndrome, vomiting
Protein, serum (albumin/globulin)	*Total:* 6.4–8.3 g/dL *Albumin:* 3.5–5.0 g/dL *Globulin:* 2.3–3.5 g/dL	Dehydration, multiple myeloma	Chronic liver disease, myeloproliferative disease, burns
Sodium, serum	138–144 mEq/L	Increased intake, either orally or IV; Cushing's disease; excessive sweating; diabetes insipidus	Addison's disease, sodium-losing nephropathy, vomiting, diarrhea, fistulas, tube drainage, burns, renal insufficiency with acidosis, starvation with acidosis, paracentesis, thoracentesis, ascites, heart failure, syndrome of inappropriate antidiuretic hormone
T₃ uptake	24%–34%	Hyperthyroidism, thyroxine-binding globulin (TBG) deficiency	Hypothyroidism, pregnancy, thyroid-binding globulin, excess
Thyroxine	5–12 µg/dL	Hyperthyroidism, pregnancy	Hypothyroidism, renal failure
Serum glutamic oxaloacetic transaminase (SGOT)—*see* Aspartate aminotransferase	—		
Urea nitrogen, serum (BUN)	10–20 mg/dL	Acute or chronic renal failure, heart failure, obstructive uropathy, dehydration	Cirrhosis, malnutrition
Uric acid, serum	*Men:* 2.1–8.5 mg/dL *Women:* 2.0–6.6 mg/dL	Gout, chronic renal failure, starvation, diuretic therapy	
BLOOD GASES Bicarbonate (HCO₃)	21–28 mEq/L	Metabolic alkalosis	Metabolic acidosis
pH, serum	7.35–7.45	*Metabolic alkalosis*–alkali ingestion, *respiratory alkalosis*–hyperventilation	*Metabolic acidosis*–ketoacidosis, shock, *respiratory acidosis*–alveolar hypoventilation
Oxygen pressure (PO₂), whole blood, arterial	80–100 mm Hg	Oxygen administration in the absence of severe lung disease	Chronic obstructive lung disease, severe pneumonia, pulmonary embolism, pulmonary edema, respiratory muscle disease

Test	Normal Values	Possible Significance	
		Increases	*Decreases*
Carbon dioxide pressure (PCO$_2$), whole blood, arterial	35–45 mm Hg	Primary respiratory acidosis, loss of H$^+$ through nasogastric suctioning or vomiting	Primary respiratory alkalosis
IMMUNODIAGNOSTIC STUDIES			
Carcinoembryonic antigen	<3 ng/mL	Cancer of colon, lung, metastatic breast, pancreas, stomach, prostate, ovary, bladder, limbs; also neuroblastoma, leukemias, osteogenic carcinoma. *Noncancerous* conditions such as: hepatic cirrhosis, uremia, pancreatitis, colorectal polyposis, peptic ulcer disease, ulcerative colitis, regional enteritis	
URINALYSIS			
pH	4.8–8.0	Metabolic alkalosis	Metabolic acidosis
Specific gravity	1.010–1.030	Dehydration, pituitary tumor, hypotension	Distal renal tubular disease, polycystic kidney disease, diabetes insipidus, overhydration
Glucose	Negative	Diabetes mellitus	
Protein	Negative	Nephrosis, glomerulonephritis, lupus erythematosus	
Casts	Negative	Nephrosis, glomerulonephritis, lupus erythematosus, infection	
Red blood cells	Negative	Renal calculi, hemorrhagic cystitis, tumors of the kidney	
White blood cells	Negative	Inflammation of the kidneys, ureters, bladder	
Color	Normal yellow	*Abnormal: red to reddish brown* —hematuria; *brown to brownish gray*—bilirubinuria or urobilinuria; *tea-colored*— possible obstructive jaundice	*Almost colorless:* chronic kidney disease, diabetes insipidus, diabetes, mellitus
Sodium	40–220 mEq/L/24 h	Salt-wasting renal disease, syndrome of inappropriate antidiuretic hormone, dehydration	Heart failure, primary aldosteronism
Chloride	110–250 mEq/24 h	Chronic obstructive lung disease, dehydration, salicylate toxicity	Gastric suction, HF, emphysema
Potassium	25–120 mEq/L/24 h	Diuretic therapy	Renal failure
Creatinine clearance	90–139 mL/min		Renal disease
Hydroxycortico-steroids	2–10 mg/24 h	Cushing's disease	Addison's disease

Test	Normal Values	Possible Significance	
		Increases	*Decreases*
Ketosteroids	*Men:* 7–25 mg/24 h *Women:* 4–15 mg/24 h	Hirsutism, adrenal hyperplasia	Thyrotoxicosis, Addison's disease
Catecholamines (vanilymandelic acid)	*Epinephrine:* 0.5–20.0 µg/24 h *Norepinephrine:* 15–80 µg/24 h	Pheochromocytoma, severe anxiety, numerous medications	
URINE TESTS **Schilling test**	Excretion of 8%–40% or more of test dose should appear in urine		Gastrointestinal malabsorption, pernicious anemia

Index to Mnemonics/ Memory Aids

Condition	Mnemonic	Page
Acid-base balance	RAMS	100
Angina: Precipitating factors	3 E's	40
Asthma: Sx, Cause, Dx, Tx	WHISTLE	77
Atelectasis: Characteristics, Tx	COLLAPSE	77
Blood Glucose: Sx, implications	(rhyme)	146
Bronchitis: Sx, Tx	COUGH	77
Cancer: Patient Care	CANCER	289
Circulation: Assessment	4 P's	125
Compartment syndrome: Assessment	5 P's	243
C.P.R.	ABC's	40
Cushing's syndrome: Signs	3 S's	208
Diabetes: Assessment	3 P's	146
Heart failure: Signs/Symptoms	OVERLOAD	40
Histoplasmosis: Characteristics	SOIL	77
Hypertension: Assessment	ELEVATED	16
Hypertension: Complications	4 C's	16
Hypoglycemia: Signs, Sx	DIRE	146
MI: Signs/Symptoms	INTENSE PAIN	40
Pain: Assessment	PQRST	129
Pain: Management	ABC's	130
Pneumonia: Signs, Sx, Tx	FRAPPÉ	77
Postoperative complications: Tx	4 W's	121
Pulmonary edema: Signs/Symptoms	FOWLERS	40
Pulmonary embolism: Signs, Dx	SUDDEN	77
Traction: Nursing care plan	TRACTION	244
Transient ischemic attacks: Assessment	3 T's	258
Tuberculosis: Cause, Dx, Sx, Tx	SPREAD	77
Varicose veins: Assessment	TWISTED	16

Index to Common Tubes

Appendix 1

For a quick reference as you study or review, use this index to locate 25 tubes that are covered throughout the book as they are used in various conditions.

Tube	Condition	Page(s)
Cantor	Intestinal obstruction	173
Catheterization	Prostatic Hyperplasia	192
Chest tubes	Hemothorax	116
	Pneumothorax	67
	Post-op cardiac surgery	24
	Sucking chest wound	67
	Thoracic surgery	69, 72–75
Endotracheal	Post-cardiac surgery	25
	Sucking chest wound	67
Three-way Foley	Prostatectomy	123, 193
Gastrostomy tube	Hiatal hernia	123, 163
Hemovac	Laryngectomy	71, 72
	Mastectomy	123
	Total hip, knee replacement	123
Jackson-Pratt	Mastectomy	123
	Total hip, knee replacement	123
	Wounds	123
Levine	Gastric surgery	112, 164
Linton	Esophygeal varices	155
Miller-Abbott	GI surgery	112
	Intestinal obstruction	173
	Paralytic Ileus	119
Nasogastric (NG)	Aneurysm	13
	Gastric distention	119
	Gastric surgery	112, 164
	Intestinal obstruction	119
	Paralytic Ileus	119
	Splenectomy	53
	Wound dehiscence, evisceration	118
Oropharyngeal airway	Post-operative	115, 116
Penrose drain	Bowel resection	122
Rectal	Gastric distention	119
Salem sump	Gastric surgery	112, 164
Sengstaken-Blakemore	Esophageal varices	155
Shunts	Dialysis	187
Suction	Post-cardiac surgery	25
Suprapubic catheter	Prostatectomy	123, 192
Swan-Ganz	Pre-op cardiac surgery	24
	Post-op cardiac surgery	25
	Shock	108

Index: Nursing Treatments

☞ Hands-On Care, Skills, Activities and Procedures)

Use this index as a quick checklist of over 100 essential skills and procedures mentioned in this book that nurses need to know about or be able to perform in giving patient care.

Index to Positioning the Patient

Appendix K

For a quick reference as you study or review, use this index to locate 40 positions of choice (or contraindications) in various conditions.

Position	Selected conditions	Page(s)
High Fowler's	Appendicitis, ruptured	124
	Asthma	64
	Autonomic hyperreflexia	265
	Cardiac dysrhythmias	29
	Chest tubes	73
	Diaphragmatic hernia (feeding)	163
	Emphysema	62
	Pneumothorax	67, 117
	Pulmonary edema	39
	Thoracic surgery (post-op)	69
Lateral, left (Trendelenberg)	Post-operative patient	115
Lateral, right	Liver biopsy	124, 155
Legs, elevated	Cast	124
	Compartment syndrome	226
	Osteoarthritis	239
	Thrombophlebitis	15
	Varicose veins	14
	Vein ligations, strippings	16
Low Fowler's	Cholecystectomy	145
	Wound dehiscence	118
Lung, affected	Flail chest	124
	Pleurisy	116
Lung, unaffected	Atelectasis	59, 116
Non-operative side	Cataract	215
Operative side	Pneumonectomy	69, 124
Prone	Amputation, lower extremity (stump care)	124, 242
	Multiple sclerosis	269
Recumbent (See Flat in Bed)		
Respiratory excursion, optimal	Iron deficiency anemia	50
Rest to affected joint	Gout	242
Retinal tear dependent	Retinal detachment	216
Semi-Fowlers (30°)	Cirrhosis	154
	Craniotomy, supratentorial	252
	Fluid overload	86, 99
	Heart failure	38
	Laryngectomy	71
	MI	37
	Pericarditis	26
	Pneumonia	116
Semi-prone	Unconscious patient	251
Sit up, lean forward	Emphysema	62
Sitting (Orthopneic)	Pulmonary edema	39
Sitting with knees flexed	Pancreatitis	139–140
Supine	Post cardiac catheterization	23
Wedge charnley pillow	Total hip replacement	239–241
William's position	Ruptured disk	261–262
AVOID:		
Chair, high	Varicose veins	14
Hip flexion/sitting	Aneurysm	13
	Ileofemoral bypass	125
	Polycythemia vera	51
	Vein ligation, stripping	16
Leg elevation	Arterial insufficiency	16
	Ileofemoral bypass	125
Standing, prolonged sitting	Varicose veins	14
	Vein ligations, stripping	16
Trendelenberg	Lobectomy	124
	Shoen	108, 117

Home Health Care

For a quick review of essential information related to health care teaching covered in this book, refer to the pages listed to locate what you need to know to provide basic home care teaching in 40 conditions/situations.

Patient Groups Most Frequently Seen By Home Health Care Nurse—Patients Who Have/Are:

1. Diabetes.
2. AIDS.
3. Skin wounds.
4. Bladder dysfunction.
5. Chronic obstructive pulmonary disease (COPD).
6. Heart failure.
7. Geriatric patients.
8. IV therapy.
9. Ventilator dependent.

Most Common Conditions Seen In Home Health Care

System/Condition	Primary Concern of Home Health Care Goals
PULMONARY SYSTEM	
Asthma	*Teaching:* medication regimen to prevent or control attacks, prevent upper and lower respiratory tract infections, p. 64.
COPD	*Teaching:* medication regimen that involves various routes, use of assistive mechanical ventilation, p. 63. Infection control.
Pneumonia	*Teaching:* antiinfective medication regimen, p. 58. Prevention of complications.
Tracheostomy/laryngectomy	Respiratory care. Patency of tube. *Teaching:* tube changes, dressing and tie changes, pp. 70–71. Prevention of complications. ↓ Emotional problems associated with artificial airway.
Tuberculosis	*Teaching:* personal hygiene, rest, nutrition, medication regimen, pp. 61–62.
CARDIOVASCULAR SYSTEM	
Coronary artery disease	*Teaching:* medication regimen, control of risk factors, compliance with exercise and diet, p. 34.
Heart failure	Assessment. *Teaching:* medical regimen to prevent congestive heart failure, p. 39.
Coronary artery bypass surgery	*Postoperative teaching:* medical regimen to prevent complications, life-style changes (i.e., limitations) made necessary by this surgery and underlying cardiac condition, p. 25.
Hypertension	*Teaching:* medication regimen to control condition, preventive measures to control risk factors, p. 11.
Myocardial infarction	Assessment. *Teaching:* medication regimen, control of risk factors to prevent recurrence or complications, measures to prevent further damage, p. 38.
Pacemaker	Monitor pacemaker function and heart rate to prevent complications, p. 30.
Peripheral vascular disease	*Teaching:* medical regimen to enhance circulation in extremities, prevent complications, pp. 12, 14.
Thrombophlebitis	*Teaching:* control of factors that contribute to thrombus formation, p. 15. Prevention of chronic venous insufficiency or pulmonary emboli.

Adapted from Jaffe, Marie S., *Home Health Nursing Care Plans,* 2nd edition, St. Louis: Mosby, 1993.

NEUROLOGIC SYSTEM

Alzheimer's disease	*Teaching:* safety.
	Preservation of cognitive, social, physical, and psychological function.
Amyotrophic lateral sclerosis	*Teaching:* preservation of muscle function and independence, p. 272.
Cerebrovascular accident	*Teaching:* medical regimen to treat underlying condition, p. 255.
	Rehabilitation and aftercare to maximize potential.
Parkinson's disease	*Teaching:* administration of medication, self-care to meet own basic needs, pp. 271–272.
Seizure disorder	*Teaching:* medication administration to control seizures, p. 253.
	Prevention of physical and psychological trauma resulting from seizures.
Spinal cord injury	Rehabilitation and aftercare to maximize function, pp. 263, 265.

GASTROINTESTINAL SYSTEM

Cirrhosis	Ongoing assessment.
	Elimination of underlying causes, if possible.
	Prevention of further liver damage and complications, p. 155.
Hepatitis	Testing and treatment to prevent spread of disease in the community.
	Teaching: care in acute stage, pp. 152–153.
	Prevention of permanent liver damage.
Ulcerative colitis/ Crohn's disease	*Teaching:* measures to prevent exacerbation, p. 172.

ENDOCRINE SYSTEM

Diabetes mellitus	*Teaching:* medication regimen, monitoring glucose level, measures to control disease and prevent complications, p. 142.

HEMATOLOGIC SYSTEM

AIDS	*Teaching:* prevention of transmission of infection, p. 132.
	Activities of daily living.
Anemias (iron deficiency and pernicious)	*Teaching:* compliance with medical regimen to control condition or prevent recurrence, pp. 50–53.

MUSCULOSKELETAL SYSTEM

Amputation	*Teaching:* stump care, prosthesis care, compliance with rehabilitation regimen, p. 242.

Osteoarthritis/rheumatoid arthritis	Care of involved joints.
	Teaching: medical regimen to prevent progression of the disease, pp. 135, 239.
	Prevention of injury to the joints.
Fractured hip; knee or hip prosthesis/replacement	Optimal mobility.
	Teaching: medical and rehabilitative regimen, pp. 240–241.
Fractures/cast care	Ensuring immobilization.
	Prevention of complications of the fracture.
	Teaching: care for the body part, p. 225.
Laminectomy/spinal fusion (lumbar or cervical)	*Teaching:* postoperative care to promote healing and function, p. 262.
	Prevention of complications.
Osteomyelitis	Symptomatic treatment.
	Prevention of secondary infection.
	Prevention of transmission of infection to others.
Osteoporosis	*Teaching:* medical regimen to prevent or control progression of bone mass loss and fractures, p. 236.

RENAL SYSTEM

Kidney transplant	*Teaching:* immunosuppressive therapy, p. 190.
	Monitor for signs and symptoms of rejection.
Prostatic hypertrophy with prostatectomy	Maintenance of urinary output pre- and postoperatively.
	Wound care postoperatively.
	Teaching: medical regimen, p. 193.
	Prevention of complications.
Chronic renal failure	Providing for activities of daily living.
	Administration of peritoneal dialysis prn.
	Teaching: fluid and diet restrictions, compliance with hemodialysis, prevention of complications, pp. 187–188.
Urinary tract infection	*Teaching:* medication regimen to prevent or control bladder infection and spread to kidneys, pp. 184, 231.

INTEGUMENTARY SYSTEM

Burns	Rehabilitation phase of burn care.
	Teaching: care of wounds, pp. 303–304.
	Support of compliance with physical therapy regimen.
Decubitus ulcer	Care of existing ulcer.
	Teaching: prevention, p. 237.

REPRODUCTIVE SYSTEM

Mastectomy

Maintaining function of the operative side (exercise regimen), p. 284.

Psychological consequences of loss of body part.

CHEMOTHERAPY AND RADIATION THERAPY

Monitoring physical and emotional effects.

Assessment of side effects.

Care for resulting needs (nausea, diarrhea, oral lesions, skin reaction, fatigue, bleeding tendency, weakness), pp. 276–282.

POSTOPERATIVE CARE

Reinforcement of hospital discharge plan.

Reduction of risk of infection.

Wound care and dressing change.

Teaching: use of incentive spirometer, pp. 116–121.

Monitoring temperature.

Administration of antiinfective therapy.

Assessment of respiratory and urinary status.

⋈ NCLEX-RN Test Plan:
Nursing Process Definitions and Descriptions

Appendix M

The phases of the nursing process include:

⋈ I. Assessment: Establishing a database.
A. *Gather objective and subjective information relative to the patient:*
  1. Collect information from the patient, significant others, and/or health care team members; current and prior health records; and other pertinent resources.
  2. Utilize assessment skills appropriate to patient's condition.
  3. Recognize *symptoms* and significant findings.
  4. Determine client's ability to assume care of daily health needs (self-care).
  5. Determine health team member's ability to provide care.
  6. Assess *environment* of patient.
  7. Identify own or staff reactions to patient, significant others, and/or health care team members.

B. *Confirm data:*
  1. *Verify* observation or perception by obtaining additional information.
  2. *Question* prescriptions and decisions by other health care team members when indicated.
  3. *Observe* condition of patient directly when indicated.
  4. *Validate* that an appropriate patient assessment has been made.

C. *Communicate information gained in assessment:*
  1. Document assessment findings thoroughly and accurately.
  2. Report assessment findings to relevant members of the health care team.

⋈ II. Analysis: Identifying actual or potential health care needs and/or problems based on assessment.
A. *Interpret data:*
  1. Validate data.
  2. Organize related data.
  3. Determine need for additional data.
  4. Determine patient's unique needs and/or problems.

B. *Formulate patient's nursing diagnoses:*

  1. Determine significant relationship between data and patient needs and/or problems.
  2. Utilize *standard taxonomy* for formulating nursing diagnoses.

C. *Communicate results of analysis:*
  1. Document patient's *nursing diagnoses.*
  2. Report results of analysis to relevant members of the health care team.

⋈ III. Planning: Setting goals for meeting patient's needs and designing strategies to achieve these goals.
A. *Prioritize nursing diagnoses:*
  1. Involve patient, significant others, and/or health care team members when establishing nursing diagnoses.
  2. Establish *priorities* among nursing diagnoses.
  3. Anticipate needs and/or problems on the basis of established priorities.

B. *Determine goals of care:*
  1. Involve patient, significant others, and/or health care team members in setting goals.
  2. Establish *priorities among goals.*
  3. Anticipate needs and/or problems on the basis of established priorities.

C. *Formulate outcome criteria for goals of care:*
  1. Involve patient, significant others, and/or health care team members in formulating outcome criteria for goals of care.
  2. Establish *priorities* among outcome *criteria* for goals of care.
  3. Anticipate needs and/or problems on the basis of established priorities.

D. *Develop plan of care and modify as necessary:*
  1. Involve the patient, significant others, and/or health care team members in designing strategies.
  2. *Individualize* the plan of care based on such information as *age, gender, culture, ethnicity and religion.*
  3. Plan for patient's safety, comfort, and maintenance of optimal functioning.
  4. Select nursing interventions for delivery of patient's care.
  5. Select *appropriate teaching approaches.*

E. *Collaborate with other health care team members when planning delivery of patient's care:*

Source: National Council of State Boards of Nursing, Inc., *NCLEX-RN Test Plan,* 1994.

1. Identify health or social resources available to the patient and/or significant others.
2. *Select appropriate health care team members* when planning assignments.
3. Coordinate care provided by health care team members.

F. *Communicate plan of care:*
   1. Document plan of care thoroughly and accurately.
   2. Report plan of care to relevant members of the health care team.
   3. Review plan of care with patient.

✉ IV. **Implementation: Initiating and completing actions necessary to accomplish the defined goals.**

A. *Organize and manage patient's care:*
   1. Implement a plan of care.
   2. Arrange for a patient care conference.

B. *Counsel and teach patient, significant others, and/ or health care team members:*
   1. Assist patient, significant others, and/or health care team members to recognize and manage stress.
   2. Facilitate patient relationships with significant others and health care team members.
   3. *Teach* correct principles, procedures, and techniques for maintenance and promotion of health.
   4. Provide patient with health status information.
   5. Refer patient, significant others, and/or health care team members to appropriate *resources.*

C. *Provide care to achieve established goals of care:*
   1. Use *safe* and *appropriate techniques* when administering patient care.
   2. Use precautionary and *preventive* interventions in providing care to patient.
   3. *Prepare patient for surgery, delivery,* or other *procedures.*
   4. Institute *interventions* to compensate for adverse responses.
   5. Initiate *life-saving interventions* for emergency situations.
   6. Provide an *environment* conducive to attainment of goals of care.
   7. Adjust care in accord with patient's expressed or implied needs, problems, and/or preferences.
   8. Stimulate and motivate patient to achieve *self-care* and independence.
   9. Encourage patient to follow a treatment regimen.
   10. Assist patient to maintain optimal functioning.

D. *Supervise and coordinate the delivery of patient's care provided by nursing personnel:*
   1. *Delegate* nursing interventions to appropriate nursing personnel.
   2. *Monitor* and follow up on delegated interventions.
   3. Manage health care team members' *reactions* to factors influencing therapeutic relationships with patients.

E. *Communicate nursing interventions:*
   1. Record actual patient responses, nursing interventions, and other information relevant to implementation of care.
   2. Provide complete, accurate reports on assigned patient(s) to relevant members of the health care team.

✉ V. **Evaluation: Determining the extent to which goals have been achieved and interventions have been successful.**

A. *Compare actual outcomes with expected outcomes of care:*
   1. Evaluate responses (*expected and unexpected*) in order to determine the degree of success of nursing interventions.
   2. Determine impact of therapeutic interventions on the patient and significant others.
   3. Determine need for modifying the plan of care.
   4. Identify factors that may interfere with the patient's ability to implement the plan of care.

B. *Evaluate the patient's ability to implement self-care:*
   1. Verify that *tests or measurements* are *performed correctly* by the patient and/or other care givers.
   2. Ascertain patient's and/or others' *understanding* of information given.

C. *Evaluate health care team members' ability to implement client care:*
   1. Determine *impact of teaching* on health care team members.
   2. Identify factors that might alter health care team members' response to teaching.

D. *Communicate evaluation findings:*
   1. Document patient's response to therapy, care, and/or teaching.
   2. Report patient's response to therapy, care, and/or teaching to relevant members of the health care team.
   3. Report and document others' responses to teaching.
   4. Document other caregivers' responses to teaching.

Notes:
1. Throughout the outline in this book, the stages of the nursing process are referred to as: assessment, analysis/nursing diagnosis, nursing care plan/implementation, evaluation/outcome criteria.
2. The practice questions in this book are coded as to the phase of the nursing process being tested; the codes are found following the answer/ rationale for each question. *Key to Nursing Process Codes:*

AS	Assessment
AN	Analysis
PL	Planning
IMP	Implementation
EV	Evaluation

For an index to questions relating to each phase of the nursing process, see Appendix N.

◾ Index: Questions Related to Nursing Process

Appendix
N

Use this index to locate practice questions throughout the book in each of the five phases of the nursing process.

	Question No.				
Chapter	**Assessment (AS)**	**Analysis (AN)**	**Planning (PL)**	**Implementation (IMP)**	**Evaluation (EV)**
1—Nursing Assessment of the Adult	1, 2, 3, 4				
2—Peripheral Vascular Disorders	3, 13, 14, 15	1, 6	9	5, 7, 11, 12	2, 4, 8, 10
3—Cardiac Structure Disorders		2	4	3	1
4—Cardiac Function Disorders	2, 8, 9, 12			1, 4, 6, 7, 10	3, 5, 11, 13
5—Hematologic Disorders	4	1	8, 10	2, 3, 5, 6, 7, 9	
6—Respiratory Disorders	1, 2, 7, 16, 18, 22, 23	10, 15, 21, 24, 27	6, 20, 25	3, 4, 5, 8, 9, 12, 14, 19, 26	11, 13, 17
7—Fluid and Electrolyte Imbalances	5, 15, 21	3, 10, 12, 14, 22, 23, 25	24	2, 4, 6, 7, 8, 9, 16, 17, 18, 19, 20	1, 11, 13
8—Shock	4	3, 5	1		2
9—Perioperative Nursing			6	1, 2, 3, 5	4
10—Pain	1, 2			3, 4	
11—Altered Immune System Disorders				1, 2, 3, 4, 5	
12—Connective Tissue Disorders		2		1, 4	3
13—Biliary and Pancreatic Disorders	1	2, 4, 5	6, 11	3, 7, 9, 10, 12	8, 13
14—Hepatic Disorders	1, 4, 5, 7	2, 3, 6, 9	8		
15—Gastric Disorders	10, 12, 13		2, 5, 7	1, 3, 4, 6, 8, 9, 11	
16—Intestinal Disorders	3, 13, 14	8	5, 7, 11	1, 2, 6, 9, 10, 12	4
17—Renal Disorders	1, 4, 17, 19	9, 14, 20	10	3, 6, 7, 8, 11, 12, 13, 15, 16	2, 5, 18
18—Endocrine Disorders	2, 4		1, 3		

Chapter	Question No.				
	Assessment (AS)	Analysis (AN)	Planning (PL)	Implementation (IMP)	Evaluation (EV)
19—Sensory Disorders	6, 8			2, 4, 5, 7, 9, 10, 11, 12	1, 3
20—Musculoskeletal Disorders	3, 6	4, 7	12	1, 2, 5, 8, 9, 10, 11, 13, 14	
21—Neurologic Disorders	1, 9	3, 6	5	2, 4, 7, 8	
22—Disorders of the Spinal Cord	3	4		1, 2, 5	6
23—Degenerative Neurologic Disorders	1	2, 3		4	
24—Neoplastic Disorders	4, 9			1, 2, 3, 6, 7, 10	5, 8
25—Emergency Nursing		1, 2, 3		4	

Index: Questions Related to Categories of Human Functions

This index lists *practice questions* for you to use in reviewing *categories of human functions* (which are *detailed* examples of what subtopics are covered by the four *broad* client needs categories).

The eight categories of human functions include:

Protective Functions client's ability to maintain defenses and prevent physical and chemical trauma, injury, and threats to health status (e.g., communicable diseases, abuse, safety hazards, poisoning, skin disorders, and pre- and post-operative complications).

Sensory-Perceptual Functions client's ability to perceive, interpret, and respond to sensory and cognitive stimuli (e.g., auditory, visual, verbal impairments, brain tumors, aphasia, sensory deprivation or overload, body image, reality orientation, learning disabilities).

Comfort, Rest, Activity, and Mobility Functions client's ability to maintain mobility, desirable level of activity, adequate sleep, rest, and comfort (e.g., pain, sleep disturbances, joint impairment).

Nutrition client's ability to maintain the intake and processing of essential nutrients (e.g., obesity, gastric and metabolic disorders that primarily affect the nutritional status).

Growth and Development client's ability to maintain maturational processes throughout the life span (e.g., child bearing, child rearing, maturational crisis, changes in aging, psychosocial development).

Fluid-Gas Transport Functions client's ability to maintain fluid-gas transport (e.g., fluid volume deficit/overload, acid-base balance, CPR, anemias, cardiopulmonary diseases).

Psychosocial-Cultural Functions client's ability to function (intrapersonal/interpersonal relationships; e.g., grieving, death/dying, psychotic behaviors, self concept, therapeutic communication, ethical-legal aspects, community resources, situational crises, substance abuse).

Elimination Functions client's ability to maintain functions related to relieving the body of waste products (e.g., conditions of GI and/or GU systems).

Chapter	Protective Functions (1) Question No.	Sensory-Perceptual Functions (2) Question No.	Comfort, Rest, Activity, and Mobility Functions (3) Question No.	Nutrition (4) Question No.	Growth and Development (5) Question No.	Fluid-Gas Transport Functions (6) Question No.	Psychosocial-Cultural Functions (7) Question No.	Elimination Functions (8) Question No.
1—Nursing Assessment of the Adult					1, 2, 4	3		
2—Peripheral Vascular Disorders						1, 2, 3, 4, 5, 6, 7, 8, 9, 10, 11, 12, 13, 14, 15		
3—Cardiac Structure Disorders						1, 2, 3, 4, 5, 6		
4—Cardiac Function Disorders				10		1, 2, 3, 4, 5, 6, 8, 9, 11, 12, 13	7	
5—Hematologic Disorders	5		3			1, 2, 4, 6, 8, 9, 10	7	
6—Respiratory Disorders						1, 2, 3, 4, 5, 6, 7, 8, 9, 10, 11, 12, 13, 14, 15, 16, 17, 18, 19, 20, 21, 22, 23, 24, 25, 26, 27		
7—Fluid and Electrolyte Imbalances	17			1, 2, 14, 15, 16, 20, 24		3, 4, 5, 6, 7, 8, 9, 10, 11, 12, 13, 18, 19, 21, 22, 23, 25		
8—Shock		2				1, 2, 3, 4, 5		
9—Perioperative Nursing	1, 3, 4, 5, 6							
10—Pain			1, 2, 4				3	
11—Altered Immune Disorders	1, 2, 4, 5							3
12—Connective Tissue Disorders			1, 2, 4	3				
13—Biliary and Pancreatic Disorders				2, 3, 4, 5, 6, 7, 8, 9, 10, 11, 12, 13				1

Chapter	Protective Functions (1) Question No.	Sensory-Perceptual Functions (2) Question No.	Comfort, Rest, Activity, and Mobility Functions (3) Question No.	Nutrition (4) Question No.	Growth and Development (5) Question No.	Fluid-Gas Transport Functions (6) Question No.	Psychosocial-Cultural Functions (7) Question No.	Elimination Functions (8) Question No.
14—Hepatic Disorders		9		1, 2, 3, 4, 7		8		5, 6
15—Gastric Disorders	3, 8, 9			2, 4, 5, 6, 7, 10, 11, 12, 13				
16—Intestinal Disorders	11		1	6				1, 2, 3, 4, 5, 7, 8, 9, 10, 12, 13, 14
17—Renal Disorders	20			10, 11		19		1, 2, 3, 4, 5, 6, 7, 8, 9, 12, 13, 14, 15, 16, 17, 18
18—Endocrine Disorders			2, 4	1, 3				
19—Sensory Disorders		1, 2, 3, 4, 5, 6, 7, 8, 9, 10, 11, 12						
20—Musculoskeletal Disorders			1, 2, 3, 4, 5, 6, 7, 8, 9, 10, 11, 12, 13, 14					
21—Neurologic Disorders		2, 3, 4, 5, 6, 7, 9		8		1		
22—Disorders of Spinal Cord		3, 4, 6	1, 2, 5					
23—Degenerative Neurologic Disorders			1, 2, 3			4		
24—Neoplastic Disorders	4, 8, 10	9	1, 2, 5			7	3, 6	
25—Emergency Nursing	4					1, 2		3

Index: Questions Related to Client Needs

Appendix P

To *practice questions* in each of the four categories of *client needs* that are tested on NCLEX-RN, refer to the questions listed.

The four broad categories of client needs include:

Safe, Effective Care Environment *coordinated care, environmental safety, safe* and *effective treatment* and procedures (e.g., client rights, confidentiality, principles of teaching/learning, control of infectious agents).

Physiologic Integrity *physiologic adaptation, reduction of risk potential, provision of basic care* (e.g., drug administration, emergencies, nutritional therapies).

Psychosocial Integrity *psychosocial adaptation; coping* (e.g., behavioral norms, chemical dependency, communication skills, family systems, mental health concepts, psychodynamics of behavior, psychopathology, treatment modalities).

Health Promotion and Maintenance *normal growth and development* from birth to death, *self-care* and *support systems, prevention* and *early treatment of disease* (e.g., newborn care, normal perinatal care, family planning, human sexuality, parenting, death/dying, life-style choices, immunity).

Chapter	Safe, Effective Care Environment (SECE) Question No.	Physiologic Integrity (PhI) Question No.	Psychosocial Integrity (PsI) Question No.	Health Promotion and Maintenance (HPM) Question No.
1—Nursing Assessment of the Adult	1, 2	3, 4		
2—Peripheral Vascular Disorders	10	1, 2, 3, 4, 5, 6, 8, 11, 13, 14, 15		7, 9, 12
3—Cardiac Structure Disorders	1	2, 4		3
4—Cardiac Function Disorders	4, 8, 10	2, 3, 5, 6, 9, 11, 12, 13	7	1
5—Hematologic Disorders	1, 3, 5, 9	2, 4, 6, 8, 10	7	
6—Respiratory Disorders	3, 6, 8, 9, 10, 13, 17	1, 2, 4, 5, 7, 11, 12, 15, 16, 18, 20, 21, 23, 24, 25, 27		14, 19, 22, 26
7—Fluid and Electrolyte Imbalances	6, 7, 8, 9, 16, 17, 18, 19, 23	1, 3, 4, 5, 10, 11, 12, 13, 14, 15, 21, 22, 24, 25		2, 20
8—Shock		1, 2, 3, 4, 5		
9—Perioperative Nursing	2, 3, 6	1, 4	5	
10—Pain		1, 3, 4	2	
11—Altered Immune System Disorders	1, 3, 4, 5	2		
12—Connective Tissue Disorders		2, 3		1, 4
13—Biliary and Pancreatic Disorders	6	1, 2, 4, 5, 7, 8, 9, 10, 11, 12, 13		3
14—Hepatic Disorders	8	1, 2, 3, 4, 5, 6, 7, 9		
15—Gastric Disorders	1, 3, 9	4, 6, 7, 8, 10, 11, 12, 13		2, 5

Chapter	Safe, Effective Care Environment (SECE) Question No.	Physiologic Integrity (PhI) Question No.	Psychosocial Integrity (PsI) Question No.	Health Promotion and Maintenance (HPM) Question No.
16—Intestinal Disorders	4, 7, 8, 11	2, 3, 5, 6, 9, 10, 13, 14		1, 12
17—Renal Disorders	5, 9, 12, 15, 18	1, 2, 3, 4, 7, 10, 11, 13, 14, 16, 17, 19, 20		6, 8
18—Endocrine Disorders		1, 2, 3, 4		
19—Sensory Disorders	1, 2, 7, 10, 11, 12	3, 4, 6, 8, 9		5
20—Musculoskeletal Disorders	1, 4, 5, 11, 14	2, 3, 6, 7, 8, 9, 10, 12, 13		
21—Neurologic Disorders	8	1, 2, 3, 5, 6, 7, 9		4
22—Disorders of the Spinal Cord	2, 3	1, 4, 5, 6		
23—Degenerative Neurologic Disorders	2, 3	1, 4		
24—Neoplastic Disorders	3, 8, 10	1, 4, 5, 9	6, 7	2
25—Emergency Nursing		1, 2, 3, 4		

Resources

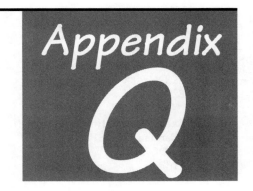

Appendix Q

Selected sources of information and services. (Every effort has been made to provide current names and addresses; however, addresses do change frequently.)

Health and Welfare Agencies/Associations

ACTION (programs for older adults)
806 Connecticut Ave. NW
Washington, DC 20525
202-254-7310

Administration on Aging
Department of Health and Human Services
200 Independence Ave. SW
Washington, DC 20201
202-245-0724

American Burn Association
Shriner's Burn Institute
University of Cincinnati
202 Goodman St.
Cincinnati, OH 45219
513-751-3900

American Cancer Society
1599 Clifton Rd. NE
Atlanta, GA 30329
404-320-3333

American Diabetes Association
National Center
1660 Duke St.
Alexandria, VA 22314
800-232-3472

American Foundation for the Blind
15 W. 16th St.
New York, NY 10016
212-620-2000

American Liver Foundation
1425 Pompton Ave.
Cedar Grove, NJ 07009
800-223-0179

American Lung Association
1740 Broadway
New York, NY 10019
215-315-8700

American Pain Society
PO Box 186
Skokie, IL 60076
312-475-7300

American Parkinson's Disease Association, Inc.
116 John St.
New York, NY 10038
212-732-9550

American Speech-Language-Hearing Association
10801 Rockville Pike
Department AP
Rockville, MD 20852
301-897-5700

American Spinal Injury Association
2020 Peachtree Rd. NW
Atlanta, GA 30309

Arthritis Foundation
1314 Spring St. NW
Atlanta, GA 30309
404-872-7100

Asthma and Allergy Foundation of America
1717 Massachusetts Ave. NW
No. 305
Washington, DC 20036
800-7ASTHMA

Centers for Disease Control
Department of Health and Human Services
U.S. Public Health Service
Atlanta, GA 30333
404-639-3534

Concern for Dying
250 W. 57th St.
New York, NY 10107
215-246-6962

Epilepsy Foundation of America
815 15th St. NW, Suite 528
Washington, DC 20005
202-638-5229

Guillain-Barré Foundation
129 North Carolina Ave. SE
Washington, DC 20003
202-387-2216

Leukemia Society of America
31 St. James Ave.
Boston, MA 02116
617-482-2256

Muscular Dystrophy Association
3561 E. Sunrise Ave.
Tucson, AZ 85718
602-529-2000

Myasthenia Gravis Foundation
61 Gramercy Park North
New York, NY 10010
212-533-7005

National Association to Control Epilepsy
22 E. 67th St.
New York, NY 10012

**National Association of Patients on Hemodialysis
and Transplantation**
211 E. 43rd St.
New York, NY 10017
212-867-4486

National Cancer Institute
Office of Cancer Communications
Building 31, Room 10A24
National Institutes of Health
Bethesda, MD 20892
800-4-CANCER

National Center for the American Heart Association
7320 Greenville Ave.
Dallas, TX 75231
214-373-6300

National Foundation for Ileitis and Colitis
444 Park Ave. South
New York, NY 10016
212-685-3440

National Head Injury Foundation
333 Turnpike Rd.
Southborough, MA 01722
508-485-9950

National Hemophilia Foundation
110 Greene St., Suite 406
New York, NY 10012
212-219-8180

National Institute of Allergy and Infectious Diseases
Building 10, National Institutes of Health
Bethesda, MD 20892
301-496-4000

**National Institute of Arthritis and Musculoskeletal
and Skin Diseases**
National Institutes of Health
Bethesda, MD 20892
301-496-4000

**National Jewish Center for Immunology and
Respiratory Medicine**
1400 Jackson St.
Denver, CO 80206
800-222-LUNG

National Kidney Foundation
30 E. 33rd St.
New York, NY 10016
212-889-2210

National Multiple Sclerosis Society
205 E. 42nd St.
New York, NY 10017
212-532-3060

National Parkinson's Foundation
1501 NW 9th Ave.
Miami, FL 33136
305-547-6666

National Psoriasis Foundation
6443 Southwest Beaverton Hwy., Suite 210
Portland, OR 97221
503-297-1545

National Safety Council
444 N. Michigan Ave.
Chicago, IL 60611
800-621-7619

National Society to Prevent Blindness
500 E. Remington Rd.
Schaumburg, IL 60173
312-843-2020

National Spinal Cord Injury Association
600 W. Cumming Park, #3200
Woburn, MA 01801
800-962-9629

Office for Handicapped Individuals
Department of Education
Room 3106, Switzer Building
400 Maryland Ave. SW
Washington, DC 20202
202-245-0080

Osteoporosis Foundation
612 N. Michigan Ave., Suite 510
Chicago, IL 60611

Paget's Disease Foundation
PO Box 2772
Brooklyn, NY 11202
718-596-1043

Phoenix Society (assistance following burn injuries)
11 Rust Hill Rd.
Levittown, PA 19056
215-946-BURN
800-888-BURN

Self Help for Hard of Hearing People (Shhh)
4848 Battery Ln.
Department E
Bethesda, MD 20814
301-657-2248

United Network for Organ Sharing
3001 Hungary Spring Rd.
Richmond, VA 23228
804-289-5380

AIDS Information and Hotlines

American Foundation for AIDS Research	212-682-7440
American Red Cross AIDS Education Office	202-737-8300
Centers for Disease Control—Statistics:	
AIDS cases and deaths	404-330-3020
Distribution-categories	404-330-3021
Demographics	404-330-3022
Hearing Impaired AIDS Hotline	800-243-7889
National AIDS Hotline	800-342-AIDS
National AIDS Information Clearing House	800-458-5231
National AIDS Network	202-293-2437
National Gay/Lesbian Crisis Line	800-767-4297
Project Inform (Drug Information)	800-822-7422
Spanish AIDS Hotline	800-344-7432

Professional Organizations/ Associations

American Academy of Ambulatory Nursing Administration
N. Woodbury Rd., Box 56
Pitman, NJ 08071

American Academy of Nurse Practitioners
45 Foster St., Suite A
Lowell, MA 01851

The American Assembly for Men in Nursing
PO Box 31753
Independence, OH 44131

American Association of Critical-Care Nurses
101 Columbia
Aliso Viejo, CA 92656

American Association of Nurse Anesthetists
216 Higgins Rd.
Park Ridge, IL 60068

American Association of Occupational Health Nurses, Inc.
50 Lenox Pointe
Atlanta, GA 30324

American Association of Office Nurses
109 Kinderhook Rd.
Montvale, NJ 07645

American Association of Spinal Cord Injury Nurses
75-20 Astoria Blvd.
Jackson Heights, NY 11370-1178

American Holistic Nurses' Association
4101 Lake Boon Tr., Suite 201
Raleigh, NC 27607

American Nephrology Nurses' Association
N. Woodbury Rd., Box 56
Pitman, NJ 08071

American Radiological Nurses Association
c/o Elaine Deutsch Plankey
2462 Stantonsburg Rd., Suite 162
Greenville, NC 27834

American Society of Ophthalmic Registered Nurses, Inc.
PO Box 193030
San Francisco, CA 94119

American Society of Plastic & Reconstructive Surgical Nurses, Inc.
N. Woodbury Rd., Box 56
Pitman, NJ 08071

American Society of Post Anesthesia Nurses
11512 Allecingie Pkwy.
Richmond, VA 23235

Association of Nurses in AIDS Care
704 Stonyhill Rd., Suite 106
Yardley, PA 19067

Association of Operating Room Nurses
10170 E. Mississippi Ave.
Denver, CO 80231

Association for Practitioners in Infection Control
505 E. Hawley St.
Mundelein, IL 60060

Association of Rehabilitation Nurses
5700 Old Orchard Rd., 1st floor
Skokie, IL 60077

Dermatology Nurses Association
N. Woodbury Rd., Box 56
Pitman, NJ 08071

Emergency Nurses Association
230 E. Ohio, 6th floor
Chicago, IL 60611

Hospice Nurses Association
PO Box 8166
Van Nuys, CA 91409

International Association for Enterostomal Therapy Inc.
2081 Business Center Dr., Suite 290
Irvine, CA 92715

Intravenous Nurses Society, Inc.
Two Brighton St.
Belmont, MA 02178

National Association of Hispanic Nurses
6905 Alamo Downs Pkwy.
San Antonio, TX 78238

National Association of Home Care (NAHC)
519 C St. NE
Washington, DC 20002

National Association of Orthopaedic Nurses, Inc.
N. Woodbury Rd., Box 56
Pitman, NJ 08071

National Black Nurses Association, Inc.
1012 Tenth St. NW
Washington, DC 20001

National Gerontological Nursing Association
3100 Homewood Pkwy.
Kensington, MD 20895

North American Nursing Diagnosis Association
3525 Caroline St.
St. Louis, MO 63104

Nurses Environmental Health Watch
33 Columbus Ave.
Somerville, MA 02143

Oncology Nursing Society
1016 Greentree Rd.
Pittsburgh, PA 15220-3125

Society of Gastroenterology Nurses and Associates, Inc.
1070 Sibley Tower
Rochester, NY 14604

Society of Otorhinolaryngology and Head/Neck Nurses
439 N. Causeway
New Smyrna Beach, FL 32169

Society for Peripheral Vascular Nursing
309 Winter St.
Norwood, MA 02062

Society of Respiratory Nursing
5700 Old Orchard Rd., 1st floor
Skokie, IL 60077

Transcultural Nursing Society
Department of Nursing
Madonna College
36600 Schoolcroft Rd.
Livonia, MI 48150

World Federation of Neuroscience Nurses
6214 Craigmont Rd.
Baltimore, MD 21228

Patient Education Materials

Abbott Laboratories
Professional Services—D383
Abbott Park
N. Chicago, IL 60064

American Cancer Society
1599 Clifton Rd. NE
Atlanta, GA 30329

American Diabetes Association
National Center
1660 Duke St.
Alexandria, VA 22314

American Liver Foundation
1425 Pompton Ave.
Cedar Grove, NJ 07009

American Lung Association
1740 Broadway
New York, NY 10019

Arthritis Foundation
1314 Spring St. NW
Atlanta, GA 30309

Eli Lilly and Company
Educational Resources Program
PO Box 100B
Indianapolis, IN 46206

National Head Injury Foundation
333 Turnpike Rd.
Southborough, MA 01772

National Kidney Foundation
30 E. 33rd St., Suite 1100
New York, NY 10016

National Multiple Sclerosis Society
205 E. 42nd St.
New York, NY 10017

National Safety Council
444 N. Michigan Ave.
Chicago, IL 60611

Nutrition Education Association
PO Box 20301
Houston, TX 77225

Phoenix Society (assistance following burn injuries)
11 Rust Hill Rd.
Levittown, PA 19056

Ross Laboratories
Creative Services and Information Department
625 Cleveland Ave.
Columbus, OH 43216

Schering Corporation
Professional Film Library
Galloping Hill Rd.
Kenilworth, NJ 07033

Skin Cancer Foundation
245 Fifth Ave., Suite 2402
New York, NY 10016

United Ostomy Association
36 Executive Park, Suite 120
Irvine, CA 92714

Bibliography

Beare P G, Myers J L. *Principles and Practices of Adult Health Nursing,* 2nd ed. St. Louis: C. V. Mosby, 1994. Focuses on all settings where nursing has a role in health care delivery—acute care, outpatient, rehabilitation, longterm and home care. The nursing science content is reinforced with information from the related sciences and humanities. All dimensions of the nurse's role are addressed as well as recent trends in health care, prevention, technologic advances, family involvement in patient education, therapeutic communication, and the needs of the aging population.

Black J M, Matassarin-Jacobs E (Eds.). *Luckmann and Sorensen's Medical-Surgical Nursing: A Psychophysiologic Approach,* 4th ed. Philadelphia: W. B. Saunders, 1993. This text offers an in-depth presentation of current medical-surgical nursing practice as well as a discussion of basic behavioral and physiologic concepts. A wide range of specific health problems are presented, and the components of the nursing process are consistently related to underlying psychophysiologic principles.

Caroline N. *Emergency Care in the Streets,* 5th ed. Boston: Little, Brown and Company, 1995. A comprehensive text on evaluating and managing various emergencies. The book uses boxed summaries, flowcharts, skill evaluation checklists, illustrations, and tables to clarify and summarize important concepts.

Deglin J H, Vallerand A. *Davis's Drug Guide for Nurses,* 4th ed. Philadelphia: F. A. Davis, 1995. Provides comprehensive, up-to-date, and practical information for the safe and effective administration and monitoring of drug therapy. Pharmacologic content is presented within a nursing process framework with appropriate nursing diagnoses.

Dudek S G. *Nutrition Handbook for Nursing Practice,* 2nd ed. Philadelphia: J. B. Lippincott, 1993. A comprehensive handbook that uses the nursing process to integrate nutrition into nursing care plans. Where applicable, possible adverse nutritional side effects of commonly used medications and appropriate interventions have been included.

Judge R, Zuidema G, Fitzgerald F. *Clinical Diagnosis,* 5th ed. Boston: Little, Brown and Company, 1989. Integrates physical diagnostic techniques with the clinical thought process, problem solving, diagnostic laboratory methods, and clinician–patient interaction.

Nelson R. *Video/Audio Review of Acute and Chronic Health Problems in the Adult.* San Francisco: Review for Nurses, 1995. Focuses on review of key concepts frequently tested on nursing exams. Available through: 1-800-345-7277.

Phipps W, Cassmeyer V, Sands J, Lehman M. *Medical-Surgical Nursing, Concepts and Clinical Practice,* 5th ed. St. Louis: C. V. Mosby, 1994. The text examines the social, cultural and environmental factors that influence nursing. The nursing process is utilized with outcome criteria clearly identified for interventions described. Common problems resulting from pathophysiological changes are presented using a systems approach.

Potter P, Perry A. *Basic Nursing, Theory and Practice,* 3rd ed. St. Louis: C. V. Mosby, 1995. A basic textbook for the beginning nursing student. A major portion of the text is devoted to skills essential to nursing practice.

Shlafer M, Marieb E. *The Nurse, Pharmacology and Drug Therapy,* 2nd ed. Redwood City, CA: Addison-Wesley, 1993. To make it feasible to learn so many drugs, this text focuses on prototype drugs as representative of their class or the drug most commonly used. Integrated throughout each chapter are nursing implications, including special sections on the elderly, children, and drug therapy during pregnancy and lactation. Each chapter ends with a nursing process summary.

Index

The Lippincott's NurseNotes Series Disk Instructions

System Requirements
- A PC compatible computer with an Intel 386 or better processor. Windows 3.1 or later.
- 4 Megabytes RAM (minimum); but recommend 8 MB RAM on Windows 3.1.
- 8 Megabytes RAM (minimum); but recommend 12 MB RAM minimum on Windows 95.
- 3 Megabytes of available hard disk space.

Installation
Installing *NurseNotes: Medical–Surgical* for Windows
1. Start up Windows.
2. Insert the *Medical–Surgical* disk into the floppy disk drive.
3. From the Program Manager's File Menu, choose the Run command.
4. When the Run dialog box appears, type a:\setup (or b:\setup if you're using the B drive) in the Command Line box. Click OK or press the Enter button.
5. The installation process will begin. A dialog proposing the directory "nnpm" on the drive containing Windows will appear. If the name and location are correct, click OK. If you want to change this information, type over the existing data, then click OK.
6. When the *Medical–Surgical* setup routine is complete, a new group called "Nurse Notes" will appear on your desktop.
7. Start the *Medical–Surgical* program by double-clicking on its icon.

NurseNotes: Medical–Surgical disk program
Lippincott's *NurseNotes* Series consists of two modes: Test Mode and Study Mode.

TEST MODE
To begin a test, click the Start Over button with your mouse cursor. As a result, the first question will appear on the screen. If you decide to stop the test before you complete it, your answers will be saved. You can resume the test by selecting the Resume button from the Main Menu screen. You may clear your answers for a test at any time by clicking on the Start Over button.

NurseNotes: Medical–Surgical—Toolbar
The Toolbar contains a series of buttons that provide direct access to all test program functions. When you move the cursor over a button, an explanation of its function displays in the Status Bar which is immediately above the ToolBar.

From left to right, the Toolbar buttons are:
- Program Help
- Pause
- Mark Question
- Table of Contents
- First Question Arrow
  (go to the first question in the section)
- Prior Question Arrow
  (go to the previous question in the test)
- Next Question Arrow
  (go to the next question in the test)
- Last Question Arrow
  (go to the last question in the section)
- Stop

To get help at any time during the test, choose the Program Help button. Program Help reviews basic functions of the program. To close the Program Help window, click on the Program Help button again. Answer each question by clicking on the oval to the left of an answer selection or by selecting the appropriate letter on the keyboard (A, B, C, or D). When an answer is selected, its oval will darken. If you change your mind about an answer, simply select that choice, by mouse or keyboard, again.

To register your answer selection and proceed to the next question, click on the Next Question Arrow button or press the Enter key.

If you are unsure about an answer to a particular question, the program allows you to mark it for later review. Flag the question by clicking on the Mark Question button. To review all marked questions for a test, click on the Table of Contents button, which is immediately to the right of the Mark button. This will open the Table of Contents window.

The Table of Contents window lists every question included on the test and summarizes whether it has been answered, left unanswered, or marked for later review. Click on an item in the Table of Contents window and the program will move to that test question, or use the Arrow buttons to move to the first, previous, next, or last question. To close the Table of Contents window, click on the Table of Contents button again.

At any time during the test or when you are finished taking the test, click on the Stop button. If you wish, you may return to the session at a later time without erasing your existing answers by selecting the Resume button.

After taking the test, you may receive your score by clicking the Results Button on the Main Menu Screen. There are four different ways to review your results: Test Results, Nursing Process, Category of Human Function, and Client Need.

STUDY MODE
After taking the test and receiving your score, you may wish to enter the Study Mode. This mode supplies you with the test questions, the answers that you chose, and the rationale for correct and incorrect answers. To enter the Study Mode, click the Study Mode button with your mouse cursor. You will not be able to modify the answers you have given; however, you can select any of the answer choices for an explanation of that answer. You may also wish to use the Table of Contents button to show you which questions you marked for review. Each of these windows may be closed by clicking again on their respective buttons.

To exit the *Medical–Surgical* program, click the Exit button on the Main Menu.